WB100 ONE

£15.95 ORD

Medici

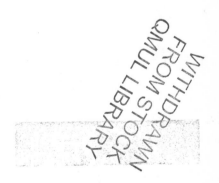

D1334293

For Churchill Livingstone

Publisher: Laurence Hunter
Project Editor: Barbara Simmons
Copy Editor: Jane Ward
Project Controller: Nancy Arnott
Design Direction: Erik Bigland, Charles Simpson
Page Layout: Gerard Heyburn
Indexer: Anne McCarthy

Churchill's Mastery of Medicine

Medicine

Paul O'Neill

BSc (Hons) MB ChB FRCP MD

Senior Lecturer in Geriatric Medicine, University of Manchester;
Hospital Dean for Clinical Studies
South Manchester University Hospitals NHS Trust
Manchester

Tim Dornan

MA BM ChB DM FRCP

Consultant Physician and Hospital Dean for Clinical Studies
Hope Hospital, Salford
Manchester

David W Denning

MB BS FRCP MRCPath DCH

Senior Lecturer and Honorary Consultant in Infectious Diseases
University of Manchester, North Manchester General Hospital
and Hope Hospital Manchester

Illustrations by
David Gardner

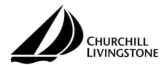

**CHURCHILL
LIVINGSTONE**

NEW YORK, EDINBURGH, LONDON, MADRID, MELBOURNE,
SAN FRANCISCO AND TOKYO 1997

CHURCHILL LIVINGSTONE
Medical Division of Pearson Professional Limited

Distributed in the United States of America by Churchill
Livingstone Inc., 650 Avenue of the Americas, New York, N.Y.
10011, and by associated companies, branches and
representatives throughout the world.

First published 1997

ISBN 0 443 050783

British Library of Cataloguing in Publication Data
A catalogue record for this book is available from the British
Library.

Library of Congress Cataloging in Publication Data
A catalog record for this book is available from the Library of
Congress.

Medical knowledge is constantly changing. As new information
becomes available, changes in treatment, procedures, equipment
and the use of drugs become necessary. The authors and
publisher have, as far as it is possible, taken care to ensure that
the information given in this text is accurate and up to date.
However, readers are strongly advised to confirm that the
information, especially with regard to drug usage, complies with
current legislation and standards of practice.

The
publisher's
policy is to use
**paper manufactured
from sustainable forests**

Printed in Great Britain by Bell and Bain Ltd, Glasgow

Acknowledgements

We would like to thank Dr Adrian Brodison, Dr Roger Chisholm, Dr John Houghton, Dr Phil Kalra, Dr Dev Mandal and Catherine Parchment for their help in reviewing the manuscript, and Julie Young, who typed large sections of it and its various revisions. We would like to thank Barbara Simmons of Churchill Livingstone for her patient and skilled editorial support.

We would also like to thank our wives, Jo, Ceri and Merian, for their patience and support without which nothing would have been written at all.

Contents

Using this book

Philosophy of the book

This chapter aims to help you:

- understand how the emphasis on self-assessment in this book can make learning easier and more enjoyable
- use this book to increase your understanding as well as knowledge
- plan your learning

How much do you know about diabetes? Are they the right things? Can you answer exam problems on diabetes? This book aims to help you with these questions. You probably have some knowledge of medicine, perhaps a bit patchy, and some clinical experience. We want to help you to be better at integrating knowledge and solving either real problems or simulated ones in examinations. We have tried to present essential information, for doctors practising in the UK, in a concise and ordered fashion. Principles are illustrated and mechanisms explained rather than simply giving you lots of facts to memorise.

Do not think though that this book offers a 'syllabus'. It is impossible to draw boundaries around medical knowledge and learning is a continuous process carried out throughout your career. As we see it in 1997, this book includes all that you *must* know, most of what you *should* know about, and some of what you *might* be aware of.

We assume that you are working towards one or more examinations, probably in order to qualify. Our purpose is to show you how to overcome this barrier. As we feel strongly that learning is not simply for the purpose of passing exams, the book aims both to help you to pass and to develop *useful* knowledge and understanding.

Layout and content

The first part of each chapter sets out the key learning objectives; those things which anyone starting a medical career needs to know and an examiner expects them to know. More detailed learning objectives are to be found at the start of each major section. One starting point might be to look at these objectives and then test yourself in the self-assessment section at the end of each chapter. This will help to steer you towards areas that you need to work on. Alternatively, you can go straight into the main body of the chapter and check that you have achieved the objectives at the end; if not then you will need to do further work and perhaps read about the topics elsewhere.

The main part of the text describes important topics in major subject areas. Within these sections, we have put down the essential information in a logical order with explanations and links. In order to help you, we have used lists to set out frameworks and to make it easier for you to put facts in a rational sequence. Tables are used to link quite complex information.

There are some situations in medicine that require you to act immediately and senior help may not be available. For some of these emergencies, we have put the steps that you must take in an 'emergency' summary box. These are based on current guidelines, but guidelines do change.

You have to be sure that you are reaching the required standards, so the final section of each chapter is there to help you to check out your knowledge and understanding. The self-assessment is in the form of multiple choice questions, case histories, short notes, data interpretation, possible viva questions and picture questions. Questions are designed to integrate knowledge across different chapters and to focus on the decisions you will have to take in a given clinical situation. Detailed answers are given with reference to relevant sections of the text; the answers also contain information and explanations that you will not find elsewhere, so you have to do the assessments to get the most out of this book.

Using the book

Your first task before using the book is to map out on a sheet of paper a series of three lists dividing the major subjects (corresponding to our chapter headings) into an assessment of your strong, reasonable and weak areas. This gives you a rough outline of your learning schedule, which you must then fit in with the time available. Clearly, if your exams are looming large, you will have to be ruthless in the time allocated to your strong areas. The major subjects should be further classified into individual topics. Encouragement to store information and to test your ongoing improvement is by the use of the self-assessment sections. You must keep checking your current level of knowledge.

Overall the aim is to help you to learn through the use of interlinked steps:

- What do you already know about the subject?
- Why do you want to learn more about the subject? Knowledge is acquired much more easily if it can be put in a framework.
- What things needs explaining? What do you not understand?
- Can you expand on these things? Explain as much as you can from different aspects.
- Set yourself goals for where your knowledge is lacking.
- Check that you have achieved these.

If you can, discuss problems with colleagues/friends. The areas which you understand least well will become apparent when you try to explain them to someone else. You will also benefit from hearing a different perspective on a problem.

Approach to examinations

The discipline of learning is closely linked to preparation for examinations. Many of us simply opt for remembering facts because full understanding is often not required, such as in multiple choice exams. We would prefer it if you acquired a deeper knowledge and understanding but, recognising constraints on your time, advocate a pragmatic approach that combines the necessity of passing exams with longer-term needs.

The hardest step is to determine what will be in the exam; medicine does not draw boundaries around knowledge either in breadth or depth. The best approach is to combine your lecture notes, textbooks (not reference) and past examination papers. From the last, for example, you may find out that not only are the pulmonary manifestations of HIV infection a possible examination topic but you will also get an indication of the depth of knowledge required.

You then have to choose what sources you are going to use for your learning and revision. Textbooks come in different forms. At one extreme, there is the large reference book, which includes extensive literature citation. At the other end of the spectrum is the condensed 'lecture note' format, which often relies heavily on lists. In the middle of the range are the medium-sized textbooks. You should choose the book(s) that suits your needs (and that of the examination!) and that you find readable.

You should now have a rough syllabus, your own lecture notes and some books that you feel comfortable in using. The next stage is to map out the time available for preparation. You must be realistic in this, allowing time for breaks and working steadily, not cramming. If you do attempt to cram, you have to realise that only a certain amount of information can be retained in short-term memory, so as the classification of the lipid disorders moves in, then the terminology of the renal tubular acidoses moves out! Cramming is simply retention of facts. If the examination requires understanding you will be in trouble.

You might be tempted to do general reading of a large textbook. Even if this was feasible in the time available (the number of pages to be read tends to increase as the exam gets closer), it is not very effective. Do you remember anything of the topic you have just covered? An analogy would be driving a car along a familiar route, arriving, but being unable to recall anything of the journey.

We advise an approach, as outlined above, based on the use of key steps, learning objectives and self-assessment. For a subject such as endocrinology, we would recommend setting out the topics to be covered and then attempting to summarise your knowledge about each in note form. By this means, gaps in your knowledge/understanding become apparent. Use of 'mind-maps' may be appropriate in helping making connections, for example between the physiological control of thyroxine secretion and thyrotoxicosis. It is much more efficient to go to textbooks having been through this exercise as you are then 'looking' for information and explanation.

Self-assessment will help in determining the time to be allocated to each system. If you are consistently scoring excellent marks in a particular subject it is not cost effective to spend a lot of time trying to achieve the 'perfect' mark. In an essay, it is many times easier to obtain the first mark (try writing your name) than the last. You should also try to decide on the amount of weight to be assigned to each subject; this should be heavily biased to the likelihood of it appearing in the exam! It is not sensible to devote large amounts of time to the ocular manifestations of systemic disease if ophthalmology is not included in the 'syllabus' you have devised.

As the examination draws near you should attempt practice questions and complete papers. It is not sufficient to have the necessary knowledge and understanding; you need to demonstrate these to the examiners. Many people pay insufficient attention to the type of question they are going to encounter. Moving the focus away from books and lecture notes to actual questions helps in identifying where knowledge is still lacking and what work is still to be done.

Methods of examination

Multiple choice questions

Unless very sophisticated, multiple choice questions test recall of information. The aim is to gain the maximum marks from the knowledge that you can remember. You should read the stem with great care, highlighting the 'little' words such as *only, rarely, usually, never* and *always*. You will often lose marks because of 'negatives', such as *not, unusual and unsuccessful*. If the stem is phrased *may occur*, this has entirely different connotations to *characteristic*. The latter may mean a feature which should be there and the absence of which (for example central chest pain in myocardial ischaemia) would make you question the correctness of the diagnosis. Alternatively, it can also be used to describe rare features which would suggest the diagnosis, for example yellow vision (xanthopsia) in digoxin toxicity. If the stem is long with several lines of text or data then you should try and summarise it by extracting the essential elements.

You must check the marking method before starting. Most employ a negative system in which marks are lost for incorrect answers. The temptation is to adopt a cautious approach answering a relatively small number of questions. However, this can lead to problems as we all make simple mistakes or even disagree vehemently with the answer in the computer! Caution may lead you to answer too few questions to pass after the marks have been deducted for incorrect answers.

Distracters are the technical term for parts of questions which sound as though they are correct but are definitely incorrect. A good example would be symptoms and signs of *hyper*natraemia being included in a question on *hypo*natraemia. This is the most common cause of losing marks even though you know the answer.

Short notes

Short notes are not negatively marked. The system is for a 'marking template' to be devised which gives a mark(s) for each important fact. You will gain nothing for style or superfluous information. Your aim is to set out your knowledge in an ordered *concise* manner. The common faults are, first, devoting too much time to a single question thereby neglecting the rest and, second, not limiting the answer to the question asked. For example, in a question about the management of diabetes mellitus, you should not list all facts about diabetes, only those relevant to management.

Essays

Similar comments apply to essays, but you may get marks for logical development of an argument or theme. Conversely, you will not obtain good marks for an essay that is a set of unconnected statements. Length matters little if there is no cohesion. Most people are aware of the need to 'plan' their answer yet few do this. It is important in an examination based on essays that you manage your time and all questions are given equal weight, unless guided otherwise in the instructions. A brilliant answer in one essay will not compensate you for not attempting another because of time. Nobody can get more than 100% (usually 75%) on a single answer!

Data interpretation

Data interpretation involves the application of knowledge to solve a problem. In your revision, you should aim for an understanding of principles; it is impossible to memorise all the different data combinations. In the exam, a helpful approach is to translate numbers into a description, for example a serum potassium of 2.8 mmol/l is *low* and the ECG tracing of a heart rate of 120/min shows a *tachy*cardia. Pattern recognition can then be attempted.

Data questions are not usually negatively marked so put down an answer even if you are far from sure that it is right. Conversely, there is no point in listing four possibilities if the question asks for one response. The examiner will not choose from your answers, the first response will be taken!

Slide/picture questions

Pattern recognition is the first step in a picture question. You should couple this with a systematic approach looking for abnormalities. For example you should check the breast shadows, bony skeleton, soft tissues, retrocardiac space, etc. in a chest radiograph. Describe in your mind what you see and try to match it with common problems. Again, even if doubtful, put an answer down. Slides often come with an accompanying statement or data. You should use this alongside the visual image as it may give a clue as to the answer required; it may be essential in distinguishing between two conditions which give a similar slide appearance.

Case history questions

A more sophisticated form of exam question is an evolving case history with information being presented sequentially; you are asked to give a response at each stage. They are constructed so that a wrong response in the first part of the question still means that you can obtain marks from the subsequent parts. Patient management problems are designed to test the recall and application of knowledge through an understanding of the principles involved. As with the data interpretation, you should always give answers unless the exam instructions indicate the presence of negative marking.

Viva

The viva examination can be a nerve-wracking experience. You are normally faced with two examiners who may react with irritation, boredom or indifference to what you say. You may feel that the viva has gone well and yet you failed, or, more commonly, you think that the exam has gone badly simply because of the apparent attitude of the examiners.

Your main aim during the viva should be to steer the questioning of the examiners so that they are constantly asking you about things you know about. Despite what is often said, you can prepare for a viva. Questions are liable to take one of a small number of types centred around subjects that cannot be examined in the traditional clinical exam:

- emergency medicine (e.g. diabetic coma)
- management of common conditions (e.g. hypertension)
- clinical sciences (e.g. control of blood pressure).

For each heading, you can prepare a list of the *common* problems.

Another approach used by examiners is to invite you to start the viva by asking what you have read recently or what do you think is an important recent medical advance: prepare something along these lines beforehand.

During the viva there are certain techniques that will help you to make a favourable impression. When discussing the management of something, it is better to say 'I would do this' rather than 'the book says this'. You should try and strike a balance between saying too little and too much. It is hard on examiners when you will not expand on any of your answers and it is equally difficult if you refuse to shut up! Remember, the longer you talk without stopping the more likely it is that you have either gone off the topic or are showing the examiners the inadequacy of your knowledge.

In a viva, the examiners are likely to want to explore the *limits* of your knowledge; do not be upset if they push you hard. It is alright to say you do not know something, most examiners will want to change tack to see what you do know about.

Normal values

In both examinations and clinical practice, most test results are given together with the normal reference range for that laboratory. However, you are expected to know certain normal ranges as they are essential for making decisions in an emergency. Furthermore, familiarity with the ranges for common indices will help you to obtain a

'feel' for data interpretation and abnormal patterns. Thus, a serum potassium of 1.9 mmol/l means much more than one of 3.1 mmol/l even though both are low.

In the list of normal values in Tables 1 and 2, we have indicated with an * the indices that you would be expected to be able to give an approximate normal range. Remember that laboratories do vary and that a normal range is simply that which 95% of the normal population served by that laboratory would fit into.

Conclusions

We have set out a framework for using this book, but you should amend this according to your own needs and the examinations you are facing. Whatever approach you adopt, the aim should be for an understanding of the principles involved rather than rote learning.

Table 1 Normal values for haematology

Index	Range	Unit
White blood cell*	4.0–11.0	x 10^9/l
Neutrophils	2.0–7.5	x 10^9/l
Lymphocytes	1.5–4.0	x 10^9/l
Eosinophils	0.04–0.4	x 10^9/l
Monocytes	0.2–0.8	x 10^9/l
Basophils	<0.1	x 10^9/l
Red blood cells		
Male	4.5–6.5	x 10^{12}/l
Female	3.8–5.8	x 10^{12}/l
Haemoglobin: male*	13.0–17.0	g/dl
Haemoglobin: female*	11.6–16.5	g/dl
Packed cell volume (PCV)		
Male	0.40–0.54	l/l
Female	0.37–0.49	l/l
Mean cell volume (MCV)*	80.0–97.0	fl
Mean cell haemoglobin (MCH)	27.0–32.0	pg
Mean cell haemoglobin concentration (MCHC)	31.0–35.0	g/dl
Red cell distribution width (RDW)	11.5–15.0	–
Platelets*	150–400	x 10^9/l
Erythrocyte sedimentation rate (ESR)		
Male*	<5	mm/h
Female*	<7	mm/h
Plasma viscosity	1.50–1.72	cp
Reticulocytes	0.2–2.0	%
Serum B$_{12}$	160–600	ng/l
Serum folate	2.0–10.0	µg/l
Red cell folate	125–600	µg/l
Ferritin		
Males	20–300	µg/l
Female premenopausal	12–250	µg/l
Female postmenopausal	20–300	µg/l
Hb$_{A2}$	1.8–3.5	%
HbF	0.2–1.0	%
Glucose b-phosphate dehydrogenase	4.6–13.5	IU/g haemoglobin
Prothrombin time (PT)*	12.0–16.0	s
Activated partial thromboplastin time (APTT)	21.0–27.5	s
Fibrinogen	2.0–4.0	g/l
Fibrin degradation products (FDP) (D-dimer)	<0.5	mg/l
Bleeding time (Adults)	1.6–8.0	min

* Values that you would be expected to know.

Table 2 Normal reference ranges for biochemistry

Index	Range	Value
Sodium*	132–144	mmol/l
Potassium*	3.5–5.0	mmol/l
Chloride	95–108	mmol/l
Bicarbonate*	24–30	mmol/l
Urea*	2.7–7.5	mmol/l
Creatinine*	50–120	μmol/l
Glucose		
Fasting	3.2–6.0	mmol/l
Random	3.3–9.2	mmol/l
Bilirubin	1–20	μmol/l
Calcium*	2.10–2.65	mmol/l
Phosphate*	0.70–1.40	mmol/l
Total protein	60–80	g/l
Albumin	33–49	g/l
Globulin	21–38	g/l
Urate		
Female	<0.38	mmol/l
Male	<0.42	mmol/l
Blood gases		
pH*	7.38–7.42	
PCO_2*	34–45 (4.5–6.0)	mmHg (kPa)
PO_2*	90–110 (12–14.7)	mmHg (kPa)
Base excess*	−2 to +2	
Enzymes		
Alkaline phosphatase (ALP) (adult)	25–110	IU/l
Amylase	10–87	IU/l
Aspartate aminotransferase (AST)	5–45	IU/l
Alanine aminotransferase (ALT)	5–45	IU/l
Female/Male	5–45	IU/l
Gamma-glutamyl transferase (GGT)	<65	IU/l
Creatine kinase (CK)	<150	IU/l
Lactate dehydrogenase (LDH)	200–500	IU/l
Cerebrospinal fluid		
Protein*	0.25–0.75	g/l
Glucose* (depends on blood sugar)	2.5–5.5	mmol/l
Hormones		
Thyroxine (T_4)	50–150	nmol/l
Triiodothyronine (T_3)	1.1–2.8	nmol/l
TSH	0.5–5.0	mU/l
Cortisol	200–650	nmol/l (07:00–09:00 h)
	60–250	nmol/l (22:00–24:00 h)
Urine free cortisol	<300	nmol/24 h
Lipids:		
Total cholesterol		
Satisfactory	<5.2	mmol/l
Borderline	5.2–6.5	mmol/l
Unsatisfactory	>6.5	mmol/l
Fasting triglycerides	0.3–2.0	mmol/l
Iron	12–30	μmol/l
Total iron-binding capacity (TIBC)	45–70	μmol/l

*Values that you would be expected to know.

Cardiovascular disease

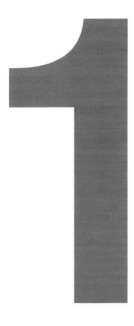

1.1 Background

Introduction

Cardiovascular disease is the most common cause of death in the western world and a preventable cause of much chronic ill-health. It will impinge on whichever branch of medicine you go into and may dominate your practice. As a general practitioner, cardiovascular disease will present some of the commonest serious situations you have to treat. As an anaesthetist, you will have to decide whether patients with it can safely be anaesthetised. As a surgeon, you will have to exclude it as a cause of abdominal pain. Cardiovascular diseases are ubiquitous, so they figure large in the 'core' knowledge and skills of the medical graduate.

Learning objectives

You should:

- be able to take with absolute confidence a history from a patient with chest pain or other major symptom of cardiovascular disease and construct a differential diagnosis
- have a good understanding of ischaemic heart disease and other forms of atherosclerotic vascular disease
- be competent at recognising heart failure and the commoner valvular lesions
- understand how to recognise and treat the common dysrhythmias
- understand how hypertension is defined and when and how to treat it
- have a clear understanding of **venous** and **arterial** thromboembolism and how to recognise and treat them
- be competent at performing cardio-pulmonary resuscitation.

Anatomy

You need a knowledge of the surface anatomy of the heart, as seen from the front, to interpret physical signs, chest radiographs and electrocardiographs (Fig. 1). The heart has a triangular projection and lies mostly behind the sternum. The base of the triangle is parallel and slightly to the right of the right sternal border. The apex is in the interspace between the left fifth and sixth ribs in the midclavicular line. The right atrium forms the right heart border. The left border is composed of the left atrial appendage superiorly and the left ventricle inferiorly. The anterior surface is composed, from right to left, of the right atrium, right ventricle, interventricular septum and left ventricle. The left atrium is at the back of the heart and, seen laterally, forms the upper posterior heart border. The lower border is formed by the left ventricle. The right ventricle forms the anterior heart border in a lateral projection (as illustrated under chest radiography in Fig. 4 below). The anatomy of the coronary circulation is described on page 13.

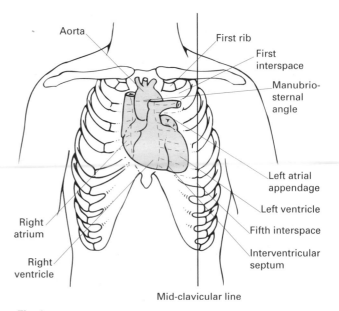

Fig. 1
Surface anatomy of the heart as seen from the front.

Physiology

Cardiac output is maintained by:

- impulse generation and propagation
- cyclical myocardial contraction
- an intact valvular system.

Impulse generation

The cardiac impulse is generated by cyclical depolarisation of the sino-atrial (SA) node, a specialised area close to the junction of the superior vena cava and the right atrium. The impulse spreads rapidly and reaches the atrio-ventricular (AV) node through the right and left atria. The ventricles are isolated electrically from the atria by the annulus fibrosus. The impulse is conducted by the His bundle, which leads into the right and left bundle branches, activating the right and left ventricles, respectively. The anatomy of impulse propagation is summarised in Figure 2. Spontaneous, rhythmic depolarisation is not unique to the SA node. It can arise lower in the conducting system. The lower in the conducting system the impulse arises, the slower the rate (e.g. atrium 80 beats/min, AV node 50 beats/min, ventricle 30 beats/min). The rate of ventricular contraction is governed by the most rapidly depolarising focus in the heart. Lower and slower pacemakers are overridden by impulses from above. Impulses can arise in diseased myocardium, often at a very fast rate (see dysrhythmias, p. 26). Impulses may pass through myocardial tissue when the conducting tissues are blocked (bundle branch block, p. 11) or through abnormal accessory pathways (p. 30).

The cardiac cycle

Atrial depolarisation causes right then left atrial contraction, corresponding to (though lagging behind) the P wave on the electrocardiograph. There is an electrical

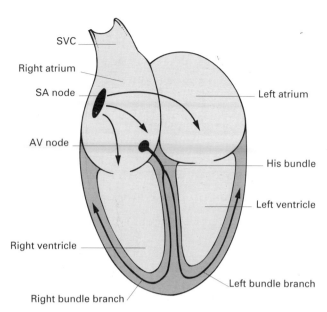

Fig. 2
The cardiac conducting system.

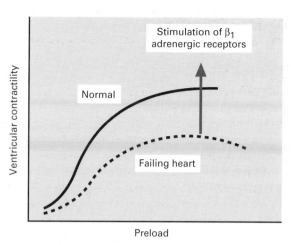

Fig. 3
The relationship between preload and cardiac contractility (Starling's relationship) and the effect of adrenergic stimulation.

pause (the PR interval) as the P wave passes through the AV node then contraction of the left and right ventricles (corresponding electrically to the QRS complex). Rising ventricular pressures close the mitral and tricuspid valves then open the pulmonary and aortic valves. At the end of systole, repolarisation occurs (T wave) and the ventricles relax. When aortic and pulmonary artery pressures exceed left and right ventricular pressures, respectively, the valves close. Closure of the mitral and tricuspid valves is heard as the first heart sound at the start of ventricular systole and aortic and pulmonary valve closure as the second sound at the end of it. Atrial systole is responsible for 20–30% of ventricular filling, the rest occurring passively. Each ventricle ejects about 80 ml blood with each cardiac cycle, or 65% of its end-diastolic volume (ejection fraction).

Cardiac output
Cardiac performance is determined by cardiac rate and stroke volume. Rate is controlled by the balance between sympathetic stimulation, which increases it, and parasympathetic (vagal) stimulation, which reduces it. Stroke volume depends on contractility and the 'afterload' or resistance against which the heart is pumping. This corresponds to peripheral vascular resistance or, in the case of aortic or pulmonary stenosis, the degree of outflow obstruction.

Stroke volume is also influenced by 'preload', the venous filling pressure. The way in which cardiac muscle responds to changes in preload is an important physiological concept, known as **Starling's law of the heart**, which states that the energy of contraction is proportional to the initial length of the muscle fibres. The heart responds to increased preload by an increased stroke volume up to a level of preload at which it is overwhelmed and decompensation occurs (Fig. 3). Sympathetic stimulation, acting on cardiac β_1-adrenoceptors, increases car-

diac performance for a given level of preload. How this relates to the pathophysiology and management of heart failure is considered on page 22.

Coronary artery perfusion occurs during diastole. A very fast heart rate increases myocardial work and reduces oxygen delivery, so it can precipitate ischaemia. Tachycardias also reduce cardiac output by shortening the time for ventricular filling.

Maintenance of blood volume
This is discussed in Chapter 4, which emphasises the close interrelationship between cardiovascular, renal and fluid/electrolyte physiology. That relationship is integral to clinical management.

Clinical assessment

History

The main symptoms of cardiovascular disease are:

- chest pain
- breathlessness
- ankle swelling
- fatigue
- palpitations
- syncope.

They result from impaired oxygen delivery to the myocardium (chest pain), brain (syncope) and all other tissues (fatigue), increased pulmonary and systemic venous pressure (breathlessness and ankle swelling) and abnormal cardiac rate and rhythm (palpitations). You should remember that chest pain may also be caused by disease of the aorta (e.g. dissection, p. 48), pulmonary circulation (pulmonary embolism/infarction, p. 47) and pericardium (pericarditis, p. 39).

Examination

Your examination should systematically test out the anatomy and physiology of the heart and circulation as described above and in Chapter 4. As with all other aspects of clinical examination, use all your senses in the order *look, feel, listen.*

Pulse rate and rhythm

Feel the radial and, if necessary, other pulses to measure the heart rate and decide if the rhythm is fundamentally regular, perhaps with superimposed ectopic or dropped beats, or chaotic (atrial fibrillation).

Arterial circulation

The arterial circulation is assessed from:

- the blood pressure, measured first sitting or lying, then standing to detect volume depletion or vasodilatation
- peripheral cyanosis and/or impaired capillary refill after blanching the nail beds, measures of impaired capillary perfusion
- the character of the carotid pulse, a crude way of detecting a reduced stroke volume or aortic valve dysfunction (p. 33).

Venous circulation

Venous circulation is assessed by examining the jugular venous pulse, auscultating the lung bases and testing for ankle and sacral oedema. There are several components to jugular venous examination:

- assessment of venous pressure as a sign of preload (p. 167)
- assessment of its response to respiration, discussed under pericardial effusions (p. 39)
- observation of the waveform, particularly important in detecting tricuspid incompetence.

Crackles at the lung bases may be a sign of pulmonary venous hypertension. Peripheral oedema indicates raised systemic venous pressure.

Heart and valves

The stethoscope allows you to detect:

- abnormalities of the first and second heart sounds
- added sounds, as in, for example, valvular heart disease (p. 31), heart failure (p. 21), or pericarditis (p. 39).

Peripheral arterial system

You should remember to examine the abdominal aorta and all peripheral pulses. Absence of pulses or bruits over large vessels signifies arterial obstruction.

Stigmata of cardiovascular disease

Infective endocarditis (p. 36) is the classical cardiovascular disease in which non-cardiac signs are as important as cardiovascular examination in making the diagnosis. Some other diseases, discussed under valvular heart disease (p. 31), have important stigmata which should be picked up by observation or general examination.

Investigation

Learning objectives

You should:
- be able to interpret the chest radiograph and electrocardiograph (ECG)
- know how other investigations can contribute to cardiovascular diagnosis and the indications for requesting them.

The chest radiograph

Echocardiography is a more sensitive and specific way of detecting most important cardiovascular abnormalities than the chest radiograph but you are unlikely to ba able to request one in the middle of the night and many patients can be managed without ever having one. Most relevant information can be obtained from a postero-anterior (PA) radiograph, but a lateral view can give extra information about individual chambers, particularly the left atrium. **Portable** films are taken antero-posterior and make the heart look larger than it is. Examine the radiograph systematically for:

- overall heart size
- changes in shape indicating disease of individual chambers
- calcification in valves (or the presence of prosthetic valves)
- abnormalities of the vessels, lung fields, and costophrenic angles.

The main patterns that you should be able to recognise are summarised in Figure 4. The cardiovascular diagnosis you will most often make is heart failure. Several features shown in the figure deserve special mention:

- increased pulmonary venous pressure causes dilatation of the upper lobe veins (>4 mm) and constriction of the lower lobe veins, termed 'upper lobe venous diversion'
- you can assess heart size by measuring the ratio of the width of the heart to the width of the thorax, expressed as the cardiothoracic ratio: a ratio >50% signifies cardiomegaly (except on an AP radiograph)
- septal ('Kerley') lines are caused by interstitial fluid; they are straight, often short (<1 cm), horizontal, peripheral and present first at the bases
- fluffy perihilar and more generalised shadowing signify fluid in the alveolar spaces, i.e. *severe* pulmonary venous hypertension.

The ECG

If you are unclear about ECG interpretation, you should read one of the excellent concise texts devoted to the subject; this description is very much revision. With increasing experience, you will start by taking a quick glance to detect any obvious abnormality. No matter

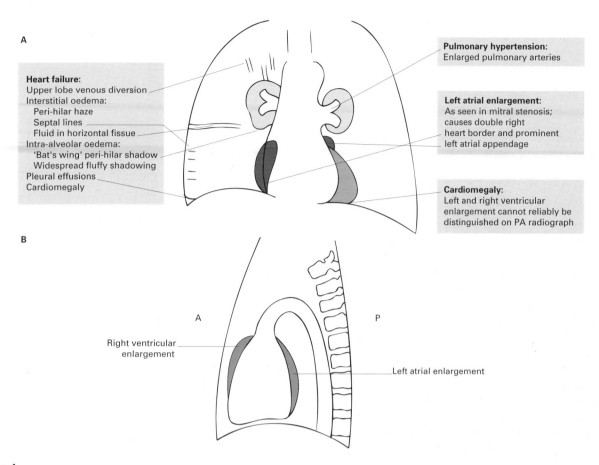

Fig. 4
Principal abnormalities that can be seen on a chest radiograph in cardiac disease. **A** PA radiograph; **B** lateral radiograph.

how experienced you are, you should also read on ECG systematically looking for:

- the cardiac rate
- the rhythm
- the electrical axis
- ventricular hypertrophy
- abnormal PQRST configurations.

You should also check the calibration, normally printed at the head of the paper. A normal paper speed is 25 mm/s. One large square (5 mm) represents 200 μs and 1 small square (1 mm) represents 40 μs. 1 mV causes a vertical deflection of 1 cm.

Rate, conduction and rhythm

Rate. First check the QRS complexes to see if they are regular or irregular. If regular, divide the number of large squares between two consecutive R waves into 300 to give the rate. If irregular, divide the number of large squares between four R waves into 900. A normal rate is 60–100 beats/min or 5–3 large squares between two consecutive R waves.

Conduction. Check for P waves as a sign that the impulses are arising within the atria. Next check the PR interval, which represents AV conduction. The PR interval (normal range 3–5 small squares) is short if the impulse is arising unusually close to the AV node or there is an electrical 'short-circuit' between the atria and ventricles ('accessory pathway'). The PR interval is

lengthened by disease of the AV node or His bundle. Finally check the width of the QRS complexes; normally this is up to 3 small squares. Complexes broader than this are being propagated by slow electrical spread through muscle rather than the conducting tissues (bundle branch block or 'intraventricular conduction delay').

Rhythm. Abnormalities are discussed under dysrhythmias (p. 26).

Axis

You cannot interpret ECGs without knowing from memory the vectors of each of the twelve leads, shown in Figure 5a, b. The highest voltage electrical activity in the normal ECG is left ventricular depolarisation, which spreads in a direction between −30° and 90° (the 'electrical axis'). This changes if ischaemic damage, hypertrophy or strain alter the net direction of depolarisation.

Axis deviation is detected by inspecting the R and S waves in leads aVL, I, II, avF and III. Movement towards increasingly large R waves is movement towards the electrical axis.

Normal axis. The R wave is larger than the S wave in I and II and lead II is usually the tallest; S may be greater than R in lead III.

Right axis deviation. The S wave is greater than the R wave in lead I.

Left axis deviation. The S wave is greater than the R wave in lead II.

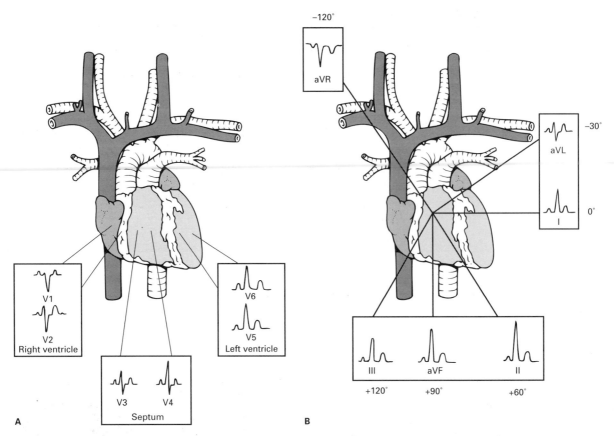

Fig. 5
The vectors of the chest leads for an ECG. **A** The chest leads are arranged radially across the pericardium. **B** The other six leads are calculated from values given by leads on the arms and legs. The electrical axis is the result of electrical activity during systole measured in the limb leads.

Ventricular hypertrophy

Muscle hypertrophy or strain causes increased electrical activity, as seen in the chest leads.

Left ventricular hypertrophy. The sum of the downwards deflection in V1 or V2, whichever is the greater, and the upwards deflection in V5 or V6, whichever is the greater, is greater than 35 small squares. This may be accompanied by downsloping ST segments or T wave inversion in left-sided leads (strain pattern). There is usually left axis deviation.

Right ventricular hypertrophy. Compared with the normal R wave (in Fig. 5a), the R wave is greater than the S wave in V1 and there is a deep S wave in V6. There is often a peaked P wave (right atrial hypertrophy) and right axis deviation in the limb leads.

The PQRST complex

Table 3 shows the normal PQRST configuration and a range of abnormal patterns, all of which you should be able to recognise. In diagnosing myocardial infarction, you should remember that it is normal to have a small Q wave in III; this disappears on deep inspiration. A Q wave must be at least 25% of the size of the R wave and 1 mm in width to be classified as 'pathological'.

1.2 Ischaemic heart disease

Any disease process which disturbs the relationship between myocardial oxygen supply and demand can cause ischaemia. This may be:

- impaired coronary artery blood flow
  — coronary atherosclerosis
  — coronary artery spasm
  — occlusion of the coronary ostia by aortic dissection
  — tachycardia causing shortened diastole (p. 9)
- impaired oxygen delivery
  — hypoxia
  — anaemia
- increased cardiac work
  — any cause of increased afterload
  — tachycardia.

Ischaemia is often multifactorial. The term 'ischaemic heart disease' (IHD) is used here to mean atherosclerotic coronary artery disease.

Learning objectives

You should:
- know the risk factors for IHD
- understand the pathogenesis
- understand how to diagnose and treat angina and myocardial infarction
- know the indications for fibrinolytic therapy and coronary revascularisation.

Table 3 Abnormalities of the PQRST complex in disease

	Pattern	Description	Comment
Disease states			
Myocardial ischaemia		Horizontal or downsloping ST segment depression	May occur at rest or, more usually, on exertion
		T wave inversion	
Myocardial infarction		Q wave; ST segment elevation; T wave inversion	Changes appear in the order ST elevation, T inversion, appearance of Q wave. They revert in the same order: T wave inversion sometimes permanent and Q waves always permanent. T wave changes alone in subendocardial infarction
Bundle branch block		'M-shaped complexes'; width >3 small squares	LBBB; M-shaped complexes in I, aVL and lateral chest leads. RBBB; 'RSR' configuration in V_{1-2}
Pericarditis		'Dished' or upwardly concave ST segments	Usually best seen in chest leads
Effect of digoxin		'Reverse tick' appearance	

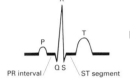

Normal PQRST complex (for comparison to others)

Coronary artery anatomy

Coronary artery anatomy is summarised in Figure 6. The right and left coronary arteries lead from the two coronary sinuses which arise from the aorta above the aortic valve. The right coronary artery supplies the right atrium and ventricle, small parts of the interventricular septum and left ventricle and often the inferior wall. It supplies the SA node in 60% of patients and the AV node in 90% so right coronary artery disease is prone to cause sinus dysfunction and AV block. The left main coronary artery divides into its major **left anterior descending branch**, which supplies the anterior left ventricle and septum, and the **circumflex branch**, which supplies the posterior and inferior left ventricular wall. There is interindividual variation in the territories of these vessels, which can influence clinical presentations.

Epidemiology

Risk factors

IHD is the single commonest cause of death in the developed world, accounting for 30% of male and 20% of female deaths in the UK. Knowledge of epidemiology is important for you as a clinician:

- to identify 'at-risk patients' and weight differential diagnoses
- to practise preventive medicine.

The incidence of IHD:

- rises progressively with age
- is higher in men than women
- rises sharply at the menopause
- is higher in patients with a positive family history.

The 'big three' remediable risk factors are:

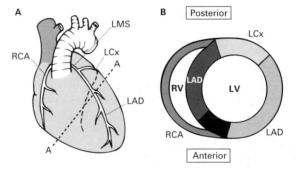

Fig. 6
A Coronary artery anatomy. **B** Section across the heart (A–A) shows the approximate distribution of blood supply. LAD, left anterior descending; LCx, left circumflex (dotted line shows its position at the back of the heart); RCA, right coronary artery. RV, right ventricle; LV, left ventricle. The section marked black is supplied by the RCA in many people. (Source: Textbook of Medicine, ed. Souhami and Moxham, Churchill Livingstone, 1997)

- hyperlipidaemia (see p. 272)
- smoking
- hypertension.

The Framingham study showed that coronary risk varies five-fold across the cholesterol distribution in the normal population. Likewise, there are 'dose–effect' relationships between coronary risk and smoking and hypertension. These risk factors are additive.

Weaker risk factors include:

- obesity
- type A personality
- inactivity
- alcohol abuse.

Alcohol has a complex effect in that low-level drinking (≤ 14 units per week in women and 21 in men) reduces coronary risk whereas higher intake increases it.

Many diseases, including chronic renal failure (p.

159), diabetes (p. 278) and gout, increase coronary risk. High levels of coagulation factors such as fibrinogen have the same effect but are not routinely measured.

Prevention

There is evidence that coronary risk can change:

- migrants adopt the IHD risk of the area they migrate to, indicating that 'environment' can outweigh genetic make-up
- the incidence of IHD fell very significantly in the USA at a time when awareness of the risk factors increased.

Persuasive evidence that cardiac mortality can be prevented has been slow to emerge from clinical trials. There is evidence that modification of lifestyle, including diet, smoking and physical activity can reduce risk. Trials of antihypertensive therapy have always shown more effect on the risk of stroke than of IHD, perhaps because some antihypertensives have atherogenic side-effects. Trials of cholesterol-lowering drugs have produced the most enigmatic results. Most show a reduced incidence of coronary *events* (though not always of coronary *mortality*) but the reduction in *overall* mortality has been poor because improvements in IHD were offset by other causes of death. Present evidence suggests that treating hypercholesterolaemia with drugs reduces the risk of non-fatal myocardial infarction by about 25%, and there is now evidence of a significant reduction in coronary mortality.

The most important practical point is that patients with established IHD stand to gain most from action against risk factors because their absolute risk of a coronary event is highest. In this context, lipid lowering can cause angiographic regression of coronary artery disease and reduce mortality.

Pathophysiology

Coronary artery stenosis and thrombosis, the causes of angina and myocardial infarction, are caused by atherosclerosis. Atherosclerotic plaques are composed of free lipid within the intima associated with smooth muscle cell and macrophage proliferation, fibrosis, and hyperplasia of the overlying endothelium. Shearing forces created by blood flow and/or contraction of the arterial wall cause fissure or rupture of the atherosclerotic plaque, exposing thrombogenic material within the plaque. Platelet thrombi form at the site of plaque rupture. These may embolise into the distal coronary artery, cause thrombotic occlusion of the artery or resolve. Despite re-endothelialisation, the lesion may progress and stenose the artery. These events cause the various clinical manifestations of IHD and provide the basis for prevention and treatment. Both angina and myocardial infarction are caused by myocardial hypoxia but only in myocardial infarction is there muscle necrosis.

Angina

Angina may be caused by:

- a fixed stenosis (>50%) of one or more coronary arteries

- coronary artery spasm
- platelet thrombo-embolism on a ruptured plaque.

Clinical presentation

Symptoms

Typical angina is an exercise-related, pressing precordial chest pain, radiating to the jaw and left arm and relieved by nitrates. It is often worse when exercising in cold air. Sometimes, angina is experienced as 'breathlessness' (resulting from transient left ventricular dysfunction) rather than pain. Anginal pain may come on when lying down at night (decubitus angina; caused by increased venous return in patients with incipient heart failure) or at rest (Prinzmetal angina; caused by coronary artery spasm). Coronary ischaemia may be painless, detected by cardiographic monitoring.

Important differential diagnoses are:

- gastro-oesophageal reflux and oesophageal spasm (p. 106)
- peptic ulcer and cholecystitis
- aortic dissection (p. 48) and pericarditis (p. 39)
- hyperventilation, air-swallowing and other psychosomatic disorders.

There is also a syndrome of uncertain cause (reflected by its name, **syndrome X**) in which patients with angiographically normal coronary arteries experience typical angina.

The term unstable angina is used to describe:

- increasing frequency, severity or duration of angina attacks (also termed 'crescendo angina')
- symptoms coming on at rest or after little provocation
- decreased responsiveness to glyceryl trinitrate.

It is caused by platelet thrombo-embolism on a ruptured plaque, spasm or a critical stenosis and may be a prelude to acute myocardial infarction.

Signs

You should examine patients carefully and keep in mind the cardiovascular and systemic diseases which can disturb the balance of oxygen supply and demand (e.g. dissecting thoracic aneurysm, aortic stenosis, anaemia). Look for risk factors such as hypertension. Patients with IHD may have signs of heart failure or peripheral vascular disease but many will have no abnormal signs at all.

Investigation

ECG

The resting ECG may show ST segment or T wave changes suggestive of ischaemia, or evidence of unsuspected previous myocardial infarction or hypertension, but it is often normal. It is most likely to be abnormal if recorded 'in pain'.

Exercise testing

Exercise can be used to provoke symptomatic or asymptomatic ECG changes which are absent at rest. After recording a baseline ECG, the patient is exercised on a treadmill or bicycle ergometer and the work load serially increased under medical supervision with resuscitation facilities immediately to hand. The following are criteria for a positive response:

- downsloping ST segment depression > 1 mm
- typical ischaemic symptoms
- dysrhythmias (e.g. ventricular ectopics)
- fall in blood pressure.

The result is expressed as a *probability* of IHD, recognising that some patients with IHD have negative tests and minor ST segment changes may develop in patients without IHD.

Exercise testing is contraindicated immediately after acute myocardial infarction and in uncontrolled hypertension, severe aortic stenosis and unstable angina.

The test must stop immediately if:

- the patient develops severe ischaemic symptoms or cannot tolerate the test
- the systolic blood pressure falls > 10 mmHg
- there is ST segment depression > 3 mm
- an arrhythmia develops.
  Indications for exercise testing include assessment of:
- severity of IHD, e.g. after myocardial infarction
- chest pain, if the diagnosis is unclear from the history and resting ECG
- a patient's capacity to exercise
- prognosis, e.g. to decide on the safety of returning to work
- response to treatment.

Other investigations

ST segment changes can be 'captured' by monitoring patients with unstable angina in the coronary care unit or, out of hospital, by ambulatory ECG monitoring. ST changes may occur with pain or 'silently'. Isotope scintigraphy may be used: a thallium scan performed at rest and after exercise can detect areas of impaired myocardial perfusion. Conventional echocardiography cannot directly assess the coronary circulation but can exclude valvular lesions as the cause of chest pain in patients with murmurs (aortic stenosis or mitral valve prolapse) and may be performed in angina to assess left ventricular function and detect abnormalities of ventricular wall motion caused by IHD.

Coronary angiography

This is the 'gold standard' investigation. Indications are:

- investigation of chest pain of uncertain aetiology
- assessment of severity of IHD in patients with positive exercise tests.

Coronary angiography can reliably assess the severity of coronary atherosclerosis and exclude its presence but cannot absolutely exclude ischaemia as the cause of chest pain. Exercise thallium scanning may be diagnostic of coronary ischaemia in patients with normal coronary arteries (syndrome X).

Management

The goals of management are to:

- prevent progression of coronary artery disease and optimise life expectancy
- relieve symptoms.

To achieve the first, you should measure fasting plasma lipids and treat them if raised (p. 273); smoking and alcohol excess should be discouraged. Life expectancy can also be improved by coronary revascularisation in selected cases and prescribing ACE inhibitors (angiotensin-converting enzyme inhibitors) in patients with coincident heart failure. Other aspects of secondary prevention are discussed under myocardial infarction (p. 17). Figure 7 summarises the treatments which relieve symptoms. Some of them are cardioprotective and can be expected to reduce mortality as well as relieve symptoms.

The four main classes of drug used to treat angina have additive effects and are prescribed stepwise. Some patients with mild angina are reluctant to take maintenance therapy and prefer to use lingual nitrate as needed. Beyond that, the choice is likely to be:

first step: beta-blocker, if not contraindicated

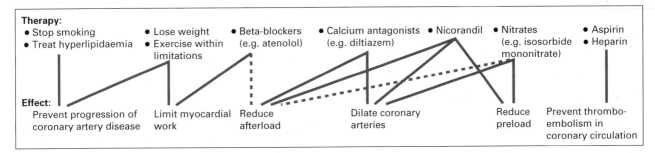

Fig. 7
The medical treatment of angina. Dotted lines indicate minor effects.

second and third steps: calcium antagonist then
   nitrate
fourth step: nicorandil
Finally: revascularisation if symptoms uncontrolled;
earlier if a strongly positive exercise test.

Aspirin and heparin

Unless contraindicated by allergy, intolerance or active
peptic ulceration, all patients should have aspirin (75 or
150 mg daily) to prevent future myocardial infarction.
Its mode of action is described on page 245. Heparin is
indicated for unstable angina.

Diet

Obesity increases cardiac work and is a risk factor for
disease progression. Obese patients should be encouraged to lose weight; a diet low in animal fat may
improve their lipid profile.

Nitrates

Nitrates work directly on vascular smooth muscle, with
three main effects:

- venodilatation, reducing preload and cardiac work
- peripheral arterial vasodilatation, reducing afterload
- coronary artery vasodilatation.

A commonly used drug is glyceryl trinitrate (GTN), dis-
solved under the tongue or sprayed onto it. It is used
either to prevent pain or to give acute relief. Long-acting oral nitrates (usually isosorbide mononitrate) or
transdermal nitrate patches are given to patients who
need GTN more than occasionally. Tolerance develops,
so any patient on maintenance nitrate must have a daily
nitrate-free interval of at least 6 hours.

Headache, palpitations and dizziness — direct
results of vasodilatation — are the main side-effects.
They are usually transient but may be intolerable.
Nitrate skin patches (chemically related to TNT) can
explode if they are between the two paddles of a defib-
rillator during resuscitation!

Beta-blockers

Beta-blockers are competitive antagonists of adrenaline
and noradrenaline at β-adrenoceptors. There are two
types of receptor: β_1 and β_2. Beta-blockers may be 'selective' to β-receptors in the heart (β_1-blockers) or non-
selective, in which case bronchial receptors are blocked
as well and bronchospasm can result. Atenolol is a commonly used cardioselective beta-blocker; propranolol is
non-selective. Beta-blockade reduces the rate and contractility of the heart, reduces cardiac work and limits
the heart rate during exercise.

A cardioselective beta-blocker such as atenolol is
often used as first-line treatment for angina, particularly
if the patient is also hypertensive or has had a myocardial infarct.

The two main side-effects/contraindications are
inherent in their mode of action: the negative
inotropic effect of beta-blockers can precipitate or
worsen heart failure and blockade of β_2-adrenoceptors
precipitates bronchospasm in patients with obstructive
airways disease. They may also cause peripheral vasoconstriction; for most patients, that just means cold
hands, but it can worsen intermittent claudication or
cause gangrene in those with peripheral vascular disease.

Calcium antagonists

There are many drugs that are calcium antagonists; all
block calcium channels but they have different tissue
specificities and, therefore, different actions. The dihy-
dropyridines (including nifedipine, nicardipine,
nimodipine and amlodipine) principally vasodilate
peripheral arterioles and the coronary arteries, lowering blood pressure, reducing afterload and relieving
coronary artery spasm. Verapamil impedes the transport of calcium across myocardial smooth muscle cells,
including the conducting tissues, prolonging the action
potential and refractory period and having a negative
inotropic effect. It is often used as an antiarrhythmic.
Diltiazem has similar cardiac effects but is less negatively inotropic.

All drugs in the class are effective antianginals and
antihypertensives. Amlodipine is often used as the first-
choice calcium antagonist. Side-effects include negative
inotropy, sinus bradycardia and atrioventricular block.
Other 'class' effects result from vasodilatation; they
include headache, flushing, hypotension and ankle
swelling.

Nicorandil

Nicorandil has a dual mode of action, leading to relaxation of vascular smooth muscle. Its potassium channel-
opening action causes coronary and peripheral
vasodilation, and its nitrate activity causes venodilatation. It therefore relieves angina by reducing preload
and afterload and relieving coronary artery spasm.

Nicorandil has vasodilator side-effects, as described
under Nitrates and Calcium antagonists, and is contraindicated in severe heart failure and hypotension.

Coronary revascularisation

Referral for coronary angiography with a view to percutaneous coronary angioplasty (PTCA) or coronary
artery bypass grafting (CABG) is indicated in:

- unstable angina
- severe IHD, even if controlled medically, to improve
  life expectancy
- stable angina uncontrolled with medical therapy.

Many factors influence selection for revascularisation,
including availability of the service and the choice of
patients and their doctors. The survival advantage is
greatest in patients with severe coronary artery disease
(left main stem or triple artery disease). The risks may
outweigh any likely benefits in patients who are grossly
obese or continue to smoke despite the presence of IHD.
Old people benefit as much from revascularisation as
the young, so age is not in itself a contraindication, particularly for angioplasty.

PTCA is less invasive than CABG, meaning that it can be performed in patients who are unfit for CABG and in acute myocardial infarction when major surgery has an unacceptably high mortality. It is also increasingly taking the place of CABG in less severe coronary artery disease, such as single or limited stenoses. About one-third of patients treated by PTCA need repeat procedures and fewer have their angina completely relieved than is achieved by CABG, but patient survival in randomised trials has been comparable with the two procedures.

Unstable angina

This is a serious problem because it may precede acute myocardial infarction and is, therefore, sometimes an indication for urgent revascularisation. The management consists of:

- hospitalisation to exclude myocardial infarction and control pain
- aspirin and i.v. heparin on the presumption of thrombosis on a ruptured atherosclerotic plaque
- nitrate i.v. to control pain
- use of other antianginals in combination, as described for stable angina.

Severe ST segment changes during attacks of pain or failure to control the pain with medical therapy are indications for angiography with a view to urgent revascularisation.

Myocardial infarction

Pathology

Angiography has shown that myocardial infarction is caused by coronary artery occlusion in at least 90% of patients. The effects of coronary occlusion can be predicted from the coronary anatomy (Fig. 6) although you should remember coronary anatomy and the sites of stenoses vary from individual to individual. Occlusion of the left anterior descending artery causes lateral, anterior or septal infarction, and this may be very extensive. Right coronary artery occlusion causes right ventricular and inferior infarcts, which tend to be smaller and may involve part of the septum, including the AV node. Posterior infarction is caused by occlusion of the distal circumflex artery. 'Subendocardial' infarction is the term given to a diffuse and concentric pattern of myocardial damage not caused by a localised coronary artery occlusion. It may occur in diffuse coronary artery disease, in association with increased ventricular wall thickness or pressure, or in conditions of reduced coronary artery perfusion or generalised hypoxia.

Clinical presentation

Diagnosis is based upon:

- history and signs
- ECG
- cardiac enzymes
- other circumstantial evidence.

History and signs

The pain of myocardial infarction differs from angina in two ways:

- duration, usually lasting > 20 min and often several hours
- lack of association with exercise and lack of relief from nitrates.

The pain varies from mild 'indigestion' to excruciating pain. It may be accompanied by a sense of impending death (angor animi). There may be breathlessness and/or palpitations. The presentation may be with syncope caused by a dysrhythmia. About 50% of patients have a previous history of angina or myocardial infarction and many of the remainder have obvious risk factors such as hypertension or cigarette smoking.

Sweating and pallor are common. There may be a bradycardia (resulting from increased vagal tone, typically in inferior infarction) or tachycardia. Blood pressure is usually normal or low. There may be basal crackles and a third or fourth heart sound, indicative of left ventricular failure. The jugular venous pressure is not usually raised at presentation; if it is, and particularly if there are no signs of left ventricular failure, think of **right ventricular infarction**.

Investigations

ECG

The patterns of injury and order in which they develop were discussed on page 13 and shown in Table 3. Examples are given in the self-assessment section. It follows from Figure 5 that:

- inferior infarction: causes changes in leads II, III and aVF
- anterior infarction: across the anterior chest leads V1–4 (termed septal if confined to leads V3–4)
- lateral infarction: I, aVL and V5–6
- posterior infarction: the subtlest change, a dominant R wave in lead V1, often associated with ST depression in the anterior leads.

Myocardial infarcts are classified into Q wave and non-Q wave types, corresponding to coronary artery occlusions with focal necrosis of the full width of the myocardium and diffuse partial thickness (sub-endocardial) damage, respectively. 'Hyperacute T waves' (increased height with a dramatic peaked appearance) are the earliest sign of full thickness myocardial infarction but are seen in only a minority of patients. The order of development of other changes is summarised in Table 3. The ST segment changes usually normalise within 1 week of infarction. T wave changes may be permanent or revert later. Q wave changes are usually permanent. The ECG signs of non-Q wave infarction are ST segment depression and T wave inversion.

Release of cardiac enzymes

Increased blood levels of enzymes typically found in heart muscle are indicative of damage to the heart. The enzyme which is most specific to cardiac muscle is the MB isoenzyme of creatine phosphokinase (CK-MB). This rises in the bloodstream within 24 hours of acute myocardial infarction and remains elevated for about 48 hours. Many laboratories measure total creatine phosphokinase activity (CK), which is a non-specific marker of muscle damage and can be increased by minor muscle damage such as an intramuscular injection. Despite its non-specificity, a CK *rise and fall* in a patient with good clinical and cardiographic evidence of myocardial infarction is diagnostic. Aspartate aminotransferase (AST) rises early after myocardial infarction but is even less specific because it is released by liver and other tissues as well as the heart. Like total CK, its lack of specificity is not a problem if there is other evidence of myocardial infarction, the concentration at least doubles and the time course of its rise and fall fits the diagnosis. Lactate dehydrogenase (LDH) is, likewise, non-specific but is raised for up to 10 days after myocardial infarction, useful if the patient presents late and the diagnosis is in doubt.

The rise in cardiac enzymes is proportional to the amount of necrotic cardiac muscle and gives a rough guide to severity. With the possible exception of CK-MB, myocardial infarction should not be diagnosed on enzymes alone. A firm diagnosis is based on two out of three of the following criteria:

- typical history
- ECG changes
- doubling of cardiac enzyme.

Other circumstantial evidence

There is often a small rise in temperature at about 12 hours, a rise in ESR and a neutrophil leucocytosis. These are non-specific signs of tissue necrosis. More specific evidence is the development of heart failure, dysrhythmias or pericarditis.

Immediate management

Faced with a patient with suspected acute myocardial infarction, your immediate responsibilities are to:

- site a venous cannula
- perform an ECG
- take a rapid history
- assess the cardiac rhythm, arterial and venous circulations (p. 167)
- give aspirin (150 mg as an immediate dose, repeated once daily) *on suspicion* of acute myocardial infarction
- relieve pain with diamorphine and an antiemetic (e.g. metaclopramide or prochlorperazine)

- give high concentration oxygen to correct any hypoxia caused by left ventricular failure
- give fibrinolytic therapy with the shortest possible 'door-to-needle' time if there are definite ECG changes
- take blood for urea, creatinine and electrolytes (particularly potassium) and cardiac enzymes
- arrange admission to a coronary care unit.

The reason for checking potassium is that catecholamines secreted in response to myocardial infarction drive potassium into cells. The patient may already be hypokalaemic as a result of previous diuretic therapy. Hypokalaemia predisposes to cardiac dysrhythmias, so you need to prescribe potassium supplements to maintain plasma potassium ≥ 3.5 mmol/l. Plasma urea and creatinine are measured to detect pre-existing renal failure, and as a baseline in case renal function deteriorates acutely.

You must also:

- ensure adequate pain relief with opiates and antianginals
- identify and treat heart failure.

These are discussed in more detail under Complications below.

Fibrinolysis

The use of drugs that break down fibrin can restore flow in the occluded artery in about two-thirds of patients. There are two main drugs: *streptokinase* works by activating free plasminogen and *alteplase* activates plasminogen bound to fibrin. Streptokinase is a foreign, antigenic protein; there is a risk of anaphylaxis if it is repeated. Alteplase (although biosynthetic) is the same as endogenous plasminogen activator and, therefore, is non-antigenic. Both drugs are given by i.v. infusion. Streptokinase is much cheaper and used as treatment of first choice. It may cause hypotension. Alteplase is indicated in patients who have previously received streptokinase and in patients who become hypotensive on streptokinase.

Contraindications to fibrinolysis include:

- recent history of haemorrhage
- trauma, surgery, recent childbirth or vascular injury
- active peptic ulceration
- recent history of stroke, particularly haemorrhagic
- uncontrolled hypertension, liver disease or varices
- active proliferative diabetic retinopathy at risk of bleeding
- pregnancy (fetal death may result).

The main side-effect of fibrinolysis is bleeding and this may cause acute haemorrhagic stroke.

Aspirin and fibrinolytic therapy, given appropriately, together reduce the acute mortality of myocardial infarction by over 40%.

Subsequent management

Patients should continue to receive aspirin (unless there is a contraindication); many will need further analgesia or nitrate therapy and some will receive diuretic therapy and an ACE inhibitor for heart failure. More specific management details are considered under the headings of complications, post-infarction prophylaxis and rehabilitation.

Complications

There is a high risk of ventricular fibrillation during the first 4 to 6 hours. Patients often respond well to resuscitation and have an excellent prognosis.

Complications developing later are more ominous. Bad prognostic signs are:

- hypotension or marked left ventricular failure
- extensive or progressive ECG changes
- massive enzyme rise (e.g. total CK > five times normal)
- acute hyperglycaemia or history of diabetes
- rise in blood urea
- greater age.

Dysrhythmias

Dysrhythmias may occur early after fibrinolytic therapy, when they are caused by reperfusion of ischaemic myocardium (reperfusion dysrhythmias). They have a benign prognosis and should not be treated unless the patient is haemodynamically compromised. Dysrhythmias are covered in detail below (p. 26). Common dysrhythmias specific to acute myocardial infarction are:

Ventricular fibrillation (VF)

Ventricular ectopic beats and tachycardia (VT). Isolated ventricular ectopics are of little significance. Ectopics which are multifocal, come in runs or occur close upon the previous complex (R on T) may precede ventricular fibrillation. They can be suppressed by lignocaine but this does not prevent ventricular fibrillation so they should not be treated unless there is haemodynamic compromise.

Sinus tachycardia. This may be caused by heart failure or anxiety. There is no specific treatment.

Sinus bradycardia. This occurs early and results from increased vagal tone. It can be treated with atropine if symptomatic.

Atrial fibrillation. This is a bad prognostic sign because it signifies severe myocardial damage. It requires cardioversion if it causes acute haemodynamic compromise. Otherwise, the treatment is digoxin. Anticoagulation is essential to reduce the risk of embolism from the fibrillating atrium.

Supraventricular tachycardia.

Complete heart block. There are two quite distinct situations. Patients with **inferior myocardial infarcts** may develop oedema of the atrio-ventricular node, which causes first-, then second-, then third-degree (complete) heart block. Complete block is usually transient with a satisfactory idioventricular rate (p. 27) because the escape pacemaker is relatively high in the conducting system. Such patients do not usually require pacing. Patients with **anterior infarcts** may develop 'bifascicular block' (an ECG diagnosis based on right bundle branch block with left axis deviation), which can progress to complete heart block. This signifies widespread myocardial damage with interruption of the conduction pathways below the His bundle. If complete heart block occurs, it causes profound bradycardia and hypotension and may not resolve spontaneously. Bifascicular block, in this situation, is an indication for prophylactic pacing.

Heart failure

Left ventricular dysfunction may cause 'forwards failure' — hypotension, renal impairment, impaired capillary perfusion — and 'backwards failure' — pulmonary oedema (p. 21). Treatment is with diuretics and nitrates, orally or i.v. Provided the patient is not hypotensive (systolic < 100 mmHg), an oral ACE inhibitor (e.g. captopril) should be started without delay.

Right heart failure may occur secondary to left ventricular dysfunction, in which case the treatment is as above. If it develops without signs of left ventricular failure, right ventricular infarction should be suspected and the treatment is the exact opposite: infusion of colloid to increase right ventricular filling pressure. Diuretic therapy worsens cardiac output in this situation, as will nitrates.

Cardiogenic shock is caused by severe left ventricular dysfunction. There is:

- hypotension
- poor capillary perfusion: cold, cyanosed nail beds with delayed capillary refill
- poor cerebral perfusion: impairment of consciousness
- impaired renal perfusion: renal failure.

Oxygen, a nitrate infusion and a diuretic are given to relieve breathlessness. Dobutamine (an inotropic agent) is infused to optimise left ventricular performance. Dopamine may also be infused in low dose to improve renal perfusion. A pulmonary artery catheter may be inserted to monitor the haemodynamic response. The mortality is up to 90% despite treatment.

Unremitting pain

The pain of myocardial infarction usually settles within hours and requires just one or two doses of opiate, but there are patients in whom anginal pain continues. Opiates should be given as needed, nitrate infused or given orally and a beta-blocker and/or calcium antagonist given. Heart failure and dysrhythmias should be controlled because they worsen angina. If pain continues and/or there are new ST segment changes on the ECG, the patient needs coronary angiography with a view to revascularisation (see Unstable angina above).

Pericarditis

Pericarditis can occur about 48 hours after full thickness myocardial infarction. The pain (p. 38) is recognisably different from the pain of the infarct and usually transient. Anticoagulants should be withheld because there is a risk of haemorrhage into the pericardial space.

Septal rupture

An acute ventricular septal defect is a rare result of ischaemic septal damage. There is acute haemodynamic deterioration and a pansystolic murmur, often accompanied by a thrill. The only effective treatment is surgery.

Ruptured papillary muscle

Rupture of a papillary muscle can vary in severity from mild mitral valve prolapse to florid mitral incompetence. If mild, it is managed medically. If severe, the treatment is valve replacement, which has a high mortality.

Left ventricular aneurysm and cardiac rupture

Full-thickness myocardial infarction causes softening and dyskinesia (impaired contraction) of the ventricular wall, which heals by fibrosis. If the dyskinetic area is large, the healing area of infarction may form an aneurysm which is non-contractile and, paradoxically, enlarges during systole. There is likely to be mural thrombus (see below). Left ventricular aneurysms are associated with:

- persistent and severe left ventricular dysfunction
- a dyskinetic 'feel' to the cardiac apex on examination
- the development of dysrhythmias
- a high risk of arterial thrombo-embolism
- persistent (> 1 week) ST segment elevation on the ECG.

Diagnosis is by echocardiography. Some left ventricular aneurysms can be treated surgically.

The area of softening may rupture before it has become fibrotic. This causes sudden death a week or more after infarction. There is electro-mechanical dissociation (complexes on the ECG with no cardiac output).

Mural thrombus

Even without aneurysm formation, thrombus can form on the endocardial surface after full thickness infarction, particularly if the left ventricle is contracting poorly. The thrombus may embolise to the brain, limbs or mesenteric circulation. Full thickness infarction, poor left ventricular performance and aneurysm formation are indications for prophylactic anticoagulation. The thrombus may be demonstrated echocardiographically.

Venous thrombo-embolism

Myocardial infarction causes:

- recumbency
- reduced cardiac output
- increased synthesis of coagulation factors, as a response to acute illness.

All these predispose to deep venous thrombosis and pulmonary embolism, classically 10 or more days after the infarct. Management is discussed on page 147. You should encourage patients to keep their legs mobile in bed, avoid unnecessarily long recumbency and give them prophylactic heparin. Patients with poor cardiac output or evidence of venous thrombosis should be fully anticoagulated.

Postinfarction prophylaxis

Prophylaxis is summarised in Box 1. Most of the treatments have been tested in clinical trials and shown to improve survival, but not in all of their possible permutations, leaving an element of choice to the clinician. The indications for and contraindications to fibrinolytics, aspirin and anticoagulants have already been discussed; hyperlipidaemia on p. 273, exercise testing on p. 15 and cardiac rehabilitation on p. 21. Diuretics, nitrates and calcium antagonists are given for specific indications but have no general role in improving life expectancy.

Box 1
An approach to improving prognosis and preventing complications after myocardial infarction

Immediate

Fibrinolysis
Aspirin — continue indefinitely
Lipid measurement — treat later if abnormal
Heparin, prophylactic use — continue throughout hospital stay

First 24–48 hours

ACE inhibitor — if full-thickness anterior MI or any evidence of left ventricular failure (LVF) (unless hypotensive); continue indefinitely
Beta-blocker — if no evidence of LVF (unless asthmatic, etc.); continue indefinitely

Rest of hospital stay

Full anticoagulation — if severe LV dysfunction or dysrhythmias
Reconsider ACE inhibitors and/or beta-blockers
Coronary risk factors — identify and discuss, e.g. smoking, inactivity

After discharge

Cardiac rehabilitation — encourage physical activity, advise about diet, smoking, alcohol
Hyperlipidaemia — treat; screen other family members
Exercise test — refer for angiography with a view to revascularisation if positive
ACE inhibitors and/or beta-blockers — reconsider use

Beta-blockers

Beta-blockers have been proven to reduce coronary mortality if given intravenously on admission and, in a separate trial, orally for up to 5 years afterwards. A reasonable practice is to introduce an oral beta-blocker in all patients without a contraindication such as asthma as soon as it is clear that they are not developing hypotension or heart failure.

ACE inhibitors

ACE inhibitors are also of proven value in left ventricular dysfunction and are most effective if introduced early. A practical policy is to start a small dose of a short-acting ACE inhibitor in any patient who has left ventricular failure (LVF) and is not hypotensive and in all patients with anterior infarcts, because they are likely to have left ventricular dysfunction.

Plasma lipids

The stress of myocardial infarction increases plasma lipids within about 24 hours, so they should be measured either immediately or 3 months later.

Cardiac rehabilitation

Patients with uncomplicated myocardial infarction are usually kept in bed for 48 hours then allowed to return gradually to normal mobility during a hospital stay of 5 to 7 days. Sensitive management by medical and nursing staff alleviates anxiety and helps them come to terms with their diagnosis. Investigations and treatment choices should be discussed and the diagnosis and its implications carefully explained, with plenty of opportunity to ask questions. They should be supplied with written material appropriate to their diagnosis and level of interest and given a chance to discuss their future plans and prospects.

After discharge, cardiac rehabilitation can improve the outcome of myocardial infarction in physical as well as psycho-social terms. It consists of supervised exercise training, education and counselling. Important points to discuss are:

- resumption of sexual activity
- return to work (a time of difficulty, particularly in patients who are self-employed or have manual jobs)
- physical activity.

1.3 Heart failure

Heart failure is common. The overall prevalence is about 1%, rising to over 10% in old people. Together with IHD it is a leading cause of acute hospital admission. It has a high mortality; the overall 5-year survival is about 50% and severe heart failure has a prognosis as bad as disseminated cancer. Its symptoms have a major impact on quality of life. On the positive side, recent clinical trials have shown how the prognosis can be improved by both traditional and new drugs.

Learning objectives

You should:
- have a clear understanding of the pathophysiology of heart failure and the range of disease processes which cause it
- be able to diagnose it from the symptoms, signs and chest radiograph
- understand its treatment and how that relates to the pathophysiological mechanisms.

Definitions

Getting to grips with some terms used to describe heart failure will help you to understand the range of clinical manifestations. First, remember that 'heart failure' is not a precise diagnosis in itself but the common end-product of a range of pathological processes. Good clinical practice is to base treatment on as precise a *pathological* diagnosis as possible.

Low-output versus high-output heart failure

Heart failure can be defined as failure to maintain a cardiac output sufficient to meet the needs of the tissues, despite an adequate filling pressure (excluding haemorrhagic shock and volume depletion). True heart failure may be caused by 'pump failure' (low-output heart failure) or increased demand (high-output heart failure), as in anaemia (p. 228).

Left versus right heart failure

Pure failure of one side of the heart is unusual because:

- disease processes do not usually affect just one side of the heart
- left heart failure increases pulmonary venous pressure and leads to right heart failure.

Pure right heart failure resulting from pulmonary hypertension is a notable exception. However, symptoms and signs may be *predominantly* related to right or left heart failure. Right heart failure causes symptoms and signs of *systemic* venous congestion whereas left ventricular failure causes *pulmonary* venous congestion. Biventricular failure is a better term than congestive cardiac failure to describe a combination of the two.

Forwards versus backwards failure

Forwards and backwards describe the effects of a reduced cardiac output on the arterial and venous circulations respectively. The relationship of forwards and backwards failure to the symptoms of heart failure is discussed on page 9 and Figure 8 (page 22) shows how these terms relate to the signs.

Severity and chronicity

Heart failure ranges from asymptomatic systolic dysfunction to a disease causing intolerable symptoms. It may be chronic or, as when caused by a cardiac arrhythmia, transient and completely reversible.

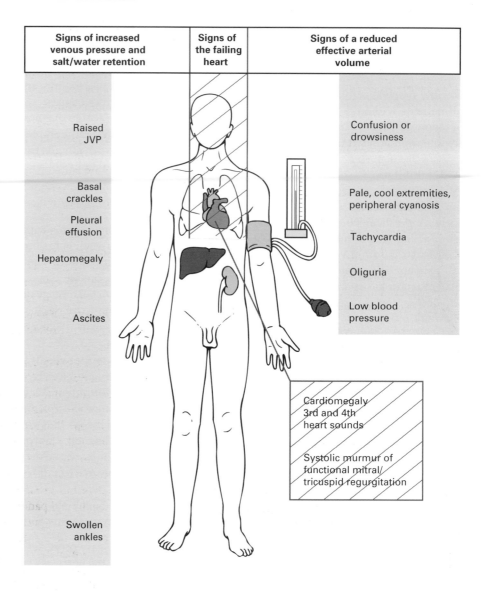

Signs of increased venous pressure and salt/water retention	Signs of the failing heart	Signs of a reduced effective arterial volume
Raised JVP		Confusion or drowsiness
Basal crackles		Pale, cool extremities, peripheral cyanosis
Pleural effusion		Tachycardia
Hepatomegaly		Oliguria
Ascites		Low blood pressure
	Cardiomegaly 3rd and 4th heart sounds	
	Systolic murmur of functional mitral/ tricuspid regurgitation	
Swollen ankles		

Fig. 8
Symptoms and signs of heart failure

Pathophysiology of heart failure

The earliest effect of impaired cardiac contractility is failure to increase cardiac output in response to exercise, experienced by the patient as exertional dyspnoea. Eventually the failing heart cannot maintain an adequate stroke volume at rest and venous pressure rises. At first, the Starling effect (p. 9) restores contractility at the cost of cardiac dilatation. As contractility progressively fails, venous pressures rise and pulmonary and systemic oedema result.

A reduced cardiac output reduces the *effective* arterial volume, and triggers compensatory mechanisms, including activation of the renin–angiotensin–aldosterone system and secretion of catecholamines and antidiuretic hormone (p. 167). Hyperaldosteronism causes salt and water retention, expanding the blood volume, further increasing venous pressure and causing oedema. Catecholamine secretion tends to restore cardiac output by increasing contractility and heart rate but also increases peripheral vascular resistance (afterload). Increased venous pressure increases secretion of atrial natriuretic peptide but insufficiently to counteract the combined

sodium-retaining effects of venous hypertension and secondary hyperaldosteronism.

Think of heart failure as a vicious circle in which these compensatory mechanisms initially maintain cardiac output but later become part of the disease process. Since contractility cannot usually be corrected, the treatment of heart failure (see Fig. 9) is directed primarily at those compensatory mechanisms.

Causes of heart failure

IHD is the most common cause, but it is only one of many. Others include:

- decreased myocardial contractility
  - heart muscle disease, e.g. alcoholic cardiomyopathy
- altered cardiac rhythm
  - tachycardia
  - bradycardia
- increased arterial resistance
  - systemic hypertension
  - pulmonary hypertension

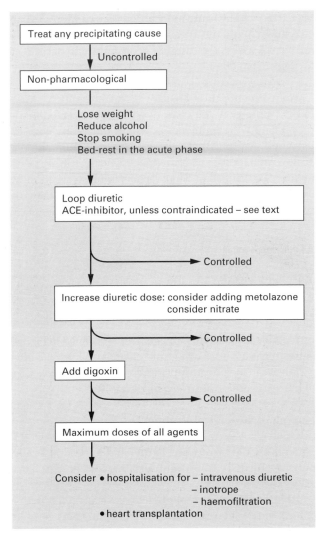

Fig. 9
Management of chronic heart failure.

- increased blood volume
  — overtransfusion
  — renal failure
- valvular lesions
  — outflow resistance, e.g. aortic stenosis
  — increased flow, e.g. mitral regurgitation
- compromised cardiac filling
  — constrictive pericarditis
  — pericardial effusion
- increased demand (high-output cardiac failure)
  — anaemia
  — thyrotoxicosis
  — left to right shunt.

There is often more than one cause.

Clinical presentation

Symptoms and signs

This section integrates symptoms and signs and lists them according to the underlying mechanisms (Fig. 8):

- increased venous pressure

- reduced cardiac output
- failing heart

Increased venous pressure
Symptoms
- Breathlessness. Increased pulmonary venous pressure causes alveolar oedema, which impairs gas exchange and reduces the compliance of the lungs. Dyspnoea occurs only after exertion in mild heart failure and at rest in more severe failure. Lying flat increases venous return and makes breathlessness worse (orthopnoea). There may be severe nocturnal episodes of left ventricular failure (paroxysmal nocturnal dyspnoea).
- Cough. This may be unproductive or productive of white frothy sputum sometimes pink-tinged or frankly blood-stained.
- Wheeze. Heart failure may cause airways narrowing with wheeze (cardiac asthma) indistinguishable from the wheeze of obstructive airways disease.
- Oedema.
Signs of left ventricular failure
- Basal crackles. Crackles which do not disappear after coughing are a sign of pulmonary oedema.
Signs of right ventricular failure
- Oedema. Fluid collects first in the most dependent parts of the body, usually the ankles, and spreads proximally. Press firmly over the medial aspect of the shin just proximal to the ankle for a few seconds to detect it. *Sacral oedema* may be more prominent in bedbound patients. Severe right heart failure causes ascites and pleural effusions by the same mechanism as ankle swelling.
- Hepatomegaly.
- Raised jugular venous pressure. This is covered in detail on page 167. Look for pulsation behind sternomastoid, observe how it varies with respiration and, if necessary, accentuate it by pressing briefly over the liver to increase venous return (hepato-jugular reflux).

Reduced effective arterial volume
Symptoms
- Dizziness and syncope. These are caused by impaired cerebral perfusion, worse on standing and often exacerbated by diuretic and vasodilator therapy.
- Fatigue.
Signs
- Low blood pressure. This results in pale cool extremities with peripheral cyanosis. Tachycardia can also occur.
- Tachycardia. This results from sympathetic activation.

Failing heart
Signs
- Cardiomegaly. Cardiac dilatation is fundamental to the pathophysiology of heart failure (p. 9). The apex beat is displaced. If you place the heel of your hand

over the sternum and your fingers over the apex, you will feel right ventricular dilatation under the heel and left ventricular dilatation under the fingers.

- Added sounds. The third heart sound is caused by diastolic filling of a diseased and non-compliant ventricle and the fourth sound by atrial contraction. Both are pathological in older adults, but a third sound may be heard in fit young people. They are heard best at the apex with the bell of the stethoscope. The way to remember how they sound is to think of Kentucky (Ken-tuck-*y*; 1, 2, 3) for the third sound and Tennessee (*Tenn*--essee; 4, 1, 2) for the fourth. If there is a tachycardia, you may not be able to distinguish between them. Both may be present.
- Pansystolic murmur. Cardiac dilatation stretches the mitral and tricuspid valve rings so you may also hear a pansystolic murmur as an *effect* of heart failure.

Investigations

It is usually possible to diagnose heart failure from the history, examination and chest radiograph (p. 11). An echocardiogram is much more sensitive and specific than the radiograph to confirm the diagnosis and identify its cause. A radionuclide scan, which measures ventricular size in systole and diastole, is more accurate than the echocardiogram at measuring the ejection fraction. The choice of other investigations is guided by a thorough history and examination. An ECG will show signs of underlying IHD and may point to other diagnoses. Do not forget to exclude systemic diseases such as alcoholism, anaemia and thyrotoxicosis.

Clinical presentations

There are two main clinical presentations of heart failure, which are different enough to be described separately:

- acute left ventricular failure
- chronic biventricular failure.

Pure right heart failure may also occur (p. 21).

Acute left ventricular failure

Acute left ventricular failure is caused by:

- acute myocardial infarction (p. 19)
- chronic IHD
- fluid overload, e.g. renal failure (p. 157)
- valve failure; e.g. bacterial endocarditis (p. 36).

The patient is sitting bolt upright, gasping for breath and often coughing up profuse pink, frothy sputum. There is a tachycardia, third and/or fourth heart sounds and bibasal pulmonary crackles. The chest radiographic appearances are as shown on page 11. Immediate management is shown in the emergency box.

Patients with severe left ventricular failure often respond gratifyingly well. Their acute attack may have been triggered by acute myocardial infarction so cardiac enzymes should be measured. Once the patient has recovered, assess the cause of heart failure to decide on further management.

Chronic biventricular failure

Heart failure is all too often overlooked or treated inappropriately with antibiotics or bronchodilators. None of its symptoms (p. 23) clearly distinguish it from chronic airflow limitation; even orthopnoea is not specific to heart failure. The distinction depends on a full history, physical examination and a chest radiograph. Patients may, of course, have both cardiac and pulmonary disease.

Management

You should aim to:

- relieve symptoms
- optimise the long-term prognosis.

A stepwise approach to management is outlined in Figure 9; treatment includes drugs and changes to lifestyle; ultimately it can include transplantation. The modes of action of the drugs are summarised in Figure 10.

Non-pharmacological treatments

Diet. Obesity increases cardiac work. Overweight patients should be advised to diet and hyperlipidaemic patients treated to prevent progression of coronary artery disease.

Abstinence from alcohol. Excessive alcohol impairs contractility and may cause permanent heart muscle damage (cardiomyopathy).

Bed rest. This improves heart failure in the short term, although, in the longer term, patients should be advised to remain active.

Emergency treatment: management of acute left ventricular failure

- Give 100% oxygen, unless there is a possibility that the diagnosis is exacerbation of chronic airflow limitation rather than LVF
- Do an ECG to exclude acute myocardial infarction or dysrhythmia
- Give diamorphine or morphine with an anti-emetic (e.g. prochlorperazine)
- Give frusemide 40–80 mg intravenously; repeat and increase dose as necessary

Depending upon response:
- Start a nitrate infusion unless the patient is hypotensive
- Consider inotrope infusion (dobutamine) if severely hypotensive
- Admit to a coronary or intensive care unit
- Repeat diamorphine as needed
- Consider ventilation for intractable pulmonary oedema

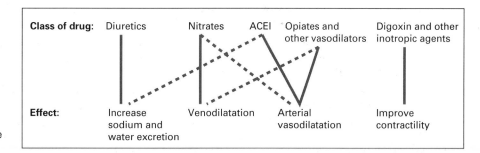

Fig. 10
The modes of action of drugs used in heart failure. Dotted lines indicate minor effects.

Limitation of salt and fluid intake. Thirst is common and may exacerbate heart failure.

Stopping smoking.

Drug treatment

Figure 9 (p. 23) summarises an approach to their use.

Diuretics

A loop diuretic (frusemide or bumetanide) is usually the first-line treatment. Hypokalaemia may occur so the diet should include plenty of potassium (e.g. from fruit). Thiazides are a relatively ineffective first-line treatment but work synergistically with a loop diuretic in severe heart failure. Metolazone is most effective in this context. Potassium-sparing diuretics (e.g. amiloride) are relatively ineffective on their own but may be given in combination with a loop diuretic or thiazide if hypokalaemia is a problem. Electrolytes should be checked several weeks after starting treatment and potassium supplements or combination therapy given as necessary.

ACE inhibitors

ACE inhibitors act:

- as vasodilators, by reducing the synthesis of angiotensin II, a potent vasoconstrictor
- as mild diuretics, by reducing aldosterone synthesis
- on the tissues to inhibit cardiac hypertrophy in hypertension.

They relieve symptoms, retard the progression of heart failure and improve mortality. An ACE inhibitor (e.g. captopril, enalapril, lisinopril) should be given (with a diuretic) unless there are contraindications. These are:

- likelihood of pregnancy, because they can cause fetal anomalies
- renal artery stenosis (p. 161)
- low blood pressure (e.g. < 100 mmHg systolic) because they can exacerbate hypotension
- severe aortic or mitral stenosis.

Patients with heart failure may have a precipitous fall in blood pressure when given an ACE inhibitor; this may be a 'first-dose' or sustained effect. You should observe the following precautions:

- in mild heart failure, omit diuretics for 24–48 hours before starting the ACE inhibitor

- In patients with low blood pressure or severe heart failure
  — start with a small dose, using a short-acting drug (e.g. captopril)
  — start treatment recumbent in hospital and monitor blood pressure closely after the first dose.

Blood pressure, renal function and electrolytes should be monitored after starting ACE inhibitors to detect hyperkalaemia (a direct effect of ACE inhibition) or worsened renal function.

Other vasodilators

Patients who cannot tolerate ACE inhibitors (e.g. because of intractable cough) can be treated with other vasodilators such as hydralazine or prazosin, which act predominantly by reducing afterload. Nitrates may be used to reduce preload but their long-term benefit is limited by tolerance. Angiotensin receptor antagonists (e.g. losartan) are likely to play an increasing role.

Digoxin

Digoxin is both an inotropic and an antidysrhythmic agent and of proven value in the long-term management of heart failure associated with both atrial fibrillation and sinus rhythm. It can be given together with diuretics and ACE inhibitors or other vasodilators. Hypokalaemia potentiates digoxin and may cause toxicity.

Cardiac transplantation

Cardiac transplantation relieves the symptoms of heart failure and has a 5-year survival of up to 70%. It is reserved for younger patients (< 50 years) with end-stage disease and a proven poor physiological response to exercise. The indications include:

- ischaemic heart disease
- cardiomyopathies
- intractable ventricular tachydysrhythmias
- congenital heart disease
- cardiac tumours.

If there is significant pulmonary vascular disease, combined heart–lung transplantation is required. This is more technically demanding and has a lower survival.

1.4 Dysrhythmias

You must be ready to manage cardiac dysrhythmias from your first day as a house officer. One per cent of the general population and 10% of old people are in atrial fibrillation. Supraventricular tachycardia is a not infrequent acute medical emergency. You must be ready to treat ventricular fibrillation or complete heart block causing sudden collapse after acute myocardial infarction.

Learning objectives

You should:

- be alert to the clinical presentations of dysrhythmias
- understand how to diagnose them from the ECG
- be prepared to tackle dysrhythmic emergencies
- know how to manage cardiac arrest
- have a good understanding of atrial fibrillation and its complications and treatment.

Causes of dysrhythmias

Many different sites within the heart can act as pacemakers. An ectopic pacemaker with a faster rate of depolarisation can override the SA node. If impulse generation or conduction fails, a slower pacemaker lower down the conducting system will take over (p. 8). Dysrhythmias can be of the following types:

- slow rate or missed beats
  - increased vagal stimulation of the SA node (sinus bradycardia)
  - slow, erratic or absent impulse generation in the SA node
  - impaired atrio-ventricular (AV) conduction (heart block)
- fast rate or extra beats
  - increased adrenergic stimulation of the SA node (sinus tachycardia)
  - impulse generation from an ectopic site
  - totally disorganised impulse generation from within the myocardium (atrial or ventricular fibrillation).

Dysrhythmias may arise:

- spontaneously
- as a result of heart disease
  - ischaemic
  - cardiomyopathy (p. 40)
- as a result of systemic disease, e.g. thyrotoxicosis.

Remember that dysrhythmias may be precipitated or exacerbated by hypokalaemia; this is particularly important because of the association of hypokalaemia with diuretic therapy for heart disease and the stress of acute myocardial infarction (p. 18). Hypoxia and acidaemia are other precipitants.

Re-entry

Impulses normally propagate through the atria, conducting tissue and ventricles in an orderly manner, followed by a refractory period before the tissues are receptive to the next impulse. Electrical circuits in diseased myocardium can allow impulses to go round in circles and repeatedly re-activate the myocardium at a greatly increased rate. Re-entrant circuits can also be formed by congenital accessory pathways which carry impulses between the atria and ventricles faster than the His bundle. The impulse passes down the accessory pathway, back up the His bundle and round in circles, setting up a tachycardia.

Ectopic impulses are propagated backwards as well as forwards through the conducting system so that, depending on the site of the ectopic pacemaker, atrial contraction may occur before, simultaneously with or after ventricular contraction. On the ECG, this determines the timing of the P wave in relation to the QRS complex. Retrograde conduction causes inversion of the P wave.

Clinical presentation

Both bradycardias and tachycardias can cause syncope and heart failure, by reducing heart rate and compromising ventricular filling, respectively. A fast heart rate can also cause angina (p. 12) and palpitations. Dysrhythmias may be a chance ECG finding.

Symptoms

The word 'palpitations' means different things to different people. The challenge is to get a clear description of what the patient actually experiences. Key features are the speed and regularity of the heart beat during the attack, its duration, precipitating and relieving factors, and associated symptoms. The state of ventricular function can modify symptoms. Thus, a patient with severe ventricular disease may have no palpitations during a dysrhythmia which would cause intolerable palpitations in someone with good myocardial contractility. Poor ventricular function can cause intolerable left ventricular failure or syncope during a dysrhythmia which would cause little more than fluttering in the chest in a patient with a healthy myocardium.

Signs

A pulse rate < 60 or > 100 beats/min or an irregular cardiac rhythm constitutes a dysrhythmia. If the rhythm is irregular, you have to decide if it is chaotic (atrial fibrillation) or added/missed beats are superimposed on a fundamentally regular rhythm. A tachycardia is more likely to be supraventricular than ventricular if the patient does not seem very ill (though this is not an absolute rule). A pulse rate over 140 beats/min is unlikely to be a sinus tachycardia unless there is a very severe and obvious systemic illness causing it. Profound bradycardia (< 40/min) is strongly suggestive of complete heart block.

Investigation

For most patients, the only way of diagnosing the dysrhythmia, and for *all* patients the 'gold standard', is the ECG. If you do not see the patient during an attack, you may be able to 'catch one' by hospital monitoring or on an ambulatory ECG. You should examine the ECG systematically for:

- the presence of P waves
- their rate and rhythm
- their relationship to the QRS complexes
- the ventricular (QRS) rate and rhythm
- the shape of the QRS complex.

You may need to use a piece of blank paper or card to mark out the position of P waves and check their regularity. Examples of ECGs are shown in the self-assessment section.

The spectrum of dysrhythmias

These are the important dysrhythmias, classified by the nature of the pulse. Unless otherwise stated, the pulse is regular.

- Cardiac arrest (no pulse)
  — asystole
  — electromechanical dissociation (EMD)
  — ventricular fibrillation
- bradycardias (slow pulse)
  — complete heart block
  — sinus bradycardia
  — sick sinus syndrome
- dropped beats
  — second-degree heart block (pulse regularly irregular)
- extrasystoles (single extra beats)
  — supraventricular (regularly irregular)
  — ventricular (regularly irregular)
- tachycardias (fast pulse)
  — sinus tachycardia
  — atrial fibrillation (irregularly irregular)
  — atrial tachycardia
  — atrial flutter
  — junctional (AV nodal) tachycardia
  — accessory pathway tachycardia
  — accelerated idioventricular rhythm
  — ventricular tachycardia.

Each type is discussed in more detail below.

Cardiac arrest

The patient is collapsed and pulseless. First, you should establish an airway and start cardio-pulmonary resuscitation. (If you are unclear about how to do so, request (re)training urgently.) Once an ECG is available, it will show:

- asystole: no QRS complexes
- electromechanical dissociation (EMD): QRS complexes but no palpable pulse

- ventricular fibrillation or tachycardia.

There are nationally agreed management guidelines, summarised in Figure 11 and you should not join a cardiac arrest team unless you know them. Lignocaine or another antidysrhythmic is given to stabilise the ventricular rhythm after ventricular fibrillation or tachycardia and/or for ventricular dysrhythmias resistant to DC shock. Emergency pacing is often required for bradycardias. Arterial blood gases should be checked as soon as possible in all patients and i.v. 4.2% or 8.4% bicarbonate given to correct the lactic acidosis which may result from anaerobic metabolism. Asystole and electromechanical dissociation have an appalling (< 10%) prognosis for successful resuscitation unless there is a rapidly treatable cause such as pericardial tamponade.

Bradycardias and dropped beats

Heart block

The SA node depolarises regularly but atrio-ventricular conduction is abnormal or absent.

First-degree heart block. There is prolongation of the PR interval to > 5 small squares (0.2 s) in every complex because of delayed conduction in the AV node.

Second-degree heart block. There are two broad subtypes:

- Wenckebach phenomenon: the PR interval lengthens progressively until a beat is missed
- dropped beats: some P waves are not followed by a QRS complex; the beats may be dropped randomly or regularly, e.g. two-to-one or three-to-one (total to conducted).

Third-degree (complete) heart block.
AV conduction is completely blocked so that the atria (P waves) and ventricles (QRS complexes) are dissociated. The rate of the P waves is faster than the QRS rate, which is determined by the level of the block in the conducting system (p. 8). A 'junctional' (high) pacemaker may produce a satisfactory ventricular rate (e.g. 50 beats/min). A lower block, as after anterior myocardial infarction (p. 19), will cause a catastrophically slow ventricular rate (20 beats/min) with broad QRS complexes (> 3 small squares) because the impulse spreads in a disorganised way through the myocardium rather than through conducting tissue.

Heart block may result from, in order of frequency:

- ischaemia or fibrosis of the conducting system
- drugs, e.g. digoxin, calcium antagonists
- congenital causes; despite complete heart block, there is often a satisfactory ventricular rate and no symptoms.

Sinus bradycardia

The heart rate is < 60 beats/min but P waves are present and each is followed by a QRST complex after a normal

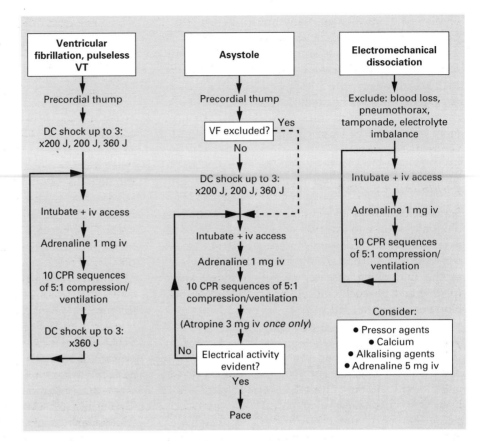

Fig. 11
Flow diagram of resuscitation procedures (based on the recommendations of the UK Resuscitation Council).

PR interval. This is common in athletes, patients on beta-blockers and after acute myocardial infarction. Less common causes are untreated hypothyroidism, obstructive jaundice and raised intracranial pressure.

Sick sinus syndrome

The P waves are slow or erratic owing to disease of the SA node, but conduction is normal. Sometimes there may be secondary tachycardias (tachy-brady syndrome). The cause is ischaemia or degeneration of the SA node.

Clinical presentation and management of bradycardias

First- and second-degree block are asymptomatic although in second-degree block the dropped beats can be felt in the pulse. Sinus bradycardia may cause hypotension and syncope after acute myocardial infarction. Severe bradycardia caused by complete heart block or sinus arrest presents with syncope which may be intermittent (Stokes–Adams attacks). If bradycardia persists, it may also cause heart failure.

You should assess a bradycardic patient as follows:

Is the bradycardia causing hypotension or heart failure? If not, no immediate action is needed. If so, give atropine immediately. This will treat sinus bradycardia and improve some forms of second- and third-degree heart block by reducing vagal tone on the AV node. If the patient is collapsed and/or does not respond to atropine, call for senior help with a view to emergency pacing. Intravenous isoprenaline (β_1-agonist) is a poor second-best emergency measure.

Is the bradycardia a warning sign? For example, heart block after myocardial infarction — call for senior help if you suspect this.

Is there a drug or other disease causing the bradycardia?

Intermittent bradycardias causing syncopal attacks or persistent, symptomatic complete heart block are indications for permanent pacing.

Extrasystoles and tachycardias

Extrasystoles are single extra beats.

Supraventricular extrasystoles

Supraventricular extrasystoles arise in the atrium or AV node and have the same QRS configuration as normally timed impulses. Depending on their origin, they may have a relatively normal P wave, one which follows the QRS complex or none at all. They are benign and need no treatment.

Ventricular extrasystoles

Ventricular extrasystoles are more sinister because they signify automaticity within the ventricles, which may predispose to malignant arrhythmias. Particularly if they are multifocal (arising from several different sites within the ventricles, as shown by multiple different QRS configurations) they are a sign of underlying ventricular disease, often with a bad prognosis. Antidysrhythmic drugs may themselves provoke dysrhythmias and clinical trials have shown them to do more harm than good when given for asymptomatic ventricular extrasystoles.

Sinus tachycardia

Sinus tachycardia is an adrenergically mediated, physiological response to exercise, volume depletion or disease. The PQRST complexes are normal and the rate rarely exceeds 140 beats/min. Treatment is aimed solely at the underlying disease, except in thyrotoxicosis (p. 259) and phaeochromocytoma (p. 271) when beta-blockers may be needed.

Other tachycardias

A sustained tachycardia > 140 beats/min is usually pathological, although pathological tachycardias may have ventricular rates < 140/min. Having excluded a sinus tachycardia, the task is to distinguish supraventricular from ventricular tachycardias because the management differs. This depends almost entirely on ECG interpretation and is summarised in Figure 12.

There are three key steps:

- is it a *narrow complex* (QRS <3 small squares) or *broad complex* tachycardia?
- are there P waves?
- are the complexes completely irregular?

Narrow and broad complex tachycardias. A narrow complex tachycardia must be 'supraventricular' (arising in the atrium or AV node) because the narrowness of the complexes indicate that they were propagated through the His–Purkinje system. A broad complex tachycardia is *probably* arising in the ventricle, its breadth being caused by slow propagation through ventricular muscle. However, the complexes may be broad in a supraventricular tachycardia if there is bundle branch block.

P waves. The presence of P waves identifies a broad complex tachycardia as supraventricular. The shape of the P waves and relationship to the QRS complexes is also important. In an atrial tachycardia, the P waves precede the QRS complex. If they are absent, immediately before or after the QRS complex, it is a nodal tachycardia. In atrial fibrillation, fibrillation waves may be seen every 1–2 small squares. In atrial flutter, there are 'saw-tooth waves' at a rate of about 300/min (1 large square between them).

Regularity. If the complexes are completely irregular, the diagnosis is atrial fibrillation.

Other clues. Other ways of identifying a broad complex tachycardia as supraventricular are:

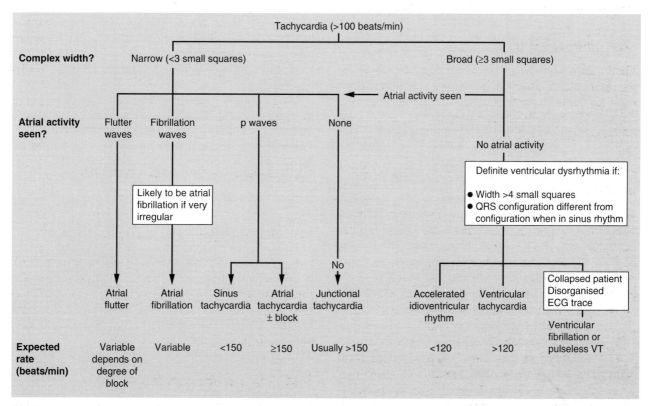

Fig. 12
Diagnosis of tachycardias.

- if ECGs during the dysrhythmia and in sinus rhythm are available for comparison, the QRS configuration will be unchanged in a supraventricular tachycardia with bundle branch block and changed in ventricular tachycardia
- very broad complexes (> 4 small squares) indicate a ventricular tachycardia.

You may be able to show up atrial activity (P waves) by performing carotid sinus massage (see below) to slow the ventricular rate.

Management of ventricular tachycardias

The management of ventricular tachycardia and fibrillation has been considered under cardiac arrest (p. 27). If the patient is collapsed, the treatment is DC shock. Recurrent ventricular tachycardia or sustained tachycardia not requiring immediate cardioversion, is treated with lignocaine or flecainide (which have a membrane-stabilising effect) or amiodarone (which prolongs the duration of the action potential).

Management of supraventricular tachycardias

If there is severe cardiovascular compromise, urgent cardioversion is needed. A DC shock is given, synchronised to the downstroke of the QRS complex to avoid precipitating ventricular fibrillation. Otherwise, the following treatments are given in the order indicated.

Vagal stimulation. Sudden immersion of the face in cold water or the Valsalva manoeuvre may restore sinus rhythm or at least slow AV conduction enough to show P waves on the ECG and aid diagnosis.

Adenosine. This transiently induces complete heart block and may correct junctional tachycardia. Like vagal stimulation, it may transiently reveal P waves.

Verapamil. This impedes the transport of calcium across myocardial smooth muscle cells, prolonging the action potential and refractory period. Given intravenously, it may restore sinus rhythm. It must never be given to patients on beta-blockers (because the combination can cause asystole) or if there is a suspicion of ventricular tachycardia.

Digoxin. Unless emergency cardioversion is needed (see above), digoxin is the treatment of choice for atrial fibrillation. It is rapidly absorbed and can be given orally as a loading dose, or 'titrated' against the heart rate. It may be used for other refractory dysrhythmias. Before using it, check that the patient is not already on it because it can *cause* dysrhythmias: classically atrial tachycardia with two-to-one block.

Amiodarone. This has a long half-life and is given i.v. for refractory supraventricular dysrhythmias.

Atrial pacing and cardioversion. Atrial pacing 'takes over' impulse generation from the ectopic focus and can restore sinus rhythm. Resistant dysrhythmias are treated by cardioversion. You should remember that patients who are digoxin-toxic (particularly if hypokalaemic) may develop asystole or malignant dysrhythmias after cardioversion. The treatment is to stop

digoxin, correct hypokalaemia and give digoxin-specific antibodies for severe, resistant toxicity.

Supraventricular tachycardia associated with Wolff–Parkinson–White syndrome

This tachycardia is caused by a congenital accessory conducting pathway between the atria and ventricles (Re-entry, p. 26). There is a short PR interval (< 3 small squares) and slurred upstroke to the R wave (delta wave). Supraventricular tachycardias may occur and can be terminated by adenosine or verapamil. Atrial fibrillation may also occur. Destruction of the accessory pathway by radiofrequency ablation may be needed as a long-term solution.

Atrial fibrillation

This is the commonest dysrhythmia. It can be intermittent ('paroxysmal') or sustained. Apart from the fibrillation waves, there is an irregular QRS rhythm caused by the haphazard transmission of atrial impulses to the ventricles. Cardiac output is impaired by loss of atrial systole (p. 9) and varies with the length of diastole, causing variability in blood pressure and strength of the peripheral pulses. The heart rate can only reliably be measured at the cardiac apex or on an ECG.

Causes

Any condition which causes atrial dilatation, such as mitral stenosis, heart muscle disease, hypertension and ischaemia, can cause atrial fibrillation. Pericarditis and systemic diseases including thyrotoxicosis and alcohol abuse are other causes. There may be no obvious cause ('lone atrial fibrillation').

Effects

Reduction of cardiac output causes dyspnoea and lethargy and may precipitate heart failure (p. 22). Uncontrolled atrial fibrillation causes palpitations, ischaemic chest pain and syncope. Intracardiac thrombus can form in the dilated atrium leading to stroke, particularly in patients with associated valvular disease. The risk is low in young people with lone atrial fibrillation but increases with:

- age
- coincident heart disease
- instability of the rhythm: conversion between atrial fibrillation and sinus rhythm may dislodge atrial thrombus.

Treatment

The priorities of treatment are to control the ventricular rate and to prevent thrombo-embolism.

Digoxin is used to slow the ventricular rate by increasing the degree of AV block and reducing the number of atrial impulses propagated to the ventricles. If digoxin alone fails to do this (especially during exercise), verapamil or a beta-blocker may be given adjunctively. Patients with atrial fibrillation of less than 12 months, duration and no underlying cause may be cardioverted. Sotalol or amiodarone (which prolong the duration of the action potential) are used to prevent paroxysmal atrial fibrillation.

Patients aged < 60 years with lone atrial fibrillation have such a low risk of stroke that anticoagulation is not needed, although aspirin is advisable. Low intensity (INR ~ 2; see p. 247) chronic anticoagulation with warfarin is indicated for those with the risk factors listed above or a history of transient ischaemic attack or non-haemorrhagic stroke, unless they have a contraindication. Beyond age 80, the risks of anticoagulation begin to outweigh the likely benefits.

1.5 Valvular and congenital heart disease

Traditional medical student teaching has strongly emphasised the bedside differential diagnosis of rheumatic and congenital heart disease. This is less important in an era when echocardiography is freely available but you must still be able to *detect* valvular heart disease. The spectrum of disease is shifting away from rheumatic disease towards endocarditis, a complication of i.v. drug abuse, and the valvular lesions of cardiac ischaemia and old age.

Learning objectives

You should:
* understand how the individual lesions cause their characteristic symptoms and signs
* approach the bedside confident in the knowledge of what you are looking and listening for
* understand the complications and management.

Clinical presentation

Symptoms and signs
Valvular heart disease impairs cardiac output and increases pulmonary and systemic venous pressure, so the symptoms are no different from other cardiac diseases (p. 23).

To understand murmurs, orientate your thinking around ventricular contraction. Incompetence of one of the AV valves causes back-flow into the atrium from the moment the valve should have shut, heard as a pansystolic murmur. A ventricular septal defect also causes a pansystolic murmur. Stenosis of the aortic or pulmonary valve causes a murmur which is loudest when blood flow is at its greatest, mid to late systole. Mitral or tricuspid stenosis cause a low-pitched rumbling murmur which is loudest when blood is flowing into the ventricle in mid-diastole. Aortic or pulmonary incompetence cause a leak back across the valve early in diastole when the pressure differential is greatest, heard as a

high-pitched 'whiff'. Thrills are palpable murmurs, most often felt with systolic murmurs. Apart from the character and timing of the murmur, there are three other features which help you in your diagnosis:

* the position (and radiation)
* relationship to respiration
* presence of other cardiovascular signs.

The physical signs of valvular heart disease are summarised in Table 4. Remember that:

* mitral murmurs are heard best at the apex
* aortic and pulmonary stenotic murmurs are heard best at the upper right and left sternal edges, respectively
* all other murmurs are heard best at the left sternal edge.

The relationship with respiration is easy to remember: during inspiration, blood is drawn into the lungs. This increases flow through the right side of the heart and reduces flow on the left side. The situation is reversed on expiration. Thus, inspiration makes tricuspid and pulmonary murmurs louder and expiration intensifies mitral and aortic murmurs. Other features, including radiation and the associated signs, are summarised in Table 4. For more detail, you are referred to a textbook of bedside diagnosis.

Causes of valvular heart disease

In the developed world, the causes of valvular heart disease are, in approximate order of frequency:

* degenerative
* secondary to disease of the heart and aorta; dilatation of supporting structures causes incompetence by stretching the valve
* rheumatic heart disease, usually affecting the mitral valve alone or mitral and aortic valves (p. 33)
* congenital, including 'floppy mitral valve' (p. 33)
* infective endocarditis, affecting the mitral valve (most common), aortic, tricuspid and pulmonary (least common).

Mitral valve disease

You should be familiar with three mitral lesions:

* stenosis
* regurgitation
* prolapse.

Mitral stenosis

Mitral stenosis is almost invariably rheumatic, is the commonest lesion of rheumatic heart disease and is more common in women than in men. There is thickening, fusion and eventually calcification and immobility of the valve cusps, which narrows the orifice and increases left atrial pressure. The principal effects of mitral stenosis are

Table 4 The physical signs of valvular heart disease: common murmurs

	Character	Best heard	Radiation	Associated signs
Systolic				
Mitral regurgitation		Apex	Left axilla	
Mitral prolapse		Apex	Left axilla or back	
Ventricular septal defect		Lower LSE		
Tricuspid regurgitation		Lower LSE		Giant V waves in jugular venous of pulse; pulsatile hepatomegaly
Aortic stenosis		Upper RSE	Carotids	Plateau pulse; narrow pulse pressure
Diastolic				
Mitral stenosis		Apex	Left axilla	Malar flush; parasternal heave; tapping apex
Aortic regurgitation		Lower LSE		Collapsing pulse; wide pulse pressure

LSE, left sternal edge; RSE, right sternal edge; OS, opening snap; I PSA, presystolic accentuation if in sinus rhythm.

left atrial hypertrophy and **pulmonary venous hypertension** leading, eventually, to right ventricular failure.

Symptoms and signs

The symptoms of pulmonary venous hypertension and right heart failure are described on page 21. Haemoptysis is a common symptom of mitral stenosis. There may be palpitations resulting from atrial fibrillation. The signs are shown in Table 4. The loud first heart sound and opening snap (caused by increased left atrial pressure) are only heard if the valve is mobile and are lost as it becomes increasingly calcified.

Investigations

The heart is usually normally sized on a chest radiograph but the following abnormal signs may be seen, in approximate order of frequency:

- left atrial hypertrophy: 'double shadow' to the right heart border
- enlargement of the pulmonary artery, pulmonary venous engorgement and septal lines (as described for left ventricular failure, p. 11)
- calcification of the mitral valve ring.

Echocardiography is needed to confirm the diagnosis and estimate severity. The gradient across the mitral valve and the valve area can be measured and signs of pulmonary hypertension identified.

Complications
Atrial fibrillation, caused by left atrial enlargement

(p. 30), is almost invariable in significant mitral stenosis. **Stroke and other forms of arterial thromboembolism** result from stasis of blood in the enlarged, fibrillating left atrium. **Pulmonary embolism** may result from reduced cardiac output and venous stasis. An abrupt increase in pulmonary venous pressure, as when the patient goes into atrial fibrillation, can cause overt **pulmonary oedema** but subacute symptoms are more common. Alveolar oedema predisposes to **infection.**

Management
Management of mitral stenosis consists of long-term anticoagulation to prevent thrombo-embolism, antibiotic prophylaxis against endocarditis (p. 38), diuretics for pulmonary oedema and right heart failure, and digoxin for atrial fibrillation. Antibiotics may be needed for chest infections.

Surgery is indicated for pulmonary hypertension (which progresses irreversibly if surgery is delayed) and uncontrolled symptoms. The options are valvotomy (closed or open) and valve replacement, which is needed if the valve is calcified and/or there is significant mitral regurgitation.

Mitral regurgitation

The common causes of mitral regurgitation, in approximate order of frequency, are:

- secondary to left ventricular dilatation, as in left heart failure

- rheumatic
- secondary to papillary muscle dysfunction or ruptured chordae tendineae
- bacterial endocarditis.

Mitral regurgitation may develop acutely as a result of papillary muscle rupture after myocardial infarction (p. 20).

As the valve becomes incompetent, the regurgitated blood is accommodated by dilatation of the left atrium. There is pulmonary hypertension but it is less severe than in mitral stenosis because the atria are able to empty during diastole. The left ventricle enlarges to accommodate the increased stroke volume but may eventually fail. These adaptive changes cannot occur in *acute* mitral regurgitation so there is left ventricular failure.

Symptoms and signs
There are no specific symptoms. The signs reflect the systolic flow across the valve, increased stroke volume and, if present, left and right ventricular failure. The murmur is described in Table 4. There may be left ventricular enlargement, a soft first heart sound because of non-apposition of the mitral valve cusps and a third heart sound from increased diastolic inflow to the left ventricle.

Investigations
The chest X-ray may show enlargement of the left ventricle and atrium, pulmonary oedema and valve calcification. The main abnormality on the ECG is left ventricular hypertrophy (p. 12). There may be atrial fibrillation. The definitive investigation is echocardiography.

Complications
Complications are heart failure, infective endocarditis and atrial fibrillation. This is less common than in mitral stenosis because the left atrium is less dilated.

Management
All patients should be advised about antibiotic prophylaxis against endocarditis (p. 38). Uncomplicated mitral regurgitation can be left untreated and observed for the development of left ventricular dysfunction, which is treated with diuretics and ACE inhibitors, or dysrhythmias. Surgery is indicated if there is progressive left ventricular enlargement which may pass a 'point of no return'; there is a need for surveillance and appropriately timed surgical referral.

Mitral valve prolapse

This may be:

- congenital: 'floppy mitral valve' (enlarged valve cusps) is common, particularly in women, and often diagnosed in young adult life. Mitral valve prolapse may also be associated with rare inherited disorders of collagen, e.g. Marfan's syndrome
- acquired: this is usually a result of ischaemic papillary muscle dysfunction.

This discussion concentrates on congenital floppy mitral valve.

There is mitral regurgitation caused by late systolic prolapse of the valve cusps into the left atrium. The regurgitation is rarely haemodynamically important.

Symptoms and signs
Patients are usually asymptomatic but may present with anginal or atypical chest pain or other complications (noted below). The signs are summarised in Table 4. There may be a mid-systolic 'click' in some cases.

Investigation
The diagnosis is made by echocardiography.

Complications
It is often an innocent, chance finding. Uncommonly, there may be myxomatous degeneration of the valve cusp causing arterial thrombo-embolism, notably strokes. Ventricular or supraventricular tachydysrhythmias may occur.

Management
Patients with chest pain and/or supraventricular arrhythmias are treated with beta-blockers. Antibiotic prophylaxis against endocarditis is indicated if there is significant mitral regurgitation. Thrombo-embolic complications are treated by anticoagulation.

Aortic valve disease

You need to know about two lesions:

- aortic stenosis
- aortic incompetence.

Aortic stenosis

Aortic stenosis may be rheumatic or congenital. If rheumatic, the mitral valve is likely to be affected as well. Congenital aortic stenosis is usually associated with a bicuspid aortic valve. Other causes are congenital supravalvular or sub-valvular stenosis resulting from malformation of the aorta and left ventricle, respectively.

Fusion of the valve cusps causes left ventricular outflow obstruction, compensatory myocardial hypertrophy and increased cardiac work. Cardiac output is limited and cannot rise in response to exercise. Coronary perfusion is impaired and myocardial ischaemia results. Ultimately, the left ventricle cannot overcome the outflow resistance and left ventricular failure occurs.

Symptoms and signs
You must be alert to the diagnosis of aortic stenosis because it may be asymptomatic until too late a stage in its natural history for good surgical results. It is easy to misattribute the symptoms to other diseases. They are **dyspnoea**, at first exercise related but later occurring at

rest, **orthopnoea** and **paroxysmal nocturnal dyspnoea** resulting from left ventricular failure, **angina**, which is caused by the imbalance between myocardial work and coronary perfusion and may occur without coronary artery disease, and **exertional syncope**, a sinister symptom of severely limited cardiac output which may presage sudden death.

A crucial point is that the intensity of the murmur (Table 4) is a poor guide to the severity of stenosis. You need to distinguish aortic sclerosis, a degenerative and innocent condition which is common in old people, from aortic stenosis. Sclerosis causes a loud murmur but has little haemodynamic effect, whereas the murmur of tight aortic stenosis may be inaudible because flow across the valve is severely limited. Other signs (absent in aortic sclerosis) are a slow rising, low-volume carotid pulse, narrow pulse pressure (systolic minus diastolic) and thrusting apex beat which is not displaced unless there is left ventricular failure. A thrill may be felt in the aortic area or over the carotid arteries. The aortic component of the second heart sound may be soft because of impaired valve mobility, and there may be a fourth heart sound.

Investigations

The chest radiograph may be normal or show:

- prominence of the left ventricle
- cardiac enlargement if there is left ventricular failure
- prominence of the ascending aorta because of 'poststenotic dilatation'
- calcification of the valve.

The ECG shows left bundle branch block or left ventricular hypertrophy and strain (p. 12). Echocardiography demonstrates the disordered anatomy of the valve, the gradient across it and the degree of left ventricular hypertrophy and dilatation.

Complications

These include **left ventricular failure** (a serious sign of decompensation), **dysrhythmias** which are triggered by exertion, presumed because of myocardial ischaemia, and may cause sudden death, **systemic embolism** from the diseased valve and **infective endocarditis**.

Management

Antibiotic prophylaxis should be recommended and patients advised against strenuous activity. **Vasodilators should not be given** because they increase the risk of syncope. Beta-blockers can be used for angina. Heart failure is treated with diuretics. Tight aortic stenosis can only be treated by valve replacement. A gradient greater than 50 mmHg is the threshold for surgery.

Aortic regurgitation

Aortic regurgitation can have acute and chronic causes (Table 5). There is back-flow of blood into the left ventri-cle during diastole, which is accommodated by dilatation of the left ventricle and an increased stroke volume. If the disease progresses slowly, the left ventricle can adapt to remarkably severe regurgitation. The cardiovascular system is 'hyperdynamic' because blood is passing to and fro across the valve. The pulse pressure is wide. Myocardial ischaemia occurs because the increased stroke volume increases myocardial work and the low diastolic pressure impairs coronary perfusion.

Symptoms and signs

Patients may be dyspnoeic and aware of a 'pounding heart beat'. The signs (Table 4) are:

Hyperdynamic circulation: a collapsing pulse, wide pulse pressure, aortic systolic flow murmur and visible, palpable or audible pulsation in the arterial or capillary circulation.

Left ventricular dilatation: a displaced, heaving apex.

Regurgitation: an early diastolic murmur heard best on expiration, with the patient leaning forwards, in the third left interspace with the diaphragm of the stethoscope. The aortic component of the second heart sound is absent because of non-apposition of the cusps.

There will always be a systolic flow murmur. To decide if the diagnosis is pure aortic incompetence or mixed aortic valve disease, you must distinguish this from the midsystolic murmur of aortic stenosis. Only diagnose aortic stenosis if the pulse pressure is not widened.

Investigations

There is left ventricular enlargement and possibly calcification of the valve on the chest radiograph and left ventricular hypertrophy and strain on the ECG. An echocardiogram shows the abnormal valvular anatomy, left ventricular dilatation and regurgitant jet.

Complications

Dilatation and ischaemia of the left ventricle cause left ventricular failure and secondary right ventricular failure. There is atrial fibrillation in about 20% of patients and angina, particularly if there is coincident coronary artery disease.

Table 5 Causes of aortic regurgitation

	Acute	**Chronic**
Dilatation of valve ring	Aortic dissection	Severe, prolonged hypertension Syphilitic aortitis Inherited disorder of collagen, e.g. Marfan's syndrome
Diseased valve cusps	Infective endocarditis	Congenital: bicuspid aortic valve Acquired: rheumatic heart disease

Management

This consists of antibiotic prophylaxis (p. 38), treatment of heart failure and dysrrhythmias, and early surgical referral. Once there is heart failure, left ventricular function is unlikely to recover.

Right heart valvular disease

This is less common than left heart disease because both infective endocarditis and rheumatic disease affect the left side more than the right. It may be congenital or, more commonly, secondary to left heart disease or pulmonary arterial disease.

If the lesion is secondary to left heart disease, there will be both left and right heart failure. If it is primary, there will only be symptoms and signs of systemic venous hypertension and a reduced cardiac output. You can work out from first principles the *cardiac* signs of right-sided valvular disease if you know how to palpate for right ventricular hypertrophy; the signs are similar to the analogous left-sided lesion but get louder on inspiration rather than expiration. The only lesion you will commonly encounter is tricuspid regurgitation resulting from pulmonary hypertension (see p. 44 for causes). You should consult a reference textbook for other lesions.

Tricuspid regurgitation

The pathognomonic feature is transmission of right ventricular systolic pressure into the systemic venous system. There are giant V waves in the JVP, pulsatile hepatomegaly and signs of right ventricular failure. Other signs include a parasternal heave of right ventricular dilatation, pansystolic murmur at the left sternal edge (Table 4), third heart sound and (often) atrial fibrillation. The diagnosis is made by recognising pulsatile venous hypertension.

Treatment is primarily aimed at underlying left heart failure or pulmonary disease. The systemic venous pressure often cannot be normalised so care is needed with diuretic therapy. If you aim for a normal jugular venous pressure, there is a danger that you will cause volume depletion.

Congenital heart disease

Some congenital lesions have been described above. Others which are rare or do not present in adulthood are not discussed in this book. Several which might be seen in adults are described briefly.

Atrial septal defect

Atrial septal defect (ASD) may be diagnosed for the first time in adult life. The septal defect allows blood to flow from the left to the right atrium. There is compensatory right ventricular enlargement and increased output. A sustained increase in pulmonary vascular flow causes pulmonary hypertension. Exceptionally, this increases right heart pressure to a level where the flow across the defect reverses and the patient becomes cyanosed from right-to-left shunting of deoxygenated blood. At that stage, the problem is irreversible, even with surgery.

An ASD may present with dyspnoea or fatigue, respiratory infections secondary to increased pulmonary blood flow, palpitations from atrial fibrillation or heart failure. The physical signs, resulting from increased right ventricular flow, are:

- right ventricular hypertrophy
- splitting of the second heart sound which does not vary with respiration ('fixed'), and a loud pulmonary second sound
- an ejection systolic murmur caused by increased flow across the pulmonary valve
- a tricuspid diastolic flow murmur.

The chest X-ray shows pulmonary plethora, enlargement of the pulmonary arteries and cardiomegaly. The ECG shows right bundle branch block. The diagnosis is confirmed by echocardiography.

Antibiotic prophylaxis against infective endocarditis is essential. Significant defects should be closed surgically before pulmonary hypertension develops.

Ventricular septal defect

Small ventricular septal defects (VSDs) may not be diagnosed until adulthood. There is flow from the left to the right ventricle in systole. Cardiac output is limited and patients may experience dyspnoea and fatigue. As with ASDs, pulmonary hypertension and right-to-left shunting may occur. Small defects may be associated with loud murmurs, so the intensity of the murmur is a poor guide to the seriousness of the lesion. With larger defects, the murmur may become softer with time as right and left ventricular pressures equalise as a result of pulmonary hypertension.

Apart from the murmur (Table 4), there is biventricular hypertrophy. The chest X-ray shows prominence of the pulmonary arteries and cardiomegaly.

Antibiotic prophylaxis is essential and haemodynamically significant defects should be closed before pulmonary hypertension develops.

Coarctation of the aorta

There is narrowing of the aorta distal to the arch and the origin of the main arteries. It is commonly associated with a congenitally bicuspid aortic valve, which predisposes to aortic stenosis. Coarctation is more common in males than females and may be associated with Turner's syndrome. Obstruction to blood flow by the coarct causes the blood pressure in the lower half of the body to be low, delays the lower body pulse wave, impairs renal perfusion and causes compensatory hypertension in the upper body.

Patients may present with (upper body) hypertension, left ventricular failure or hypertensive subarachnoid haemorrhage. Other physical signs include radio-femoral delay, a midsystolic murmur caused by blood flow across the coarct and left ventricular hypertrophy. The chest radiograph shows dilatation of the aorta, left ventricular hypertrophy and rib notching (caused by collateral arteries bypassing the coarct).

The diagnosis is confirmed by echocardiography and CT or MR scanning or aortography. Treatment is by balloon dilatation or surgical resection. The longer the patient has been hypertensive, the less the likelihood that surgery will be curative so it should be performed without delay.

1.6 **Infective endocarditis**

Infective endocarditis is infection of one or more of the heart valves or other endocardial structures. There are probably only 500 cases in the UK each year, but it is nevertheless important because it is hard to diagnose, treatable and fatal if you miss it.

Learning objectives

You should:
- be able to distinguish between the different forms of infective endocarditis and the diagnostic and therapeutic approach to each
- know the indications for prophylaxis of infective endocarditis and where to find current information on appropriate regimens.

Predisposing cardiac defects

These include:

- prosthetic valves
- congenital heart disease, especially ventricular septal defect, bicuspid aortic valve
- rheumatic heart disease (usually mitral valve disease)

- degenerative valve disease, e.g. calcified mitral annulus.

About 30% of patients, particularly i.v. drug abusers, have no underlying valve defect. Some cardiac defects, including ASD and mitral valve prolapse without regurgitation, carry virtually no risk of endocarditis.

Microbiological diagnosis of endocarditis

The cardinal microbiological feature is *persistent* bacteraemia. To confirm this, you should take three cultures at different times (e.g. separated by 1–3 hours). If the patient has recently received antibiotics, cultures may need to be drawn over 2–3 days.

The important microbial causes of endocarditis together with features specific to individual organisms are shown in Table 6. Most cases (around 80%) have positive blood cultures. False-negative cultures occur in patients previously treated with antibiotics, if bacteraemia is below the level of detection or the organism is non-culturable (e.g. Q fever). The rare bacteria grow slowly so blood cultures may take 10–20 days to become positive. Most laboratories discard blood cultures after 7 days so it is important to speak to your local microbiologist if you are seriously considering the diagnosis of endocarditis.

Clinical features

The clinical features of endocarditis depend on whether it is acute, subacute or associated with a prosthetic valve.

Acute endocarditis
The patient is almost always febrile and seriously ill. A loud murmur is usually apparent unless severe aortic incompetence has resulted from perforation or rupture of the valve leaflets. The systemic features of subacute infective endocarditis are absent (see below). A regurgitant murmur is much more likely to represent endocarditis than an aortic systolic or mitral diastolic

Table 6 Microbial causes of infective endocarditis (IE) in approximate order of frequency.

Organism	Particular features
Viridans group streptococci	Archetypal subacute IE
Staphylococcus aureus	Acute IE with rapid valve destruction, common in drug abusers, and then often on tricuspid valve
Enterococcus faecalis	Variable course, may be fulminant; difficult to treat successfully
Streptococcus bovis	Usually subacute, may be associated with colonic carcinoma
Staphylococcus epidermidis	Particularly associated with prosthetic valves, often subacute
Candida spp.	One cause of culture-negative IE, with large vegetations, requires surgery for cure
Rare bacteria	Unusual causes of subacute IE with slow growing (1–3 weeks) organisms, very responsive to treatment
Q fever endocarditis	Always culture negative, subacute IE with positive serology, difficult to treat

murmur. In staphylococcal endocarditis, Janeway lesions are common (see below).

The white cell count is usually elevated. Blood cultures are usually positive within 12–48 hours.

Subacute infective endocarditis

Subacute bacterial endocarditis (SBE) can be a difficult diagnosis. About 30% of patients present with a stroke, transient ischaemic attack or peripheral embolic episode. Most are chronically ill with few distinctive features. Weight loss, malaise, fatigue and anorexia are typical. Patients often do not report febrile episodes but are usually febrile on hospital admission. Vascular phenomena, mostly caused by immune complex deposition, are relatively common but may only be found by repeated examination. These are:

- petechiae, without marked thrombocytopenia
- splinter haemorrhages of the nails
- conjunctival haemorrhages
- Roth's spots in the fundi (small 'bull's eye' haemorrhagic lesions)
- Osler's nodes (tender, erythematous lesions of the finger or toe pads)
- Janeway lesions (small, painful vasculitic lesions)
- glomerulonephritis (with red cells, casts and proteinuria)
- finger clubbing
- splenomegaly.

Characteristically, if you listen repeatedly, you will hear changing murmurs in SBE. As with acute endocarditis, a regurgitant murmur is more specific than a simple flow murmur.

Many other abnormalities may accompany SBE. Oral hygiene may be poor or there may be a history of dental extraction without prophylaxis. Other portals of entry may be apparent such as skin sepsis, clinical features suggesting a large bowel cancer, signs of i.v. drug abuse, evidence of exposure to a likely source of Q fever or prior bacteraemia.

Often the white cell count is raised, usually the patient has a normochromic, normocytic anaemia and the ESR or plasma viscosity is almost always elevated. However, these laboratory features are non-specific. A positive rheumatoid factor is commonly associated with vascular phenomena.

Prosthetic valve endocarditis

Prosthetic valve endocarditis occurs in two forms:

- early (up to 2 months after surgery)
- late (≥ 2 months after surgery).

Early infections are probably acquired during surgery whereas late cases are either acquired after discharge from hospital or caused by organisms of 'low pathogenicity' such as *Staphylococcus epidermidis*. Clinically, these infections range in severity from fulminant to chronic. You will find the diagnosis difficult, especially if you do not take blood cultures prior to treatment or in cases caused by unusual organisms. A new regurgitant murmur or valve dysfunction should raise the question of endocarditis.

Investigations

Echocardiography

Echocardiography is often helpful in diagnosis. Three features are useful. These are regurgitation, the presence of vegetations and a periannular abscess (Table 7). Valve thickening is not specific enough to confirm the diagnosis. Transthoracic scans have about a 40% sensitivity for vegetations; therefore, a negative scan does not rule out the diagnosis. Transoesophageal echocardiography is considerably more sensitive (90%) than the transthoracic technique although more difficult. Echocardiography is also important in assisting decision-making with regard to surgical intervention.

Management

Once blood cultures have been obtained, you should start empirical treatment if the diagnosis is strongly suspected, particularly if the patient is acutely ill. Acute endocarditis on a native or prosthetic valve is rapidly fatal unless urgently treated. Do not wait for blood culture results or take more than three sets when the patient is ill.

Antibiotic treatment

Empirical treatment regimens are shown in Table 8. Culture results will determine the best therapy and appropriate duration. You will be guided in this by a microbiologist.

Table 7 Typical abnormalities on echocardiography of infective endocarditis.

Acute	Subacute	Prosthetic
Regurgitant valve	Small or large vegetations on left	Periannular abscess
Periannular abscess	side of heart	Regurgitant valve
Tricuspid vegetation (IVDA)	Regurgitant valve	Improperly functioning valve
Small vegetations		

IVDA, intravenous drug abusers.

Table 8 Initial antibiotic treatment of infective endocarditis.

	Antibiotic regimen
Acute endocarditis	
Native valve	Ampicillin + flucloxacillin + gentamicin[a]
Prosthetic valve	Vancomycin + ceftazidime + gentamicin[a]
Subacute endocarditis	Ampicillin + gentamicin[a]

[a] Some units prefer other aminoglycosides such as netilmicin.

The duration of antibiotic therapy varies. The shortest courses are for viridans streptococci (2–4 weeks). Fully 6 weeks of i.v. therapy are required for staphylococcal and enterococcal endocarditis as they are difficult to cure. Longer courses of therapy (months) are required for fungal and Q fever endocarditis and even then these are difficult or impossible to cure.

Supervising treatment
During the treatment of endocarditis, you must be constantly searching for signs of worsening valvular disease by listening for new regurgitant murmurs and by repeating echocardiography. Persistent or recurrent fever is quite common and represents one or more of:

- worsening endocarditis with myocardial abscess formation
- drug fever, often with eosinophilia or skin rash
- another complication, such as urinary tract infection, deep vein thrombosis or splenic or liver abscess, etc.

Surgery
Surgery is indicated in the following circumstances:

- large vegetation (e.g. ≥ 1 cm) still present after 2 weeks of medical therapy (to prevent stroke or peripheral embolus)
- enlarging myocardial (periannular) abscess, especially if near conducting system and if fever persists
- heart block
- severe valvular dysfunction leading to cardiac failure
- fungal endocarditis
- prosthetic valve endocarditis.

Prevention of endocarditis
Good dental hygiene. This is the most important means of prevention in at-risk individuals. You should stress this to your patients.
Antibiotic prophylaxis of endocarditis. Antibiotic prophylaxis is indicated for the following valvular or vascular defects:

- any prosthetic valve or arterial dacron graft
- all congenital heart disease except atrial septal defect
- any acquired valve defect

- rheumatic valve disease
- mitral valve prolapse, but only if valve is regurgitant
- hypertrophic obstructive cardiomyopathy
- prior infective endocarditis.

Procedures that justify antibiotic prophylaxis include dental work that leads to bleeding of the gums, respiratory tract surgery including tonsillectomy and adenoidectomy, vaginal, bladder or GI surgery and sclerotherapy of oesophageal varices. Current guidelines on which procedures require prophylaxis and the recommended antibiotics are available from many sources, including the British Heart Foundation and the British National Formulary.

1.7 Pericardial and heart muscle disease

Learning objectives

You should:
- be able to recognise pericarditis and construct an appropriate differential diagnosis
- be able to recognise pericardial tamponade and understand how to manage a pericardial effusion
- understand how to recognise myocarditis and other heart muscle diseases.

The pericardium is a fibrous sac surrounding the heart. There is a potential space between it and the heart. Pericarditis is inflammation of the pericardium, usually causing an accumulation of fluid in the pericardial sac. Large pericardial effusions can obstruct cardiac filling (tamponade).

Pericardial disease causes characteristic symptoms and signs. The pain is described as sharp or burning, often radiating to the back and relieved by leaning forwards. It is similar to the pain of pleurisy and the two types of pain may coexist. Pericardial inflammation causes a distinctive 'friction rub', which is distinguished from a murmur by its 'scratchy' character, making it sound 'close to your ears'. It may be there one minute, gone the next and present in both systole and diastole. Pericardial rubs are very positional. If you suspect pericarditis, listen to the heart with the patient lying flat, at 45°, sitting up and lying on the left side.

Pericarditis

Aetiology

There are many causes of pericarditis (Box 2). In young people in the UK, viral pericarditis is by far the most common cause. Systemic lupus erythematosis (SLE, see p. 310) is a rare cause and pericarditis can be a complication of tuberculosis and Hodgkin's disease. In older patients, a full thickness myocardial infarct, bronchogenic or breast carcinoma are more common. Tumour, infection and uraemia may also present with effusions.

Viral pericarditis

Young and middle-aged otherwise healthy adults are most often affected by viral pericarditis. The presentation is sudden, with typical pericardial pain (see above), dysrhythmias and/or breathlessness. The pain may be severe enough to require morphine. Sometimes there is a recent personal or family history of a viral illness.

There is a characteristic pattern of ST segment elevation across the chest leads of the ECG (Table 3). An echocardiogram may reveal pericardial fluid. The disease resolves spontaneously over 3–10 days. Most cases are caused by viruses, such as Coxsackie virus.

Purulent pericarditis

Although purulent pericarditis is fortunately uncommon, it is fatal if not recognised and treated. It presents with:

- features of bacterial infection (fever, night sweats, chills)
- chest symptoms (dyspnoea, cough and chest pain)
- hypotension.

It is not immediately distinguishable from a chest infection but there is usually a pericardial or pleural rub and signs of tamponade. An echocardiogram reveals an effusion and the diagnosis is established by aspirating pericardial fluid (pericardiocentesis). The fluid is examined in the same way as pleural fluid.

Pericardial tamponade

Large pericardial effusions can obstruct blood flow through the heart. The patient is breathless and lying still with a sinus tachycardia (e.g. > 125/min). The heart sounds are quiet. The jugular venous pressure (JVP) is greatly raised. Unlike the raised JVP of heart failure, this *rises* on inspiration (Kussmaul's sign). The absence of signs of left ventricular failure (no crackles or wheeze on auscultation of the chest) helps to differentiate tamponade from left ventricular failure. In severe cases, the systolic blood pressure falls > 10 mmHg on inspiration and peripheral pulses may disappear completely, reappearing on expiration. This is because cardiac filling is limited by external compression and the inspiratory fall in intrathoracic pressure critically drops cardiac output. Confusingly, both the inspiratory *rise* in JVP and the *fall* in blood pressure are termed 'paradoxical'. Only the

---

> **Box 2**
> **The causes of pericarditis**
>
> - Infections
>   — purulent (e.g. bacterial)
>   — tuberculous
>   — viral
>   — other infections, e.g. *Aspergillus*, amoebic, etc.
>
> - Inflammatory
>   — full thickness myocardial infarction
>   — autoimmune disease, e.g. SLE
>   — contiguous inflammatory process (e.g. pulmonary infection)
>
> - Malignant
>   — for example, bronchogenic carcinoma with direct spread, Hodgkin's disease
>
> - Other
>   — uraemic pericarditis
>   — postoperative pericarditis

---

rise in JVP is truly paradoxical; the fall in blood pressure is an exaggeration of normal physiology.

If the patient is moribund with severe hypotension and other features of pericardial tamponade, a long (e.g. lumbar puncture) needle should be inserted into the pericardium alongside the xiphisternum as an emergency procedure. You may have to do this yourself although you should get senior help quickly.

Constrictive pericarditis

In chronic pericarditis (particularly tuberculous) the continuous inflammatory process leads to pericardial fibrosis. The pericardium may become calcified and visible on a chest radiograph or CT scan. As fibrosis usually leads to tissue contraction, the pericardium becomes too small for the heart leading to cardiac failure. These patients benefit substantially from pericardiectomy.

Myocarditis

Myocarditis is infection of the myocardium leading to cardiac dysfunction. It may be associated with pericarditis.

Causes

Most cases are caused by viruses such as Coxsackie virus. Myocarditis may also be produced, rarely, by Epstein–Barr, mumps or rubella viruses. In AIDS and cardiac transplant recipients, *Toxoplasma* myocarditis is a problem. Rare instances of myocardial dysfunction are caused by poisons such as ethylene glycol (antifreeze). A few bacterial toxins also reduce myocardial contractility substantially, in particular streptococcal toxins in the context of severe streptococcal disease.

Clinical features

Viral myocarditis varies in severity from an ECG abnormality in a patient with a viral illness to a fulminating illness causing heart failure and death in 5–10 days despite intensive care. It is characterised by fever, chest pain (which may be pericardial in character), dyspnoea and cardiac dysrhythmias. Signs include tachycardia, a third heart sound, a friction rub (if there is pericardial involvement) and evidence of heart failure.

Investigations

There may be cardiomegaly and signs of heart failure on the chest radiograph, non-specific ST segment and T wave changes on the ECG and raised cardiac enzyme levels, indicative of myocardial damage. Echocardiography shows cardiac enlargement and impaired contractility. A tissue diagnosis, if needed, can be made by cardiac biopsy.

Management

This consists of strict bed rest, treatment of dysrhythmias and anticoagulation if there is significant heart failure. The likelihood is complete recovery, although patients may die in the acute phase or progress to chronic disease. Cardiac transplantation may have to be considered.

Cardiomyopathy

This is a broad pathological term which covers many individual diseases. It is subclassified into:

- **dilated cardiomyopathy**, in which the primary problem is poor contractility leading to dilatation, usually of both sides of the heart, increased filling pressures and reduced cardiac output
- **hypertrophic cardiomyopathy**, in which there is hypertrophy of the myocardium, reducing the size of the cardiac chambers and sometimes obstructing cardiac outflow; contractility is maintained or increased
- **restrictive cardiomyopathy**, in which there is poor contractility and poor compliance of the wall, usually because of an infiltrative process which impedes inflow and reduces stroke volume.

A feature which the various heart muscle diseases have in common is an increased risk of thrombo-embolism and dysrhythmias. The mainstays of treatment, together with the management of heart failure, are anticoagulant and antidysrhythmic therapy. Most cardiomyopathies are rare diseases. You are referred to a reference textbook for more details.

Cardiac tumours

The neoplastic disease of the heart which you are most likely to encounter is external invasion by a malignant tumour such as carcinoma of the bronchus. This can cause tamponade, dysrhythmias and other cardiac complications. *Primary* tumours are rare and usually benign. One which deserves mention is **cardiac myxoma**. This is a gelatinous, polypoid lesion which usually develops in the left atrium and can obstruct the mitral valve, simulating mitral stenosis. There are three features to cardiac myxoma:

Systemic. Patients are systemically unwell and have a high ESR and finger clubbing. These are reactions — presumed immunological — to the tumour tissue.

Thrombo-embolism. The tumour provides a focus on which intracardiac clot can form and from which it can embolise.

Haemodynamic. The tumour prolapses through the mitral valve during diastole. This can cause left heart failure and pulmonary hypertension. Prolapse of the tumour can be heard as a diastolic 'plop' at about the time of a third heart sound. There may be a mid-diastolic and/or systolic murmur.

Left atrial myxomas are rare but should be considered in a patient with an unidentified source of arterial emboli. Right atrial myxomas are even rarer and cause pulmonary rather than systemic embolism. The diagnosis is made by echocardiography and treatment is surgical.

1.8 Hypertension

Essential hypertension is a condition of uncertain aetiology in which peripheral vascular resistance is increased and blood pressure 'reset' to a higher level. Hypertension may also be secondary (see Box 3) to diseases which:

- increase blood volume by reducing sodium and water excretion
- increase peripheral vascular resistance.

The endocrine causes of hypertension listed in Box 3 are discussed in Chapter 7, renal artery stenosis in Chapter 4 and coarctation of the aorta on page 35.

Whatever its cause, high blood pressure thickens the arterial media and intima and accelerates atherosclerosis. In the kidney, this arterial damage can cause a vicious circle of worsening renal function, sodium/water retention and hypertension by impairing glomerular perfusion and causing secondary aldosteronism (p. 167). Another important pathological feature is left ventricular hypertrophy caused by the increased cardiac load of hypertension. In the severest ('accelerated' or 'malignant') hypertension, there is fibrinoid necrosis in the arterioles and loss of capillary autoregulation leading to widespread haemorrhage, ischaemia and tissue necrosis, clinically important in the eyes, kidneys and brain (p. 196).

Epidemiology

Systolic and diastolic blood pressure are normally distributed. The distribution varies from population to population and is higher in blacks than whites. Blood pressure increases with age. Pulse pressure also

---

> **Box 3**
> **Causes of secondary hypertension**
>
> - Increased catecholamine secretion
>   phaeochromocytoma
> - Increased aldosterone
>   renal artery stenosis
>   primary aldosteronism (Conn's syndrome)
> - Increased glucocorticoid
>   Cushing's syndrome
>   steroid therapy
> - Other cases of sodium/water retention
>   renal failure of any cause
> - Other vascular diseases
>   coarctation of the aorta
> - Neurogenic
>   raised intracranial pressure

increases so that the systolic pressure increases disproportionately to the diastolic. There is no clear cut-off which defines 'abnormal' blood pressure. With increasing systolic and diastolic pressure, there is a progressive increase in the risk of stroke and cardiovascular disease. World Health Organization criteria define a blood pressure over 140/90 mmHg as borderline and over 160/95 as hypertension. These criteria are, however, points drawn on a line of increasing risk.

Risk factors for hypertension are:

- a positive family history
- obesity
- alcohol abuse
- non-insulin-dependent diabetes (50% of patients are hypertensive)
- high salt intake (more a 'population' than an 'individual' risk factor).

Only 5–10% of cases of hypertension are secondary, but the possibility must always be considered, particularly in patients below the age of 40 who have a low prevalence of essential hypertension.

Complications

Cardiac complications

These are:

- left ventricular hypertrophy, an effect of a sustained increase in cardiac work. Particularly if complicated by IHD, this may lead to left ventricular failure
- IHD (p. 12), for which hypertension is one of the three main risk factors
- atrial fibrillation (see p. 30).

Cerebrovascular disease. Hypertension is strongly associated with stroke because it:

- causes cerebral atherosclerosis and predisposes to cerebral thrombosis
- directly causes intracerebral haemorrhage through its effects on the cerebral vasculature

- increases the risk of subarachnoid haemorrhage.

Renal disease. The chicken/egg relationship between hypertension and renal disease has been mentioned above and is discussed in more detail on page 158.

Retinal disease. This includes retinal artery thrombosis and retinal vein thrombosis.

Aortic aneurysm. Aortic dissection results from cystic medial necrosis in the arterial wall and is an effect of hypertension.

Clinical approach

The diagnosis is made by opportunistic blood pressure measurement or screening high-risk patients (see risk factors, above).

Blood pressure measurement

Blood pressure varies minute-to-minute, especially on sight of a doctor ('white coat hypertension'). It should be measured under as relaxed conditions as possible, repeated after a few minutes if high and (unless *very* high) repeated days or weeks apart before a decision is made to treat.

Important points of technique are to:

- measure blood pressure sitting; repeat it standing if the patient is old, has risk factors for orthostatic hypotension or a history of it
- use a large cuff if the patient has a fat arm; a normal one will over-read
- raise pressure in the sphygmomanometer 20 mmHg above the palpated systolic blood pressure before lowering it so that you are not caught out by the 'auscultatory gap'
- lower the column of mercury in the sphygmomanometer at a rate of 2 mm per heart beat to ensure accuracy.

History

Having established that the blood pressure is high, consider the following.

Why is it high? Ask about family history of hypertension, history of renal disease, prolonged enuresis in childhood or urinary infection. Take a careful alcohol and drug history. Be alert to the triad of headache, sweating and palpitations. These are the symptoms of phaeochromocytoma, an uncommon cause of hypertension but all too often diagnosed in the postmortem room rather than the clinic.

Is there target organ damage? Take a careful cardiovascular history, with particular attention to angina and previous strokes or transient ischaemic attacks.

How high is the patient's cardiovascular risk? Ask about diabetes, smoking and family history of IHD.

Examination

Your examination should answer the same three questions: Why? Is there target organ damage? How high is the risk?

General appearance. Uncommon though it is,

Cushing's disease will only be diagnosed by an alert clinician who spots the characteristic appearance. Remember, also, the more common association between hypertension and obesity; measure the patient's body mass index. Take note of breathlessness.

Retinal examination. Sustained hypertension causes atherosclerotic changes in the retinal arterioles (irregularity, increased light reflex and attenuation of the veins at arterio-venous crossings — nipping). Similar changes occur with age. It is now clear that these changes cannot be interpreted precisely enough to be used as an index of hypertensive tissue damage, particularly given the better information available from investigations (see below). However, *severe* hypertension can cause quite specific changes:

- cotton wool spots, signs of retinal ischaemia
- flame haemorrhages, caused by vessel rupture and extravasation of blood into superficial nerve fibre layers
- papilloedema or swelling of the optic disc, a sign of cerebral oedema.

Papilloedema is an imprecise sign but to be taken very seriously as evidence of accelerated hypertension (p. 44) if unequivocally present. Cotton wool spots and haemorrhages are easier to identify and always a sign of serious microvascular disease.

The heart. Examine carefully for atrial fibrillation or other dysrhythmia, left ventricular hypertrophy and signs of heart failure. The aortic component of the second heart sound may be loud, reflecting increased pressure on the valve.

Kidneys. Even if renal disease is present, the kidneys are more likely to be small than large but there is a chance you might feel an enlarged hydronephrotic or polycystic kidney.

Peripheral vascular system. Examine for:

- radio-femoral delay; uncommon though coarcts may be, they will only be diagnosed at a treatable stage if alert clinicians routinely check this sign in new hypertensives, particularly young people
- signs of a thoracic or abdominal aneurysm; inequality of the blood pressure in the two arms with signs of aortic valve dysfunction and a pulsatile abdominal mass, respectively
- renal or aortic bruits and signs of peripheral vascular disease, pointers to renal artery stenosis.

Investigation

Ambulatory blood pressure monitoring is now widely used to:

- confirm the diagnosis of hypertension
- assess severity
- monitor the response to treatment.

It is particularly useful in white coat hypertension.

Other investigations are done to answer the same three questions as the history and examination.

Mandatory tests

Test urine. Test for proteinuria as a sign of primary renal disease or hypertensive nephropathy. Examine the urine under the microscope for cells and casts and culture it if there is proteinuria or other evidence of renal disease.

Measure serum creatinine and electrolytes. These are to detect underlying renal disease and Conn's syndrome (p. 270). Conn's is rare but easily diagnosed and, unlike essential hypertension, curable; it will only be detected if every new case of hypertension is screened by measuring serum potassium *before a drug is prescribed*.

ECG. Look for signs of left ventricular hypertrophy and strain or IHD, both of which constitute target organ damage and strengthen the case for treatment.

Chest radiograph. This is to exclude cardiac hypertrophy, left ventricular failure and rib notching caused by coarctation of the aorta.

Other optional tests. These may be indicated in individual cases.

Echocardiography. This is more sensitive than either the ECG or chest radiograph for left ventricular hypertrophy and dysfunction. Arguably, it should be done in every case.

Renal ultrasound scan and i.v. urography. Examination of the renal tract is indicated if the history, physical examination or urinalysis point to renal disease. Ultrasound is the first-line test.

Fasting glucose and lipids. Diabetes and hyperlipidaemia are associated with hypertension and increase the risk of cardiovascular disease. They increase the likely benefits of treatment.

Management

When to treat hypertension
If the blood pressure is very high (> 110 mmHg diastolic) more than transiently, there is an imminent risk of stroke and you should treat without delay. You should remember, however, that:

- high blood pressure can be an *effect* of raised intracranial pressure, for example after acute stroke
- the cerebral circulation adapts to sustained hypertension by 'autoregulation', an upwards shift of the range of blood pressures over which cerebral circulation is unaffected by a drop in blood pressure. Lowering blood pressure too far and too fast in a patient with severe, sustained hypertension can abruptly lower perfusion and cause cerebral ischaemia.

Blood pressure must, therefore, be lowered cautiously and with consideration of its likely causes and complications even in the severest cases. The management of hypertensive emergencies is considered on page 44. In most cases, you are treating a well patient to prevent strokes, heart attacks, heart failure, renal failure and death in the distant future. You need to understand the 'pros and cons' of treatment and explain them to the patient.

Clinical trials have consistently shown that treating hypertension is more effective at preventing strokes than heart attacks. For a blood pressure reduction of 5–6 mmHg diastolic over 5 years, you can expect a 40% reduction in the risk of stroke and a 15% reduction in coronary risk. These are *relative* risks, so the benefit to an individual depends on his/her absolute risk. That risk increases with age, the presence of other risk factors (e.g. smoking and hyperlipidaemia), the presence of established complications and the level of blood pressure. Therefore, more than 500 patient-years of treatment are needed to prevent one stroke in a group of 50-year-olds compared with 300 patient-years in 70-year-olds. Given the inconvenience and possible side-effects of treatment, it is clear that patients must be well informed to help them make the decision. The treatment recommendations of the British Hypertension Society are summarised in Figure 13.

A simple approach is to remember three diastolic thresholds:

- 90 mmHg: below this level, treatment is given only in exceptional circumstances (e.g. in children or to prevent progression of renal disease)
- 100 mmHg: below this level, treatment is discretionary; above it, treatment is indicated
- 110 mmHg: in all but exceptional circumstances, treatment is mandatory.

Elderly people may have **isolated systolic hypertension** (i.e. high systolic with normal diastolic blood pressure) as an effect of atherosclerotic, poorly compliant arterial walls. Treating this reduces cardiovascular risk. Thiazide diuretics are most effective. Over the age of 80, there are no data to guide treatment. The same guidelines can be applied as to 'young elderly' people, tempered by good clinical sense and the avoidance of polypharmacy.

Treatment

Non-pharmacological treatment
Non-drug treatments can be introduced at borderline levels of hypertension and as part of a general 'healthy living' policy. These are to:

- aim for 'ideal' body weight
- drink alcohol in moderation (p. 41)
- avoid added salt in cooking or at the table
- take regular exercise.

These alone can lower blood pressure enough to avoid drug treatment and should be coupled with general lifestyle advice to reduce cardiovascular risk.

Drug treatment
The choice of antihypertensive drug is very much a matter of physician and patient preference because the disease has such a long natural history that completed clinical trials relate to 'yesterday's drugs'. Once-daily treatment is convenient and improves compliance. Side-effects, even if they seem trivial to you, are a significant disadvantage in the treatment of an asymptomatic disease. The presence of target organ disease, other cardiovascular risk factors and contraindications all influence choice. Drugs act in different ways to achieve their antihypertensive result (Fig. 14). The aim of treatment is to achieve a blood pressure as near normal as possible, taking into account the patient's age. A general target is < 160/90 mmHg but the goals should be individualised for each patient.

Thiazide diuretics. In *low dose* (e.g. bendrofluazide 2.5 mg daily) these are a proven effective first-line therapy for mild hypertension. Impotence is their main side-effect. In higher doses (which are no more effective

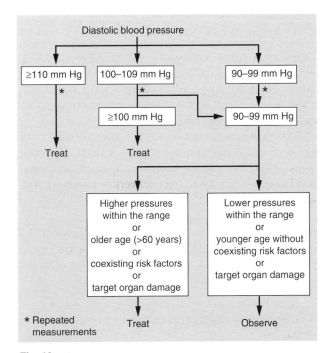

Fig. 13
British Hypertension Society recommendations for the decision to start treatment.

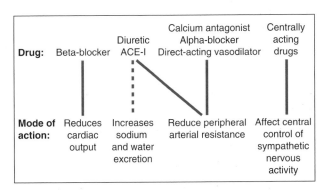

Fig. 14
Modes of action of anti-hypertensive drugs. Dotted lines indicate minor effects.

at lowering blood pressure), they may cause gout, glucose intolerance and hypokalaemia.

Loop diuretics. These are less effective than thiazides in essential hypertension but more effective in salt-retaining states (e.g. renal failure). They are indicated in hypertensive heart failure. They may be combined with ACE inhibitors or other antihypertensive drugs.

Beta-blockers. They are a proven effective first-line treatment for mild–moderate hypertension and can be given in combination for more severe hypertension. They are cardio-protective and relieve angina. They improve survival after myocardial infarction. They are contraindicated in heart failure, asthma and peripheral vascular disease and may cause impotence.

Calcium antagonists. Particularly the once-daily preparations are a suitable first-line treatment for moderate hypertension and may be given with other drugs for more severe hypertension. They relieve angina. They are preferable to beta-blockers in heart failure but should nevertheless be used cautiously because of their negative inotropic effect.

ACE inhibitors. They generally produce fewer side-effects than other antihypertensives. ACE inhibitors may be used as monotherapy in moderate hypertension and are strongly indicated in hypertensive patients with heart failure, in whom they improve life expectancy. They have an important role in the management of *severe* hypertension. They act synergistically with loop diuretics. They may precipitate acute renal failure in renovascular disease (p. 161). Their other main side-effect is cough, which affects up to 20% of patients. The newer angiotensin receptor antagonists may be equally effective without this side-effect.

Alpha-blockers. Newer agents like doxazosin are better tolerated than older members of the class. They are usually used as second-line agents for more severe hypertension, often in combination with other drugs.

Accelerated hypertension

Diagnosis

Accelerated hypertension is rare in the days of widespread screening for hypertension and effective, well-tolerated drugs. The clinical signs are **proteinuria**, resulting from fibrinoid necrosis in the renal vasculature, **retinal haemorrhages** and **exudates** caused by similar changes in the retinal microcirculation and **papilloedema** caused by cerebral oedema. There may be left ventricular failure due to cardiac overload. Unlike mild–moderate hypertension, accelerated hypertension may be symptomatic, even before major complications develop. The symptoms include:

- visual disturbance
- headache
- breathlessness.

Physical signs include:

- diastolic blood pressure usually over 130 mmHg
- left ventricular hypertrophy and, possibly, failure

- retinal changes.

Patients may present with impaired consciousness, focal neurological signs or fits (hypertensive encephalopathy) and are at high risk of cerebral haemorrhage. They may develop acute renal failure.

Management

Blood pressure must not be lowered too quickly or too far. The aim is to reduce it no lower than 100 mmHg diastolic within 12–24 hours. The patient should be admitted to hospital for bed rest. Oral treatment should be used if possible; for example, sub-lingual nifedipine combined with an oral beta-blocker such as atenolol or any other commonly used antihypertensive. If seriously ill (encephalopathy or left ventricular failure), treatment is usually with an i.v. infusion of labetalol (a combined alpha- and beta-blocker). Always ask yourself if the patient could have a phaeochromocytoma. If one is suspected, the first-line treatment is an infusion of phentolamine (an alpha-blocker). If you see severe hypertension with major neurological signs, ask yourself if the patient could have hypertension *secondary* to an intracranial haemorrhage and arrange an urgent CT scan.

Hypertension in pregnancy

Mild–moderate hypertension is a common complication of pregnancy, usually treated with methyldopa, nifedipine, oral labetolol or another beta-blocker. ACE inhibitors increase the risk of congenital malformations and are contraindicated. Hypertension may be a sign of pre-eclampsia, other signs of which are proteinuria, oedema and hyperuricaemia. Severe hypertension associated with pre-eclampsia necessitates delivery.

1.9 Pulmonary vessel disease

Learning objectives

You should:
- understand the range of causes
- be able to work out from simple physiological principles the symptoms, signs, radiological and electrocardiographic features
- understand the principles of treatment.

Causes of pulmonary hypertension

Pulmonary hypertension may be caused by left heart disease transmitted through the pulmonary vein and capillaries or by disease of the pulmonary circulation itself (Box 4). While *acute* left heart failure causes pulmonary oedema, there are adaptive changes to *chronic* pulmonary venous hypertension which minimise pulmonary oedema and transmit pressure into the pulmonary arteries. This is well exemplified by mitral stenosis (p. 31). Disease of the pulmonary circulation is

Box 4
Some causes of pulmonary hypertension

Acute
  Pulmonary embolism
  Left ventricular failure

Chronic
  Increased pulmonary venous pressure
    Left ventricular failure
    Mitral incompetence or stenosis

  Increased flow
    Atrial or ventricular septal defect
    Patent ductus arteriosus

  Pulmonary arterial disease
    Recurrent pulmonary embolism
    Autoimmune disease
    Primary pulmonary hypertension

  Secondary to parenchymal lung disease
    Chronic obstructive pulmonary disease
    Pulmonary fibrosis; sarcoidosis

  Secondary to hypoxia
    Alveolar hypoventilation

usually secondary to lung disease. This may be direct obliteration of the pulmonary vascular bed or a reflex vasoconstriction to hypoxia. An extreme example of the latter is alveolar hypoventilation associated with gross obesity (Pickwickian syndrome) in which there is diminished alveolar ventilation, hypoxia and secondary pulmonary hypertension. Cor pulmonale describes right heart failure secondary to chronic airflow limitation. Pulmonary hypertension may be secondary to increased flow, as in chronic left-to-right shunting of blood. *Primary* pulmonary hypertension is a rare disease of unknown aetiology, chiefly affecting young women.

It follows from the pathophysiology that:

- pulmonary venous hypertension or left-to-right shunts should be corrected as early as possible, before irreversible changes have occurred
- hypoxic vasoconstriction may be a reversible factor at all stages in the natural history of pulmonary hypertension and oxygen therapy has an important place in treatment.

Clinical presentation

The symptoms and signs result from 'forwards' and 'backwards' heart failure. They include dyspnoea, chest pain, lassitude and syncope. Signs include the parasternal heave of right ventricular hypertrophy and a loud pulmonary second heart sound. There may be the pansystolic murmur of functional tricuspid regurgitation (from right ventricular dilatation) and the early diastolic murmur of pulmonary regurgitation (secondary to increased pulmonary artery pressure).

Investigations

The chest radiograph shows enlargement of the pulmonary arteries at the hila with reduced peripheral vascular lung markings (pruning). On the ECG, there are a tall and peaked P wave in lead II (P pulmonale, caused by right atrial hypertrophy) and signs of right heart hypertrophy and strain; a dominant R wave in V1, T wave changes in leads V1-3 and right axis deviation. Blood gases should always be checked to detect hypoxia. Other relevant investigations include radionuclide lung scanning to detect pulmonary embolism, echocardiography, pulmonary function tests, right heart catheterisation with pulmonary angiography and lung biopsy.

Management

The principles of management are:

- Correct any underlying cause. For mitral stenosis, ventricular septal defects and other structural cardiac diseases, that means surgery.
- Avoid hypoxia. That often means domiciliary oxygen therapy.
- Treat heart failure. This relieves breathlessness and, in the case of left heart failure, directly relieves pulmonary hypertension. Diuretics must not be over-used because an adequate right heart filling pressure is essential to maintain cardiac output.
- Consider anticoagulation. Pulmonary embolism may be the primary cause of pulmonary hypertension. It may also result from a reduced cardiac output and exacerbate pulmonary hypertension of some other cause.

Intravenous prostacyclin (a potent vasodilator) may be effective in primary pulmonary hypertension.

1.10 Venous thrombo-embolism

It is important to distinguish clearly between **venous** and **arterial** thrombo-embolism. The lungs provide such an effective filter that the venous and arterial systems are separate from the point of view of thrombo-embolism. It is a good intellectual discipline to use the rather cumbersome terms 'venous thrombo-embolism' and 'arterial thrombo-embolism'.

Learning objectives

You should understand:
- the causes, in terms of Virchow's triad
- how to investigate and treat a deep venous thrombosis or pulmonary embolism.

Deep venous thrombosis

Always keep in mind Virchow's triad, the three factors which predispose to thrombosis:

- stasis
- increased coagulability of blood
- disease of the blood vessel wall.

Diseases which cause venous thrombosis may do so by more than one mechanism. A patient convalescing after surgery is both immobile and hypercoagulable. A tumour can increase blood coagulability, compress the vessel wall and cause stasis. The reason *in situ* thrombosis is more common in veins than in arteries is that blood flows slower in veins. An important point in relation to the first member of the triad is that, whatever its cause, venous thrombosis *causes* stasis and so tends to propagate. An important predisposing factor in women is oestrogen, either during pregnancy or as the contraceptive pill. Thrombophilia is discussed on page 247.

Deep venous thrombosis (DVT) is common and often 'silent'. It has been shown, for example, that one third of patients develop venous thromboses after acute myocardial infarction and over 80% of old people develop them after hip fractures. A DVT may be the presenting feature of malignant disease. Your understanding of the natural history and causes is valuable both in making the diagnosis and in deciding whether or not there is likely to be a sinister underlying cause. The peak time for the development of a DVT is a week or more after an acute insult. A swollen leg the day after a fracture is unlikely to be caused by a DVT but is very likely to be caused by it when it occurs after a week or more. By the same logic, a DVT 2 weeks after a long air flight or a broken leg in an otherwise healthy young person is probably the result of immobility while the same problem developing out of the blue in a middle-aged person with no history of immobility should be considered the presentation of an occult tumour until proven otherwise. Thrombo-embolism which recurs or responds poorly to anticoagulation is a particularly sinister sign.

Only leg vein thrombosis is discussed here because it is the commonest and the potentially most serious form of venous thrombosis but you should remember that thromboses may occur in other sites, including the axillary and renal veins. The principles of diagnosis and management are similar whatever the site.

Clinical presentation

The symptoms of DVT of the leg are:

- pain
- swelling
- heaviness or a bursting sensation in the affected limb.

The signs are:

- swelling and 'turgor' (heaviness to palpation)
- mild cyanosis or reddening

- tenderness over the affected veins
- increased warmth
- dilated superficial veins.

Your ability to detect swelling can be improved by measuring limb girth above and below the knee. Asymmetry > 1 cm is taken as significant. Although the whole leg may feel painful, tenderness is often localised to the affected vein. In calf vein thrombosis, there is tenderness over the back of gastrocnemius and pain may be elicited by sharply dorsiflexing the foot ('Homan's sign'). Femoral vein thrombosis may cause tenderness over the antero-medial aspect of the thigh. However, physical signs have serious limitations:

- pelvic vein thromboses may occur with no symptoms or signs at all; the deep venous thrombosis of a fatal pulmonary embolism may be clinically 'silent'
- involvement is often more extensive than the clinical signs suggest
- compared with venography, physical signs are unreliable in diagnosing DVT.

Differential diagnosis

DVTs have to be distinguished from superficial thrombophlebitis and cellulitis. Thrombophlebitis is inflammation in a superficial vein (often varicose) with secondary thrombosis; it is tender, palpable as a hard 'knot' and often visibly inflamed and red. It is treated with non-steroidal analgesia. Cellulitis, like DVT, causes diffuse swelling and pain. Features which favour a diagnosis of cellulitis are:

- no localised tenderness over veins
- more reddening in cellulitis, sometimes with a clear demarcation line
- obvious portal of entry and spread of infection from it.

A ruptured popliteal cyst is another condition which mimics DVT; it usually occurs in patients with rheumatoid arthritis or other joint disease and can be diagnosed by arthrography. DVT can complicate all of these diagnoses.

The most important point to emphasise is that clinical examination is unreliable in the diagnosis of DVT. Unless there is an absolutely obvious DVT, further investigation is needed.

Investigation

The 'gold standard' is venography; however, it is painful and expensive. Duplex ultrasound scanning is a less invasive investigation. An extremely sensitive technique, used for research rather than clinical practice, is ^{131}I-labelled fibrinogen scanning. Most patients have an ultrasound scan first, then venography if the ultrasound scan is equivocal or negative and there is a strong index of suspicion.

Management

Patients who are immobile or have cardiovascular disease should have *prophylactic* heparin (p. 246) and/or compression stockings, which divert blood flow into the deep veins. In established DVT, the aims are to:

- relieve pain and swelling
- prevent further propagation of the clot
- prevent pulmonary embolism
- allow healing and minimise the chances of permanent venous damage
- prevent recurrence.

Established DVT is treated by anticoagulation unless there are strong contraindications. Heparin should be given intravenously and continued for 5 days to prevent propagation and initiate healing. Warfarin is introduced once the clinical diagnosis is certain. Bed rest and elevation of the limb relieve swelling. Compression stockings divert blood from the superficial to the deep veins and relieve swelling.

Anticoagulants are continued for 4–6 weeks when DVT complicates short periods of immobility, 6 months in cases of spontaneous DVT and lifelong for recurrent DVT. Anticoagulation is discussed on page 246.

Complications

There may be permanent damage to the veins, resulting in a 'post-phlebitic limb' which is permanently swollen, uncomfortable and prone to cellulitis and further episodes of thrombosis. Even without that complication, thrombosis may recur, particularly at times of illness or immobility. Pulmonary embolism is the most serious complication.

Pulmonary embolism

Pulmonary emboli usually come from the iliac, femoral or distal leg veins but may arise elsewhere in the venous system or right side of the heart. Risk factors and causes are as for DVT. Pulmonary embolism, like DVT, may be clinically 'silent' and found postmortem. Individual small pulmonary emboli are not haemodynamically significant but a large embolism or multiple small emboli cause pulmonary hypertension, which may become chronic (p. 44).

A key point in understanding treatment is that pulmonary embolism is a dynamic situation. Emboli are quickly removed by the fibrinolytic system; unless the patient succumbs to the initial event, the threat is from further embolism. Anticoagulation, the mainstay of treatment, works by limiting the formation of new clot in the deep veins. Fibrinolytic therapy is not usually given because there is a risk of dislodging further emboli and the endogenous fibrinolytic system is effective at removing emboli.

Embolism and infarction

An important conceptual point is the distinction between pulmonary embolism and infarction. Emboli may cause infarction of the affected lung if there is severe and lasting ischaemia but not if the embolus is small, dissolution is rapid and/or there is an adequate collateral blood supply from the bronchial arterial system. Clinically, embolism can be inferred from its cardiovascular effects and infarction from its effects on the lungs, chiefly pleurisy if the infarct extends out to the pleural surface.

Clinical presentation

A typical history of pulmonary embolism is a sudden onset of tight chest pain and dyspnoea, often followed by haemoptysis. Pulmonary emboli can be asymptomatic or present purely with right heart failure. There may be syncope caused by an abrupt reduction in cardiac output. If there is pulmonary infarction, the pain may change in character, becoming sharp and related to respiration. Pleurisy may be the sole presenting symptom. Patients may present with infection in an area of infarcted lung. Often, the circumstances give a clue to the diagnosis, e.g. recent immobility or treatment with the contraceptive pill.

On examination, there may be a parasternal heave, increased splitting of the second heart sound and a raised jugular venous pressure. There is tachypnoea, tachycardia and there may be cyanosis, a pleural rub and signs of an effusion. The patient may or may not have signs of a deep venous thrombosis.

Massive pulmonary embolism presents as an emergency with collapse, severe dyspnoea, hypotension, pallor, cyanosis, tachycardia and signs of right heart strain or failure.

Investigations

The initial diagnosis of pulmonary embolism usually has to be made on clinical suspicion because readily available investigations are unhelpful. The **chest radiograph** is usually normal but may show oligaemia (reduced lung markings in the affected area), consolidation, loss of volume and a raised hemidiaphragm, a pleural effusion and one or more linear opacities representing areas of atelectasis. The **ECG** may show signs of right ventricular strain, seen as right axis deviation, right bundle branch block or an 'SI, QIII, TIII pattern' (S wave in lead I, Q wave in lead III and T wave inversion in lead III). The **blood gases** show hypoxia with a reduced pCO_2.

The specific investigation is a **ventilation:perfusion radionuclide scan**. A technetium isotope is given intravenously to detect areas of non-perfusion; labelled xenon is inhaled to demonstrate non-aerated lung. Areas which are aerated but not perfused suggest embolism. Infarction may affect aeration as well as perfusion, but pulmonary emboli are often multiple, so it is usually possible to demonstrate some areas of ventilation:perfusion mismatch in addition to 'matched' defects corresponding to areas of infarction.

Pulmonary arteriography by pulmonary arterial catheterisation is the definitive investigation; if it is positive, the catheter can be left in place and used to infuse streptokinase directly into the pulmonary artery.

Venography is sometimes performed on the basis that demonstration of DVT is strong presumptive evidence of embolism, although a negative result is unhelpful. Diagnostic aspiration of a pleural effusion may be helpful; typically it will be a blood-stained exudate.

Management

Apart from analgesia and oxygen, the treatment is anti-coagulation, as described for DVT. Massive pulmonary embolism may be treated by surgical embolectomy and systemic or pulmonary fibrinolytic therapy. It is tempting to treat right heart failure in pulmonary embolism with diuretics, but that is inappropriate because a high filling pressure is needed to maintain right heart output. If there is severe hypotension, inotropic support may be given.

1.11 Arterial disease

Diseased arteries can expand and rupture or narrow and occlude. They may be occluded by disease in their wall, thrombosis on a diseased wall or embolism from elsewhere in the arterial system. The arterial wall may, itself, be a source of emboli. The causes of arterial disease are atheroma, other degenerative processes and inflammation (vasculitis). There are many causes of inflammation, including infection and autoimmunity. Arteritis is considered under the individual diseases (Chapter 10). You are referred to a textbook of surgery for information about occlusive peripheral arterial disease. Thoracic and abdominal aneurysms may present to you as emergencies so they are discussed briefly here.

Learning objective
- You should understand the causes and clinical presentations of aortic aneurysms at their various sites.

Thoracic aortic aneurysm

Atheroma is by far the most common cause of thoracic aortic aneurysm. Syphilis, once common as a cause of aortic incompetence and aneurysm, is now rare. Arteritides of the aorta are also a rare cause. Aneurysms may develop in patients with Marfan's syndrome, a congenital disorder of collagen whose other stigmata are a high, arched palate, 'spidery', long fingers, tall stature, and dislocated lenses. Atheromatous aneurysms occur most often in middle-aged or elderly men and are strongly associated with hypertension and generalised arterial disease. They involve the ascending aorta, arch and descending aorta in roughly equal proportions. They may:

- expand, be painful and have pressure effects
- dissect
- rupture.

Expanding thoracic aneurysm

An expanding aneurysm may be found by chance on a chest radiograph, or it may stretch the aortic valve ring and present with aortic incompetence or present with pain or pressure symptoms. The pain is central or to one side of the chest and radiates to the back. Pressure symptoms include:

- dysphagia
- hoarseness
- dyspnoea
- superior vena caval obstruction.

The most important radiographic sign is widening of the mediastinum. Further investigation is by transthoracic or transoesophageal echocardiography, MR or CT scanning.

Surgery for acute dissection has an extremely high mortality and rupture is terminal so early diagnosis and elective surgery give the best prognosis. Marfan's syndrome causes thoracic aortic aneurysms in young people and is an important indication for elective surgery. Elderly patients may be unfit for surgery, in which case treatment is symptomatic.

Ruptured thoracic aneurysm

This presents with sudden death or collapse associated with chest pain and shock. It is untreatable.

Dissecting thoracic aneurysm

Dissection occurs when there is a breach in the intima and blood tracks into the media. It may arise in the ascending or descending thoracic aorta.

Clinical presentation
Dissection is an uncommon cause of chest pain and can be difficult to diagnose but you must consider it because to give fibrinolytic therapy for a presumed myocardial infarct may kill your patient. The problem is made more difficult by the fact that a dissecting aneurysm can occlude a coronary ostium and actually present with myocardial ischaemia. Depending on its location in the aorta, the pain is felt in the centre or to one side of the anterior chest, radiating to the back, neck and arms. The patient may describe a sudden tearing sensation and the pain may be excruciating.

About 50% of patients with a dissection are hypertensive at the time of presentation. They may have a difference of systolic blood pressure > 20 mmHg between the two arms because of occlusion of the subclavian arteries. There may be signs of spinal or carotid artery occlusion. Aortic regurgitation may develop as a result of stretching of the valve ring or pericarditis as a result of blood tracking into the pericardial sac.

Investigation
The chest radiograph may show mediastinal widening, a left-sided pleural effusion or enlargement of the

aortic knuckle. The ECG may be normal, non-specifically abnormal or show signs of acute myocardial ischaemia. Transoesophageal echocardiography is the investigation of choice to confirm the diagnosis and locate the intimal tear. CT or MR scanning may also be used.

Management and prognosis

Pain should be controlled. The mortality during acute aortic dissection is 1% per hour. It can be reduced by lowering blood pressure to <110 mmHg systolic with i.v. labetalol. If the ascending aorta is involved, immediate surgery is indicated. Dissection of the descending aorta is treated by strict bed rest and blood pressure control because surgery has a higher mortality than medical management.

Abdominal aortic aneurysm

Abdominal aortic aneurysm is the most common aneurysm encountered in clinical practice. The causes are similar and the mechanisms which lead to symptoms and signs are analogous to thoracic aortic aneurysm.

Clinical presentation

The cardinal symptom is abdominal pain radiating to the back and the cardinal sign a pulsatile abdominal mass. Sometimes the mass may be found by chance on physical examination. It is important to distinguish between tender and non-tender pulsatile masses because tenderness is a sign of impending rupture. Apart from pain, an expanding aneurysm may present with complications, including obstruction of a ureter (caused by an inflammatory reaction to the aneurysm) or embolism into the peripheral arterial system. Rupture presents with pain and hypotension together with the tender abdominal mass. There may be involvement of the renal arteries causing renal failure and involvement of the distal arteries causing leg ischaemia.

Investigation

Ultrasound, CT or MR are first-line investigations. Small aneurysms are unlikely to rupture but those over 5 cm are at high risk.

Management

Risk factors, including hypertension, should be treated. Small aneurysms are observed by serial scanning to detect expansion and impending rupture. High-risk aneurysms should be treated surgically before they rupture. Emergency surgery has a better outlook than for thoracic aneurysms but still a high mortality.

Self-assessment: questions

Multiple choice questions

1. The anatomy of the heart:
   a. If you stand on the patient's right side with your right hand across the sternum and cardiac apex, the left ventricle lies under the sternum
   b. On a PA chest radiograph, the left heart border is mostly formed by the left ventricle
   c. In an ECG, disease of the interventricular septum causes changes in chest leads V3–4
   d. When examining the heart, the cardiac apex is the point where the heart beat can be felt most strongly
   e. Occlusion of the left anterior descending coronary artery causes infarction of the anterior wall of the left ventricle and interventricular septum.

2. Cardiac physiology/physical examination:
   a. Bedside examination of the jugular venous pressure gives an estimate of cardiac preload
   b. A pulse rate < 30 beats/min is probably a **sinus** bradycardia
   c. Heart rates > 160 beats/min are usually initiated by a pacemaker other than the SA node
   d. The mitral and tricuspid components of the second heart sound can usually be heard as two separate sounds during inspiration
   e. An increased pulse pressure (systolic–diastolic BP) does not necessarily signify an increased stroke volume

3. The ECG:
   a. The T wave corresponds to atrial contraction
   b. If the S wave is greater than the R wave in lead I, there is right axis deviation
   c. If the S wave is greater than the R wave in lead II, there is left axis deviation
   d. ST segment depression may be a sign of cardiac ischaemia
   e. A tall R wave in V1 may be a sign of right ventricular hypertrophy

4. Endocarditis:
   a. It is important to take blood cultures over at least a 24 hour period to make the diagnosis
   b. Transthoracic echocardiography is a sensitive means of making or confirming the diagnosis
   c. Most patients with *Staphylococcus aureus* bacteraemia have endocarditis
   d. Viral endocarditis leads to valvular abnormality
   e. In patients with a new stroke, endocarditis can be ruled out if the patient is afebrile

5. Treatment of endocarditis:
   a. Intravenous antibiotics for 6 weeks are necessary to cure *viridans* type streptococcal endocarditis
   b. Staphylococcal endocarditis on the tricuspid valve in a drug addict is treated with flucloxacillin and valve replacement
   c. Large vegetations are an indication for surgery
   d. Combination antibiotic therapy is almost always appropriate for endocarditis
   e. If gentamicin is used for treatment, it should not be used for more than 2 weeks

6. Pericardial disease:
   a. A normal heart size on chest radiography rules out pericardial disease
   b. In tamponade, crackles at the lung bases and peripheral oedema are usual
   c. A low-voltage ECG is a clue to the presence of a large pericardial effusion
   d. Hard-to-hear heart sounds are typical of a large pericardial effusion
   e. Almost all cases of purulent pericarditis have a pericardial friction rub

7. In a patient with a raised jugular venous pulse:
   a. A further increase on expiration is characteristic of pericardial tamponade
   b. Giant V waves suggest tricuspid stenosis
   c. Facial engorgement and lack of pulsation in the jugular venous pressure are characteristic of superior vena caval obstruction
   d. The cause could be pulmonary embolism
   e. Diuretic therapy is indicated, whatever the cause

8. In acute myocardial infarction:
   a. The diagnosis should be questioned if the jugular venous pressure is not raised
   b. Streptokinase should not be given until the diagnosis has been confirmed by two sets of raised cardiac enzymes
   c. Dysrhythmias in the early hours after presentation carry a poor prognosis
   d. Lignocaine should routinely be given to prevent dysrhythmias
   e. Rupture of the interventricular septum is an uncommon but serious complication

9. The following are true of valvular/congenital heart disease:
   a. Mitral stenosis is usually caused by rheumatic heart disease
   b. An indication for surgery in mitral stenosis is worsening pulmonary hypertension
   c. A patient with rheumatic aortic valve disease is likely also to have mitral valve disease
   d. Coarctation of the aorta may be associated with a chromosomal abnormality
   e. ACE inhibitors are the treatment of choice for dyspnoea caused by aortic stenosis

10. In the treatment of hypertension:
    a. Spironolactone is an appropriate drug for patients with primary aldosteronism (Conn's syndrome)
    b. Ankle swelling is a side-effect of ACE inhibitors
    c. Intravenous propranolol is the usual emergency treatment for severe hypertension
    d. Loop diuretics work synergistically with ACE inhibitors
    e. A beta-blocker is a logical first choice in a patient who also has angina

11. In acute dissection of the thoracic aorta:
    a. The operative mortality is about 30%
    b. Spinal cord ischaemia may occur
    c. Hypertension should be treated aggressively
    d. Acute aortic stenosis may occur
    e. The patient may develop myocardial ischaemia

12. Heart failure:
    a. ACE inhibitor therapy is reserved for patients whose symptoms are uncontrolled by large doses of diuretics
    b. May be caused by alcohol abuse
    c. Previous tuberculous pericarditis could cause it
    d. The presence of a wheeze discriminates asthma from heart failure
    e. A suspected diagnosis of heart failure in a 23-year-old woman is supported by hearing a third heart sound

13. Hypertension:
    a. Treatment is of no proven benefit in patients over the age of 70
    b. The symptoms of phaeochromocytoma include headache, sweating and palpitations
    c. Oral treatment producing a fall in diastolic blood pressure of 20 mmHg over 24 hours might be regarded as successful treatment of accelerated hypertension
    d. ACE inhibitors are the drugs of choice for hypertension in pregnancy
    e. Addison's disease should be considered a possible cause in a hypertensive patient with hirsutism

14. In ischaemic heart disease:
    a. Prevalence is increased in chronic renal failure
    b. Untreated hypothyroidism predisposes to it
    c. Polycythaemia may precipitate myocardial ischaemia
    d. An alcohol intake of 18 units per week in a man increases the risk of ischaemic heart disease
    e. A high plasma fibrinogen reduces the risk

15. In the treatment of angina:
    a. An ACE inhibitor is the treatment of first choice if the patient is also hypertensive
    b. Of treatments which relieve symptoms, only revascularisation has been proven to improve life expectancy
    c. Heparin is indicated in the treatment of unstable angina
    d. Revascularisation is only indicated for patients aged <60 years
    e. Treating hyperlipidaemia is valueless once a patient has developed angina

16. Cardiac dysrhythmias:
    a. Digoxin toxicity may cause supraventricular tachycardia
    b. A patient with a completely irregular pulse of 180 beats/min is likely to be in atrial fibrillation
    c. Complete heart block may be asymptomatic
    d. Digoxin is effective in preventing paroxysms of atrial fibrillation
    e. A QRS width less than 3 small squares on the ECG indicates that a tachycardia is supraventricular

17. Venous thromboembolism:
    a. Heparin treatment for deep venous thrombosis should be continued for 5 days
    b. The recommended duration of warfarin treatment for a first pulmonary embolism with no obvious precipitating cause is 6 months
    c. Ultrasound is a reliable way of excluding calf vein thrombosis
    d. Intravenous streptokinase should be given without delay once pulmonary embolism is diagnosed
    e. Measurement of fibrin degradation products is a sensitive way of detecting venous thromboembolism

Case histories

History 1

You are a cardiologist who receives a referral letter as follows:
'This rather awkward 73-year-old woman has had good health in the past apart from some wheeziness and chest infections for which she has needed courses of antibiotics most winters. She visited her brother in America last summer and had a health check. Her blood pressure was 190/94. When she came back, she demanded treatment. I explained that, at her age, it was quite inappropriate to treat her hypertension but she was insistent. I prescribed atenolol which she took for a few days but she claimed it made her breathless. She is asking for a second opinion. I am sorry to waste your time but would be grateful if you could see her.'

1. Are there any points in the referring doctor's assessment and management with which you disagree?

2. How would you assess her?
3. You confirm that she is hypertensive; how would you manage her?

History 2

> A 58-year-old woman presents with biventricular failure. She admits to drinking a bottle of sherry and smoking 20 cigarettes per day. Echocardiography reveals a dilated, poorly contracting left ventricle.

1. Suggest two causes for her heart failure
2. Name two complications of her cardiac disease which might develop

> It is suggested she should be anticoagulated.

3. List two contraindications either suggested by her history or which you might identify on a more detailed history/examination

History 3

> Mr Shah is a 59-year-old bus driver admitted under your care with anginal chest pain. His previous health has been good, he is on no treatment and he does not smoke. Examination is normal. His ECG shows sinus rhythm, rate 80/min and is normal apart from some T wave flattening in leads V3–5. He is pain-free by the time you see him.

1. How should he be managed?

> You are called to see him 6 hours later. He has had another attack of pain. His ECG shows ST segment elevation and T wave inversion in leads V2–5.

2. How should he be managed?

> After a further 2 hours, the nursing staff call you again because his monitor shows many ectopic beats, different from one another in size and shape. His BP is 130/78 and his pulse 80 beats/min.

3. What action should you take?

> You see him the next morning. His BP is 132/82. He is in stable sinus rhythm. He now has bilateral fine basal crackles and has had some more anginal chest pain. His ECG now shows Q waves in leads V2–5.

4. How should he be managed?

> The next morning, he complains of a sharp pain in the chest, relieved by lying in certain positions in bed and leaning forward

5. What is the likely diagnosis? How could you confirm your diagnosis at the bedside?

> Mr Shah makes a good recovery and becomes mobile around the ward. Ten days after admission, and just after being given the all-clear to be discharged, he collapses and the cardiac arrest team are called. The ECG shows complexes but no pulse can be felt.

6. What is the diagnosis?
7. What is the management?

> Sadly, resuscitation is unsuccessful. He has a postmortem.

8. What is the pathologist likely to find?

History 4

> A 68-year-old man has had difficulty managing his garden for some time because of breathlessness. Recently, he has not only been breathless when he exerts himself but he has noticed precordial tightness radiating to the neck and left arm. He has used his wife's bronchodilator spray but it hasn't helped at all. On one occasion 2 weeks ago he found himself lying on the lawn after attempting to mow it. He has been brought up to the emergency department after a particularly severe attack of pain. His blood pressure is 106/82, pulse 80/min sinus rhythm, the apex beat has a thrusting character and he has a soft midsystolic murmur. His chest radiograph shows cardiomegaly and his ECG shows an R wave in V5 of 35 mm. He is on no treatment.

1. Suggest a differential diagnosis.
2. How would you investigate him?

Short notes

Write short notes on:

1. Indications for antibiotic prophylaxis against infective endocarditis
2. Diagnosis and management of infective endocarditis in an i.v. drug abuser
3. You examine a patient's retinae and see cotton wool spots; write notes on what other retinal features could tell you if the appearances were caused by diabetes or hypertension

Viva questions

1. An elderly man is admitted under your care because of immobility. He has two swollen legs, one larger than the other.

   a. What explanations can you think of?
   b. What other physical signs would you look for?

2. A patient of yours is being considered for a renal transplant. The surgeon wishes to know if he has ischaemic heart disease. How would you tell?

Data interpretation

1. Each of the following signs is strongly suggestive of a cardiovascular diagnosis; what is the diagnosis and what is the cause/mechanism of the sign?
   a. Splinter haemorrhages
   b. Absent A wave in the jugular venous pulse
   c. Septal lines on a chest radiograph
   d. M shaped QRS complex > 3 small squares on the ECG
   e. A midsystolic click and late systolic murmur
   f. Unmatched perfusion defect on a ventilation:perfusion lung scan
   g. Diastolic opening snap
   h. Pulsatile hepatomegaly
   i. Collapsing pulse
   j. Rib notching on chest radiograph

2. What cardiac rhythm is shown in each of the short rhythm strips given as Picture 1a–n?

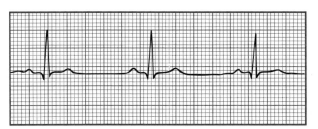

Picture 1a

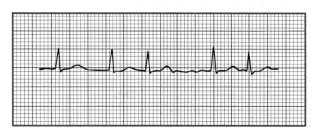

Picture 1b

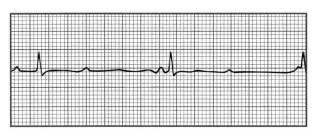

Picture 1c

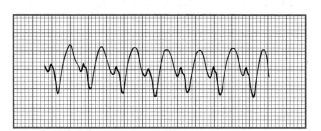

Picture 1d

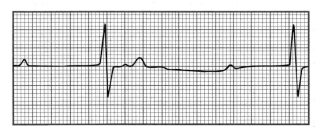

Picture 1e

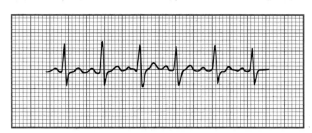

Picture 1f

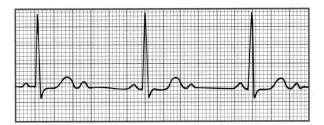

Picture 1g

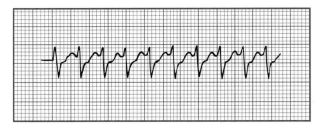

Picture 1h

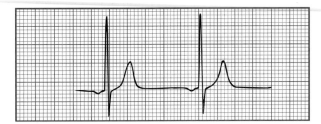

Picture 1i

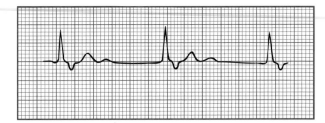

Picture 1j

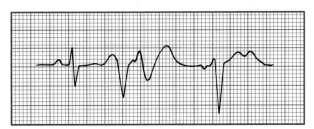

Picture 1k

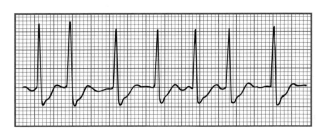

Picture 1l

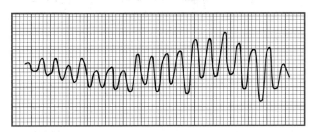

Picture 1m

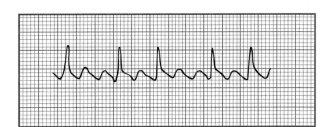

Picture 1n

3. Interpret the 12-lead ECGs given as Picture 2a–j.

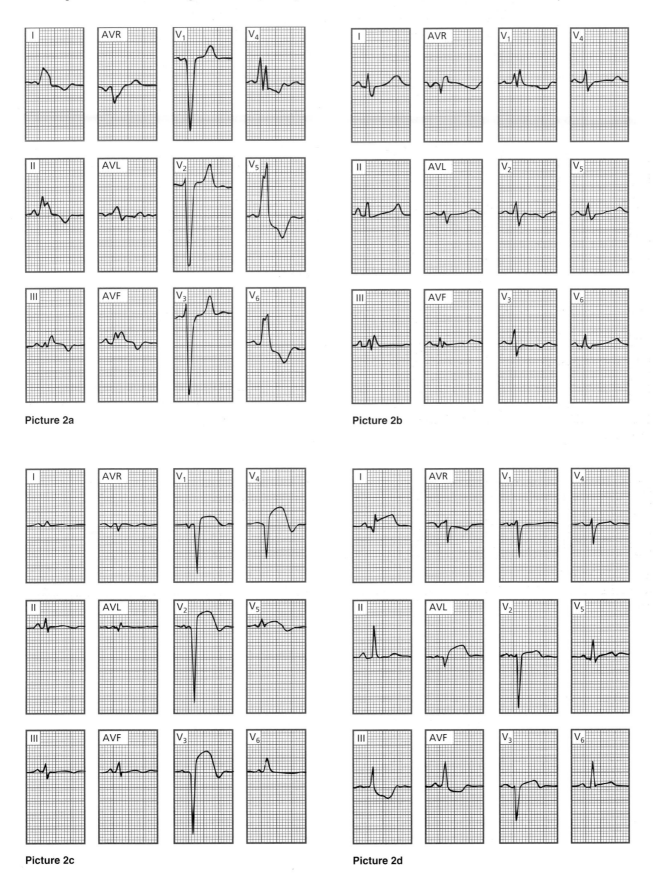

Picture 2a

Picture 2b

Picture 2c

Picture 2d

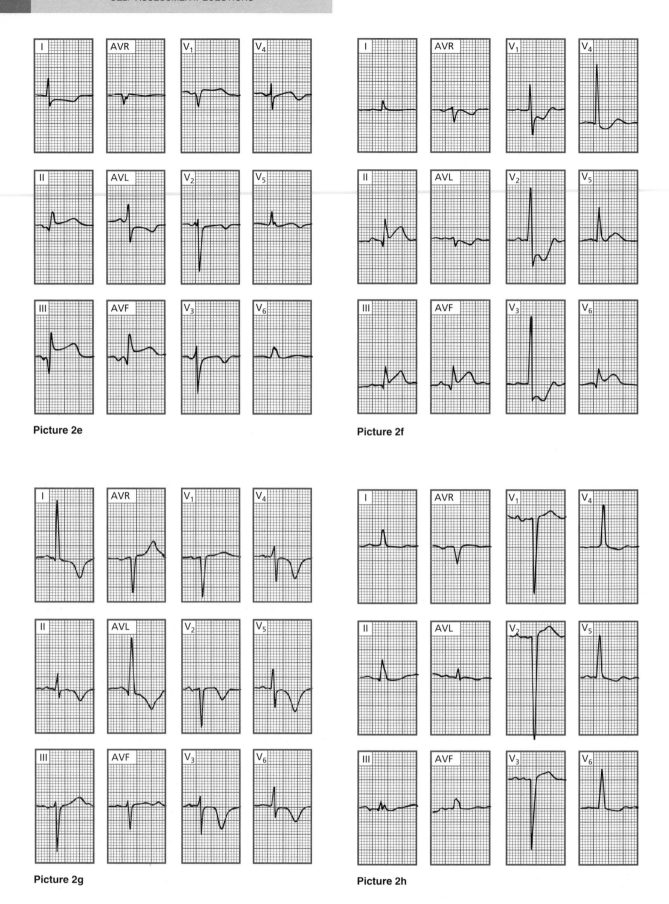

Picture 2e

Picture 2f

Picture 2g

Picture 2h

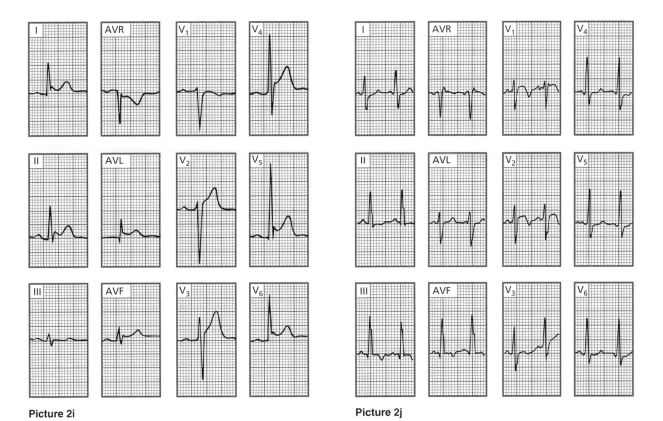

Picture 2i

Picture 2j

4. The two traces shown in Picture 3 were taken from a patient in a coronary care unit. At the time of the first (Picture 3a), she was free of pain. The second (Picture 3b) was taken after she complained of chest pain. Interpret the first ECG; what new changes are shown in the second?

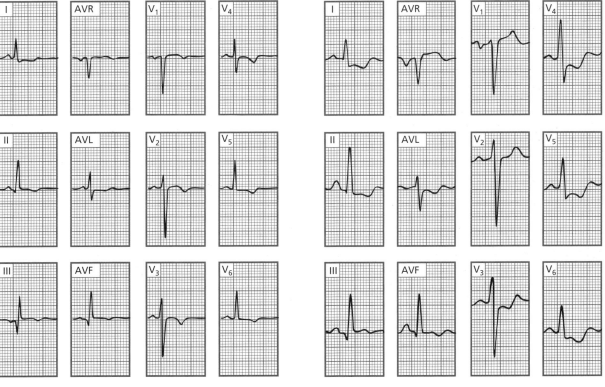

Picture 3a

Picture 3b

Self-assessment: answers

Multiple choice answers

1. a. **False.** The *right* ventricle presses against the sternum; the left ventricle constitutes the apex and is felt under the fingers.
   b. **True.**
   c. **True.**
   d. **False.** The apex is the downmost, outermost point at which pulsation can be felt, not the point of maximum impulse.
   e. **True.** Anterior myocardial infarction is caused by disease of the left anterior descending artery.

2. a. **True.**
   b. **False.** Parasympathetic slowing of the SA node would not be expected to cause such a slow pulse rate. The likely explanation is conducting tissue disease with an 'idioventricular' pacemaker relatively low in the conducting system, i.e. complete heart block.
   c. **True.** This is faster than would be expected for a sinus tachycardia.
   d. **False.** This is nonsensical because the mitral and tricuspid sounds make up the *first* heart sound.
   e. **True.** Lack of compliance of the arterial walls is a feature of ageing. Old people may have a high pulse pressure despite a normal or reduced stroke volume.

3. a. **False.** See Table 3.
   b. **True.**
   c. **True.**
   d. **True.** It may also be a digoxin effect.
   e. **True.**

4. a. **False.** Three sets taken separately over a maximum of 12 hours (and preferably less if the patient is acutely ill) are necessary.
   b. **False.** Specific yes, but not sensitive. Transoesophageal echocardiography is better.
   c. **False.** Older, hospitalised patients are less likely to have endocarditis than younger patients from the community.
   d. **False.** Viruses have not been reported to cause endocarditis alone.
   e. **False.** Fever is unhelpful in this situation. Many patients with strokes have fever without endocarditis and the opposite is also true. Patients admitted with a new stroke or TIA should have a blood culture if they have a valvular defect and/or fever.

5. a. **False.** These organisms are usually exquisitely susceptible to penicillin and gentamicin and 2 weeks of therapy suffices.

   b. **False.** Flucloxacillin (with gentamicin or rifampicin) is the medical treatment of choice but valve replacement is not appropriate. Insertion of a prosthetic heart valve into a drug addict is very likely to lead to prosthetic valve endocarditis subsequently because of their continuing habit.
   c. **True.**
   d. **True.** For two reasons; first, the selected combinations are usually additive or synergistic. Second, to prevent the development of resistance.
   e. **False.**

6. a. **False.** Although this would be unusual unless very acute.
   b. **False.** Rare; the clues to pericardial tamponade are (i) raised jugular venous pressure, (ii) quiet heart sounds, (iii) absence of chest signs, (iv) pulsus paradoxus.
   c. **True.**
   d. **True.**
   e. **False.** About 50% have a rub, which is one reason the diagnosis is difficult.

7. a. **False.** It is normal for the jugular venous pressure to rise on expiration; Kussmaul's sign of pericarditis is for it to rise on *inspiration.*
   b. **False.** This is a sign of tricuspid incompetence.
   c. **True.**
   d. **True.** Pulmonary embolism may cause acute right heart failure.
   e. **False.** In some situations, e.g. right ventricular infarction and acute pulmonary embolism, diuretic therapy worsens cardiac output by reducing the abnormally high filling pressure.

8. a. **False.** It is not usually raised at presentation, exept in right ventricular infarction.
   b. **False.** It should be given without delay on the basis of symptoms and ECG changes.
   c. **False.** (Reperfusion) dysrhythmias at this stage have a benign prognosis and may signify a satisfactory response to fibrinolysis.
   d. **False.** This is of no proven value.
   e. **True.**

9. a. **True.**
   b. **True.**
   c. **True.**
   d. **True.** Turner's syndrome, 45X0.
   e. **False.** Because the cardiac output is fixed and cannot rise with exercise, vasodilator therapy is dangerous.

10. a. **True.** Spironolactone is an aldosterone antagonist.
    b. **False.** Because they inhibit the

renin–angiotensin–aldosterone system, they are mildly diuretic. Other vasodilators can cause ankle swelling

c. **False.** If a parenteral drug is given, it is usually labetolol. More often, treatment is oral.

d. **True.**

e. **True.** A calcium antagonist would also be logical.

11. a. **False.** It is much higher.
    b. **True.**
    c. **True.** Nitroprusside or labetolol infusion is a recommended treatment.
    d. **False.** Aortic *regurgitation* may occur.
    e. **True.** The coronary ostia may be occluded by the dissection.

12. a. **False.** An ACE inhibitor is indicated early in almost every patient with heart failure because it improves life expectancy.
    b. **True.** Alcoholic cardiomyopathy.
    c. **True.** Tuberculosis may cause constrictive pericarditis in later years.
    d. **False.** Wheeze may occur as a result of heart failure alone (cardiac asthma).
    e. **False.** Third heart sounds may be heard in healthy young people.

13. a. **False.** There is well-proven benefit, particularly in the prevention of stroke.
    b. **True.**
    c. **True.**
    d. **False.** ACE inhibitors are contraindicated in pregnancy.
    e. **False.** Cushing's syndrome, not Addison's disease.

14. a. **True.**
    b. **True.** Hypothyroidism causes hypercholesterolaemia and atherosclerosis.
    c. **True.** By increasing blood viscosity and impairing blood flow.
    d. **False.**
    e. **False.**

15. a. **False.** ACE inhibitors are not antianginals; a beta-blocker or calcium antagonist would be an appropriate choice.
    b. **False.** Beta-blockers are cardioprotective, at least in patients who have had myocardial infarcts.
    c. **True.**
    d. **False.**
    e. **False.** Lipid-lowering may cause regression of coronary atherosclerosis; presence of coronary artery disease is an *indication* for lipid-lowering treatment.

16. a. **True.** Typically, paroxysmal atrial tachycardia.
    b. **True.**
    c. **True.** Particularly congenital complete heart block.

d. **False.** Digoxin slows the ventricular rate during paroxysms of atrial fibrillation but does not prevent them; sotalol or amiodarone may prevent them.

e. **True.**

17. a. **True.**
    b. **True.**
    c. **False.** Ultrasound is not a reliable technique to exclude venous thrombosis below the knee.
    d. **False.** Streptokinase does not have a clearly defined role in the management of pulmonary embolism; it may be given by infusion into the pulmonary artery after massive pulmonary embolism.
    e. **False.** FDPs are only able to detect massive fibrin deposition, as in disseminated intravascular coagulation.

Case history answers

History 1

1. Important points are:
   - the diagnosis of hypertension is not proven by a single measurement
   - it is wrong to say that age is a contraindication to anti-hypertensive therapy
   - the previous history is strongly suggestive of chronic airflow limitation which appears to have been made worse by a beta-blocker, albeit a cardioselective one.

2. Is she hypertensive? Measure blood pressure on several different occasions, including standing measurements to exclude postural hypotension. Does she have evidence of target organ damage?
   - Examine her
   - Chest radiograph
   - Test urine for protein, measure creatinine and potassium
   - Record ECG.

3. Explain and negotiate management with her (something it seems her doctor did not do). Discuss lifestyle measures to control blood pressure and coronary prevention. Avoid beta-blockers, which she cannot tolerate, probably because it worsens her airways obstruction. Consider low-dose thiazide diuretic, calcium antagonist or ACE inhibitor.

History 2

1. Most likely causes are alcoholic cardiomyopathy and IHD. Possible causes are hypertension and valvular heart disease.
2. The most likely complications are arterial thromboembolism and dysrhythmias.
3. Likelihood of continued drinking, which could

cause dangerously unstable anticoagulation. Peptic ulcer and/or oesophageal varices are likely in view of severe alcohol abuse.

History 3

1. His history is suggestive of IHD but there is no definite evidence of acute myocardial infarction. He should be admitted, ideally to a coronary care unit, and observed. Give aspirin but no fibrinolytic therapy
2. He now has evidence of an evolving antero-septal myocardial infarct. He definitely needs the coronary care unit and should be given oxygen, analgesia (diamorphine with anti-emetic) and fibrinolytic therapy (streptokinase). Prophylactic subcutaneous heparin is advisable. A beta-blocker may also be given.
3. These are probably reperfusion arrhythmias caused by fibrinolytic therapy. Even if they are not, he is haemodynamically stable and the management is to observe him.
4. He has signs of left ventricular failure. ACE inhibitor definitely indicated, he may also be given a diuretic; nitrate is indicated for pain. Beta-blockers should be avoided because of heart failure. Continue aspirin.
5. Pericarditis. Auscultate for pericardial rub.
6. He is in electro-mechanical dissociation.
7. Figure 11 shows the resuscitation procedures.
8. An antero-septal full thickness myocardial infarct in the territory of the left anterior descending artery, probably resulting from a recent coronary thrombosis. It is likely that his terminal collapse was caused by cardiac rupture, given the electro-mechanical dissociation, although massive pulmonary embolism and a further infarct should also be considered

History 4

1. The history and signs strongly suggest aortic stenosis; he has exertional dyspnoea, angina and syncope. His pulse pressure is narrow and he has left ventricular hypertrophy. He may have IHD. He is not hypertensive so an aortic aneurysm is unlikely. You should exclude anaemia.
2. He needs an urgent echocardiogram. If the diagnosis of tight aortic stenosis is confirmed, he needs referral to a cardiac surgeon urgently. If not, he should be investigated for IHD

Short notes answers

1. Indications are discussed on page 37.

2. **Clinical features** are
   - fever, tricuspid murmur (or occasionally left-sided murmurs), Janeway lesions, evidence of i.v. drug abuse.

- assess cardiac status carefully for failure.

Investigations include:

- blood culture (two or three samples at different times), ECG, chest radiograph, urea and electrolytes (to manage antibiotics), FBC.
- hepatitis BsAg, hepatitis C antibody (and liver function tests) and possibly HIV.
- echocardiogram
- label all blood specimens 'High risk'.

Management depends on status:

- cardiac status poor and left-sided lesions: commence antibiotics immediately after taking blood cultures and consider transfer to regional cardiothoracic unit immediately
- cardiac status reasonable and left-sided lesion: commence antibiotics after taking blood cultures and arrange urgent echocardiogram
- right-sided lesion clinically, commence antibiotics immediately after blood cultures taken and monitor carefully to check no other complications of sepsis and you have not missed a left-sided lesion.

    You will probably need a central line. Give ampicillin 2 g 4 hourly, flucloxacillin 2 g 4 hourly and gentamicin 1.5 mg/kg 12 hourly (or equivalent) if renal function normal. The drugs and dosages may need to be altered when the results of cultures are known. Surgical referral is not necessary unless left-sided endocarditis occurs.

3. Both diabetes and hypertension cause retinal ischaemia, seen as cotton wool spots. Both can also cause hard exudate formation and flame haemorrhages.

    Diabetic retinopathy. The earliest abnormality is microaneurysm (small red dot) formation, so a diabetic patient with cotton wool spots (a more advanced feature) should have these; their absence is strongly against the diagnosis. New vessel formation would confirm the diagnosis but is an advanced feature of diabetic retinopathy so its absence does not exclude diabetes.

    Hypertensive retinopathy. The abnormalities are less specific. Marked arterio-venous nipping would be consistent with a diagnosis of hypertension but the sensitivity and specificity of this sign is very poor. The presence of papilloedema would be informative. It is not a feature of diabetic retinopathy. Together with cotton wool spots, it could signify accelerated hypertension but this is a rare disease.

Viva answers

1. a. Swollen legs may be caused by
   - cellulitis
     raised venous pressure, systemically or locally
   - lymphoedema
   - hypoalbuminaemia.

This man has a process affecting both legs so think first of a disease process which is systemic or proximal to the legs. It could be heart failure, lymphoedema, hypoalbuminaemia or vena caval compression or thrombosis; but why is the swelling asymmetrical? Perhaps he has dual pathology. Patients with bilateral swollen legs for those reasons may develop a secondary venous thrombosis or cellulitis within one leg. The patient could also have bilateral DVTs or bilateral cellulitis affecting one leg more than the other.

b. You should examine the legs for the signs of DVT and cellulitis (p. 46), look for signs of heart failure (Fig. 8) and do a careful abdominal and rectal examination because lymphoedema, caval compression/thrombosis and bilateral DVTs could be caused by abdominal malignancy. Although you were not directly asked this, it would show that you are thinking through the problem logically if you state that you would like to know the patient's plasma albumin.

2. You should structure your answer and, ideally show your depth of knowledge by indicating the weight of each piece of information.

History. History of myocardial infarction and symptoms of angina or heart failure; suggestive of IHD if present but unable to exclude IHD.

Examination. Signs of heart failure might indicate underlying IHD and signs of peripheral vascular disease would be presumptive evidence of widespread arterial disease but physical examination is relatively insensitive for IHD.

Investigations. Resting ECG may show evidence of old myocardial infarction or ischaemia; informative if abnormal but relatively insensitive;

Ambulatory ECG may show 'silent' ischaemic changes at rest or precipitated by exertion.

Exercise ECG is much more sensitive than the resting ECG but lacks the sensitivity and specificity of coronary angiography.

Coronary angiogram is the 'gold standard', both sensitive and specific for IHD.

Exercise thallium scan is a sensitive investigation to detect areas of impaired coronary perfusion.

Data interpretation

1. a. Infective endocarditis. Caused by a small vessel vasculitis.
   b. This indicates loss of atrial contraction, typically seen in atrial fibrillation.
   c. Pulmonary venous hypertension. Caused by interstitial oedema.
   d. Bundle branch block or intraventricular conduction delay. The width of the complex indicates that the impulse has spread slowly through ventricular muscle rather than conducting tissues.

e. Mitral valve prolapse. Caused by the valve cusps sliding over one another during systole and prolapsing back into the left atrium.
f. Pulmonary embolism. Signifies non-perfusion of an aerated segment of lung.
g. Mitral stenosis. Caused by high left atrial pressure and the opening of a stenotic mitral valve in early diastole; this sign is lost when the valve is calcified and immobile.
h. Tricuspid incompetence. Pressure is transmitted back into the venous system from the right ventricle through the incompetent valve.
i. Aortic regurgitation. Incompetence of the valve causes a low diastolic pressure and increased stroke volume causes a high systolic pressure; the increased pulse pressure is felt as a collapsing pulse.
j. Coarctation of the aorta. Caused by collateral intercostal vessels bypassing the coarct.

2. a. Sinus bradycardia, rate 52/min. Each QRS complex is preceded by a P wave with a normal PR interval.
   b. Atrial fibrillation, rate 105/min. The QRS complexes are completely irregular; fine fibrillation waves can be seen between the third and fourth complexes
   c. Complete heart block with junctional escape rhythm. The ventricular rate is 42 beats/min. P waves can be seen at a rate of 75/min; the fifth P wave can just be seen before the upstroke of the R wave. The atria and ventricles are beating independently of one another. The complexes are less than three small squares in width indicating that ventricular depolarisation is propagating through the normal conducting pathways. The ventricular rate, though slow, is not catastrophically slow. Contrast this with Picture 2e.
   d. Broad complex tachycardia (> 3 small squares), rate 166/min. On this rhythm strip alone, you cannot distinguish between ventricular and supraventricular tachycardia (see text).
   e. Complete heart block with left ventricular escape rhythm. The ventricular rate is 29/min; P waves can be seen at a rate of 53/min, again completely independent of the ventricular complexes. The complexes are broader than in Picture 2c, confirming their origin within the ventricles.
   f. Sinus tachycardia, rate 143/min. P waves clearly visible before each QRS complex.
   g. Second-degree (Mobitz type) heart block, rate 52/min. Each QRS is preceded by a P wave with a normal PR interval but for every conducted P wave there is one which is not conducted. Contrast this with Picture 2c in which the atria and ventricles are completely dissociated.
   h. Supraventricular tachycardia, rate 250/min. The fact that it is a narrow complex tachycardia (< 3 small squares) indicates that it is supraventricular.

It is absolutely regular, excluding atrial fibrillation. There is a 'saw tooth' appearance to the complexes, suggesting atrial flutter with 1:1 conduction of the flutter waves to the ventricles.

i. (High) junctional rhythm, rate 56/min. There are small P waves at the same interval before each QRS complex. The PR interval is short and the P waves are inverted. The impulse is arising in the region of the AV node, spreading backwards through the atrium (hence the inverted P wave) and causing atrial depolarisation just ahead of ventricular depolarisation.

j. (Low) junctional rhythm. Similar to picture 2i but the inverted P waves are coming between the R and the T wave. The site of impulse generation is closer to the ventricle than the atrium and the order of depolarisation is reversed.

k. Multifocal ventricular ectopic beats. There is a sinus beat followed by two bizarre, broad complexes (their breadth indicating that they arise within the ventricle) which differ from one another in shape, showing that they arise from different foci. The configuration of the P wave and the electrical axis of the fourth complex have changed from the first beat but the complex is of supraventricular origin.

l. Fast atrial fibrillation, rate 140/min. Narrow complexes with an irregular rhythm are diagnostic of atrial fibrillation. The faster the rate, the harder it may be to detect the irregularity. Mark out the complexes with a piece of paper and slide it along the rhythm strip to detect irregularity.

m. Ventricular fibrillation. Broad, rapid, disorganised impulses are diagnostic of ventricular fibrillation.

n. Atrial flutter with variable block, rate 113/min. This is a narrow complex tachycardia with obvious flutter waves. The timing of the QRS complexes is irregular because of variable conduction of the flutter impulse.

3. a. Left bundle branch block. There are P waves and a normal PR interval but the QRS complex is > 3 small squares because of slow spread through the ventricular muscle. M-shaped complexes in the lateral chest leads are the characteristic of *left* bundle branch block.

b. Right bundle branch block. Like Picture 3a, a sinus rhythm, but in this case the M-shaped complexes are in V1. The right-sided chest leads are normally predominantly negative; in this case, most of the deflection is in a positive direction.

c. Acute anterior myocardial infarct. There are Q waves (indicating full thickness infarction), ST segment elevation and T wave inversion in leads V1–5, characteristic of anterior infarction. ST segment elevation usually does not persist more than a few days, showing that it is a recent event.

Note also that the T waves are flat or inverted in the lateral (I, AVL) and inferior (II, III, AVF) leads suggesting widespread ischaemia.

d. Acute lateral infarct. There are Q waves and ST segment elevation in leads I and AVL. There is also some ST segment elevation in the anterior chest leads. There is ST segment *depression* in leads III and AVF. Misleadingly termed 'reciprocal ST segment depression', this is a sign of ischaemia extending beyond the area which has actually infarcted.

e. Acute inferior infarct. There are Q waves in III and AVF and ST segment elevation in II, III and AVF. Reciprocal ST segment depression is seen in I and AVL. There is T wave inversion in V2–5, suggesting widespread ischaemia. Note also the short PR interval and inverted P waves suggesting a junctional rhythm.

f. Inferior infarct with posterior and lateral extension. The changes of inferior infarction are similar to Picture 3e, including reciprocal ST depression in the anterior chest leads. There is ST elevation in V6 indicating lateral extension. Note that V1 is predominantly positive, without the M-shaped complex of right bundle branch block. This is the appearance of posterior infarction.

g. Subendocardial (non-Q wave) infarct. There is deep T wave inversion in V2–6, I, AVL and II but no Q waves. This suggests extensive partial thickness (subendocardial) myocardial infarction.

h. Left ventricular hypertrophy. The maximum downwards deflection is in V2 (37 small squares). The maximum upwards deflection is in V5 (15 small squares). The sum (52 small squares) is very much increased. There are widespread downsloping ST segments. There are also Q waves across the septal leads (V1–3) suggesting a previous myocardial infarct.

i. Pericarditis. There is ST segment elevation in leads I, II, AVL, V2–6. The shape of the ST segment ('dished', or upwardly concave) seen well in V4–6 (contrast with ECG C) is characteristic of pericarditis, as is the wide distribution of the ST segment elevation.

j. Pulmonary embolism. There is a sinus tachycardia (115/min) with T wave inversion in V1–3, an S wave in lead I and a Q wave and T wave inversion in lead III ('SI, QIII, TIII'). These changes result from acute right ventricular strain.

4. The first ECG (Picture 4a) shows an inferior myocardial infarct. There are Q waves and T wave inversion in III and AVF. There is also T wave inversion in V1–6 compatible with anterior ischaemia. The second ECG (Picture 4b) shows myocardial ischaemia. ST segment depression has developed in V3–6, I and AVL. This is characteristic of ischaemia. Her chest pain is probably caused by unstable angina, an indication for urgent angiography with a view to revascularisation.

Respiratory disease

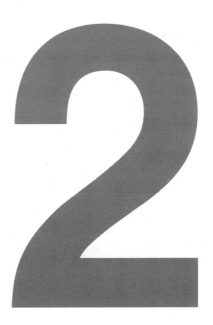

2.1 Clinical aspects

Learning objectives

You should:
- understand the important principles of respiratory anatomy and physiology as applied to the common respiratory diseases
- be able to interpret the common respiratory symptoms and signs and construct a differential diagnosis based on probabilities
- be able to use investigations in respiratory medicine appropriately to the clinical problem
- understand the principles of management of the common respiratory diseases and the immediate treatment of the common respiratory emergencies.

Anatomy

You must know the important anatomy of the respiratory tract as this influences the ways in which clinical problems present or diseases develop.

The right main bronchus is more vertical and foreign bodies or aspirated material are more likely to pass down it. There is then a division into the upper and intermediate bronchi, with the latter dividing into the middle and lower lobe bronchi.

On the left side, the main bronchus divides into the upper and lower lobe bronchi. The **lingular** branch of the upper lobe bronchus is sometimes affected by bronchiectasis (p. 74). All bronchi divide into segmental and sub-segmental branches until the acinus is reached, where a terminal bronchus sub-divides into bronchioles supplying alveoli.

The divisions of the major bronchi are linked to the lobes of the lungs. The left lung is divided into upper and lower lobes by the **oblique** fissure, which runs from the fourth vertebra to the sixth costochondral junction anteriorly. The right lung is subdivided into upper, middle and lower lobes, by the addition of the **horizontal** fissure, which begins at the oblique fissure in the midaxillary line running anteriorly to the sternal end of the fourth costochondral cartilage.

Diaphragm

The diaphragm is a muscular sheet with a central tendon on which the pericardium sits, hence the cardiac shadow is narrowed and elongated when the patient inspires (diaphragm *descends*) and is broadened when the person *expires*. Cardiomegaly may, therefore, be erroneously diagnosed on a radiograph if the patient fails to breathe in adequately. Conversely, cardiac enlargement may be missed in hyperinflation. The nerve supply to the diaphragm is the phrenic nerve (C3, 4, 5). Paralysis causes *paradoxical* movement, i.e. on inspiration, the diaphragm on that side ascends.

Interpretation of examination and radiographic findings

In any patient with a possible respiratory (or cardiac) problem, a chest radiograph is a useful investigation. You need to be able to relate the anatomical relationships to your clinical findings or radiographic abnormalities. Important points to note are:

- if possible, you should always request postero-anterior (PA) films. AP (portable) films may give a false impression of cardiomegaly
- abnormalities posteriorly on clinical examination point to pathology in the lower lobes
- you should describe masses on PA radiographs as being in the upper, mid or lower zones (*not lobes*)
- a lateral radiograph will localise an abnormality
- upper lobe collapse causes *tracheal* deviation
- lower lobe collapse causes *mediastinal* shift and the *left* lobe collapses behind the heart
- the *middle* lobe collapses as a triangle adjacent to the right heart with loss of the border.

Pulmonary vasculature and lymphatics

The divisions of the pulmonary arteries follow those of the bronchi to the lung parenchyma. The pulmonary venules eventually drain into the four pulmonary veins. In heart failure, 'upper lobe diversion' is reported on radiographs, meaning that the upper lobe veins are visible and distended (p. 10).

In pulmonary hypertension, the peripheral arteries become narrowed. On a radiograph, this is seen as 'pruning' of the pulmonary arteries, with little flow to the periphery (oligaemia). In a major pulmonary embolus, blocking one of the large arteries may limit the oligaemia to one zone of the radiograph.

There is an extensive lymphatic network which may be infiltrated by cancer cells causing blockage. Usually the lymph channels are not visible on a radiograph, but in **lymphangitis carcinomatosis** they can be seen as fine lines adjacent to the peripheral lung borders — **Kerley B lines**. The lymph network drains into the **thoracic duct**, which runs posteriorly to the root of the neck. *Trauma* and *malignancy* may cause blockage of the duct and leak of lymph — **chylothorax**.

Pulmonary physiology

The main function of the lung is gas exchange and to achieve this efficiently there needs to be:

- adequate ventilation of the alveoli
- matching between ventilation ($\dot{V}$) and perfusion ($\dot{Q}$)
- adequate diffusion of gases between the alveoli and the capillary bed
- carriage of gases in the blood.

Other functions of the lungs include the modification of drugs and hormones (e.g. conversion of angiotensin I) and a physical and immunological (e.g. cilia, macrophages, IgA) barrier to noxious agents, including pathogens.

Ventilation

Mechanics

Inspiration is an active process whereas expiration depends mainly on elastic recoil. The ribs move up and out (think of a bucket handle) and the diaphragm descends. If resistance to airflow increases (*obstruction*, as in chronic bronchitis and emphysema), the accessory muscles and the abdominal musculature are utilised.

Conditions which affect these structures may interfere with ventilation. For example:

- respiratory muscle weakness: Guillain–Barré syndrome
- diaphragmatic weakness: phrenic nerve palsy
- thoracic spine and rib disorders: kyphoscoliosis.

When ventilation is impaired, the cardinal abnormality is a raised pCO_2.

Control

The respiratory centre in the brainstem controls respiration. Neurogenic stimuli (pain, anxiety, volition) may affect respiration. The major function of the centre is to match respiration with metabolic needs, maintaining:

- PaO_2 11–13 kPa (80–100 mmHg)
- $PaCO_2$ 4.8–6.0 kPa (35–45 mmHg)
- pH   7.35–7.44
- bicarbonate   22–30 mmol/l.

These values are maintained, at rest, by a pulmonary blood flow of 5 l/min and a ventilation of 6 l/min. In any single breath, the tidal volume ($\simeq$ 500 ml) can be divided into alveolar ventilation and dead-space ventilation; the latter is where no gas transfer takes place. In health, this is predominantly in the large airways ($\simeq$ 150 ml), but pulmonary emboli, for example, can cause increase in dead-space ventilation.

There are strong chemical stimuli (PaO_2 and H[+]) to breathe via the carotid and aortic bodies and the respiratory centre in the medulla. The most potent stimulus is an increase in $PaCO_2$. In patients with chronic bronchitis and emphysema, sensitivity to changes in $PaCO_2$ can be lost such that reliance is placed on *hypoxic* drive ($PaO_2 < 8$ kPa). Correction with high inspired oxygen can then be dangerous (p. 81).

An increase in H[+] concentration (acidosis) stimulates ventilation, as in **Kussmaul's** respiration seen in **metabolic acidosis** (p. 172). The respiratory centre can be depressed (e.g. opiates, sedatives) or stimulated (e.g. aspirin) by drugs. Other stimuli include pulmonary embolism and sepsis.

Match of ventilation and perfusion

There is a wide variation in matching between alveolar ventilation ($\dot{V}$a) and perfusion ($\dot{Q}$). Towards the apices, ventilation tends to dominate with the reverse towards the bases. Where there is perfusion without ventilation, **shunting** occurs producing **hypoxaemia**, which is the hallmark of $\dot{V}/\dot{Q}$ mismatching. Normally, where ventilation is inadequate, the local control of blood flow causes vasoconstriction of arterioles. In diseases affecting the lung parenchyma, e.g. fibrosing alveolitis, this control breaks down and perfusion still occurs causing hypoxia. It can also occur in atelectasis or collapse. In certain non-respiratory conditions such as sepsis or chronic liver disease, pulmonary arterioles can open up, again bypassing the alveoli and causing a shunt (and hence hypoxia).

In contrast to the change in blood-flow mechanisms causing hypoxia, increases in $PaCO_2$ tend to occur where global (mechnical) ventilation is inadequate, e.g. in respiratory muscle weakness.

The match between ventilation and perfusion is used in the diagnosis of pulmonary emboli (p. 47). A ventilation/perfusion scan can show areas of the lung which are being ventilated but not perfused. Multiple defects are often seen in areas remote from a chest radiograph abnormality or the side with the pleuritic pain.

Oxygen transport

Oxygen is carried within the blood predominantly as oxyhaemoglobin. The shape of the dissociation curve is sigmoid and its position can be shifted by change in other variables (Fig. 15). This ability is important as it can facilitate the transfer of oxygen to the tissues. Furthermore, the steepness of the middle part of the curve ensures that at PO_2 of ≤ 5.3 kPa (40 mmHg), as it is in the tissues, the haemoglobin readily gives up its oxygen. You need to be aware of the shape of the curve because of the widespread use of oxygen saturation monitors as a proxy for PaO_2. Whilst the arterial partial pressure is varying widely at the top part of the curve, the oxygen saturation will not change very much.

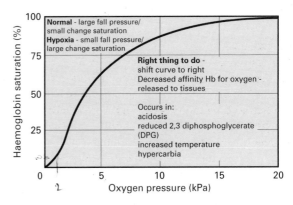

Normal - large fall pressure/small change saturation
Hypoxia - small fall pressure/large change saturation

Right thing to do -
shift curve to right
Decreased affinity Hb for oxygen - released to tissues

Occurs in:
acidosis
reduced 2,3 diphosphoglycerate (DPG)
increased temperature
hypercarbia

Fig. 15
Haemoglobin dissociation curve and the variables that affect it.

However, on the steep part of the curve, a change in saturation can indicate a large fall in PaO_2. A common pitfall is to equate the two measurements, but a saturation of 80% may indicate a PaO_2 of only 8 kPa.

Common symptoms

Breathlessness

Breathlessness is a subjective description of the sensation experienced by the patient. It is not dyspnoea, which is difficulty with breathing deduced from your observations, nor is it tachypnoea (rapid rate of breathing).

You should clarify how much the patient is limited by shortness of breath. Two patients may answer 'quite a lot' meaning for one the inability to climb the stairs without stopping, for the other being unable to complete his daily 2–3 mile stroll. The onset of breathlessness may give a clue to the underlying pathological process. A smoker who has had worsening exercise tolerance over many years is likely to have chronic bronchitis and emphysema. If, however, the same person had experienced a rapid deterioration coupled with general malaise and a productive cough, the problem is probably an acute infective exacerbation.

The variation in breathlessness needs to be assessed. How long have they experienced breathlessness? How does it vary with time? What affects their breathing? For example, asthmatic patients may be worse in the summer or when they wake ('morning dipping').

Wheeze

Wheezing is a frequent symptom of patients with airflow obstruction. As with breathlessness, diurnal or seasonal variation would suggest asthma. Heart failure may present with wheezing — 'cardiac asthma'. A further consideration is whether the patient is not describing wheezing, but rather inspiratory stridor implying extrathoracic airflow obstruction.

Cough

Either in association with breathlessness or on its own, cough is an important symptom. In most people, it is simply caused by a recent infection. Some infections, such as mycoplasma, can cause a prolonged dry cough (< 4 weeks), but persistence may reflect bronchial hyperactivity resulting from asthma. You should initiate basic investigations (e.g. chest radiograph, PEFR) in any patient with a persistent cough.

A productive cough is commonly seen in smokers, with the production of clear mucoid sputum. In patients with infection, the sputum colour changes to yellow or green. In patients with bronchopulmonary aspergillosis, yellow mucus plugs may be expectorated. Bronchiectasis is typically associated with a large volume of sputum that is frequently coloured, implying infection.

Haemoptysis

Coughing up blood is a frightening symptom. Your framework for management is:

- confirm that the problem is haemoptysis and not haematemesis or bleeding from the nasopharynx
- investigate thoroughly to exclude the possibility of a bronchial carcinoma; being a smoker will increase the likelihood of this
- consider other possible causes, for example, dry bronchiectasis (p. 74). Other causes are rupture of a small bronchial vein during a coughing bout (particularly in severe airflow obstruction) and pulmonary infarction.

Chest (non-anginal pain)

Chest pain is a common symptom. As with haemoptysis it is useful to have a framework:

- is it pleuritic?—Sharp pain, worse on inspiration or coughing
- is it caused by a rib fracture?—Sudden onset (prolonged coughing in a patient with chronic bronchitis); history of trauma; pain is worse on movement but may be increased by breathing/coughing; localised chest wall tenderness
- is it musculoskeletal?—Very common; history similar to rib fracture but often lacking definite onset; strong relationship to movement; not particularly worsened by inspiration; often diagnosis by exclusion
- other causes?—for example, herpes zoster can present with severe chest wall pain and is often misdiagnosed until the characteristic rash appears. Pericardial pain is covered on page 39.

Respiratory investigations

Imaging

Plain radiographs have been considered above. Computer tomography (CT) is useful in:

- diagnosis and staging of primary and secondary tumours
- detecting pulmonary infiltration, e.g. sarcoid or occupational lung disease
- assessing mediastinal masses including percutaneous lung biopsies.

Magnetic resonance imaging (MRI) is still being evaluated. Radioisotope scanning (ventilation/perfusion) is used in the diagnosis of pulmonary embolism (p. 47).

Respiratory function

For most patients, very simple tests are all that are required to assess respiratory function. **Peak expiratory flow rate (PEFR)** is a standard test for airflow obstruction; low values can also be obtained with poor technique or respiratory muscle weakness (e.g. in myasthenia gravis, p. 212). Normal or increased values may be seen in restrictive lung disease. You should be able to demonstrate the technique to the patient:

1. hold the spirometer and take a deep breath in
2. place the mouthpiece in the mouth and wrap your lips around it
3. breathe out *as hard and as fast as you can*

Repeat the measurement three times with the patient and record the best value.

The PEFR is dependent on age, height and gender. You should always interpret a test result by comparing it with the predicted value. There is a *diurnal* variation in bronchomotor tone, with it being greatest in the early hours of the morning (i.e. bronchoconstriction). In asthma, this variation is often exaggerated, producing **morning dipping** which can be severe (p. 82).

Spirometry provides more information, giving measurement of **forced expiratory volume in one second** (FEV$_1$), and **forced vital capacity** (FVC). Normal values are again dependent on age, height and gender. Different traces are obtained depending on the pathophysiology present (Fig. 16).

Transfer factor is a measure of gas transfer in the alveoli. In most patients, reduction reflects mismatching of ventilation and perfusion ($\dot{V}/\dot{Q}$). For example, in pulmonary fibrosis the cause of hypoxia is not because of difficulty of oxygen passing across a thickened alveolar–capillary barrier, but because of the distortion of the pulmonary architecture such that part of the lungs are being perfused and not adequately ventilated. In patients with increased amount of functioning haemoglobin in the lungs (polycythaemia, p. 238), shunts, fresh haemorrhage, transfer factor may be increased.

Fibreoptic bronchoscopy

Fibreoptic bronchoscopy may be of use in:

- visualising and taking biopsies, brushings and washings (cytology) of possible endobronchial malignancies
- culture of secretions, brushings and washings for microbiological diagnosis (particularly for tuberculosis (p. 72) and *Pneumocystis carinii* (p. 72)
- **transbronchial biopsy** for diffuse parenchymal disease, e.g. fibrosing alveolitis
- **broncho-alveolar lavage** for parenchymal disease; usually the cells in the washings are predominantly macrophages: in sarcoidosis, a lymphocyte is found (T helper cells); in fibrosing alveolitis, an increase in polymorphs is seen in active disease.

Pleural aspiration and biopsy

See page 87.

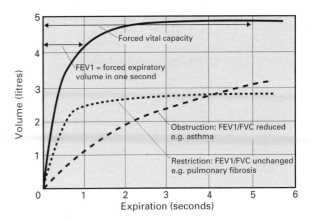

Fig. 16
Spirometric traces showing normal FEV$_1$ and FVC and those in obstructive and restrictive defects.

Blood gas analysis

In all patients with suspected respiratory disease, blood gas analysis should be undertaken. In certain circumstances, for example acute asthma, it is negligent not to do so. Normal values are given in Table 2.

Interpretation of the results is important as further action will be based on this. Patients with acute $\dot{V}/\dot{Q}$ mismatching, e.g. acute asthma, pneumonia, are hypoxic, with a respiratory alkalosis. This is type 1 respiratory failure (remember type 1: *low* PaCO$_2$). If the mismatching continues, then renal excretion of bicarbonate over several hours/days will compensate (respiratory alkalosis with *compensatory* metabolic acidosis).

Patients with ventilatory failure (e.g. respiratory muscle weakness as in Guillain–Barré syndrome) are both hypoxic and hypercarbic with a respiratory acidosis. This is type 2 respiratory failure (remember type 2: *high* PaCO$_2$). In this, the kidney will retain bicarbonate and excrete H$^+$ to compensate (respiratory acidosis with *compensatory* metabolic alkalosis). Acid-base disturbances are discussed on page 172. Later in this chapter, there is discussion of the patterns of blood gas abnormalities found with specific respiratory diseases.

Common drugs
Bronchodilators

The β$_2$-adrenoceptor agonists
The common agonists used are salbutamol and terbutaline. They work by direct stimulation of the extensive numbers of β-adrenergic receptors in the airways, causing smooth muscle relaxation. The preferred route of administration is inhalation. Metered dose inhalers (MDI) are commonly used and an important aspect of patient management is education in the use of these devices and checking that technique is satisfactory. The basic technique is:

1. shake the inhaler
2. fully expire

3. place inhaler in mouth and 'fire' at the start of inspiration
4. continue to full inspiration
5. hold breath, then repeat if prescribed.

If the patient finds this difficult, spacer systems should be tried (e.g volumatic, nebuhaler), or dry powder systems (e.g. rotacaps, turbohalers). Occasionally, oral administration is necessary, but large doses must be used to produce the same effects on airway smooth muscle, in which case toxic side-effects (tremor, anxiety and palpitations) may occur. In severe chronic asthma, home nebuliser therapy can be effective.

Theophyllines

Theophyllines have a complex mechanism of action. A primary effect is antagonism of intracellular phospho-diesterase, thereby preventing the breakdown of cyclic AMP. As with β-adrenoceptor stimulation, this promotes smooth muscle relaxation. Oral theophyllines are available in a variety of forms. Physicians are divided as to their usefulness in chronic airflow limitation (e.g. chronic bronchitis and emphysema, chronic asthma). Nocturnal administration may alleviate early morning 'dipping' in asthmatic subjects. Monitoring of blood levels is advisable (see treatment of acute asthma). Side-effects include GI (nausea, abdominal pain), cardiac (palpitations, arrhythmia) and CNS (insomnia, anxiety and, occasionally, convulsions) symptoms. Overdose, particularly with i.v. therapy (acute management), may cause convulsions and arrhythmias.

Anticholinergics

There is a cholinergic nerve supply to the bronchial tree, stimulation of which causes bronchoconstriction. Ipratropium bromide is a cholinergic antagonist that blocks this effect. It has a place in the management of some patients with chronic airflow limitation. Ipratropium is poorly absorbed orally. It is given as an MDI or, in severe cases, home nebuliser.

Prophylaxis and anti-inflammatory drugs

Corticosteroids

Corticosteroids work by suppressing the inflammatory response. Inhaled fluorinated corticosteroids (beclo-methasone, budesonide) should be administered as an MDI on a regular basis for patients who have reversible airflow limitation *and* require *regular* treatment with bronchodilators. One problem you will encounter is oropharyngeal candidiasis with dysphonia. Oral corticosteroids should be reserved for patients with chronic asthma unresponsive to inhaled treatment. The dose of prednisolone should be kept, where possible, to under 10 mg to reduce adrenal suppression and long-term problems such as osteoporosis and cataracts. Inhaled and oral steroids can be combined.

Corticosteroids are used in other respiratory conditions, such as vasculitis, or sarcoidosis. Again, the dose of prednisolone should be kept to a minimum to decrease the risk of side-effects. The use of other immunosuppressive drugs is considered in the relevant sections.

Disodium chromoglycate

A primary action of disodium chromoglycate is to stabilise the mast cell preventing histamine release. It is used as prophylaxis in (predominantly) young people with asthma and/or atopy. It is administered as a dry powder inhaler. There are no major side-effects.

Antitussives

You should always consider why the patient has a cough; is there an underlying mechanism that can be treated, for example left ventricular failure or asthma? The consequences of suppressing a cough should also be considered; would it cause the pooling of secretions and a hypostatic pneumonia?

Many proprietary antitussives work predominantly by the soothing nature of the liquid carrier. For this reason 'simple linctus' is the most appropriate starting point for a mild irritative cough. Opioids are the best cough suppressants, working both on lung and central brain receptors. Codeine or pholcodeine elixir are reasonable first-line treatments; use morphine if there is another indication (e.g. pain).

Antibiotics

Antibiotics are discussed on page 375.

2.2 Infective disorders

Learning objectives

You should:
- understand the classification of pneumonia and other forms of respiratory infection
- know the major causes of respiratory infection and their treatment
- be familiar with the clinical presentation and appropriate investigations for respiratory tract infection
- be aware of which patients require specialised advice and/or procedures.

Classification of infective disorders

Pneumonia and respiratory infection are classified as follows:

Pneumonia

An acute, presumed infective, respiratory illness typified by fever, cough, dyspnoea and a new infiltrate on a chest radiograph. The term bronchopneumonia is subsumed under pneumonia and implies the production of purulent sputum in addition to the above features. Lobar pneumonia refers to infection located in one circumscribed area of the lung with sharp edges radiologically and is most likely caused by *Streptococcus pneumoniae* infection.

Pneumonia may be community-acquired or hospital-acquired.

Atypical pneumonia. This is linked with two imprecise meanings:

- erythromycin- or tetracycline-responsive pneumonia (which includes *Legionella* pneumonia)
- non-bacterial pneumonia (which includes viruses, *Mycoplasma*, etc. but excludes *Legionella* spp).

Often atypical pneumonia presents with extrapulmonary manifestations such as headache, jaundice, diarrhoea, etc.

Aspiration pneumonia. Following vomiting or reflux, gastric contents may enter the lungs leading to both an infective and a chemical (acidic) pneumonia. Common in alcoholics, patients with stroke and those with impaired mental function.

Pneumonitis. An imprecise term meaning a new diffuse pulmonary process, which may or may not be infective. It implies fine bilateral shadows on the chest radiograph. Infections are typically caused by viruses such as adenovirus, or cytomegalovirus in immuno-compromised patients.

Acute bronchitis. An acute infection of the bronchial tree characterised by a productive cough usually with mucopurulent sputum, with or without fever, with no new chest radiograph abnormalities. Usually caused by bacteria that cause pneumonia.

Acute tracheitis or tracheobronchitis. Typically viral (e.g. parainfluenza), the patient complains of a painful rasping cough, with pain in the anterior chest, commonly without fever. The chest radiograph is usually normal. It must be distinguished from stridor caused by a foreign body and bacterial epiglottis.

Community-acquired pneumonia

Epidemiology

Community-acquired pneumonia is increasingly common with age and is also more common in debilitated patients. Mortality varies between 6 and 20%.

Pathophysiology

The vast majority of pneumonias follow microscopic aspiration of bacteria from the nasopharynx, throat and oesophagus. Radioisotope tracer studies of normal adults has shown that 45% aspirate during sleep. Pneumonia develops when enough bacteria enter the trachea, reproduce and cause bronchial and/or parenchymal infection. The implication is that the bacterial flora of the nasopharynx and throat determines the causative organism.

Causes of pneumonia and clinical syndrome

There are many different causes of pneumonia (Table 9). However, some are more common in the community, others in hospital.

Pneumococcal and *Haemophilus* pneumonia

Pneumococcal pneumonia is the most common cause of community-acquired pneumonia (50–80%), partly because it is a frequent inhabitant of the nasopharynx. Many cases occur in young or middle-aged adults, but elderly people, those with chronic chest disease, alcoholics and AIDS/HIV patients are at higher risk.

Although a frequent pathogen in patients with chronic airflow limitation (CAFL), *Haemophilus influenzae* is an uncommon cause of pneumonia.

Clinical features. Onset is usually abrupt in lobar pneumonia, but bronchopneumonia may be more gradual in onset. Other features include:

Table 9 Aetiology of pneumonia

	Community-acquired		Hospital or community-acquired	
Aetiological agent	Bronchopneumonia	Lobar	Aspiration	Hospital-acquired / ventilator pneumonia*
S. pneumoniae	+++	+++	+	+
Haemophilus spp.	+	±	+	+
Legionella spp.	+	+	−	+
Staphylococcus aureus	±	+	+	+
Gram negative	±	+	+	++
Anaerobes	±	−	++	+
Mycoplasma	±	+	−	
*Chlamydia*** spp.	+	+	−	−
Coxiella burnetii	+	+	−	−

*Usually a bronchopneumonia in pattern, occasionally lobar
**Chlamydia includes *C. trachomatis* (pneumonitis in babies), *C. pneumoniae* (adults) and *C. psittaci* (adults, related to bird exposure)

Table 10 Investigations in pneumonia

Test	Reason
Chest radiograph	For type and extent of involvement
Blood gases	To determine oxygen therapy
Blood count	May help with initial differential diagnosis
Blood culture	To isolate relevant bacteria
Urea and electrolytes	Hyponatraemia is typical of *Legionella* infection; raised urea level is a poor prognostic feature
Liver function tests	Often abnormal in atypical pneumonia
Serum for acute serology	For later aetiological diagnosis (1st specimen is often positive for influenza)
Sputum for microbiology (Gram stain and culture)	For diagnostic purposes, especially if very ill or hospital-acquired infection
Pneumococcal antigen (sputum and urine)	To diagnose pneumococcal pneumonia
Legionella antigen (urine)	To diagnose *legionella* infecton

- fever, usually high, is almost always present
- shaking chills or rigors initially are common but rigors imply bacteraemia as well as pneumonia
- cough is virtually universal and is usually productive
- pleuritic chest pain is common
- dyspnoea is usual
- an acute confusional state is common, particularly in elderly patients
- headache is unusual (cf. atypical pneumonias).

Clinical signs. The clinical signs of pneumococcal (lobar) pneumonia represent the archetype for all bacterial pneumonias. The signs include:

- pyrexia and toxic appearance (flushed and distressed)
- raised respiratory rate and use of accessory muscles of respiration
- central cyanosis (if severe)
- unilateral (or bilateral) crackles over affected lung area, usually with bronchial breathing
- pleural rub (occasional)
- labial herpes simplex reactivation.

Investigations. The investigations required to manage patients are listed in Table 10.

Treatment. You should administer high concentrations of humidified oxygen. Tracheal aspiration and physiotherapy in patients with sputum production are important general measures. The rising incidence of penicillin resistance means that penicillin and ampicillin cannot be relied upon as agents of choice for ill (e.g. hospitalised) patients with pneumonia. Third-generation cephalosporins (e.g. cefotaxime or ceftriaxone) are preferred. The quinolones (ciprofloxacin or norfloxacin) are not active against *S. pneumonia*. Erythromycin is a reasonable first choice in the community but there is increasing resistance (10–15%).

Outcome. Pneumococcal pneumonia carries a 5% mortality rate but if patients need admission to an intensive care unit, this approaches 75%. Several factors are predictive of high mortality regardless of age in community-acquired pneumonia. These are:

- respiratory rate > 30/min
- diastolic blood pressure < 60 mmHg
- serum urea > 7 mmol/l.

Complications. The most common complication is respiratory failure. Indications for ventilation include a rising pCO_2, a low pO_2 (e.g. ≤ 70 mmHg) on oxygen or an exhausted patient. Other complications include empyema, pericarditis, meningitis, endocarditis, arthritis or bacterial peritonitis. You should carefully examine any patient with a persistent fever despite antibiotics.

Patients who are asplenic, including sickle cell anaemia patients, are at risk of overwhelming pneumococcal infections (mortality > 60%). Immunisation and lifelong antibiotics are appropriate prophylactic measures.

Staphylococcal pneumonia
This occurs usually as a superinfection following influenza and has an extremely high mortality. Patients rapidly become extremely ill with respiratory failure, high fever and general features of sepsis. A Gram stain of sputum or tracheal aspirate will show Gram-positive cocci in clusters, usually intracellularly, and this alone is enough evidence in a very ill patient to treat with maximal antistaphylococcal antibiotics (e.g. flucloxacillin 2 g 4 hourly or vancomycin for MRSA; p. 377).

Legionnaire's disease (infection by *Legionella*)
Legionella are found in hot water systems of all sorts including showers, especially large ones such as hotels and hospitals.

Legionnaire's disease accounts for 1–15% of community-acquired cases and 1–5% of hospital-acquired cases of pneumonia. Chronic chest disease and smoking, together with increasing age, are the greatest risk factors, although immunosuppression is important. In hospital-acquired cases, surgery is an important risk, especially transplant surgery.

Clinical features. It varies in severity from a mild cough and fever to a multisystem disease with severe pneumonia and unconsciousness. The symptoms are often misleadingly vague with malaise, headache, myalgia and anorexia. Important clinical features are:

- cough (often mild) and minimally productive
- chest pain (non-specific)
- high fever (usually)
- diarrhoea
- change in mental status (in severe cases).

Investigations. Multiple laboratory abnormalities are common, but only hyponatraemia is useful in distinguishing Legionnaire's disease from other pneumonias. Chest radiograph abnormalities are often more marked than you would suspect from examination. A pleural effusion is common. Progression of radiological findings despite appropriate antibiotics is typical. Culture of the organism is possible but requires specialised techniques. Immunofluorescence on sputum or urine is a useful rapid diagnostic procedure. The urine may contain *legionella* antigen. Convalescent serology is the usual diagnostic method.

Treatment. The treatment of choice is erythromycin 2–4 g daily. In severe cases, the addition of rifampicin is appropriate. Ciprofloxacin is also clinically useful. A delay in starting treatment is the most important factor leading to a poor outcome. Mortality in the UK is about 20%.

Mycoplasma pneumonia

Mycoplasma pneumonia is the archetypal atypical pneumonia with constitutional features (fever, malaise and headache) preceding respiratory symptoms. It is most common in the 5–20 year age group and tends to occur in 4-yearly cycles. It may affect whole families concurrently. The term atypical pneumonia refers to the constitutional features, with cough without lobar involvement.

Clinical features. The cough is usually non-productive, although haemoptysis (usually mild) is sometimes seen. Mycoplasma may cause tracheobronchitis and/or pharyngitis (sore throat and retrosternal chest pain). Fever is usually moderate (37.5–38.0°C).

Treatment. Both tetracycline and erythromycin are effective therapy.

Complications

- myringitis — inflammation of the eardrum (15%)
- maculopapular skin rashes (15%)
- meningoencephalitis and other neurological problems (≤ 10%).

Up to half of patients develop cold haemagglutinins (cross-reaction with the I antigen of red cells) around the end of the first 10 days of illness.

Influenza

Influenza is caused by influenza viruses A and B. It is a common infection and individuals may suffer from it multiple times in their life because of the remarkable antigenic variation of the viruses. The incubation period is 1–3 days. Only immunisation or antiviral prophylaxis with amantadine reduce attack rates, apart from segregation of infectious individuals.

Clinical features. Influenza is distinctive in its more severe forms. The onset is abrupt. Systemic symptoms of feverishness, chills, headaches, myalgia, malaise and anorexia predominate. Painful movement of the eye muscles together with a burning sensation in the eyes and tearing can create an impression of photophobia. A dry cough and clear nasal discharge are typical. The illness usually lasts 3 days. The patient appears toxic and flushed with watery reddened eyes. The throat may be reddened and small lymph nodes are often palpable in the neck.

Severe influenza. Pneumonia is uncommon in influenza, but influenza outbreaks lead to increased deaths from 'pneumonia' among elderly people. In most instances, this results from secondary bacterial pneumonia complicating influenza. If infected with *Staphylococcus aureus*, there is a high mortality. In unusual circumstances, a primary influenzal pneumonia can occur in young people and this has a high mortality. It is more common in pregnancy and in those with cardiovascular disease.

Other viruses

In adults other viral causes of pneumonia are uncommon. Adenoviruses are perhaps the most common together with measles. In immunocompromised patients, viral pneumonia, especially caused by cytomegalovirus, is relatively common and often life-threatening.

Hospital-acquired pneumonia

Hospital-acquired pneumonia is a common cause of death. It particularly affects elderly people, those with chronic chest disease, ventilated patients and following major abdominal or thoracic surgery (splinting of the diaphragm).

Pathogenesis

Hospital-acquired pneumonia is usually caused by Gram-negative organisms. A number of factors influence this. The use of broad-spectrum antibiotics for other infections change the flora of the nasopharynx to a predominantly Gram-negative one. This alteration also occurs without antibiotics in ill patients; particularly those with nasogastric or endotracheal tubes. A further factor is the use of H_2-receptor antagonists, which increases stomach pH significantly. This allows the proliferation of Gram-negative bacteria in the stomach.

Clinical features

The symptoms are similar to those of community-acquired pneumonia. Lobar pneumonia is rare and, apart from Legionnaire's disease, atypical pneumonia is very rare.

Management

Antibiotic management should be directed to Gram-negative pathogens. A typical choice is cefotaxime, or ceftazidime if *Pseudomonas* is suspected.

Aspiration pneumonia

Aspiration pneumonia is a relatively common problem in hospital. In a sense, all pneumonias are aspiration pneumonias (see above), but the term implies a sudden, large volume inhalation of gastric or pharyngeal contents. Clinically, it is similar to other pneumonias and varies substantially in severity. Involvement of the superior or basilar segment of either lower lobe or the posterior segment of the upper lobes suggests the diagnosis.

The management is the same as community-acquired pneumonia except for one point. Anaerobes are more commonly implicated and you should use metronidazole or another antibiotic with good anti-anaerobic activity (e.g. a carbapenem).

Pneumonia in the immunocompromised patient

Pneumonia, pneumonitis or respiratory infection in the immunocompromised patient includes all the above considerations for community- and hospital-acquired pneumonia, but has some additional distinctive features. The key points are:

- any new respiratory symptom or new radiological infiltrate must be urgently investigated; for example, the time from first cough to death with cytomegalovirus pneumonitis or *Aspergillus* pneumonia is typically 5–7 days.
- Important organisms to consider include *Pneumocystis, Pseudomonas, Aspergillus* and other fungi, *Nocardia*, cytomegalovirus and *Mycobacterium tuberculosis*. It is, therefore, *much* more important to reach an aetiological diagnosis in an immunocompromised patient than in one with a community-acquired pneumonia
- helpful investigations (if done rapidly) include bronchoscopy and bronchoalveolar lavage, CT scanning of the chest and percutaneous lung biopsy
- empirical treatment is virtually always appropriate, based on a best guess, but with modification following the results of specific investigations
- expert advice is essential.

Lung abscess

Some pneumonias will develop into a lung abscess, particularly following aspiration. Typical causative organisms are *Staphylococcus aureus*, anaerobes, *Klebsiella pneumoniae* and fungal infections such as *Aspergillus*. On chest radiographs and CT scan, you will see a large circular lesion with cavitation and an air/fluid level.

Management consists of long-term (e.g. 2–4 months) antibiotics or antifungals with postural drainage.

Tuberculosis

Learning objectives

You should:

- be able to diagnose pulmonary and extrapulmonary tuberculosis
- be aware of the limitations of diagnostic tests
- understand the implications of a positive or negative Heaf or Mantoux test
- know how tuberculosis is transmitted and how to interrupt transmission
- understand the principles of management of tuberculosis, including the importance of resistance.

Microbiology

Tuberculosis is caused by *Mycobacterium tuberculosis*. Infection can also be caused by so-called atypical mycobacteria. Pulmonary infections with atypical mycobacteria are similar to those caused by *Mycobacterium tuberculosis* (classical tuberculosis) but are much rarer and in general more resistant to treatment.

Epidemiology

Approximately a third of the world's population are currently infected with *M. tuberculosis*. In the developed world, tuberculosis rates are rising as a result of two major factors: AIDS and deteriorating social conditions in the inner cities. Infection can occur at any age, though in the underdeveloped world, it most commonly occurs in childhood. In the UK, the majority of cases occur in otherwise healthy persons originating from the Indian subcontinent. People particularly at risk include:

- the very old
- immunocompromised patients (especially AIDS)
- homeless and displaced persons
- alcoholics.

The vast majority of infections are acquired by droplet inhalation from an infected person who coughs. It follows that the most infectious group of patients is those with cavitary pulmonary tuberculosis with sputum containing visible acid-fast bacilli (smear positive) who are coughing; followed by those whose sputum is culture-positive but smear-negative (much less infectious). *Patients who do not cough are essentially non-infectious.*

The risk of a contact acquiring tuberculosis depends on the closeness of the contact and on the infectiousness of the patient.

Clinical features

Patients with pulmonary tuberculosis present with:

- a chronic mildly productive cough

- fever (often present but not always)
- weight loss.

Diagnosis

A simple chest radiograph is virtually always abnormal; the only exceptions are patients with miliary tuberculosis. Usually, the chest radiograph shows asymmetrical upper lobe (sometimes apex of the lower lobe) infiltrates with cavitation.

The essential diagnostic test is sputum collection for microscopy and culture of *Mycobacteria* (acid-fast bacilli). Three sputum samples should be obtained; preferably early in the morning and on separate days. If these are negative or the presentation is atypical in any way, a bronchoscopy (with washings or brushings) is appropriate to verify the diagnosis.

Skin testing

Tuberculin skin tests were developed to detect infection with *M. tuberculosis*. There is very little cross-reactivity with other atypical organisms. In the UK at present, the most common skin tests used are the Heaf and the Mantoux tests. Skin testing is used for three reasons:

1. population surveys for the prevalence of exposure to *M. tuberculosis*
2. to assess whether contacts of a patient with tuberculosis are themselves infected
3. as a diagnostic aid for tuberculosis.

Grading of the response is essential for correct interpretation (Fig. 17). The Heaf test is easier to apply, although it requires specialised equipment and is done with a

specially prepared concentration of mycobacterial protein. There are three strengths of Mantoux reagent available. In the investigation of suspected cases of tuberculosis, the *intermediate* strength (1 in 1000) is the best. Use of the lowest strength is more likely to be falsely negative and may lead to a booster effect when a higher strength is used subsequently (false positive). Use of the maximum strength (1:100) is more likely to lead to a severe subcutaneous reaction.

A tuberculin skin test result is not foolproof. An immunocompromised patient will often have a false-negative response or an inappropriately mild response, which may be misleading. This is also true in some patients with miliary tuberculosis, sarcoidosis or malnourished patients. By comparison, a florid positive response implies not simply prior exposure to *M. tuberculosis* but also disease.

Treatment

It is essential to treat tuberculosis with multiple drugs because of resistant organisms. At present in the UK, 10% of patients show frank resistance to one first-line drug and about 4% have resistance to two or more drugs. Generally rifampicin, isoniazid and pyrazinamide are used together. As isoniazid can cause pellagra (mixed peripheral neuropathy and hyperpigmentation), pyridoxine (vitamin B$_6$) is generally given as well and is essential in patients whose diets are sub-optimal.

The indications for a fourth drug (ethambutol) are:

- life-threatening disease, e.g. meningitis
- immunocompromised patient (e.g. AIDS, renal transplant)
- previously treated tuberculosis with relapse
- region of origin has high resistance problem, e.g. Philippines, Vietnam, Cambodia, New York, etc. (seek advice)
- contact with patient known to have resistant tuberculosis.

In patients with susceptible organisms who respond to therapy promptly (e.g. in 1–4 weeks) and who are not immunocompromised, 6 months of therapy is appropriate. After 2 months of treatment, pyrazinamide (and ethambutol if used) can be stopped, leaving the patient on rifampicin and isoniazid for the last 4 months of therapy. Assuming the patient is compliant (which is a major problem in some), the relapse rate following a 6-month course is less than 3%. Much higher relapse rates are seen in those who only complete 2–4 months of therapy.

Expert advice should be sought for infections caused by resistant *M. tuberculosis* or other mycobacterial infections.

Outcome

The outcome from tuberculosis depends in part on how early treatment is initiated and how ill the patient is. In

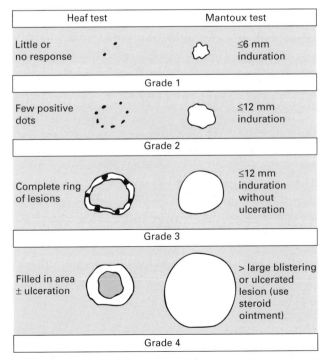

Fig. 17
Tuberculosis skin testing: graded results.

the UK, 500–750 people die each year of or with tuberculosis. The mortality rate is around 10–15%.

Chronic pulmonary and bronchial sepsis

Cavities in the lung or dilatation and deformity of the bronchi provide friendly environments for bacteria and fungi to live, almost in harmony with the patient. Cavities are caused by tuberculosis, sarcoidosis, lung cysts, ankylosing spondylitis and a few other unusual lung pathologies. These cavities usually communicate with the bronchial tree and so organisms can get in and pus can get out.

Aspergilloma

The most common long-term inhabitant of a tuberculous cavity (especially if large) is *Aspergillus*. This airborne fungus is breathed in, reproduces and causes a fungus ball (aspergilloma). Although not invasive, *Aspergillus* produces toxins which cause symptoms. Most commonly, these are productive cough and haemoptysis, which become increasingly common with time. Clubbing is found in 30% of patients. Treatment is difficult because drugs do not penetrate well into the aspergilloma, and surgery can lead to many complications.

Bronchiectasis

Literally this term means dilatation of the bronchi. There are many causes of bronchiectasis:

- congenital or genetic, e.g. cystic fibrosis
- childhood infection, e.g. whooping cough
- bronchial obstruction, e.g. overlooked foreign body
- allergic disease, e.g. allergic bronchopulmonary aspergillosis
- autoimmune disease, e.g. primary biliary cirrhosis.

Clinical features
In clinical terms, bronchiectasis occurs in 'wet' or 'dry' forms.

Dry bronchiectasis. Dry bronchiectasis is usually asymptomatic. It may be identified on a chest radiograph as curly or ring shadows in the lung. The commonest presentation is haemoptysis. Often the patients are young or middle-aged and unheralded haemoptysis leads to immediate suspicion of cancer. However, bronchoscopy is usually normal and the diagnosis can be confirmed, if necessary, with a high-quality CT scan of the chest.

Wet bronchiectasis. Wet bronchiectasis is quite different in its manifestations. These patients present with chronic productive cough. The sputum volume is large and it is grossly purulent. Despite this large amount of purulent material, fever is usually absent. Symptoms are most marked in the morning. Clubbing is usual when the disease is chronic and well established. Coexisting sinusitis is also common. Bacteriology

shows the same organisms that cause pneumonia, although *Pseudomonas aeruginosa* may appear later in antibiotic-treated patients.

Management
The principle management of bronchiectasis is:
- antibiotics for exacerbations (with occasional admissions for i.v. antibiotics)
- physiotherapy with postural drainage
- mucolytics.

Occasionally only one lobe is involved and respiratory function is good; in these patients surgical resection is feasible. Cor pulmonale from pulmonary fibrosis and brain abscess are occasional complications.

2.3 Tumours

Learning objectives

You should:
- know the importance of bronchial carcinoma in the community
- know the different pathological types of lung cancer, how they differ in their presentation and progression and understand the aetiological variation
- understand the principles of investigation, management and treatment
- be aware of how other tumours can affect the respiratory system.

Bronchial carcinoma

Bronchial carcinoma is the most common malignancy in the UK in males and is second to breast cancer in females. The male to female ratio is 3–4:1. The incidence has plateaued in males but is still rising in females because of changing smoking habits. It is more common in urban areas and is associated with atmospheric pollution.

Aetiology

The vast majority of cases are related to smoking, linked to duration and intensity of exposure (expressed as pack/years). Passive smoking slightly increases the risk for nonsmokers. Tumours associated with occupation/chemical exposure are usually adenocarcinomas; though these are still associated with cigarette smoking. Asbestos (see below) and radon are aetiological factors in a *small* number of tumours.

Pathology

Non-small cell (squamous) carcinoma
The commonest tumour is the squamous carcinoma, which accounts for just under half of all primary malig-

nancies. Squamous metaplasia leads to carcinoma in situ and then to invasive carcinoma. The tumour is usually central in origin and frequently cavitates. If peripheral, it may invade the chest wall. Distant metastasis occurs frequently. Squamous cell carcinomas commonly cause hypercalcaemia either through bone destruction or production of parathyroid hormone-related peptide (PTHrP).

Adenocarcinoma

Adenocarcinomas account for approximately 10% of lung cancers. They occur peripherally or in areas of lung scarring. The tumours are seen in non-smokers as well as smokers. The risk is increased by asbestos exposure. Cavitation is *not* a feature. If biopsied, the differentiation from a primary adenocarcinoma arising elsewhere may be difficult (e.g. GI tract). Local invasion, notably of the pleural space, is a dominant feature.

Large cell carcinoma

Large cell carcinomas are undifferentiated tumours which account for approximately one quarter of all lung cancers. They tend to arise centrally, metastasise early and carry a poor prognosis when compared with squamous cell tumours.

Small cell carcinoma

Small cell (oat cell) carcinomas arise from the APUD (amine precursor uptake decarboxylase) system. Neurosecretory granules are frequently seen and these tumours secrete peptides with hormonal activity, e.g. ADH, ACTH. They arise centrally and are rapidly growing with early dissemination. They constitute around 30% of lung tumours.

Clinical features

Generally, if you suspect a patient might have a bronchial carcinoma, you should take a detailed smoking and occupational history. For specific symptoms and signs a useful framework is:

- local problems (chest wall, lung, etc.)
- distant problems
- non-metastatic manifestations.

Local symptoms

Visualising the chest contents enables you to deduce the possible symptoms and signs of local invasion, but many patients have coexistent chronic bronchitis and emphysema. The most common presentation of bronchial carcinoma is with persistent cough or breathlessness. Alternatively, infection may be the first manifestation with signs of collapse/consolidation. There may be superadded cavitation. Your suspicions should be raised if infection is slow to clear or recurs. Chest pain may occur, often ill defined or pleuritic in nature, associated with an effusion. Local invasion of the chest wall, ribs and/or vertebra are seen in some patients with severe unremitting pain.

Occasionally haemoptysis may be the first symptom, with endobronchial erosion into blood vessels. There are other benign causes of haemoptysis, but you must always take the symptom seriously and adequately investigate it.

Apical tumours may infiltrate the lower portion of the brachial plexus (C7, 8, T1) causing pain along the medial border of the hand and arm together with weakness of the muscles of the hand, including the thenar and hypothenar eminences (**Pancoast's syndrome**). A **Horner's syndrome** may also occur as a result of damage to the sympathetic outflow through T1. The subclavian veins may be infiltrated causing thrombosis.

A central tumour with hilar involvement can obstruct the superior vena cava, presenting with facial fullness/swelling, headache and dilated chest wall veins. Central tumours can also damage the phrenic nerve producing an elevated diaphragm with paradoxical movement (elevation on inspiration).

Distant symptoms

The first manifestation of a bronchial carcinoma may be a distant metastasis. Secondary disease may become apparent in the brain (fits, hemiparesis, etc.), bone (pain, pathological fracture), liver (hepatomegaly), lymph nodes or elsewhere. Small cell carcinomas are more likely to present with distant metastases, but are seen with all tumours.

Non-metastatic manifestation of malignancy

It is often forgotten that symptoms such as anorexia and weight loss may be classified as 'non-metastatic', i.e. general effects of malignancy. Quite often bronchial carcinoma presents in this way.

The classical **paraneoplastic** syndromes are shown in Figure 18.

Investigations

The main principles you should adopt are:

- to try to achieve a histological diagnosis
- if curative treatment appears feasible, then to stage the tumour accurately

The main investigations are:

Radiology. If an abnormality is seen on a plain PA radiograph a lateral film should be taken. Sometimes, the diagnosis is suspected because of an abnormality on a film done for another purpose (e.g. preoperatively). Some worrying appearances on a chest radiograph are:

- irregular pulmonary mass, possibly with cavitation
- partial or complete collapse of a lobe
- a hilar mass
- a pleural effusion often combined with the above.

Many abnormalities are highly suggestive of a malignant process (such as sequential enlargement of a mass) but not absolutely diagnostic. You should *always* try to obtain previous films to compare with the most recent

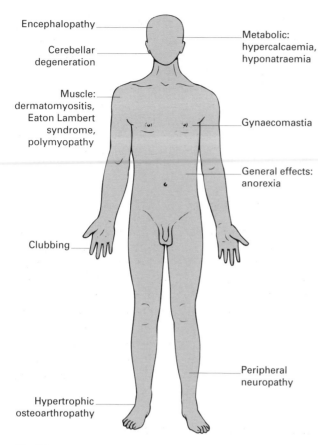

Fig. 18
Classical paraneoplastic syndromes.

one. A CT scan may be helpful both in diagnosis and staging.

Sputum cytology. Sputum cytology may be helpful in up to half of patients. The difficulty is the patient providing a useful sample; nebulised saline and physiotherapy may help. Remember that a negative sample does not exclude the diagnosis, rather a positive sample *makes* the diagnosis.

Bronchoscopy. This is the single most useful investigation, allowing visualisation of an endobronchial tumour that is centrally located (i.e. in the major bronchi) as well as biopsy, brushings or lavage for malignant cells.

Other techniques. If pleural disease is present, then fluid may be aspirated (exudate and may be blood-stained, see Table 11) and pleural biopsies taken, preferably under direct vision (fibreoptic). Peripheral or even central masses may be sampled by percutaneous needle biopsy under ultrasound or CT guidance. Thoracoscopy may be used in mediastinal disease.

Management

The use of the different modalities of treatment according to cell type is shown in Table 11.

Surgery
Unfortunately, only 20–30% of patients are fit for surgery, but, of these, resection may cure a small percentage (25%, 5 years). Your assessment of the patient's fitness and suitability for surgery should include several factors.

What is the cell type? Non-small cell carcinoma may be amenable to surgery. However, debulking operations are occasionally carried out on small cell tumours as an adjuvant to chemotherapy.

Is the tumour confined to the lung? Staging is very important. Evidence of metastases precludes surgery (plain radiographs, CT or ultrasound scanning may demonstrate dissemination). Non-metastatic manifestations are not a contraindication; these may respond to resection.

Is the tumour technically resectable? A tumour that is located close to the carina or involving more than one lobe is unsuitable for surgery.

What is the patient's lung function? An FEV_1 of < 1.5 l is against a successful outcome.

What is the patient's quality of life and general health like? Concomitant disease, for example coronary artery disease, increases the operative risks.

Radiotherapy
Radiotherapy is mainly used in palliation, but some patients with non-resectable squamous cell carcinoma

Table 11 Treatment of bronchial carcinoma

Type	Radiotherapy	Surgery	Chemotherapy
Non-small cell (squamous)	Curative 20% 5-year survival, Used in palliation	25% 5-year survival, higher in confined disease	No good response
Large cell, undifferentiated	Palliation	Less benefit compared with squamous cell	No good response
Adenocarcinoma	Poor response, some palliation	Poor survival	Poor response
Small cell (oat) to	Used in reducing tumour bulk	Used in debulking	Good response, relative no-treatment; median survival < 1 year

achieve long remission after treatment. Intraluminal radiotherapy can be of help in bulky endobronchial disease that is causing obstruction. Haemoptysis, bone metastases and SVC obstruction often respond well. In high doses, radiation pneumonitis may occur and, in the long term, progressive fibrosis can develop with breathlessness.

Chemotherapy

Chemotherapy has improved the outlook in small cell carcinoma, with a median survival of 2 months without treatment and approaching a year with combination chemotherapy. Some patients achieve much longer remission.

Terminal care

Patients throughout their illness need psychological support and access to counselling. Help for your patients can be provided by the MacMillan nurses (some of whom are involved in multidisciplinary palliative care teams) and, outside of hospital, the hospices or local patient support groups as well as community MacMillan nurses and the primary care team.

You must always be alert to the patient becoming depressed and, if so, involving the psychiatry services. As the disease progresses, re-evaluation of treatment goals is required, allowing the switch to palliation to be made at the appropriate time. At any stage, radiotherapy and occasionally chemotherapy may be helpful in alleviating symptoms. Pain, breathlessness, haemoptysis, etc. may all require specific intervention.

Other tumours

Alveolar cell carcinoma

Alveolar cell carcinoma is a very rare slowly growing tumour that is not related to smoking. It often arises in areas of damaged lungs and the characteristic histological appearance is of malignant cells growing along bronchi. It can have a single focus or may be multifocal. Presentation is usually with breathlessness, occasionally large volumes of sputum are produced (**bronchorrhoea**). A chest radiograph may show single or multiple areas of 'consolidation' with an **air bronchogram** meaning that the surrounding lung is opaque (non-aerated) and is outlining the air-filled bronchi. Diagnosis can be difficult, sputum cytology may be positive, but differentiation from adenocarcinoma may not be possible. Needle or surgical biopsy may be required. Surgical resection in the early stages gives good results.

Bronchial adenoma

Bronchial adenomas are uncommon benign tumours. The vast majority arise from the amine precursor uptake and decarboxylation system (APUD), like small cell carcinomas. Most present in young adults, with an equal sex incidence. As endobronchial tumours, they produce local effects — airway obstruction, collapse and distal infection. Common presentations are with a cough, haemoptysis, unilateral wheeze or recurrent non-resolving infection. Rarely the carcinoid syndrome may be produced. Malignant transformation is rare. The tumour is *not* usually visible on a chest radiograph, though there may be collapse. Most can be diagnosed on bronchoscopy. Surgical resection is curative with a good prognosis.

Metastatic disease

The lung is the site of metastases in many carcinomas, with lymphangitis carcinomatosis (see below), multiple or single secondaries, pleural deposits and associated effusions. Single or multiple metastases, particularly from certain tumours (e.g. hypernephroma) may have a 'cannon ball' appearance, implying a smooth rounded opacity as opposed to the ill-defined border of a primary bronchial cancer with streaky shadowing.

Lymphomas can affect the lung with diffuse infiltration, blockage of the thoracic duct (chylothorax) or mediastinal lymph node enlargement.

Solitary pulmonary nodule

An important differential diagnosis is the solitary pulmonary nodule which has been picked up as part of 'routine' investigation. Approximately 40% represent a malignant process (the majority being bronchial carcinomas, the next commonest are metastatic deposits). However most are benign, for example either infective (tuberculous) or non-infective (Wegener's) granulomas. The larger the lesion, the more likely it is to be malignant.

Your ability to trace previous radiographs will greatly help in determining the probability of a malignant process. A CT scan may show other metastases. As nodules are parenchymal, bronchoscopy is usually unhelpful. A fine needle biopsy is of much greater value but surgical resection is often required to establish the diagnosis.

Lymphangitis carcinomatosis

In lymphangitis carcinomatosis, malignant cells grow along the lymphatic channels of the lungs. Bronchial carcinoma can disseminate via this route, but other tumours may be responsible, notably breast (in females, always look for both breast shadows when examining a chest radiograph), stomach and pancreas.

Patients usually present with intense breathlessness and a dry cough. Physical signs may be absent, or there may be a few fine basal crackles. A chest radiograph may be normal or may show streaky fine basal shadowing with Kerley B lines (p. 64). There is no specific treatment; opiates may help the breathlessness.

2.4 Chronic airflow obstruction

Learning objectives

You should:
- be able to diagnose and assess the severity of airflow obstruction
- know the importance of looking for reversibility of airflow obstruction in terms of treatment
- be able to plan management both as an emergency and in the long term.

Introduction

The diagnosis of chronic airflow obstruction (CAO) (or chronic airflow limitation: CAL) is based on:

- reduced peak expiratory flow
- reduced FEV_1:FVC ratio.

The history and clinical findings are central in deciding the cause of airflow obstruction. The main possibilities are:

- chronic bronchitis and emphysema
- chronic asthma
- bronchiectasis (p. 74).

Chronic bronchitis and emphysema

The terms chronic obstructive airways disease (COAD), chronic obstructive pulmonary (COPD) or lung (COLD) disease are often used synonymously with chronic bronchitis and emphysema; however, they simply describe the pathophysiological abnormality. The danger is by using these terms, you may not consider other causes of airflow limitation and your treatment will be misguided.

Chronic bronchitis

Pathologically in chronic bronchitis, there is an increase in bronchial wall thickness with hyperplasia and hypertrophy of the mucous glands. The excess mucus secretion and wall thickening produces airflow limitation. *Clinically*, the definition requires a history of at least 2 years of a productive cough on most days for a minimum of 3 months of each year.

Emphysema

Emphysema commonly accompanies chronic bronchitis, but these do *not* always occur together. Emphysema is a *pathological* diagnosis characterised by destruction of the acinus. The commonest type is **centrilobular**, affecting the proximal part of the acinus and associated with cigarette smoking. It is seen predominantly in the upper part of the lung. You should be aware of the panacinar type which occurs in association with α_1-**antitrypsin deficiency**. It is inherited as an autosomal recessive (1:5000 population) disease and homozygotes (ZZ, normal is MM) may develop severe emphysema with progression to respiratory failure in the fourth and fifth decade. Cigarette smoking, by activating proteases, exacerbates this. The disease predominantly affects the *lower* zones (cf. the common centrilobular type in the upper lobes). Panacinar emphysema is also seen in cigarette smokers.

Prevalence and aetiology

The major association of chronic bronchitis and emphysema is with cigarette smoking. There is a clear relationship between the exposure to cigarette smoking, expressed as *pack years*, and the risk of death. Other interlinked associations of chronic bronchitis and emphysema include:

- male sex
- living in urban areas
- low social class
- air pollution.

In women, there is a rising prevalence of chronic bronchitis and emphysema that is almost certainly a *cohort* effect related to smoking habits of different generations.

There is large international variation in the prevalence of chronic bronchitis and emphysema. In the UK, the highest rates are seen in the northwest. Over the whole country, 17% of men and 8% of women aged 40–64 years fulfill the definition of having chronic bronchitis and emphysema. Fortunately, the rates are *decreasing*, which is probably related to changing smoking habits, including low tar brands and less atmospheric pollution.

Clinical features

Symptoms

The hallmark of chronic bronchitis and emphysema is a productive 'smoker's cough' with clear mucoid sputum and gradually increasing breathlessness over many years. People often complain of 'colds going onto the chest', with infective exacerbations, particularly during the winter months, associated with purulent (green/yellow) sputum. Patients may complain that their symptoms are worsened by:

- cold weather
- pollution (poor air quality)
- fog
- on waking up (*but you should always consider chronic asthma if there is marked diurnal variation*).

Signs

The signs that may appear on examination are shown in Figure 19. The symptoms and signs cannot be used to predict accurately whether the pathological changes are predominantly emphysema or chronic bronchitis.

Diagnosis

A patient will usually be a life-long heavy smoker with a chronic productive cough. He/she will have noticed gradually increasing breathlessness over a number of years. *Family history* may be important for the rare α_1-antitrypsin deficiency. Your examination findings will be a mixture of the signs set out in Figure 19. Investigations will show airflow limitation. The main differential diagnoses are compared in Table 12.

Investigations

The main investigations are:

- **Chest radiograph.** This may show hyperinflation, upper zone bullae (lower in α_1-antitrypsin deficiency) and evidence of pulmonary hypertension (prominent pulmonary conus, pruning of pulmonary vasculature).
- **Haemoglobin level.** This may be increased (secondary erthyrocytosis).

- **Electrocardiogram.** 'P' pulmonale, right ventricular hypertrophy.
- **Lung function tests.** These will show reduced PEFR, low FEV_1, normal or reduced FVC, low FEV_1/FVC ratio (Fig. 16). Increased or normal total TLC, reduced or normal transfer factor (depends on degree of emphysema) may also be seen.
- **Blood gases.** These may be:
— normal
— hypoxia with low $PaCO_2$ (high respiratory drive: pink puffer)
— hypoxia with high $PaCO_2$ (low respiratory drive: blue bloater).

Management

Once the diagnosis of chronic bronchitis and emphysema is established and its severity assessed, then the aims of management are:

- preventing progression of the condition

Pink puffer	Blue bloater
High respiratory drive	Low respiratory drive
Hypoxic	Hypoxic
Hypocarbic	Hypercarbic
Desaturates on exercise	Right heart failure (oedema)
Type 1 respiratory failure	Type 2 respiratory failure

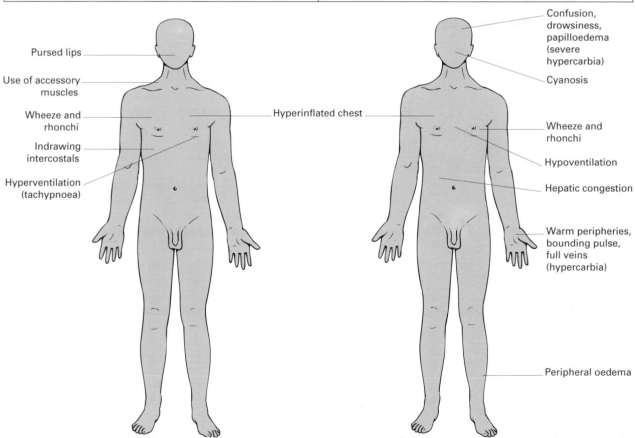

Fig. 19
The signs of chronic bronchitis and emphysema. The 'pink puffer' and 'blue bloater' are two ends of a spectrum. Patients may move from type 1 to type 2 respiratory failure and any patient with severe airflow limitation may develop cor pulmonale.

Table 12 Comparison of the three main aetiological types of chronic airflow obstruction

	Chronic bronchitis and emphysema	Chronic asthma	Bronchiectasis
Smoking	+++	+/–	+/–
Diurnal variation	+/–	+++	+/–
Cough	++	+/–	+++
Sputum	Mucoid/purulent	Mucoid/scanty	Purulent/mucoid
Wheeze	++	+++	+
Crackles (crepitations)	–	–	+++ localised
Clubbing	–	–	+++
Reversibility (>15%)	+/–	++	+/–

- relieving symptoms
- treating complications.

The biggest factor governing progression is continued smoking. Over a long period, regular exercise may maintain function. Influenza vaccination should be offered to reduce the risk of acute deterioration. In people under 70 years of age with stable severe disease, low-flow (2 1/min ≈24%) oxygen therapy may be of benefit in relieving symptoms and prolonging survival. Oxygen therapy must be administered for > 15 hours per day long term and the patient has to stop smoking.

The relief of symptoms is similar to that of chronic asthma and the drugs used are summarised on page 84. In chronic bronchitis and emphysema the following drugs are important.

Bronchodilators

Subjective benefit may be derived from regular inhalation of β_2-agonists (salbutamol) or cholinergic antagonists (ipatropium bromide). There may be little objective improvement in airflow limitation.

Theophyllines

Aminophylline formulations can be used orally. The dose may have to be higher in smokers, heavy drinkers and patients being treated with anticonvulsants (because of enzyme induction); lower doses may be needed in hepatic or cardiac failure, elderly patients and in patients taking cimetidine, allopurinol, erythromycin and propranolol (enzyme inhibition).

Corticosteroids

All patients should have a trial of corticosteroids to make sure that they do not have a reversible element to their airflow obstruction. Your aim is to show an objective benefit as opposed to the subjective increase in well-being that many patients will report. Your criteria are a more than 15% improvement of PEFR and/or FEV_1/FVC after a 2-week course of prednisolone 30 mg/day. If so, then regular therapy with inhaled (e.g. beclomethasone) or oral corticosteroids should continue.

The efficacy of inhaled therapies depend on delivery. You should know how the devices are ideally used and to be able to educate and test patients in the techniques (p. 67, for metered dose inhalers). There are a range of devices that may help to coordinate aerosol release/inhalation; e.g. spacers or breath-actuated devices. When inhaler technique is very poor, oral preparations may be of help. In severe airflow limitation, home nebulisers may be useful; these predominantly work by delivering large doses of bronchodilator (e.g. salbutamol inhaler 200 µg per puff, c.f. nebuliser 2.5–5 mg).

Complications

Acute infective episodes

Learning objective
- You should know how to distinguish the patients with an acute exacerbation of chronic airflow limitation and who require antibiotics from those who will not benefit.

Each day hundreds of patients are admitted to hospital in the UK with an exacerbation of 'COAD'. Most are treated with antibiotics. Controlled studies have failed to show a convincing benefit for antibiotics compared with placebo. There are several possible reasons for this:

- exacerbation related to other problems, e.g. pneumothorax, heart failure, stress, non-compliance with medication
- infective exacerbation caused by viruses
- although sputum cultures are often positive for *Streptococcus pneumoniae* and *Haemophilus influenzae*, these are very common colonising organisms
- yellow or green sputum production is normal in some patients (especially in the morning) and does not imply infection
- a slightly raised white cell count may reflect water depletion and stress rather than infection.

Therefore your approach to these patients should be to ask:

1. Is there any evidence for pneumonia, e.g. a new chest radiograph abnormality?
2. Is this a severe exacerbation (e.g. worsening dyspnoea *and* increased sputum volume *and* purulent sputum)?

If the patient has either of these features, the benefits of antibiotic treatment outweigh the dangers. Remember though that the patients will be at substantial risk of antibiotic-associated diarrhoea caused by *Clostridium difficile* (p. 113).

The principles of management of acute exacerbation of chronic bronchitis and emphysema are:

- positive early diagnosis (see above)
- appropriate antibiotics: options include oral cephalosporins, amoxycillin or coamoxiclav; erythromycin should be used if the patient is allergic to penicillin or if atypical infection is suspected (p. 377)
- maintain or increase bronchodilator therapy (i.e. use of a nebuliser)
- short course of or increase in corticosteroids
- consider admission to hospital if not responding.

In hospital, re-assessment is required to exclude other causes for the deterioration and whether appropriate and adequate antibiotics have been given. The major complication is **respiratory failure.**

Respiratory failure

Blood gas analysis is discussed on p. 67. Patients with a high respiratory drive (pink puffers) may have type 1 respiratory failure with hypoxia and a low $PaCO_2$ at rest. When the airflow limitation is not severe, the may appear only on exercise.

Blue bloaters with a low respiratory drive may develop type 2 respiratory failure with hypoxia and high $PaCO_2$. If the patient is stable, the pH will be normal because retention of bicarbonate will have compensated for the rise in $PaCO_2$. In acute deterioration, this compensation will not have had time to occur and the pH will be low (respiratory acidosis).

Your major aims of management of acute respiratory failure are:

- treat the underlying cause
- improve arterial and tissue oxygenation ($PaO_2 > 8$ kPa)
- avoid further deterioration of acidosis (pH <7.25).

You should always treat heart failure (p. 21) and correct any hypovolaemia as it will help the delivery of oxygen to the tissues and correction of local acidosis. Other problems may also require specific intervention, e.g. infection or a pneumothorax. Any sedatives should be discontinued.

The principal treatment of respiratory failure is continuous oxygen administration. In patients with acute type 2 respiratory failure, correction of the hypoxia may reduce respiratory drive with worsening hypercarbia and acidosis. Blood gas analysis should be repeated after 1 hour of 28% oxygen and, if necessary, the inspired oxygen reduced to 24%. In a *small* number of patients, even this is not tolerated. Clinical signs of rising $PaCO_2$ are drowsiness, warm peripheries, dilated veins and a bounding pulse. Occasionally, a respiratory stimulant (e.g doxapram) may be used short term under close supervision (overdose causes convulsions). Rarely, mechanical ventilation may be indicated if major correctable factors can be identified. Unfortunately, many patients who are ventilated are subsequently unable to breathe spontaneously.

Cor pulmonale

Cor pulmonale means heart failure developing secondary to lung disease. It is most commonly seen with chronic bronchitis and emphysema because of their high prevalence in the UK. In the early stages, pulmonary hypertension occurs with consequent right ventricular and right atrial hypertrophy. Eventually the heart fails with marked fluid retention, giving peripheral oedema, an elevated jugular venous pressure and worsening breathlessness. Although the load is predominantly on the right side of the heart, you should remember that both ventricles eventually fail.

Other problems

Patients can be severely compromised by even small **pneumothoraces** (p. 88). A **pulmonary embolus** may also occur in *immobile* patients (p. 47).

Prognosis

Only 30% of patients with severe airflow limitation and cor pulmonale will survive 5 years. Patients are also at risk of developing other smoking-related diseases, notably carcinoma of the bronchus (p. 74) and ischaemic heart disease (p. 13).

Asthma

Learning objectives

You should:
- understand the importance of asthma in terms of prevalence, morbidity and mortality
- know how to diagnose, assess and treat acute asthma
- understand the principles of long-term management in the community.

A useful definition of asthma has been produced by the American Thoracic Society: 'The disease is characterised by increased responsiveness of the bronchi to various stimuli, manifested by widespread narrowing of the airways that changes in severity either spontaneously or as a result of treatment.' This description incorporates all the key features of asthma from which you can deduce the symptoms and signs. Asthma is a common condition that causes considerable morbidity and results in approximately 2000 deaths per year in the UK.

Commonly, asthma is subdivided into intrinsic and extrinsic types, with differing features (Table 13). You must realise that these represent extremes of a spectrum and should only be used as guidance; in reality considerable overlap exists.

Table 13 Differences between intrinsic and extrinsic asthma; in reality there is considerate overlap

	Intrinsic asthma	Extrinsic asthma
Atopy	None	Yes, including family history
Skin tests	Negative, normal IgE	Positive, raised IgE
Onset	Late	Early
Character	Chronic, little seasonal variation	Intermittent, seasonal, sputum
Blood tests	No eosinophilia	Blood eosinophilia
Nasal polyps	Yes	No
Sensitivity to aspirin	Yes	No
Beta agonists	Variable response	Good response
Disodium cromoglycate	No value	Valuable

Epidemiology

Up to 5% of children and 2% of adults are affected. There is some geographical variation.

Occupational asthma is an important cause of work-related disease. For example, workers in the polyurethane industry (toluene diisocyanate) or in textiles (cotton; byssinosis) may be affected. The hallmark of occupational disease is work-related symptoms.

Pathophysiology

Remember that the total cross-sectional area of the large airways is much less than that of the small airways. Therefore, it is in the larger bronchi that most of the airflow resistance (limitation) occurs. The common factor in asthmatics is bronchial hyper-reactivity, which can be demonstrated by provocation testing. Asthmatics bronchoconstrict at much lower concentrations of the stimulus (e.g. methacholine, histamine) than normal subjects. Many factors may initiate an asthmatic attack:

- irritants: smoke, paint, chemicals
- exercise (cold, dry air)
- respiratory infections
- drugs: aspirin, beta-blockers.

Immune mechanisms, immediate and delayed, are important in the pathogenesis. An immediate hypersensitivity reaction is produced by binding of IgE fixed to mast cells to antigen (p. 345). Degranulation releases a variety of mediators (e.g. histamine, eosinophil chemotactic factor of anaphylaxis). Subsequently, through the action of phospholipase A_2, arachidonic acid and further metabolites are generated (cyclooxygenase pathway—prostaglandins and lipoxygenase pathway—leukotrienes). Leukotriene D_4 is the most potent bronchoconstrictor isolated. Non-mast cell-derived mediators such as platelet-activating factor may also have a role. These substances cause bronchoconstriction as well as chemotaxis and inflammation. Infiltration with eosinophils and activation of T lymphocytes (p. 345) and macrophages occur. Intracellular mechanisms are important, with a key role for calcium regulation in mediating smooth muscle contraction.

In addition to the local release of various mediators, imbalance may be present in the neural control mechanisms. The pathogenesis of asthma is complex and no single mediator is responsible; it is caused by summative and synergistic mechanisms.

The final pathological features are: severe mucus plugging (yellow tenacious secretions packed with eosinophils and epithelial cells), basement membrane thickening in the bronchi with mucosal and sub-mucosal oedema, eosinophil/neutrophil infiltration, vasodilatation and mucous gland hyperplasia. In patients with chronic disease, irreversible changes occur.

Clinical features

Symptoms

The predominant symptoms are shortness of breath and wheeze. Commonly, the symptoms are much worse in the early morning (diurnal variation). There may be seasonal variation, with attacks coinciding with high pollen counts. Cough may be the only problem and, if so, you may miss the underlying diagnosis. If the cough is productive of mucus plugs, you should consider allergic bronchopulmonary aspergillosis (p. 84). Triggers to attacks should be sought, including home environment and work. In some patients, particularly where the asthma has developed later in life, there may be little variation in symptoms, with chronic shortness of breath and wheeze.

Signs

The signs depend on the severity of the asthma and its chronicity. You will often see patients in an acute attack, where observation will show the patient to be distressed, centrally cyanosed, tachypnoeic and using their accessory muscles. Tachycardia is usually present; this partly reflects the overuse of β_2-agonists. You may find pulsus paradoxus, together with widespread inspiratory and expiratory wheezes. It is important to be able to assess the severity of an attack (see box, p. 83).

Inability to speak. This should not *substitute* for measuring the peak flow, but its presence should alert you.

Disturbance of conscious level. This implies muscle fatigue, profound hypoxia and rising carbon dioxide.

A silent chest. Where the asthma is severe, mucus plugging compounds the airflow obstruction and the breath sounds diminish and disappear.

Response to signs. If any of the above signs are present or if you are worried then you should ask for help with a view to immediate intervention and admission to intensive care. Remember that deaths in asthmatics in hospital are associated with *inadequate assessment* (no chest radiograph, no blood gases) and *poor treatment* (no steroids, discharge from casualty).

Diagnosis

In order to make the diagnosis of asthma you need to demonstrate a variation in airflow obstruction of at least 15%. A history of episodic wheeze, shortness of breath and cough makes the diagnosis easy; it is much more difficult in chronic asthma where there may be little variation in symptoms over time and no obvious triggers. You need a high index of suspicion, backed up by measurement of airflow limitation and reversibility. The last may require a 1–2 week trial of corticosteroids.

Wheeze does not necessarily indicate asthma; first, other common medical conditions should be considered, particularly heart failure and pulmonary emboli. Obstruction either from tumour or foreign body may occasionally be the cause. Other rare conditions may cause airflow obstruction, e.g. eosinophilic syndromes (p. 84) (tropical eosinophilia and Churg–Strauss syndrome. Carcinoid syndrome may present with wheeze.

Investigations

You should know how to assess a patient with either acute or chronic asthma. Spirometry (FEV_1, FVC) may show a reduced ratio, though in many people it is normal between attacks. The patient should be encouraged to monitor their disease by symptom diaries linked to peak flow recording. More detailed lung function may show hyperinflation with increased total lung capacity and residual volume. Transfer factor is normal. Blood gas analysis is commonly normal; though hypoxaemia is sometimes found in severe asthmatics even between attacks.

A chest radiograph is often normal, though it can show hyperinflation and, occasionally, atelectasis (segmental/lobar) or lung collapse caused by mucus plugging.

In young subjects, mild blood eosinophilia may be seen in association with atopy (hay fever, eczema). Skin tests to common allergens commonly show multiple reactions (p. 345).

Management

Emergency treatment is outlined in the box on this page.

Acute asthma (status asthmaticus)
The patient usually presents with progressive deterioration over several hours or days, sometimes associated with a definite trigger such as a chest infection or ingestion of aspirin (or another NSAID). Occasionally *brittle* asthma is present, when the onset is abrupt and life-threatening. The clinical signs in acute asthma are given above. The key to management is proper assessment. You *must* perform the following investigations on all patients in the accident and emergency department:

- peak expiratory flow rate
- chest radiograph
- blood gases.

Peak expiratory flow rate is grossly reduced (<100 l/min), and may be unrecordable. Chest radiograph shows hyperinflation. Atelectasis and/or collapse caused by mucus plugging may be seen. Evidence of infection may be present. A **pneumothorax** must be excluded on a chest radiograph; even small ones may compromise patients with airflow obstruction.

Blood gases commonly show hypoxaemia with hypocarbia and alkalosis, reflecting increased respiratory drive. In severe airflow limitation, **normocarbia** is a bad sign, signalling failing alveolar ventilation. You must continue to monitor the patient's condition, documenting improvement or worsening of the airflow obstruction.

Emergency treatment: acute asthma (bronchoconstriction)

- **Assess severity quickly:**
  — examination (severe: inability to speak, tachycardia (< 115/min), pulsus paradoxus (> 10 mmHg), cyanosis, reduced consciousness, 'silent chest')
  — measure peak expiratory flow rate (severe: < 130, may be unrecordable)
  — take a detailed history when appropriate
  — oximetry (severe: saturation < 93%)
  — take arterial sample for blood gas analysis (severe: PaO_2 < 60 mmHg (8 kPa); $PaCO_2$ > 41 mmHg (5.5 kPa))

- **Treatment**
  — give high-flow oxygen
  — give nebulised β_2-agonist (5 mg salbutamol)
  — give intravenous steroids (200 mg hydrocortisone)

- **Investigation**
  — request a chest radiograph: particularly to exclude pneumothorax

- **Reassess frequently, ask for help early**

You should ensure that a high concentration of oxygen (> 60%) is administered to all patients on arrival; hypercarbia will *not* occur. A β_2-agonist, such as salbutamol (2.5–5 mg), should be administered via a nebuliser and can be repeated 3–6 hourly. Nebulised ipratropium bromide can be used. In all cases of asthma that require admission, corticosteroids should be given as a bolus of hydrocortisone i.v. (3–6 mg/kg) followed by oral prednisolone 40–60 mg in divided doses.

Aminophylline may be used; if the patient is not receiving regular treatment then 5 mg/kg can be given over 20–30 minutes, followed by an infusion of 0.5 mg/kg. If the patient is already on oral theophyllines, the bolus is omitted and the infusion started. It is important that theophylline levels are measured and the dose adjusted to remain within the therapeutic range of 10–20 mg/l. Liver or heart disease or age over 55 years are indications for reduced dosage.

Supportive therapy is essential. Fluid intake must be maintained and dehydration corrected. Appropriate antibiotics should be prescribed *if* there is evidence of infection (p. 375). Sedation *must* be avoided.

A small percentage of patients will continue to deteriorate. You should seek expert help urgently. Worrying signs are exhaustion, with disturbance of consciousness and blood gas analysis showing respiratory alkalosis being replaced by worsening hypoxia, hypercarbia and acidosis, as alveolar ventilation decreases and fails. Early intervention with intubation and mechanical ventilation is mandatory.

Chronic asthma

Patients with chronic asthma should be seen regularly either in hospital outpatients or in specialist clinics in primary care. Severe asthmatics are often given open access to a specialist service. *Education* is an important principle, with the person being encouraged to monitor their disease, understand its basis and the use of various treatments and delivery systems.

The drugs used in the treatment of chronic asthma can be divided into:

- symptomatic: β_2-agonists, theophyllines and anticholinergics
- prophylactic: corticosteroids, disodium cromoglycate.

A patient with anything but mild symptoms *must* receive regular prophylactic treatment; undue reliance should not be placed on symptomatic treatment. You need to have a clear grasp of these drugs (p. 80).

For a patient following an acute attack, you should:

- prescribe a reducing course of steroids over a few weeks to the patient's maintenance dosage or substitute inhaled steroids
- ensure that this is done in conjunction with the patient carefully monitoring their symptoms and airflow limitation (they should be given a peak flow meter and taught how to use it)

- tell the patient that if their asthma deteriorates they should contact a doctor and not reduce the steroids any further (may increase back to higher dose).

Disodium cromoglycate. Often disodium cromoglycate is effective prophylaxis in young atopic asthmatics, including the prevention of exercise-induced bronchoconstriction. There are no serious side-effects. The drug can be administered as a dry powder or MDI.

Complications

Apart from those discussed above, pneumothorax, together with lung collapse (mucus plugging), are the most important complications of acute asthma. You should always consider whether a pneumothorax has been excluded in a deteriorating asthmatic.

Prognosis

Most asthmatics are children in whom the condition improves or disappears with maturity. Onset later in life is often associated with chronicity and difficulty in treatment. One-third of deaths occur within a couple of hours of the onset of the attack. However, in at least two-thirds, the death is potentially preventable; audit has shown that many asthmatics are inadequately assessed (PEFR, blood gases, radiographs not taken), or undertreated (discharged, no corticosteroids). You have to take great care not to make these mistakes.

Pulmonary eosinophilia

Pulmonary eosinophilia is defined as a blood eosinophilia with pulmonary infiltrates, which are often transient and peripheral on the chest radiograph. Most patients are asymptomatic, but they can present with breathlessness and a cough.

In chronic asthma, the diagnosis of allergic bronchopulmonary aspergillosis should be borne in mind. Hypersensitivity to the fungus (which is ubiquitous) *Aspergillus fumigatus* develops. Patients usually have pre-existing asthma and present with a cough productive of green 'rubbery' plugs together with fever. Recurrent pulmonary infiltrates with a blood eosinophilia (if not on steroids) are the hallmarks. A chest radiograph may show shadowing (often upper lobe). Patients have high IgE levels and positive precipitins to *Aspergillus*. Treatment is with oral corticosteroids in acute attacks.

Other causes of pulmonary eosinophilia

You should be aware of other forms of pulmonary eosinophilia:

- drug-induced, e.g. sulphonamides, nitrofurantoin
- helminthic infection, e.g. *Ascaris lumbricoides* (Loeffler's syndrome)

- fungi, e.g. *Aspergillus*, *Candida*
- cryptogenic, e.g. eosinophilic pneumonia
- granulomatosis, e.g. Churg–Strauss syndrome.

2.5 Interstitial lung disease

Pulmonary fibrosis is a description of the final patho-logical effect of several different disease processes. It may be focal or diffuse. In the end-stage, the latter is often described as *honeycomb*.

Learning objectives

You should:
- understand how different disease processes can cause pulmonary fibrosis
- be able to integrate the clinical features and investigations into a list of possible diagnoses
- be aware of rarer causes of the problems.

Cryptogenic fibrosing alveolitis

Cryptogenic fibrosing alveolitis is a disease of unknown aetiology which typically occurs in middle age. It is more common in males. The pathological features are an inflammatory response within the alveoli. Polymorph leucocytes predominate in the bronchial washings. Subsequently, progressive fibrosis super-venes. A rare acute form (**Hamman–Rich syndrome**) occurs with rapid progression to death within a few months. More typically, patients present with a gradual onset of breathlessness and a dry cough. On examina-tion, clubbing is common, and fine late inspiratory crackles are heard at the bases. Respiratory rate may be increased and cyanosis occurs in the end-stage of the disease. Pulmonary function shows a *restrictive* pattern (p. 67 and Fig. 16) and arterial hypoxia with a reduced $PaCO_2$ (high respiratory drive all seen on blood-gas analysis). The chest radiograph characteristically has *bilateral basal* shadowing with honeycombing. Auto-antibodies (e.g. rheumatoid factor) are frequently found. There is no effective treatment; corticosteroids and immunosuppressives are used but have no proven benefit.

Other conditions causing pulmonary fibrosis are listed in Table 14.

Extrinsic allergic alveolitis

There are many rare examples of conditions causing extrinsic allergic alveolitis, for example maple bark stripper's lung! You need to be aware of the much more common, but still quite rare, **bird fancier's lung** from keeping either pigeons or budgerigars. Pathologically, the condition is characterised by the formation of gran-uloma with subsequent fibrosis. The damage is initiated by a specific antibody. Lung function shows a restrictive pattern with progressive reduction in lung volumes and transfer factor. Precipitins are positive.

In **pigeon fancier's lung** exposure is often episodic. Therefore, the picture is an acute illness several hours after exposure to the antigen. Patients have fever, myal-gia, cough, breathlessness and, on examination, crack-les. In budgerigar fancier's lung there is often constant exposure, with progressive breathlessness and cough.

Table 14 Causes of pulmonary fibrosis other than cryptogenic fibrosing alveolitis

Type	Examples	Special features
Sarcoidosis		Hilar lymphadenopathy; significant radiograph abnormalities; few symptoms
Drugs	Cytotoxics, e.g. bleomycin, busulphan, methotrexate, etc. Others: amiodarone, nitrofurantion	First indication is reduction of transfer factor
Autoimmune disease	Rheumatoid arthritis (RF almost invariably strongly positive)	Three types: (i) diffuse fibrosis (ii) nodular: particularly with pneumoconiosis — *Caplan's syndrome* (iii) focal fibrosis
	Systemic sclerosis Mixed connective tissue disease SLE Ankylosing spondylitis	Pleurisy, vasculitis Upper lobe fibrosis
Occupational	Pneumoconiosis	Spectrum of fine mottling to progressive massive fibrosis; may be nodular (with RA)
	Asbestosis	Basal, pleural calcification Other associations: mesothelioma, bronchial carcinoma
	Silicosis	Eggshell calcification in hilar nodes
Extrinisic allergic alveolitis	Pigeon fancier's lung Budgerigar fancier's lung	Upper lobe, episodic symptoms Insidious; precipitins strongly positive
	Paraquat, oxygen, radiation	May progress slowly

The final picture is severe *upper lobe* fibrosis with cavitation. Auscultatory findings are a mixture of inspiratory crackles and wheezes. Finger clubbing is *uncommon*. The first line of management is to stop the exposure to the antigen. Some patients may be helped by corticosteroids.

Sarcoidosis

Sarcoidosis is important both in its own right and as a major differential diagnosis with respiratory tuberculosis. The aetiology of sarcoidosis is unknown. It usually occurs in young adulthood, with a slight female preponderance. It is more common in temperate zones and in Afro-Caribbeans more than Caucasians.

Pathology

There is activation of T cells with granuloma formation in the organ affected. There is no central necrosis, unlike tuberculosis. In the lungs, broncho-alveolar lavage may contain a large number of T lymphocytes. In the fluid, or in the serum, increased levels of **angiotensin-converting enzyme** may be found, but is of little value in diagnosis or monitoring the response to treatment. **Anergy** is found with depressed peripheral T cell immunity (p. 335; delayed hypersensitivity). As the disease progresses, fibrosis occurs.

Clinical features

The clinical manifestations of sarcoid depend on the organ affected. In the eye, blindness can occur secondary to uveitis. Erythema nodosum, keloid and lupus pernio are skin manifestations. The CNS can be involved with neuritis, space-occupying lesions and sterile meningitis. In the heart, the characteristic manifestation is conduction disturbance. Sarcoidosis is one cause of a pyrexia of unknown origin (p. 373).

The most common site of sarcoid is the lung, where sarcoidosis is classified into three stages:

I.   hilar lymphadenopathy alone: may have erythema nodosum
II. hilar lymphadenopathy and pulmonary infiltrate
III. pulmonary infiltrate with fibrosis.

Stage I is usually asymptomatic and self-limiting, whereas stage III implies some irreversible changes.

Investigations

Most patients in stage I are picked up by a routine chest radiograph showing hilar shadowing. In stage II and III, parenchymal shadowing is apparent in both lung fields. Serum angiotensin-converting enzyme is more likely to be elevated. Pulmonary function testing shows a reduced transfer factor and a restrictive defect. Where the disease is very active, a gallium lung scan will show widespread uptake in the lung tissue. Hypercalciuria may be present and, occasionally, hypercalcaemia.

Immunologically, there is an increase in cells (predominantly T lymphocytes) in broncho-alveolar lavage fluid and anergy to intradermal tuberculin testing. The diagnosis can be made with a Kveim test. Sarcoid tissue is injected intradermally and biopsied 6 weeks later. A positive test shows typical non-caseating granuloma. The Kveim test may be negative in stage I disease.

Management

Most stage I thoracic cases resolve spontaneously. With progressive disease and deteriorating pulmonary function, corticosteroids should be given. They should also be prescribed for extrathoracic involvement.

Vasculitis

Wegener's granulomatosis

In Wegener's granulomatosis, there is a widespread granulomatous angiitis affecting the lungs, kidneys and upper respiratory tract. It is more common in men and commonly presents with haemoptysis, breathlessness, pleuritic pain, general malaise and low-grade pyrexia.

Investigations show bilateral pulmonary nodules that may cavitate. There is *no* hilar lymphadenopathy. **Antineutrophil cytoplasmic antibodies** (ANCA) are usually present, consistent with vasculitis. The extent of the renal involvement determines survival. Treatment is with corticosteroids and cyclophosphamide. Fortunately, with treatment, the prognosis is good with remission in most patients.

Goodpasture's syndrome

Goodpasture's syndrome is predominantly a disease of young men, presenting with pulmonary haemorrhage and glomerulonephritis (p. 152); either may dominate the clinical picture. The diagnostic hallmark is the presence of **antiglomerular basement membrane antibody**. Proven treatments are dialysis, plasma exchange (to remove the antibody) and cytotoxic therapy.

2.6 Miscellaneous respiratory disease

Learning objectives

You should:
- be aware of a range of conditions that may affect the lung
- know the specific features of some of the different conditions.

Sleep apnoea syndrome

In the last few years, the importance of respiratory control during sleep has been highlighted with the characterisation of the sleep apnoea syndromes. These are defined as absence of gas flow at the mouth/nose for 10 seconds. Sleep apnoea is present when > 30 episodes occur per night. There are two types:

- obstructive apnoea: no airflow despite chest wall movement
- central apnoea: no chest wall movement.

Obstructive apnoea is the more common type you will see and is associated with obesity, hypertension and daytime somnolence. The patient almost always gives a long history of noisy snoring. Those with central apnoea snore less, complain of night-time wakening and are not usually obese. Other symptoms are morning headaches and intellectual deterioration. Pulmonary hypertension and right heart failure may supervene.

People with suspected sleep apnoea syndrome need investigation and management in specialist units where they can be monitored asleep. The initial approach often involves weight reduction and protryptilline (tricyclic antidepressant).

Adult (acute) respiratory distress syndrome

Adult (acute) respiratory distress syndrome (ARDS) is characterised by:

- progressive hypoxaemia
- reduced lung compliance
- normal left atrial pressure
- widespread bilateral pulmonary infiltrates.

The initial damage is to the pulmonary capillary endothelium, causing an increase in permeability with a leak into the interstitium/alveoli of plasma and red cells. The precise mechanisms are complicated.

The causes of ARDS are numerous and are linked to those of shock (see p. 356). They include sepis, trauma, aspiration, smoke inhalation and disseminated intravascular coagulopathy. Management is by specialists and requires admission to intensive care. The principles include the maintenance of tissue oxygenation using ventilatory methods that minimise the ongoing damage to the lungs. The initial trigger should be removed/treated. Fluid balance requires that the patient is not overloaded and inotropic support is often used. ARDS has a high mortality once established.

2.7 Pleural disease

The pleural space is bounded by the **parietal** pleura, lining the thoracic cavity and mediastinum. The **visceral** pleura covers the lungs and is rich in blood vessels and lymphatics. Unlike the parietal pleura, it has no pain fibres. The pressure within the space is *negative*, approximately –5 cm H_2O.

Learning objectives

You should:
- be able to diagnose patients as having disease of the pleura/pleural space
- be able to outline the investigation and management.

Pleuritic pain

The major causes of pleuritic pain are infection, pulmonary embolus, malignancy and trauma. The last may be caused by fractured ribs, which may occur during bouts of coughing (**cough fracture**) particularly in elderly people. Your approach to solving the problem must involve combining information from the history, examination and investigations.

Pain should always be relieved, not only because of the distress to the patient but also because of the associated splinting of the ribcage; the poor respiratory effort and cough may lead to hypostatic pneumonia or respiratory failure (in a compromised patient). Non-steroidal anti-inflammatory drugs (NSAIDs) are useful to relieve bone pain and inflammation. Strong opiates may be needed; if so, beware of respiratory depression.

Pleural effusion

The layers of the pleura are usually separated by a thin layer of fluid acting as a lubricant. Clinically, an effusion cannot be detected below 500 ml. Effusions may be loculated (for example in the transverse fissure) and it may be difficult to determine whether the opacity is caused by fluid or pleural thickening. Ultrasound examination may help.

There are many different causes of a pleural effusion; your first step in determining the aetiology is to set it in the context of the patient's general history and examination. A diagnostic aspiration is often of value (Table 15). Fluid should always be sent for biochemical analysis (protein and, possibly, glucose and amylase), microbiology (Gram stain, culture and possible examination/culture for tuberculosis) and cytology (malignancy, including lymphoma and mesothelioma). Often, the aetiology will be clear simply on the clinical findings. In trying to establish the diagnosis from the aspiration results, it is useful to divide the causes into:

- transudates (protein <20 g/l): usually result from cardiac failure; may be caused by hypoalbuminaemia
- exudates (protein >30 g/l): multiple causes; consider infection (including tuberculosis), malignancy, connective tissue disease (rheumatoid disease) or pulmonary infarction.

Further information, particularly in suspected tuberculosis (p. 72) and malignancy (p. 74) can be gained from a pleural biopsy. If the patient has been exposed to asbestos, even slightly, you should consider a mesothelioma (p. 89).

Initial management of an effusion is aimed at making an aetiological diagnosis, then treating as appropriate. Small effusions may be aspirated to dryness. A **haemothorax** (trauma) must be aspirated to prevent subsequent organisation and fibrosis. A further reason is that blood is a good culture medium. If the fluid is chyle, this is most likely caused by a malignant block of the thoracic duct, though trauma should be excluded.

Large symptomatic effusions of whatever aetiology require insertion of an intercostal drain. Rapid aspiration is contraindicated; it may distress the patient and, rarely, may precipitate pulmonary oedema. Malignant effusions often reaccumulate; these should be drained, then a sclerosing agent such as tetracycline instilled to achieve adhesion of the pleural layers (pleurodesis) and consequent obliteration of the pleural space.

Infection of the pleural space

There are four major types of infection in the pleural space:

- pleurisy
- parapneumonic effusion
- empyema — grossly purulent pleural effusion
- tuberculous empyema.

Occasionally pleural infection is a marker of sub-diaphragmatic disease or systemic disease such as endocarditis.

Pleurisy. Pleurisy refers to a sharp chest pain on inspiration, with features of infection. It may be a manifestation of lobar pneumonia or caused by a virus infection (e.g. Coxsackie virus). Management requires a chest radiograph and white cell count. If these are abnormal, then the patient should be managed as if they have pneumonia, with adequate analgesia. If normal, analgesia alone will suffice.

Parapneumonic effusions are divided into:

- simple: negative on culture and resolves without loculation or drainage
- complicated: positive culture or Gram stain, loculates and requires drainage.

Parapneumonic effusions follow documented pneumonia in the majority of patients. For example, more than 50% of patients with pneumococcal pneumonia develop pleural effusion. In these cases, the most important action is to determine whether it is a simple parapneumonic effusion or a complicated one. This can best be done by assessing the pH or glucose of the pleural fluid following aspiration; if low (pH < 7.2 or glucose < 2.5 µmol/l), it is likely to be a complicated effusion.

Empyema. Occasionally patients develop anaerobic empyema without a clear-cut preceding chest infection. These patients present with a subacute course over several weeks with weakness, anorexia and weight loss and few signs referable to the chest, and little or no fever. Pleural fluid from these patients is foul-smelling and purulent and a good recovery follows antibiotic and chest tube drainage. The most common organisms include Gram-negative aerobes such as *Escherichia coli* and anaerobes.

Treatment of complicated parapneumonic effusions and empyemas

Early drainage of empyemas and complicated parapneumonic effusions is important to minimise loculation and a subsequent restrictive respiratory defect by reduced lung movement. Occasionally chest tube drainage is unsatisfactory and open surgical drainage is necessary for resolution.

Tuberculous empyema

Pleural effusion is a relatively common manifestation of post-primary tuberculosis. These patients usually present with breathlessness, fever, weight loss and occasionally chest pain. Sometimes the effusions are very large, rendering the patient breathless at rest.

Diagnosis. The characteristics of a tuberculous pleural effusion are shown in Table 15. Drainage of large amounts of fluid may yield rapid temporary relief from breathlessness. Mycobacteria are isolated from pleural fluid in up to 20% of patients and a pleural biopsy is usually necessary to confirm the diagnosis (95%); the granulomata are seen histologically. Only occasionally do patients have concurrent parenchymal pulmonary tuberculosis. Sputa for smear and culture for tuberculosis are usually negative.

Pneumothorax

You will see young males (occasionally females) with sudden breathlessness and pleuritic chest pain caused by a spontaneous pneumothorax. You may find reduced breath sounds and increased percussion note may occur, though the diagnosis is more frequently confirmed by the radiograph, not by the examination findings. Management is often by aspiration, as the leak usually closes spontaneously. In patients with asthma or chronic bronchitis and emphysema, even a small pneumothorax may compromise ventilation and requires insertion of an intercostal drain. Pneumothorax secondary to trauma is managed similarly. Insertion of a chest drain is *mandatory* if a patient with a pneumothorax, however small, requires ventilation.

A *tension* pneumothorax, with increasing ventilatory embarrassment, is a medical emergency requiring immediate reduction in the intrathoracic pressure. The patient will have a combination of:

- increasing/severe breathlessness
- cyanosis
- deviated trachea
- absence of breath sounds on one side.

Table 15 Diagnostic information from pleural fluid (transudate = < 20g/dl protein, exudate = > 30 g/dl)

Diagnosis	Blood	Protein	Sugar	Amylase	Culture	Cytology
Heart failure		Transudate				
Hypoproteinaemia		Transudate				
Tuberculosis		Exudate	Low		Bacilli: low yield	Lymphocytes
Malignancy, including mesothelioma	Blood-stained	Exudate		High: pancreatic form		Malignant cells
Pulmonary embolus	Blood-stained	Exudate				
Rheumatoid disease		Exudate	Low			Lymphocytes
Pneumonia (parapneumonic)	Clear or purulent	Exudate	Normal		Usually negative	Leucocytes
Empyema	Opaque pus (offensive)	Exudate	Low		Bacteria, especially anaerobes	Pus cells
Chylous	White	Exudate			Negative	
Pancreatitis	May have blood	Exudate		High		

Asbestosis

In patients exposed to asbestos over a period of years, basal pulmonary fibrosis occurs together with pleural plaques and calcification. You must take a careful occupational history including working in the shipyards, with boilers, in demolition or as laggers. The patient is usually clubbed, breathless and has a cough. A chest radiograph shows predominantly basal changes, including plaques and sheet calcification. Asbestos bodies are usually present in the sputum in severe disease. Frequently those with asbestosis succumb to bronchial carcinoma; the effect of cigarette smoking is synergistic.

Mesothelioma may occur after only minimal exposure to blue asbestos (**crocidolite**). It develops many years later and presents with chest wall pain, which may be ill-defined and is often intractable. Breathlessness is common. A chest radiograph shows the lung being gradually encased with malignant tissue and fibrosis. An effusion is often present. An ultrasound or a CT scan will help to delineate tumour from fluid. A biopsy will confirm the diagnosis; some patients develop nodules along the course of the biopsy track. The tumour can spread through the diaphragm, though distant metastases are rare. There is no curative treatment. Pain control may require specialist advice.

Self-assessment: questions

Multiple choice questions

1. Hypoventilation occurs in the following:
   a. Central sleep apnoea syndrome
   b. Severe kyphoscoliosis
   c. Anxiety
   d. Benzodiazepine overdose
   e. Exercise

2. The following shift the oxygen haemoglobin curve to the right:
   a. Increase in temperature
   b. Fall in hydrogen ion concentration
   c. Increase in carbon dioxide concentration
   d. Hypothermia
   e. Hyperventilation

3. Pneumothorax is a recognised complication of:
   a. Rib fracture
   b. A bulla
   c. Kyphoscoliosis
   d. Cystic fibrosis
   e. *Pneumocystis carinii* pneumonia

4. The following are features of fibrosing alveolitis:
   a. Cough
   b. Clubbing of the fingers in the majority of cases
   c. Cyanosis in the early stages
   d. Circulating antibodies to alveolar tissues
   e. Haemoptysis

5. Mesotheliomas of the pleura:
   a. Only occur after prolonged heavy exposure to asbestos
   b. Respond to radiotherapy
   c. Pain is often the major symptom
   d. Metastasise early
   e. An ultrasound examination may be useful

6. Radical surgery for carcinoma of the bronchus is contraindicated with the following:
   a. Peripheral neuropathy
   b. Hypertrophic pulmonary osteoarthropathy
   c. Superior vena caval obstruction
   d. Obstruction of the bronchus
   e. FEV_1 of 0.8 litres

7. A 35-year-old man with atopic asthma is admitted with an acute attack:
   a. High-dose oxygen should be avoided
   b. A normal pCO_2 always indicates a mild attack
   c. The patient should be sedated

   d. Green sputum almost always implies bacterial infection
   e. You should not give nebulised salbutamol if his pulse rate is > 100/min

8. In a patient with restrictive lung disease:
   a. The FEV_1 is usually within normal limits
   b. The ratio of FEV_1:FVC is reduced
   c. A raised $PaCO_2$ is common in the early stages
   d. Occupation of the patient is important in the differential diagnosis
   e. Clubbing may be found

9. Useful drugs for tuberculosis include:
   a. Piperacillin
   b. Isoniazid
   c. Ciprofloxacin
   d. Ethambutol
   e. Streptomycin

10. Causes of life-threatening pneumonia or pneumonitis in adults include:
    a. *Pneumocystis carinii*
    b. Influenza A virus
    c. Respiratory syncytial virus
    d. *Staphylococcus aureus*
    e. *Legionella pneumophila*

11. Important causes of pneumonia in immunosuppressed patients include:
    a. Cytomegalovirus
    b. *Legionella*
    c. *Mycoplasma pneumoniae*
    d. *Aspergillus fumigatus*
    e. *Streptococcus pneumoniae*

12. Chronic bronchial sepsis:
    a. Is an uncommon feature of cystic fibrosis
    b. Typically is caused by unusual, difficult-to-grow bacteria
    c. May lead to haemoptysis
    d. Can usually be cured with oral antibiotics
    e. May lead to pulmonary fibrosis

13. Pleural aspiration is useful in the following situations:
    a. In diagnosing mesothelioma
    b. Pleural tuberculosis
    c. Viral pleurisy
    d. Empyema
    e. Relieving breathlessness in patients with malignant effusions

Case histories

History 1

At an insurance medical examination, a 56-year-old boiler worker was found to have finger clubbing and had recently noticed that he was short of breath on exertion. He was a long-standing smoker and had had a cough for a number of years. His hobbies included keeping and breeding budgerigars. He had never been in hospital.

On examination, the only other findings were bilateral basal crepitations. He was not cyanosed. His chest radiograph showed bilateral basal fine reticular shadowing.

Lung function testing showed:

Vital capacity	2.5 l (reduced)
FEV_1	1.9 l (reduced)
FEV_1/FVC	68% (normal)
Total lung capacity (TLC)	4.4 l (reduced)
CO diffusion	6.5 ml CO/min per mmHg (reduced)
PaO_2	10.3 kPa (77 mmHg)
$PaCO_2$	5.1 kPa (38 mmHg)

1. Intepret the abnormalities present on his investigations
2. Give two possible diagnoses
3. What further investigations may be helpful?
4. What would happen if the patient exercised?

History 2

You are a surgical house officer and are called at the weekend to see a 65-year-old patient on the orthopaedic ward who had a left hip replacement 5 days before. Apart from being a smoker and having a regular cough, she was previously well. The nurses report that she has a low-grade fever (38°C), is coughing and seems 'not herself'. She is alert but slightly confused, with a respiratory rate of 28/min and with crackles and bronchial breathing at the left base.

1. Your immediate clinical diagnosis(es) is(are):
   a. left ventricular failure
   b. diabetic ketoacidosis
   c. atypical pneumonia
   d. smoker's cough and chronic airflow limitation
   e. hospital-acquired pneumonia

2. The following data are *essential* in your immediate management plan:
   a. whether she keeps birds at home
   b. an old chest X-ray film
   c. the antibiotic prophylaxis she received for her hip operation
   d. the result of a V/Q lung scan or pulmonary arteriogram
   e. arterial blood gas result

3. Appropriate management steps in the first hour after seeing her are:
   a. arterial blood gases
   b. chest radiograph
   c. blood culture
   d. discussion with the microbiologist on call about antibiotic therapy
   e. administration of oxygen

4. Subsequent steps over next 8 hours should include:
   a. rechecking arterial gases while patient is breathing oxygen
   b. consideration of full anticoagulation with more senior physician and orthopaedic team
   c. repeat chest radiograph after 6–8 hours for signs of improvement
   d. explanation of condition to anxious relatives
   e. consideration of transfer to ITU if condition deteriorates

History 3

A 48-year-old female presents with a 2-week history of haemoptysis. In the recent past, she has had two episodes of left upper lobe pneumonia. On examination, there are no systemic signs of disease, the trachea is slightly deviated to the left, tactile fremitus is reduced at left apex and wheeze is localised to left side of chest. Chest radiograph shows loss of volume in the left upper lobe.

1. What is the likely diagnosis?
2. What is the definitive diagnostic test?

History 4

The following results are obtained from a pleural aspirate:

Straw-coloured
protein 35 g/l
cells: predominantly lymphocytes
glucose 0.5 mmol/l
culture: no growth
cytology: no malignant cells seen.

1. What are your differential diagnoses?
2. What further investigations would you request?

History 5

A 40-year-old man is referred to a chest clinic because of increasing shortness of breath of gradual onset. He has a family history of respiratory disease. Pulmonary function tests (predicted values in parentheses) show:

FEV_1 (l) 1.2 (3.7)
FVC (l) 3.0 (4.2)
TLC (l) 7.2 (5.3)
Transfer factor 12.5 (26)

1. What is the diagnosis?
2. What further investigations should be carried out?

History 6

A 44-year-old man presents with a 6-month history of a dry cough and increasing dyspnoea. On examination he is clubbed, has a normal cardiovascular system, is short of breath at rest and has showers of fine crepitations at both bases. Blood gases show:

pH 7.4
pO_2 48 mmHg
pCO_2 28 mmHg
HCO_3 15 mmol/l.

1. What is the likely diagnosis?
2. Explain the blood gas result.

History 7

A 60-year-old man presents with a few weeks' history of a severe dry cough and rapidly increasing shortness of breath. He had a resection for carcinoma of the stomach 18 months previously. There is no previous respiratory or cardiac history. On examination, he is markedly tachypnoeic at rest, but his chest is clear on auscultation. There are no other signs. He has the following pulmonary function results (predicted values in parentheses):

FEV_1 (l) 1.8 (3.1)
FVC (l) 2.0 (4.2)
TLC (l) 3.0 (5.0)
Transfer factor 12 (22)

1. What do the pulmonary function tests show?
2. What is the likely diagnosis?
3. Give two investigations you would do and explain why.

History 8

A 28-year-old female with a known psychiatric history presents with her relatives to casualty. She refuses to give a history but has marked hyperventilation and the following blood gases:

pH 7.58
pO_2 115 mmHg
pCO_2 26 mmHg
HCO_3 18 mmol/l.

1. What do the gases show?
2. Give three urgent investigations that should be carried out.

Picture questions

1. Look at Picture 2.1a, b. Describe the abnormalities and give the diagnosis. What might be the underlying cause?

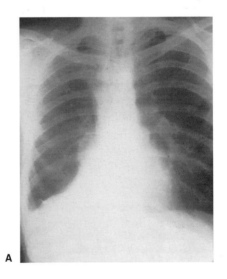

A

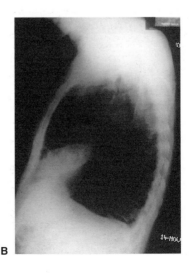

B

Picture 2.1

2. Look at Picture 2.2a,b. Describe the abnormalities and give the diagnosis. What might be the underlying cause?

3. Picture 2.3 is a PA chest radiograph from a man with a 6-month history of progressive breathlessness. Describe the abnormality. What would be your differential diagnosis? What would you look for on examination?

4. This 67-year-old man presented with haemoptysis and weight loss over a few months. What does the PA radiograph (Picture 2.4) show? What is the likely diagnosis and what other causes would you consider and (possibly) discount?

5. Picture 2.5 is a PA chest radiograph of a 58-year-old cockney schizophrenic man who sleeps rough in London.
   a. Give three abnormalities you can see
   b. What investigations would you now do? (Give at least four)
   c. What would you expect to find and/or grow in his sputum?
   d. Where should he be looked after initially?
   e. What treatment would you prescribe?
   f. Do you foresee any problems with his treatment?

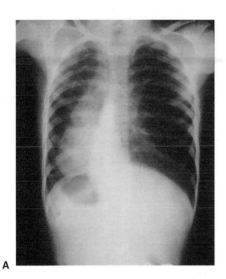

A

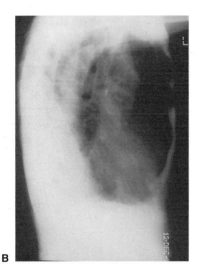

B

Picture 2.2

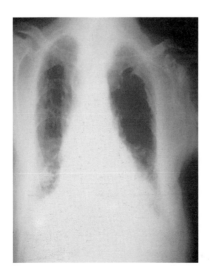

Picture 2.3

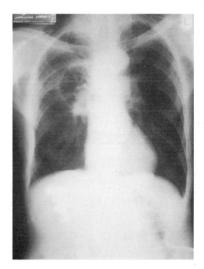

Picture 2.4

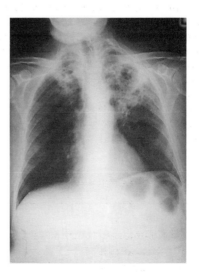

Picture 2.5

6. A 25-year-old man was out jogging when he developed chest tightness and shortness of breath. This rapidly progressed and he collapsed on the pavement. An emergency ambulance was called and he was brought to casualty. The radiographer was in casualty and did the AP chest film shown in Picture 2.6.
   a. What does it show?
   b. What signs might the man have?
   c. What would be your immediate management?

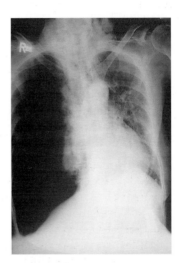

Picture 2.6

Short note questions

Write short notes on the following:

1. Ten facts you know about asthma (*without consulting any books*). List three important

principles of management of acute asthma and their rationale
2. The causes of chronic airflow limitation; make a table, giving differences and similarities.
3. Describe how you would instruct a patient in measuring a peak flow rate
4. Atypical pneumonia
5. Respiratory infection in the immunocompromised patient
6. Management of oxygen therapy and analgesia in pneumonia
7. Indications for physiotherapy in chest disease

Data interpretation

1. Table 16 is a peak flow chart on a paint factory worker.
   What is the diagnosis?
   What is the most likely cause in this person?
2. A 49-year-old smoker who has a central abdominal scar presents acutely ill and breathless with these vital signs: temperature, 39.2°C; respiratory rate, 40/min; pulse, 125/min; blood pressure, 100/70. His hands are cold and he is peripherally cyanosed. The pulse oximeter shows an oxygen saturation of 78%. His arterial blood gas results return within a group of five different samples (Table 17).
   a. Which of the group of five samples is likely to be his and why?
   b. Give a differential diagnosis
   c. What underlying diseases might you reasonably expect?
   d. List four key investigations
   e. Suggest an immediate management plan

Table 16 Peak flow chart for data interpretation 1.

Peak flow								
Work	Work	Work	Work	Work	Hols	Hols	Hols	Hols
Mon	Tues	Weds	Thurs	Fri	Sat	Sun	Mon	Tues
550	300	250	200	200	200	300	450	500
450	480	400	350	300	380	420	520	520

Table 17 Arterial blood gas results for data interpretation 2.

	1	2	3	4	5
pH	7.43	7.55	7.22	7.40	7.20
pO_2 (mmHg)	88	95	56	83	51
pCO_2 (mmHg)	34	25	25	30	50
HCO_3 (mmol/l)	18	33	16	19	22

Self-assessment: answers

Multiple choice answers

1. a. **True**. Alveolar hypoventilation is a key feature.
   b. **True**. Severe kyphoscoliosis can produce mechanical ventilation problems because of the changed curvature of the spine.
   c. **False**. Anxiety is associated with hyperventilation.
   d. **True**. Drugs such as benzodiazepines depress the respiratory centre.
   e. **False**. Alveolar ventilation is increased during exercise in normal people.

2. a. **True**. In working muscle, there is an increase in temperature which moves the curve to the *right* which is the *right* thing to do.
   b. **False**. An acidosis not alkalosis shifts the curve to the right.
   c. **True**. CO_2 retention produces an acidosis.
   d. **False**.
   e. **False**. Hyperventilation produces an alkalosis which shifts the curve to the left.

3. a. **True**. Pneumothorax can occur secondary to trauma.
   b. **True**. Any cavitating or cystic/bullous lung lesion can cause a pneumothorax. Bullae can be single or multiple. They are particularly common in emphysema including α_1-antitrypsin deficiency.
   c. **False**.
   d. **False**. Pneumothoraces are uncommon in cystic fibrosis because repeated infection causes pleural adhesions.
   e. **False**. But lung abscesses (e.g. *Staph. aureus*) can lead to pneumothorax.

4. a. **True**. Patients usually present with cough and breathlessness.
   b. **True**. Clubbing occurs in about 60% of patients but is not essential for the diagnosis.
   c. **False**. Cyanosis is a relatively late sign.
   d. **False**. The aetiology is unknown and circulating antibodies are not found.
   e. **False**. If a patient has haemoptysis you should think of another cause.

5. a. **False**. Exposure may be trivial with a long delay before appearance of the tumour.
   b. **False**. The tumour is resistant to radiotherapy and chemotherapy.
   c. **True**. Pain is often a very troublesome symptom.
   d. **False**. The tumour can spread through the diaphragm; distant metastases are rare.

   e. **True**. It may show the irregular pleural thickening.

6. a. **False**. Peripheral neuropathy is a non-metastatic complication and may respond to curative resection.
   b. **False**. As with 6a, it may respond to surgical resection. There are other non-metastatic manifestations which you should know (Fig. 19).
   c. **True**. SVC obstruction usually denotes extensive mediastinal invasion.
   d. **False**.
   e. **True**. A very low FEV_1 would be a contraindication because of inadequate respiratory reserve following resection.

7. a. **False**. A high concentration of oxygen should be administered to all patients on arrival at hospital.
   b. **False**. Normocarbia is a bad sign signalling failing alveolar ventilation.
   c. **False**. Sedation *must* be avoided.
   d. **False**. Green sputum is normal in some patients.
   e. **False**. A β_2-agonist such as salbutamol should be administered via a nebuliser immediately.

8. a. **False**. FEV_1 is often low.
   b. **False**. The ratio is usually unchanged in restrictive disease.
   c. **False**. The early pattern is type 1 respiratory failure with hypoxia and low $PaCO_2$.
   d. **True**. A number of restrictive lung diseases are caused by environmental factors, relating to occupation and hobbies.
   e. **True**.

9. a. **False**. Piperacillin has no activity.
   b. **True**. Isoniazid is a major, first-line agent.
   c. **True**. Ciprofloxacin is a useful agent, less active than rifampicin; it may obscure infection in patients treated before diagnosis considered.
   d. **True**. Ethambutol is another major, but second-line agent.
   e. **True**. Streptomycin is another major, first-line agent.

10. a. **True**. *Pneumocystis carinii* infection is usually seen in AIDS, but also in lymphoma, steroid-treated, transplant and hypogammaglobulinaemic patients.
    b. **True**. Primary influenzal pneumonia or complicated by bacteria, e.g. *S. aureus*.
    c. **False**. Respiratory syncytial virus is a problem in immunosuppressed children and bone marrow transplant patients.

d. **True**. *S. aureus* pneumonia is often rapidly fatal, especially following influenza.

e. **True**. *L. pneumophilia* pneumonia carries a high mortality if not treated appropriately.

11. a. **True**. Cytomegalovirus pneumonia occurs primarily in transplant patients.
    b. **True**. *Legionella* infection is associated with solid organ transplant patients.
    c. **False**. *M. pneumonia* is very rarely a problem.
    d. **True**. *A. fumigatus* is an increasing problem in all immunocompromised groups. May be fatal in 7 days.
    e. **True**. *S. pneumoniae* is primarily a problem in chronic chest patients, children and the community. It is not a major problem in immunosuppressed patients except in AIDS, when it is 100 times more common, but with a lower mortality.

12. a. **False**. It is the primary feature of cystic fibrosis.
    b. **False**. It is usually caused by common organisms.
    c. **True**. Haemoptysis is also seen with dry bronchiectasis, chronic bronchial sepsis and with aspergillomas.
    d. **False**. It may be ameliorated but not cured. Some patients require i.v. antibiotics for improvement.
    e. **True**. It produces a fibrotic reaction.

13. a. **False**. For the diagnosis of mesothelioma, a pleural biopsy/surgery is required.
    b. **False**. A pleural aspirate may show lymphocytes but is rarely culture positive.
    c. **False**. Viral pleurisy does not cause an effusion, just pain.
    d. **True**. An empyema will require tube or surgical drainage for treatment.
    e. **True**. Drainage in malignant effusions is often very helpful if litres of fluid are removed.

Case history answers

History 1

1. He has a moderate restrictive lung defect with hypoxia and impaired transfer factor.
2. Given the history, there are several possibilities:
   a. cryptogenic fibrosing alveolitis (p. 85)
   b. lymphangitis carcinomatosis (p. 77)
   c. asbestosis (p. 89)
   d. extrinsic allergic alveolitis: bird fancier's lung (p. 88)
   e. miscellaneous conditions such as sarcoidosis, rheumatoid disease, SLE (p. 310). No other findings suggestive of these.

3. Avian precipitins, antinuclear factor, rheumatoid factor, bronchoscopy and lavage (asbestosis fibres), transbronchial biopsy. Pleural plaques may sometimes be visible on CT scanning. It is important to diagnose occupational disease as he may be eligible for compensation.
4. The patient would become more hypoxic and he would develop hypocarbia. These are caused by ventilation:perfusion mismatching (p. 47). On exercise, this worsens with perfusion of non-ventilated lung areas and a consequent increase in alveolar:arterial oxygen gradient. The increased respiratory drive caused by the hypoxia stimulates excess loss of carbon dioxide.

General discussion. The patient is a smoker, has a short history, with occupational and social exposure to possible hazardous agents. Important points on the radiograph shadowing are shown in Table 18.

History 2

1. a. **False**. Unlikely for two reasons: bronchial breathing and fever. However, a myocardial infarction during or after surgery is not uncommon and this is a major cause of deteriorating pulmonary function postoperatively.

Table 18 Comparison of chest radiograph findings and physical signs and symptoms

Possible diagnoses	Radiograph Findings	Symptoms and Signs
Asbestosis	Linear pleural calcification	
Lymphangitis carcinomatosis	Minimal abnormalities	Cough, very breathless
Cryptogenic fibrosing alveolitis	Basal shadowing, honey-combing	Late fine inspiratory crepitations, clubbed
Extrinsic allergic alveolitis	Upper lobe mainly	Pigeons — acute symptoms; budgies — chronic symptoms
Sarcoidosis	Severe x-ray changes	Moderate symptoms
Aspergilloma	Upper zone, cavitation with marked pleural thickening	Often no symptoms; occasionally haemoptysis
Post-primary tuberculosis	Upper zone, cavitation, bilateral	May have few physical signs

b. **False**. Unlikely as no clues in history, but if she were diabetic then an infection with or without surgery could certainly have precipitated this. The patient needs blood sugar measurement.

c. **False**. Unlikely, but possible. Many hospitals have *Legionella* in the water systems and this comes in the differential diagnosis of hospital-acquired pneumonia.

d. **False**. Too ill for these alone.

e. **True**. The most common infection postoperatively, especially in the elderly and immobile patient, and more likely in smokers.

2. a. **False**. Desirable but not essential.

b. **False**. Desirable but not essential.

c. **True**. Use the BNF. Every surgeon has a different regimen. Your prescription of antibiotics should *not* be the same class of antibiotic(s) as used for prophylaxis as the bacteria causing pneumonia are much more likely to be resistant to it.

d. **False**. Although a pulmonary embolism and/or infarction is possible, you should initially manage her without these data.

e. **True**. Vital for management, to assess oxygenation, carbon dioxide retention and pH. Blood gases are essential in the management of all patients in hospital with pneumonia.

3. a. **True**. See answer to 2e.

b. **True**. For features of pneumonia.

c. **True**. Some patients are bacteraemic with pneumonia, but she may have bacteraemia from another cause and a separate pulmonary problem.

d. **True**. Unless you recently discussed a very similar case, their advice about appropriate antibiotics is usually invaluable.

e. **True**. The best level depends on the arterial blood gases.

4. a. **True**. This is vital. If you started the oxygen because the patient was hypoxic, the gases should be rechecked.

b. **True**. In postoperative patients such as this, they are usually on subcutaneous heparin anyway. The risk of bleeding into the operative site is high and so a senior medical opinion is appropriate.

c. **False**. No use at all. Radiographic resolution follows clinical improvement and in the case of *Legionella* pneumonia can take 4–6 weeks to clear.

d. **True**. This needs to be done judiciously as this patient is not under you, but the orthopaedic team, and you do not yet know how the patient will respond. But as a 'medical expert' for the surgeons, your broad outline of the problem as you observe it with cautious optimism about outcome would be appropriate.

e. **True**. This is the key reason for *you* to reassess the patient again including blood gases.

History 3

1. Common things being commonest, the most likely diagnosis is a bronchial carcinoma. The patient is in the right age group, she has had two episodes of *upper* lobe pneumonia (rare, mostly lower lobe) and has haemoptysis. You are not told whether she is a smoker and when the episodes of pneumonia occurred. The examination findings are consistent with a partial collapse of the left upper lobe and the wheeze implies local obstruction. An alternative, but much rarer, diagnosis would be a bronchial adenoma. A further possibility is that the lobe was damaged by tuberculosis sometime in the past and the recent problems result from complications of this (e.g. bronchiectasis, pneumonia, aspergilloma). You should always consider active tuberculosis (treatable) and that adenocarcinomas occur at the site of lung scarring.

2. The definitive diagnositic test is a bronchoscopy (p. 67). Other tests would be sputum for acid-fast bacilli, culture for *M. tuberculosis* and cytology (malignant cells).

History 4

1. Note the lymphocytes and the low sugar. This pattern is consistent with either tuberculosis (common; p. 72) or rheumatoid disease (relatively rare; p. 306) (Table 12). Further information from the history may help, though an effusion may be the first manifestation of rheumatoid disease.

2. Rheumatoid factor can be measured. Culture for acid-fast bacilli should be undertaken and Mantoux testing. A pleural biopsy will be more likely to give a positive result for tubercle than simply culture of the fluid. Caseating granulomata may be seen on histology. A thoracoscopy may be carried out in a specialist unit; this allows biopsy of the pleura under direct vision and gives the highest diagnostic yield.

History 5

1. The pulmonary function tests should be analysed and put into the context of the description of the patient. The patient has marked airflow limitation with reduced transfer factor and increased total lung capacity. The family history in a relatively young man points to α_1-antitrypsin deficiency (p. 78).

2. A chest radiograph may show marked lower lobe changes with bullae. The serum level of α_1-antitrypsin can be measured.

History 6

1. The history of progessive breathlessness, clubbing and showers of fine crepitations is consistent with a diagnosis of cryptogenic fibrosing alveolitis.
2. Analysis of the blood gases shows hypoxia with a compensated respiratory alkalosis.

History 7

1. The patient has a restrictive pattern and a reduced transfer factor with a previous history of carcinoma of the stomach. The present problem is one of rapidly worsening respiratory symptoms but, apart from the tachypnoea, there are no abnormal physical signs.
2. The overall picture is lymphangitis carcinomatosis.
3. Blood gases may show hypoxia with a respiratory alkylosis. A chest radiograph may show fine basal shadowing with honeycombing. A transbronchial biopsy may give a definitive tissue diagnosis.

History 8

1. You will see similar patients in casualty. The blood gases show a primary respiratory alkalosis (pH 7.58) and a metabolic acidosis. The history of a psychiatric illness is supportive of a diagnosis of salicylate overdose. In the early stages this stimulates the respiratory centre giving hypocarbia. Later a metabolic acidosis (falling pH) supervenes and finally the respiratory centre is depressed giving a combined respiratory and metabolic acidosis.
2. Confirm the diagnosis with a blood salicylate level. Above 500 mg/l indicates severe poisoning. The aim of treatment is to make the patient fluid replete (with hyperventilation, sweating and possible vomiting, it is likely that she is hypovolaemic) and then alkalinise the urine. The latter is because salicylate is a weak acid and can exist in its ionised or its unionised form within the range of pH found in the body. If the pH is high (alkaline) in the urine, salicylate is ionised and cannot diffuse back across the tubule once it has been filtered at the glomerulus. Apart from checking the salicylate levels and the blood gases, check the blood glucose (may get either hypo- or hyperglycaemia), urea and electrolytes (hypo/hypernatraemia, hypokalaemia), prothrombin time/bleeding time (may be prolonged) and a chest radiograph (non-cardiogenic pulmonary oedema in late stages). You could also request lactate levels and take blood for a subsequent toxicology screen.

    If in any doubt over a deliberate or accidental poisoning, you should contact one of the National Poison Units urgently for advice.

Data interpretation

1. a. The peak flow values indicate occupational asthma with worsening pulmonary function during the working week and improvement when not at work.
   b. In a paint factory, the most likely trigger is toluene diisocyonate.
2. a. Blood gas sample 3. Hypoxia with metabolic acidosis caused by sepsis syndrome. You already know that he is hypoxic, because of the low oxygen saturation on the pulse oximeter. He is shocked (low blood pressure, and cold, cyanosed peripheries) and likely to have a metabolic acidosis.
   b. Septic shock, probably gram positive, but could be gram negative. Possibly meningococcaemia.
   c. A previous splenectomy (pneumococcal sepsis), AIDS (pneumocystis pneumonia) (unlikely as septic shock is infrequent), alcoholism (pneumococcal sepsis).
   d. Blood cultures, chest radiograph, differential white cell count, bronchoscopy (if oxygen corrects the hypoxia), ultrasound of abdomen to look for a spleen, urea and electrolytes (as renal failure likely) and blood sugar (as he has a metabolic acidosis).
   e. High flow oxygen (as he has a low CO_2 and is severely hypoxic do not be too concerned about a rising CO_2 — it is more important to correct hypoxia rapidly); i.v. broad spectrum antibiotics, such as cefotaxime and a single dose of gentamicin (acute renal failure is likely, so beware amino glycoside toxicity); i.v. fluids; refer to intensive care unit (see septic shock, p. 356).

Picture answers

1. The PA film shows a wedge-shaped opacity adjacent to the right heart border that is indistinct. The lateral film confirms that this is caused by right middle lobe consolidation with the abnormality visible in the anterior mediastinum between the horizontal and oblique fissure. The most likely cause is a pneumonia, but trigger by a carcinoma should also be considered. Rarely it can be caused by a bronchial adenoma in a young person giving rise to secondary infection behind an obstruction.
2. These radiographs are harder to interpret. The PA film shows a shift of the lower mediastinum (heart) to the left. There is a narrow triangular opacity behind the heart adjacent to the spinal column. The lateral film shows this to be in the posterior part of the chest. The appearances are classical of a left lower lobe collapse. Remember the location of the lower lobe posteriorly. The most likely cause is a

carcinoma, but it could be the result of mucus plugging in, for example, asthma (perhaps complicated by bronchopulmonary aspergillosis).

3. He has hazy opacification of the lower (predominantly) lung fields bilaterally. Given the history, the most likely diagnosis is fibrosing alveolitis. Lymphangitis carcinomatosis could give a similar picture, but the length of the history is too long. Occupational lung disease (for example asbestosis) should be considered, though there are no calcified plaques and autoimmune disease should also be considered, e.g. SLE or rheumatoid disease. Check the relevant autoantibodies; remember there is a high prevalence of false positives, but these are not usually of a high titre. Extrinsic allergic alveolitis predominantly affects the upper zones.

On examination, the patient may be tachypnoeic at rest or after minimal exertion (getting onto the examination couch). In the late stages, cyanosis may be evident. Look for clubbing (most likely in *cryptogenic* fibrosing alveolitis). On auscultation, there will be the typical showers of late inspiratory crepitations.

4. The patient has a cavitating lesion adjacent to the upper mediastinum with increased density of the hila (lymphadenopathy). There are increased lung markings in the right upper zone, suggesting a partial collapse. The most likely cause, given the history, is a cavitating bronchial carcinoma. However, there are other possibilities. The walls of the cavity are too dense for a simple bulla and the hilar abnormality is against this. Sometimes, a bulla becomes infected with an aspergilloma, which can cause haemoptysis and may be expectorated. Again the hilar lymphadenopathy is against this. In a lung abscess, the history would be much shorter, with severe constitutional disturbance.

5. a. Cavitary disease at both apices and an elevated left diaphragm consistent with substantial left upper lobe contraction.
   b. (i) Three sputa for tuberculosis smear and culture; (ii) sputum for routine microbiology; (iii) full blood count and ESR; and (iv) biochemistry, including liver function tests and albumin; Heaf or Mantoux tests are probably unnecessary. Most other tests can await the outcome of the AFB smear.
   c. Positive smear for acid-fast bacilli. In gross cavitary disease, the smear is usually strongly positive. If negative, he should undergo bronchoscopy as soon as possible.
   d. In a single room with negative pressure ventilation in hospital.
   e. Rifampicin, isoniazid, pyrazinamide and pyridoxine. He does not fit the criteria for a fourth agent (p. 73). It is imperative to prescribe pyridoxine in a malnourished patient, otherwise

the isoniazid may induce pellagra.
   f. As he is unlikely to be compliant, he will need directly supervised treatment on discharge.
6. a. The chest radiograph shows a right pneumothorax, with mediastinal shift to the left (demonstrated by tracheal deviation and displacement of the heart) and compression of the left lung. He has a tension pneumothorax.
   b. The signs would be: (i) respiratory embarrassment (cyanosis, tachypnoea, tachycardia); (ii) signs of the pneumothorax (reduced breath sounds, increased percussion note on the right; and (iii) signs of 'tension' (pulsus paradoxus, tracheal deviation, displaced apex beat).
   c. Your management would be: (i) high concentration of oxygen ('100%' — not really achievable); and (ii) *immediate* insertion of intercostal drain (or any means of releasing the 'tension').

Short notes answers

1. Refer to text (p. 81).
2. Refer to text (Table 12).
3. The patient should be you on the peak flow meter what to do. You should be able to give clear instructions in the steps (see p. 67). Similar to the above, you should be able to explain to a patient how to use an MDI.
4. See the sections on *Mycoplasma, C. psittaci,* Q fever, *Legionella, C. pneumonia* and viral pneumonias.
5. Major pathogens include:
   a. Ordinary bacteria and Gram-negative bacteria, *Pneumocystis carinii* (p. 339).
   b. Cytomegalovirus is a major problem in bone marrow transplant, heart and lung transplant patients and is life-threatening. Infection with cytomegalovirus presents with cough and breathlessness, usually with fever and a pneumonitis; it is diagnosed by bronchoscopy and treated with ganciclovir intravenously. Infection has a high mortality, especially if diagnosed late.
   c. *Aspergillus.* Invasive aspergillosis is the invasion of tissue by *Aspergillus* spp. Therefore, it develops in previously normal lung or sinuses. It is common (5–25%) in leukaemia, bone marrow, liver, heart and lung transplant patients and now in advanced AIDS. Symptoms are usually minor: cough, mild fever and chest pain are typical. CT scans are more sensitive than plain chest radiographs in diagnosis. It may spread to the brain. It is fatal if untreated and is relatively resistant to treatment with amphotericin B or itraconazole.
6. **Oxygen.** All patients with pneumonia in hospital require supplemental oxygen. The percentage required depends on their needs and whether they

retain carbon dioxide. *The greatest danger is in leaving a patient with a low oxygen.* Patients with chronic respiratory disease, exhausted patients or those with major neuromuscular problems require monitoring of blood gases to ensure that there is not a significant rise in carbon dioxide. This may require you to make small changes in oxygen concentration and repeat arterial gases an hour later. Previously well patients should be given high oxygen concentrations (e.g. $\geq 60\%$ oxygen) and can be monitored simply with pulse oximetry.

Analgesia. In pneumonia this is only required for patients with pleurisy. Be careful that your choice will not suppress the respiratory drive and allow carbon dioxide to accumulate.

7. Physiotherapy is indicated as a treatment in:
   a. wet bronchiectasis
   b. cystic fibrosis
   c. productive lobar and bronchopneumonia
   d. aspiration pneumonia
   e. ventilator pneumonia
   f. infective exacerbations of CAFL
   g. palliative care for carcinoma of bronchus
   h. pneumothorax with drain in situ.

It is also used to help in investigation:

a. induced sputum in AIDS for *Pneumocystis* and tuberculosis, and
b. sputum production for assessment of infection.

Physiotherapists should also be involved in patient education:

a. in management of acute asthma (e.g. postural advice, breathing pattern, inhaler technique)
b. in cystic fibrosis and bronchiectasis (postural drainage).

Gastrointestinal, hepatobiliary and pancreatic disease

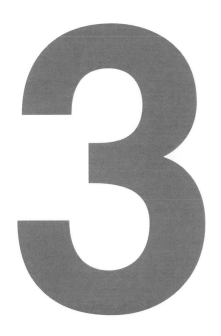

3.1 Clinical aspects

Learning objectives

You should:

- be able to link the common symptoms and signs in gastrointestinal (GI) disease with disease processes
- be able to construct a logical investigation plan based on the symptoms and signs
- be able to outline principles of management of the common problems and diseases.

Common symptoms

Dysphagia

You must take swallowing difficulties seriously. The first step is a careful history. Patients will often localise the difficulty to high (i.e. throat/pharynx) or lower areas (oesophageal). Dysphagia is a common accompaniment of neurological disease (p. 186), but usually there will be other symptoms and signs. A very important discriminating feature is difficulty with different consistencies of food:

- in neurological disease — liquids
- in local disease — solid food.

In a patient with longstanding heartburn (see below), with dysphagia over several months then a **stricture** may have occurred. However, you must exclude oesophageal carcinoma. Rarer causes of dysphagia include: **achalasia** and **systemic sclerosis** (p. 312). Always be very wary of making the diagnosis of **globus hystericus**; it is very rare and there should be other evidence of psychological disturbance.

Heartburn

Heartburn is a common symptom and is caused by reflux oesophagitis. It increases with age and is often severe in pregnancy because of relaxation of the oesophageal sphincter. Patients complain of an ill-defined burning sensation behind the sternum. It may be worsened by stooping or lying flat, which increases the reflux. Less commonly, heartburn may be caused by oesophageal **candidiasis**.

Indigestion/dyspepsia

Most patients do not give a 'classical' description of dyspepsia, but rather one of many variations. The typical description of ulcer pain is epigastric discomfort that is relieved by eating and occurs a few hours after meals or during the night. A valuable question is whether they take regular antacids. There is no reliable way of differentiating between gastritis, gastric or a duodenal ulcer at the bedside.

Abdominal pain

The following framework is useful in abdominal pain.

Is the pain of recent onset? If acute and severe, it suggests an acute problem such as perforation or acute pancreatitis; if longstanding, it might suggest a peptic ulcer (periodicity) or chronic pancreatitis.

Where is the pain? If epigastric, it suggests a peptic ulcer, if right hypochondrial, biliary disease; if periumbilical, peritoneal irritation.

Where does it radiate to? Shoulder tip pain suggests diaphragmatic irritation; pain going through into the back is linked to pancreatic disease.

What helps/worsens the pain? Local heat (hot water bottle) may help chronic pancreatic pain. Diaphragmatic irritation may be worsened by deep breathing/coughing.

What is the character of the pain? Intestinal obstruction may cause typical colic pain. Biliary colic is not typically 'colicky' as it comes in waves lasting about 30 minutes. Chronic pancreatitis causes a severe unremitting pain described as 'boring' through into the back.

Are there any associated features? Intestinal obstruction may be accompanied by vomiting and abdominal distension. Weight loss is always worrying, but it may be associated with malabsorption.

Abdominal distension

Many people complain of abdominal distension, but it is usually a subjective feeling. It is associated with functional bowel disease/irritable bowel syndrome. Rarely, you will see patients with true distension caused by ascites or intestinal obstruction.

Vomiting

The vomiting centre is in the medulla close to the **chemoreceptor trigger zone** (CTZ). It is stimulated through the CTZ by the vestibular apparatus, central connections (e.g. olfactory) or by vagal afferents from the GI tract.

Vomiting has three phases:

1. nausea and excess autonomic activity with sweating, salivation and pallor
2. retching with closure of the glottis, cessation of respiration and contraction of the diaphragm and abdominal muscles
3. expulsion of the gastric contents with relaxation of the lower oesophageal sphincter and cardia, and contractions of the abdominal muscles.

In a patient with nausea and vomiting, you should consider:

- GI disease, including food poisoning (common)
- drugs (common in hospitals)
- systemic disease, including neurological problems.

You have to consider whether the patient is compromised by the loss of fluid and electrolytes as well as by reduced intake. The principles of management are:

- treat the underlying cause; sometimes this is not possible
- symptomatic relief.

You should know the mechanisms of action of the common antiemetics (Table 19).

Haematemesis

Haematemesis is common. First, you should make sure that the patient is not shocked through reduced blood volume. Remember that patients may have *bradycardia* (rather than a tachycardia) as a result of vagal stimulation.

After this, take a history. It can be difficult to estimate the volume of blood lost as it is a frightening symptom. The history may suggest peptic ulceration and you should enquire about the use of NSAIDs. Occasionally, a **Mallory–Weiss tear** is indicated by violent retching followed by vomiting fresh blood.

The patient may be known to have liver disease/portal hypertension (varices) or a history of chronic heavy alcohol ingestion may be given. A bleeding diathesis is possible and the appropriate investigations (clotting, fibrin degradation products, platelets) should be made. Sometimes, the most difficult story to unravel is vomiting 'coffee grounds'. It is better to be cautious and assume upper GI bleeding.

Diarrhoea

People use different terms to describe their bowel habit. With any possibly abnormal bowel habit, you need to find out its time course, variability and associated symptoms. To some people, diarrhoea means a single explosive bowel movement, to others it means increased frequency of passing stools.

Passing large volumes of watery faeces is indicative of organic bowel disease. Bloody diarrhoea points to a colonic problem. *Steatorrhoea* means a motion with high fat content. It is usually described as being bulky, offensive and difficult to flush away.

Constipation

Many people complain of constipation with the usual yardstick of passing a motion once per day. In reality, the range of normality is much greater. As with diarrhoea, it is a recent change in bowel habit that is worrying. You need to have a clear idea of the person's diet (roughage) and medication; many drugs cause constipation, including narcotic analgesics (e.g. codeine) and tricyclic antidepressants (anticholinergic).

Melaena

The passage of a black, offensive tarry motion indicates high GI tract bleeding. The major diagnostic pitfall is the concurrent treatment with iron preparations (which also cause either diarrhoea or constipation).

Faecal incontinence

Faecal incontinence is very distressing. It may be associated with tenesmus (urgency) and a clear history of an acute bowel problem. More commonly it occurs in elderly, often disabled, people. There are two chronic types:

- neurogenic faecal incontinence
- overflow.

In neurogenic incontinence, the patient passes formed motions with no adequate warning. It is often linked to eating (**gastro-colic reflex**). The underlying process is usually cerebrovascular or degenerative neurological disease. Management is either by the carers anticipating the bowel habit or by promoting constipation (e.g. codeine) together with regular enemas.

In overflow incontinence, the patient is constipated. Examination confirms that the rectum is full of faeces and there is leakage of faeculent material. The management is regular enemas, remove any predisposing factors and prescribe a laxative. If the faeces are soft, then a stimulant should be used such as senna. If the faeces are hard, then a high roughage diet should be advised, with the addition of bulking agents (fibrogel) and softeners (co-danthrusate — also is a mild stimulant).

Table 19 Mechanism of action of common antiemetics

Drug	Action	Comments
Metoclopramide	Dopamine antagonism	Crosses blood–brain barrier; Parkinsonism
Domperidone	Dopamine antagonism	Peripheral receptors
Perchlorperazine	Dopamine and cholinergic antagonism	Parkinsonism, constipation
Ondansetron	5-HT$_3$ antagonism	Useful in cancer chemotherapy

Rectal bleeding

Patients with haemorrhoids or anal fissures (often painful) may complain of the passage of bright red blood. However, you should be cautious about assigning bleeding to a minor problem and failing to consider serious disease such as inflammatory bowel disease or malignancy, especially as they are treatable.

Jaundice

Jaundice becomes clinically detectable at around double the upper limit of the bilirubin concentration in the blood (30–40 μmol/l). Consider an infective cause and ask about recent exposure, such as blood transfusion or travel abroad. In obstructive jaundice, the patient may volunteer that the urine has been dark and that the motions are pale. Carefully palpate for an enlarged gall bladder (**Courvoisier's sign — pancreatic carcinoma**). Remember that, in an older person, gall stone obstruction is at least as common as malignant blockage.

Jaundice may signify decompensated chronic liver disease and you should examine accordingly. In long-standing problems such as **primary biliary cirrhosis**, the pigmentation may be deep with evidence of pruritus — excoriation of the skin (irritation by skin deposition of bile salts).

Weight loss/anorexia

Weight loss is a common presenting problem, either in association with other features or alone. The first task is to try and quantify the loss. You should always weigh the patient as a baseline. A framework for diagnosis is:

- inadequate intake — e.g. depression
- malabsorption — e.g. coeliac disease
- disturbed metabolism — thyrotoxicosis
- malignancy — e.g. GI or remote disease
- systemic disease — e.g. tuberculosis.

Investigations

Learning objective
- You must be able to utilise appropriately the range of investigations for the GI tract, particularly endoscopy and imaging.

Plain radiographs

There is limited usefulness for plain radiographs in GI disease. Chronic pancreatitis is associated with calcification. In a suspected perforated viscus, an erect film may show gas under the diaphragm. Gas is also seen in patients who have had recent surgery and it may outline the biliary tree. In the absence of a surgical explanation, the sign may point to a cholangitis.

Erect and supine films should be ordered in a patient with possible bowel obstruction. Fluid levels may be observed and there may be clues to the level of the obstruction.

Barium studies

Barium swallow
If a patient has severe heartburn or if food is 'sticking', a barium swallow may be useful to show a stricture (benign or malignant), a hiatus hernia, oesophagitis (better to request endoscopy) or filling defects caused by varices.

Videofluoroscopy
Videofluoroscopy (VF) is useful in non-obstructive dysphagia. It will show any abnormalities within the three phases of swallowing (oral, pharyngeal and oesophageal) and aspiration.

Barium meal
Although endoscopy has become the investigation of choice for suspected gastroduodenal disease, a good quality barium meal interpreted by an experienced radiologist can give structural and motility information, complementary to biopsy/culture.

Barium follow-through/small bowel enema
Visualisation of the small bowel can be achieved in one of two ways. Either the barium is taken orally and followed as it moves through the small intestine, or a catheter is placed in the upper jejunum and barium is administered direct. The latter approach will give better imaging but is more invasive.

Barium enema
The main indications for a barium enema are:

- a recent change in bowel habit
- to delineate the extent of suspected inflammatory bowel disease
- unexplained iron-deficiency anaemia
- rectal bleeding.

A significant proportion of barium enemas fail to exclude pathology because of poor bowel preparation. This requires strong laxatives and some patients find it unpleasant. Many old people are unable to retain the enema. The alternative investigation is colonoscopy (see below), but this has similar drawbacks.

CT scanning

CT imaging is useful in suspected hepatobiliary or pancreatic disease; in most centres, ultrasound is the first investigation. CT scanning can be used to guide biopsy. Contrast media can outline the GI tract.

Endoscopy

Many hospitals offer open-access endoscopy, so you must know its indications and limitations. Detailed discussion of the different types of endoscopy are with the relevant GI problems.

Laparoscopy

In place of the laparotomy, which is a major surgical procedure, suspected GI pathology is increasingly investigated using a laparoscope. Insufflation of the peritoneal cavity with carbon dioxide is required. This means that, like instrumentation of the biliary tree or laparotomy, gas may be seen subsequently on plain radiographs.

Ultrasound

Ultrasound scanning is a central investigation of GI (intra-abdominal) disease. Like CT imaging, it is particularly useful in hepatobiliary or pancreatic disease, but there is interest in its role in bowel disease. Ultrasonography is dependent on the experience of the operator and the clinical information given to them. The latter allows the operator to direct the examination to the appropriate area and to give a more definite report as to the likelihood of disease being present.

Biopsy

A key investigation may be histological examination or culture. For example, in gastric disease, culture of *Helicobacter pylori* is important, particularly in those with relapsing peptic ulceration. Histological examination is required in gastric ulcers to exclude an adenocarcinoma. In other parts of the bowel, biopsy is essential, for example in coeliac or inflammatory bowel disease. A biopsy is often taken using ultrasound or CT guidance. Alternatively, direct endoscopic visualisation may be preferable.

3.2 The oesophagus

Learning objectives

You should:
- be able to use an understanding of oesophageal pathophysiology in assessing a patient with one or more of the three common symptoms
- able to construct a differential diagnosis
- able to plan investigation and management.

The major symptoms of oesophageal disease are:

- dysphagia
- heartburn
- painful swallowing: this is unusual and is linked to infections such as candidiasis or herpes simplex.

Disorders of motility

Normal motility

The function of the oesophagus is to convey food from the pharynx to the stomach. There are two muscular layers, circular and longitudinal, with a gradual transition from striated to smooth muscle. Normally, there is a resting tone in the lower pharyngeal constrictor muscles producing an upper oesophageal sphincter; similarly, there is a lower oesophageal sphincter preventing reflux of stomach contents. When swallowing is initiated, a **primary peristaltic wave** causes relaxation of the upper sphincter and a coordinated wave of contraction moving the bolus of food down to the lower sphincter, which relaxes and allows passage into the stomach. Secondary peristaltic waves strip the oesophagus of any residual foodstuffs.

Achalasia

Rarely, the ganglionic cells controlling the coordinated peristalsis and the relaxation of the lower oesophagus degenerate, causing achalasia. The person presents with progressive dysphagia with regurgitation of undigested food several hours after eating. Recurrent aspiration pneumonias occur. Plain chest radiography may show a fluid level behind the heart. On a barium swallow, there is a mega-oesophagus with a smooth outline tapering down to the lower oesophageal sphincter.

Other disorders of motility

In older people, spasm of the oesophagus causes chest pain that may mimic angina. A barium swallow may show a *corkscrew* oesophagus and manometric recordings demonstrate the disordered motility. The difficulty is these features may be present without symptoms, and in symptomatic patients, the relationship may not be causal. Treatment is with nitrates and calcium antagonists, which relax smooth muscle.

In systemic sclerosis (p. 312), there is commonly gross disturbance of oesophageal motility, which may produce dysphagia and heartburn. Occasionally, an autonomic neuropathy (diabetes mellitus) may affect the oesophagus.

Hiatus hernia and oesophagitis

Clinical presentation

A sliding hiatus hernia is increasingly common with age. Much more rare is the rolling hiatus hernia, in which the stomach rolls up into the chest cavity alongside the oesophagus. In a sliding hiatus hernia, reflux causes the problems. The person may be obese and the symptoms may be worsened by substances that relax the lower oesophageal sphincter, such as alcohol. Similarly, the hormonal changes of pregnancy may precipitate severe heartburn. If the symptoms are long-standing, then it is reasonable to assume that they are caused by reflux oesophagitis, but recent onset in a middle-aged or older person is treated as suspicious.

Occasionally, reflux oesophagitis presents with a haematemesis or anaemia. Again, be wary of assuming that the cause of an iron-deficiency anaemia is a mild oesophagitis, thereby missing a large bowel carcinoma.

Investigation

Often no investigation is required, providing the probability of other causes is low. A full blood count will show any anaemia. A barium swallow will demonstrate a hiatus hernia, but this does not prove causation. Some mucosal irregularity may help to confirm the presence of oesophagitis. The investigation of choice is endoscopy, which allows direct visualisation of the oesophagus and biopsy of any suspicious area.

Management

There are three steps in management:

- symptomatic relief
- reducing acid to promote healing
- increasing lower oesophageal sphincter tone and gastric emptying.

For many people, a simple antacid such as Gaviscon will suffice, together with advice about weight loss and avoiding tight clothing or excessive bending. Coupled with this, in more severe cases, you should advise patients to sleep with the head of the bed elevated or propped up.

In patients with marked oesophagitis with severe symptoms, acid secretion should be reduced. A histamine receptor (H_2) blocker such as cimetidine or ranitidine will produce healing in about 50% of people. A proton pump inhibitor such as omeprazole will cause almost immediate relief in virtually all patients, together with quick healing.

In the long term, if the simple measures described above do not suffice, prokinetic agents such as domperidone (a peripheral dopamine antagonist) or cisapride will help to prevent recurrence. It is rare that patients with reflux require surgery.

Complications

There are two long-term complications of reflux that you should be aware of.

Strictures. The years of inflammation from reflux can produce scarring and constriction at the lower end of the oesophagus. Patients present with increasing dysphagia, poor nutrition and aspiration pneumonia. Endoscopy is mandatory to exclude malignancy and is therapeutic as dilatation produces dramatic relief. The stricture tends to recur, but can be mediated.

Metaplasia. The other consequence of long-term inflammation is metaplasia of the epithelium. Normally, the oesophagus is lined with stratified squamous epithelium, but there may be change in the lower part over a variable length into columnar epithelium (**Barrett's oesophagus**). This is premalignant and repeated surveillance endoscopy may be required.

Oesophageal carcinoma

Most cases of oesophageal carcinoma occur in the middle and lower third of the oesophagus and are squamous cell carcinomas with varying degrees of differentiation. Most cases occur in the sixth and seventh decades of life. The incidence shows considerable worldwide variation. In the UK, the main associations are with smoking and heavy alcohol intake. *Barrett's oesophagus* (see above) is premalignant for adenocarcinoma.

Clinical presentation

Any middle-aged or elderly person with progressive dysphagia may have carcinoma of the oesophagus. Sometimes, people develop retrosternal pain as a result of local infiltration and may have a haematemesis or anaemia. You must enquire about general well-being and any weight loss. Eventually, aphagia occurs both for solids and liquids, with a high probability of aspiration pneumonia. On examination, you may find some enlargement of the cervical lymph nodes and hepatomegaly.

Investigation

Basic investigations may show an iron-deficiency anaemia, a high alkaline phosphatase indicative of hepatic metastases and, on a chest radiograph, involvement of the hilar nodes. In a severely malnourished and water-depleted patient, hypoproteinaemia, high urea and hypernatraemia may occur.

A barium swallow will show the level of the lesion and, characteristically, the stricture is irregular in outline. Sometimes the carcinoma is ulcerated or polypoid. Endoscopy allows direct visualisation with biopsy. An ultrasound scan of the liver will demonstrate hepatic metastases. If curative surgery is being contemplated, CT or MR scanning will show the extent of any spread.

Management

Initially, management is directed towards adequate hydration and improving the patient's nutritional state. Overall, the long-term prognosis is very poor with less than 5% of people surviving 5 years. In the lower part of the oesophagus, curative surgery is sometimes attempted. In the upper part, radiotherapy is used. Survival may be improved by combining radiotherapy and chemotherapy, sometimes to reduce tumour bulk as a prelude to surgery.

Often, the only approach is palliation, in which the major aim is to preserve swallowing. Laser therapy can be used for debulking, and radiotherapy may be useful.

Stents may be inserted endoscopically to protect the lumen. Alternatively, if the lumen cannot be opened or if the patient is finding it difficult to sustain eating and drinking, a percutaneous endoscopic gastrostomy (PEG) tube may be inserted.

3.3 The stomach and duodenum

Normal structure and function

The stomach has three functions:

- acting as a reservoir, mixing the food and passing it into the duodenum in small volumes
- secreting acid and pepsinogen to aid digestion
- secreting intrinsic factor for B_{12} absorption.

Food is passed down into the 'C' shaped duodenum, in the second part of which there is the **ampulla of Vater** with opening of the pancreatic and common bile ducts.

The stomach consists of three parts: the fundus, the body and the antrum, which extends into the pylorus. There are waves of muscular contraction that aid in mixing food and moving it down towards the pylorus. The pylorus (hypertrophy of the circular muscle layer) acts as a sphincter governing passage of food into the duodenum.

The upper two-thirds of the stomach contains parietal cells, which secrete acid, and chief cells, secreting pepsinogen. The antrum contains mucus-secreting cells and G cells producing gastrin. Acid secretion is under neural (vagal) and hormonal (gastrin — stimulatory; VIP, somatostatin — inhibitory) control. Common to both is the release of histamine, which stimulates hydrogen ion production and secretion. The sites of action of inhibitory drugs are shown in Figure 20.

Gastritis

Gastritis can be divided into acute and chronic forms.

The presentations of acute gastritis are:

- dyspepsia
- bleeding from acute mucosal ulceration (occasionally)
- as an incidental finding at endoscopy.

Acute gastritis is associated with NSAID ingestion (including aspirin) and heavy alcohol (binge) drinking. Very sick patients in intensive care can develop acute ulceration with bleeding. This relates to disturbance in gastric blood flow.

Chronic gastritis is seen in association with *H. pylori* infection (see below), chemical irritation (for example bile reflux) or as an autoimmune response. In the last, antibodies are directed against gastric parietal cells and intrinsic factor, which may produce pernicious anaemia. There are different histopathological stages that may culminate in atrophic gastritis. If this occurs,

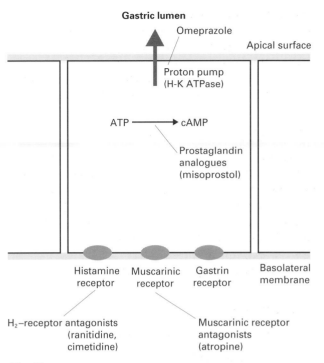

Fig. 20
The sites of action of drugs that inhibit hydrogen ion secretion by a gastric parietal cell.

premalignant changes may be found, with an increased risk of gastric carcinoma.

Most cases of acute gastritis respond to simple antacids and removal of the cause. Sometimes, in both acute and chronic gastritis, H_2-receptor antagonists can alleviate dyspepsia.

Peptic ulcer

Peptic ulceration is a common disease, affecting approximately 1 in 6 people in the UK at some time, with increasing incidence with age. It shows considerable worldwide variation. It is more common in men. Associated factors are smoking, ingestion of NSAIDs, hyperparathyroidism and blood group O as well as *H. pylori* infection.

Pathogenesis

The mechanisms leading to a peptic ulcer include:

- factors acting against the mucosal barrier — acid secretion
- Factors weakening the mucosal barrier — composition of the mucus, impaired production of prostaglandins, *H. pylori* infection and reduced blood flow (acute).

You should not simply consider excess acid secretion; most people with a gastric ulcer have normal or low acid secretion. In duodenal ulceration, many people are hypersecretors, but other factors play a role (e.g. *H. pylori* infection). Rarely ulcers are associated with the

Zollinger–Ellison sydrome: a pancreatic tumour producing large quantities of gastrin.

Clinical presentation

Patients may present with 'indigestion'. You should always explore what is meant by this, rather than simply translating it into dyspepsia. The pain is usually in the epigastrium and can be described as a gnawing or a hunger pain. It may come on several hours after eating or wake the person during the night. Eating may relieve the pain. You must enquire about *periodicity*, that is the pain will be present (not continously) over a few months/weeks and then subsides, before returning after an interval. You should always ask about smoking/alcohol and NSAID ingestion.

Frequently, the ulcer will present with a complication, particularly in older people when the resulting mortality may be high. Complications are:

- a perforation causing peritonitis and shock; corticosteroid therapy may mask these signs
- GI haemorrhage, causing either a haematemesis or melaena (see below)
- anaemia: either symptomatic or diagnosed on a full blood count
- outflow tract obstruction resulting from severe scarring of the pylorus. Rarely seen now, the history is of repeated vomiting over several months, weight loss and severe electrolyte and fluid disturbance.

Investigation

You should always request full blood count and, if abnormal, measure iron status. In all emergency patients with upper abdominal pain, you should request serum amylase estimation. An ECG may be needed if there is a possibility of a myocardial infarction. If the patient has been compromised by severe vomiting, you should check urea and electrolytes.

Your aim is to confirm the suspected diagnosis. A good quality barium meal may be all that is required, but biopsy is necessary in a gastric ulcer. Endoscopy will allow this, as well as visualising the source of any bleeding and enabling specimens to be taken for culture of *H. pylori*. A repeat endoscopy (or barium meal) may be needed to assess response to therapy, diagnose relapse or confirm healing — particularly in gastric ulcers.

Management

Patients should be advised on smoking and alcohol ingestion. The necessity of continuing with NSAID therapy should be carefully considered. Many patients can be switched to simple analgesics. Some people will need a course of iron supplements, others may need antimicrobials for *H. pylori* (see below).

The need for surgery has dropped dramatically since the introduction of the H_2-antagonists and the subsequent development of the proton pump inhibitors. The main indication for surgery is management of complications, particularly perforation and the rare outflow tract obstruction. Occasionally, surgery is required in patients who continue to have severe haemorrhage.

Specific drug therapy

Antacids

Antacids are often used by people with intermittent mild dyspepsia. It is often worth enquiring about use of 'white medicines', as this may give you a clearer idea of a longer-term problem. Antacids give symptomatic relief but have no role in healing or prophylaxis.

The H_2-receptor antagonists

The mainstay of therapy is an antagonist that acts at the histamine H_2-receptor, e.g. cimetidine or ranitidine. These can be given in divided doses, though a single dose at night may be preferable in suppressing nocturnal acid secretion. Their main uses are:

- *healing proven peptic ulcers:* very effective in duodenal ulcers, less with gastric ulcers
- *chronic therapy to prevent relapse:* moderately effective
- *chronic non-ulcer dyspepsia:* some use
- *severe oesophagitis:* heal about half of cases
- prevention of ulceration in patients who need NSAIDs: a limited role.

The H_2-receptor antagonists have no effect on the outcome from acute bleeding.

All of the H_2-receptor antagonists are well tolerated, with no proven long-term problems. You should be aware of some of the side-effects and potential drug interactions specific to cimetidine. It is an enzyme inhibitor at the cytochrome P450 system, which is a heterogeneous group of enzymes involved in the metabolism of many drugs. Cimetidine significantly inhibits the metabolism of *phenytoin, warfarin* and *theophylline*. Toxic effects may appear and the drug dosage reduced. Cimetidine has some antiandrogenic effects, with gynaecomastia and loss of libido.

Proton pump inhibitors

Omeprazole is well tolerated, has a long half-life (once-daily dosage) and no major side-effects. It will heal almost all cases of reflux (cf. 50% success with H_2-antagonists). In peptic ulceration, most patients are symptom-free within a couple of weeks and healed by 1 month. There is a risk of relapse once therapy is discontinued.

Prostaglandin analogues

Misoprostol is an analogue of prostaglandin E_2; it acts by reducing gastrin and acid secretion as well as by promoting the mucosal barrier. The main side-effect is diarrhoea. It can be used as prophylaxis against gastric damage by NSAIDs, but the first consideration is to stop these if possible.

Drugs acting on the mucosal barrier

Sulcralfate is occasionally used as it helps to preserve the mucosal barrier. It is a complex of aluminium hydroxide and sucrose. The main side-effect is constipation.

Bismuth also promotes the mucosal barrier and is bactericidal with antibiotics for *H. pylori* infection. It causes an unpleasant taste and constipation.

Helicobacter pylori

The link between *H. pylori* and gastroduodenal disease is important not simply because of understanding the basic mechanisms, but also for choice of therapy.

Many people are infected with *H. pylori* and more than half the population over the age of 50 have evidence of gastritis. However, in the absence of peptic ulceration, you should not try to eradicate the organism, unless on specialist advice.

Antimicrobial therapy may be used in peptic ulceration. Currently, many units do not routinely culture for *H. pylori* in patients presenting for the first time, but do so when the ulcer fails to heal or recurs. There are also diagnostic serum antibody tests available. The management is a combination of a specific antiulcer drug together with one or more antimicrobials. A reasonable management is triple therapy with bismuth, metronidazole and tetracycline. Alternatively, a combination of omeprazole and amoxycillin may be used.

In addition to the proven association with peptic ulcer disease, there may be links between *H. pylori* infection and development of gastric carcinoma and lymphoma.

Gastrointestinal bleeding

Learning objective

- You must be able to assess a patient, arrange the appropriate investigations and construct a suitable management plan; all of these may require consultation with senior staff.

Acute bleeding

Acute GI bleeding can present with haematemesis, coffee ground vomiting, or melaena. The causes of an acute bleed are shown in Figure 21. Most cases result from peptic ulceration or duodenitis/gastritis, but other possible causes may be suggested by the history or examination, e.g. *a Mallory–Weiss tear* or *varices* (p. 132).

The management of severe haematemesis is shown in the box. Mortality from acute GI haemorrhage is increased with:

- age (> 65 years)
- hypotension
- pre-existing anaemia.

> **Emergency treatment: management of severe haematemesis**
>
> *Put on latex gloves (as the patient may have hepatitis B or C or HIV)*
>
> 1. Assess for hypovolaemia: BP, heart rate, peripheral perfusion
> 2. Establish venous access, preferably into a large central vein with large bore cannula
> 3. Take blood for urgent cross-match (8 units whole blood)
> 4. Give a plasma expander such as gelofusin or haemacell rapidly
> 5. Ask for senior help urgently
> 6. If possible, give high inspired oxygen concentration
> 7. Gather information (from patient, carer, ambulance personnel, etc.) for cause
> 8. Examine patient: cause, other problems (e.g. ascites)
> 9. If delay in cross-match, consider transfusing O negative blood (universal donor)
> 10. Take blood for:
>   - haemoglobin (possibly pre-existent anaemia)
>   - clotting (bleeding diathesis)
>   - urea and electrolytes (renal function)
>   - blood gases in severely shocked patients.

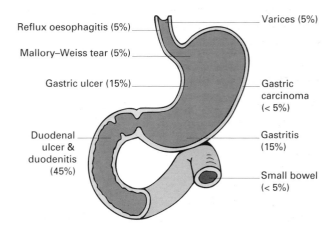

Fig. 21
The sites and frequencies of upper GI tract bleeding, together with frequencies.

The surgical team on call should be informed of the admission of a patient with severe acute bleeding. This allows time for assessment and intervention before the patient becomes moribund.

Most patients should have an endoscopy on the next available list, preferably the day following admission. If the haemoglobin is < 10 g/dl, a transfusion should be started. One unit of blood will raise the haemoglobin by approximately 1 g/dl. If the patient is not anaemic, the haemoglobin should be repeated as haemodilution takes place over the following 48 hours. Renal function should be monitored. All patients with haematemesis should receive iron therapy to replenish the iron stores.

The ongoing management is dependent on the cause and is discussed in the relevant sections. Investigation and management of chronic iron-deficiency anaemia is discussed on page 232.

Gastric tumours

Most gastric tumours are malignant. Occasionally, smooth muscle benign tumours are found (leiomyoma). A small proportion of malignant tumours are lymphomas (< 5%) and these carry a better prognosis. Most gastric tumours are adenocarcinoma.

Adenocarcinoma

The incidence of gastric adenocarcinomas is falling but is still high in the UK. It is more common in men. The tumours are associated with chronic atrophic gastritis and pernicious anaemia.

Presentation
Most tumours present late, commonly with epigastric pain, anorexia and weight loss. The pain can be indistinguishable from that of a peptic ulcer. They often bleed, leading to an iron-deficiency anaemia and, occasionally, a brisk haematemesis. Sometimes, the presentation is with metastatic disease: enlarged lymph node on the left side of the neck (Virchow's node), ascites, hepatomegaly, and bone or brain metastases. Non-metastatic manifestations (paraneoplastic syndromes) are seen, e.g. thrombophlebitis migrans or thromboembolic disease. The cachexia may be striking. Lymphadenopathy may be present and, in the abdomen, an epigastric mass is common. Other findings may be irregular hepatomegaly and ascites.

Investigation
Adenocarcinomas commonly arise in the antrum and may cause outlet obstruction. They often take the form of an ulcer with raised edges, but sometimes they are polypoid and occasionally may be diffusely infiltrative, producing **linitis plastica**.

Endoscopy is the diagnostic investigation of choice, allowing direct visualisation and biopsy. Sometimes the biopsies, may be negative and may have to be repeated. A barium meal, can give high diagnostic probability but cannot provide histopathological confirmation. It is the better investigation in diffuse infiltrating carcinoma as it will demonstrate the shrunken, non-relaxing stomach.

A full blood count should be requested and a chest radiograph and liver function tests (metastatic disease). If curative resection is being considered, further staging with ultrasound and CT scanning will be done.

Management
Because of the late presentation, curative resection is not possible for most tumours. Of all patients with gastric carcinoma, around 10% will survive 5 years. Early diagnosis and resection of mucosa and submucosal tumours may be curative, but few in the UK are identified early. There is no definite evidence that chemotherapy or other treatment modalities offer a great deal. A palliative resection with bypass may be feasible.

3.4 The small intestine

Learning objectives

You should:
- understand the interrelationship between the structure and function of the small intestine, which is the key to the common symptoms
- know about the common disease processes affecting the small intestine and how these affect the normal structure and function.

Small intestinal disease should be considered in any person with one or more of:

- weight loss
- nutritional deficiencies
- abdominal pain
- diarrhoea including steatorrhoea.

Normal function

The prime functions of the small intestine are to break down and absorb nutrients. It also provides a barrier against noxious agents.

Motility
Peristaltic action (controlled by the innervation of the bowel and gut hormones) continues the mixing of food started by the stomach and moves the contents through the small bowel, allowing absorption along its length.

Disruption of peristalsis can lead to stasis (permitting bacterial overgrowth), ileus (e.g. postoperative) or colicky pain (e.g. obstruction). The prime innervation of the gut is through the parasympathetic system, and gut motility is affected by commonly used drugs. For example, tricyclic antidepressant drugs have an anticholinergic effect and cause troublesome constipation. Ask about drugs in any patient with a disturbed bowel habit.

Secretion and breakdown
Coordinated with the movement of food through the small intestine is the secretion of bile, and of fluids from the pancreas and intestinal mucosa. The secreted fluids:

- manipulate the pH: high bicarbonate concentration. Excess loss of small intestinal fluid (e.g. fistula) may cause a metabolic acidosis
- produce a semi-liquid to facilitate the digestive process. This means that a total of 8l has to be

(re)absorbed by the small intestine every day. Interference with this results in watery diarrhoea

- break down and absorb fat, by the action of lipase (pancreas) and by the formation of micelles (bile); lipase deficiency may result in steatorrhoea
- digest protein through the action of proteolytic enzymes; pancreatic disease may cause protein malnutrition
- break down carbohydrates through a combination of pancreatic amylase and oligo/disaccharidases.

Absorption

The small intestine has a very large surface area in contact with the bowel contents, which facilitates transport. The mucosa is folded and there are projections of villi, each of which are covered by microvilli. Within the core of the villi are capillaries and lymphatic channels. The absorptive columnar epithelial cells are formed at the base of the villi and migrate to the top before being shed. The turnover time is 3–4 days and accounts for the sensitivity of the gut mucosa to antimitotic drugs or radiotherapy.

Absorption takes place through three mechanisms:

- passive diffusion, dependent on concentration gradients
- active transport, requiring a carrier protein and energy
- facilitated transport, requiring a specific mechanism but with no energy requirements.

Glucose absorption is linked to sodium transport into the intestinal lumen. There are specific transport systems for different classes of amino acids. Fat is more complicated, with breakdown into monoglycerides and fatty acids and formation with bile salts into micelles. The fat products are absorbed across the the cell and, after re-esterification, triglycerides, cholesterol and phospholipids are incorporated into chylomicrons for transport in the lymph.

Other than the major nutrients, the small intestine absorbs water, fat-soluble vitamins, essential metals and trace elements. Calcium, iron and folic acid are absorbed in the duodenum and upper jejunum, whilst vitamin B_{12} and bile salts are absorbed in the terminal ileum. All other nutrients are absorbed throughout the length of the small intestine. Damage to the mucosa may grossly impair the absorptive capacity of the gut and lead to global malnutrition or to particular deficiencies.

Defence

The intestinal mucosa forms a barrier to potential harm from a large range of different antigens. Lymphoid tissue is present throughout the small intestine (GALT: gut associated lymphoid tissue) and is either scattered or aggregated (**Peyer's patches**). There are mechanisms whereby antigens can be recognised and lymphocytes either sensitised or activated. Secretory IgA is an important element in defence (p. 333).

Malabsorption

Coeliac disease

Coeliac disease is also known as gluten-sensitive enteropathy (better description) and non-tropical sprue.

Aetiology and epidemiology

Coeliac disease is caused by sensitivity to the protein gluten, which is contained in wheat. Gluten is split into a number of peptides of which α-gliadin is the main antigenic component.

Geographically, there is a wide variation in prevalence. An association with antigens HLA-B8 and DRW3 is seen. A bimodal age-related incidence exists, with peaks in young children and in the third and fourth decade of life, but people present at any age and it should be considered in anyone with malabsorption.

Pathological features

The dominant problem is villous atropy. Alongside this, there is a thickening of the mucosa and a chronic inflammatory cell infiltrate with a predominance of T lymphocytes. The disease tends to be most severe in the proximal small bowel, less so in the terminal ileum.

Clinical features

The dominant features are simply those of malabsorption rather than any specific pointers to coeliac disease. You may find evidence of bowel problems (abdominal distension, diarrhoea) or nutritional deficiencies (weight loss, oedema). There is an association with a rare condition called **dermatitis herpetiformis**, which is an intensely pruritic, vesicular skin eruption.

Investigation

Weight. The most important initial task is to record the weight of the patient.

Haematology. Most patients will have anaemia. Both folate and iron deficiency occur so the picture may be dimorphic, meaning that some red blood cells are microcytic and some are macrocytic. Vitamin B_{12} deficiency is less common, as the terminal ileum tends to be relatively spared.

Biochemistry. The patient may have marked hypoproteinaemia and hypoalbuminaemia.

Tests of malabsorption. Although many tests of malabsorption are described, they are difficult to perform with an acceptable degree of diagnostic accuracy and are not of great help in most patients with possible malabsorption.

Jejunal biopsy. If coeliac disease is suspected, a jejunal biopsy should be arranged. The characteristic features of villous atrophy will be seen, and, when on a gluten-free diet, the changes will resolve.

Management

The main treatment is a gluten-free diet. The dietician will advise the patient on this, but you need to support the patient as the changes in lifestyle enforced by a strict diet may cause difficulties. Often young people will be reasonably well on a low-gluten rather than a gluten-free diet. Dietary supplements may be required in the initial stages of treatment to replenish stores. The disease activity should be monitored by general wellbeing, weight, basic haematology and biochemistry.

There is a small risk of lymphoma.

Blind loop/bacterial overgrowth

Malabsorption caused by bacterial overgrowth occurs by an entirely different mechanism to coeliac disease. Normally, the upper small intestine is almost sterile because of its high acidity. Bacterial counts increase through its length, with a faecal pattern in the terminal ileum. If structural integrity is disturbed or motility is impaired, bacteria can multiply. This occurs in:

- surgery: 'blind loops'
- multiple diverticula
- disturbed motility: autonomic neuropathy (diabetes), systemic sclerosis
- achlorhydria: colonisation of the upper small intestine.

The bacteria may cause some mucosal damage, but the main effects are in cleaving conjugated bile salts (interfering with fat absorption) and metabolising B_{12} and impairing its binding to intrinsic factor. Folate may be produced, so blood levels are usually normal.

From the above, you can predict that the main clinical features are:

- steatorrhoea
- diarrhoea
- vitamin B_{12} deficiency (usually mild, no neurological features).

You should consider bacterial overgrowth in any patient with the above symptoms/signs who has a history suggestive of a predisposing factor.

Investigation

[^{14}C]-Glycocholate breath test. [^{14}C]-labelled bile salts are given orally. Deconjugation by the bacteria releases [^{14}C]-glycine, which is measured through its breakdown into [^{14}C]-carbon dioxide in the small intestine. In healthy people, this occurs in the large intestine much later, so the important feature is the *timing* of the [^{14}C]-carbon dioxide peak.

Hydrogen breath test. Oral lactulose is degraded by the bacteria, releasing hydrogen. As with the [^{14}C]-bile salt test, breakdown occurs in healthy people, but in the large intestine. An early rise of hydrogen in the breath indicates production in the jejunum.

Management

The first aims in management are to restore normal bowel function and motility. These may be very difficult to achieve and the mainstay of treatment is the use of broad-spectrum antimicrobials such as metronidazole and tetracycline. Repeated courses may be needed.

Short bowel

Short bowel syndrome is simply a descriptive term implying that a considerable length of the small bowel has been lost and that the remainder is insufficient for digestion and absorption. The most common causes are surgical resection, e.g. in Crohn's disease, and bowel infarction. If the terminal ileum is resected, absorption of vitamin B_{12} is impaired together with the enterohepatic circulation of bile salts. Otherwise, the major problem is global malabsorption. Depending on the length of bowel lost, the person may manage with dietary adjustment and supplementation, otherwise parenteral nutrition is required supervised by a specialist unit.

Food poisoning and intestinal infection

Learning objectives

You should:
- be able to distinguish clinically between predominantly vomiting and predominantly diarrhoeal illnesses and understand the significance of the distinction
- be aware of the many causes of vomiting that are *not* food poisoning
- be able to construct an aetiological differential diagnosis for diarrhoea so as to be able to manage the patient appropriately.
- understand rehydration management

Food poisoning is defined as any disease of an infectious or toxic nature proven or likely to be caused by consumption of food or water. Food poisoning is extremely common, with over 75 000 cases notified annually in the UK. About 10% are acquired abroad. Poor food handling is the reason for most cases. Outbreaks (two or more people) are common.

The clinical presentation can be divided into two groups: predominantly vomiting and predominantly diarrhoea. There is some overlap between the two.

Fever, nausea and vomiting may be the initial features, even though the illness becomes primarily diarrhoea over the next day or two. Consequently, you need to follow the course of the illness over about 24 hours before deciding that the predominant symptom is vomiting. It is exceptionally rare for vomiting to be the predominant symptom of an intestinal infection for more than 48 hours.

Vomiting illnesses

There are many causes of vomiting (p. 102). However, food poisoning is the most common in previously well people, the major causes of which are (with little or no diarrhoea):

- small round structured viruses (SSRVs) including calcivirus, rotavirus and Norwalk viruses
- *Bacillus cereus* toxin
- *Staphylococcus aureus* toxin.

The toxins are produced in food and it is these, rather than the bacteria, that cause vomiting. In most cases of food poisoning, the causative bacteria reproduce in the GI tract, but in *B. cereus* and *S. aureus* food poisoning, bacterial reproduction in the gut is irrelevant.

Clinical presentation

The patient is often doubled over the toilet repeatedly vomiting or lying prostrate in bed. Upper abdominal cramping is severe. Fever is usually absent or low grade. The abdomen is soft and apart from a sinus tachycardia there are usually no abnormal signs. Occasionally, patients will have one or two loose stools, especially if it is caused by an SSRV.

Investigations

The most useful investigation is to send the implicated food (if not all consumed), some vomitus and diarrhoea to the laboratory for toxin and viral analyses. Stool cultures should also be done.

Management

You should admit the patient to hospital for intravenous fluids if the vomiting is severe or diagnosis unclear (possible surgical abdomen, etc.). Otherwise, the patient should be encouraged to drink small volumes of fluids frequently, such as oral rehydration fluid, thin soups and water. You should review the patient again after 12–24 hours if the episode has not resolved.

Diarrhoeal illness

There are many causes of infectious and non-infectious diarrhoea. The challenge is to distinguish one from another, for three primary reasons:

- correct management of the patient
- protection of other patients or family
- for public health reasons

Aetiology

Some diarrhoeal diseases are clinically distinguishable, such as haemorrhagic colitis and cholera. Others are sometimes characteristic, such as giardiasis, amoebic dysentery and *Campylobacter* enteritis. The travel or antibiotic history may be the clue to the diagnosis.

Toxins. Both *B. cereus* and *Clostridium perfringens* produce toxins that cause self-limited diarrhoea for up to 24 hours. The former is often found in cooked, stored rice and the latter in contaminated meat.

Salmonella **spp.** Infection is usually community-acquired, about 10% of cases are contracted abroad and some institutional outbreaks have been reported. Salmonellosis has a short incubation period (12–48 hours). Clinically it is not easily distinguishable from *Shigella* or *Campylobacter* infections. It is invasive and often fatal in elderly people and AIDS patients. It is difficult to eradicate carriage in some people. Carriers are occasionally a source of infection in the community.

Shigella **spp.** *Shigella sonnei* infection is common in the UK. The other three species (*S. dysenteriae*, *S. flexneri* and *S. boydii*) are usually imported. The organism can survive on door and toilet flush handles and is commonly transmitted by children in school or by flies. Excretion in stools is shortened by antibiotic therapy.

Campylobacter **spp.** Infection is common and is often associated with poultry and milk products; infection with campylobacter has a long incubation period (2–5 days). It causes more abdominal pain than other causes of intestinal infection. It is invasive in hypogammaglobulinaemic and AIDS patients.

Traveller's diarrhoea. Often referred to colloquially as 'Delhi belly' or 'Montezuma's revenge', traveller's diarrhoea is common in visitors to the developing world. It is often attributable to enteropathogenic and other *Escherichia coli* isolates. Patients usually have watery, non-bloody diarrhoea without fever; if they have either bloody diarrhoea or fever, an invasive infection (such as *Salmonella*) is more probable. Usually traveller's diarrhoea is self-limiting over 1–5 days. Careful selection of food and drink substantially reduces the risk.

Haemorrhagic colitis. Haemorrhagic colitis is caused by the same toxin-producing *Escherichia coli* as is haemolytic uraemic syndrome (E. coli 0157). It is characterised by sudden onset, extremely bloody diarrhoea, without fever. Person-to-person spread is well documented. Mortality rates are high in elderly people (40%).

Clostridium difficile. *C. difficile* causes a severe form of antibiotic-associated diarrhoea. At its worst, a necrotic membrane overlies the colonic mucosa (pseudomembranous colitis). *Clostridium* spores are acquired from other patients. During or after antibiotic therapy, spores germinate in the gut producing *C. difficile* toxin. The toxin causes a non-bloody, watery diarrhoea in which millions of spore-forming bacteria are found. Patients may be mildly or extremely ill and toxic. Ileus and toxic dilatation of the colon is occasionally seen. Isolation of patients together with restriction of antibiotic prescribing are the keys to controlling an outbreak.

Cholera. Caused by *Vibrio cholerae*, cholera is a rare imported cause of severe watery diarrhoea that can lead to hypovolaemic shock in 12 hours. Fluid requirement in the first 24 hours is typically 30–40L. Special cultures are required in the laboratory for identification.

Viral diarrhoea. Rotavirus infection occasionally affects adults. Stools do not contain blood or white cells. The viruses are spread by fomites (e.g. inanimate objects such as toys or door handles). Other viruses are sometimes implicated.

Entamoeba histolytica. *E. histolytica* causes several infectious syndromes including asymptomatic cyst passage, acute amoebic dysentery, chronic non-dysenteric colitis, amoeboma and amoebic liver abscess (p. 125).

The first two are most common. In amoebic dysentery, blood, mucus and white cells are passed in the stool by a patient who is otherwise not particularly ill. As it may be relatively chronic, it can be mistaken for ulcerative colitis, with fatal consequences if corticosteroids are given. There is an antibody test for amoebiasis. Treatment with metronidazole followed by diloxanide furoate is curative.

Giardia lamblia. G. lamblia is a protozoa that is usually acquired abroad, occasionally in the UK. The typical patient complains of three to five bulky stools a day, pale in colour with much griping abdominal pain and wind. They may lose weight. Symptoms fluctuate. The cysts appear in the stool intermittently, making diagnosis difficult; empirical therapy with metronidazole is warranted. There is a 10% relapse rate.

Other protozoa. Several other protozoa cause diarrhoea, which is usually acute in onset but may become chronic. Almost all patients have a travel history, except those with *Cryptosporidium* diarrhoea, which is often acquired in the UK. Treatment differs depending on the protozoa.

Clinical presentation

The spectrum of illness in infectious diarrhoea ranges from the trivial 'upset stomach' with a few loose stools over 1 to 3 days to the life-threatening. You must distinguish those patients, which can be difficult, particularly in elderly people, who have a higher mortality. You may need to see and examine the patient repeatedly to decide the best course of action.

History. You will find it helpful to consider the following features to arrive at an early presumptive diagnosis (see Table 20).

1. Has the patient been abroad? If so, consider traveller's diarrhoea, amoebic and shigella dysentery and other protozoal causes (e.g. *Giardia, Cyclospora,* etc.).
2. Has the patient been in hospital or a nursing home recently. If so, consider *C. difficile* or *Salmonella.*
3. Is the patient receiving antibiotics or just finished a course? If so, consider *C. difficile.*
4. Is the diarrhoea frankly bloody? If so, consider haemorrhagic colitis, *Shigella* or amoebic dysentery, or ulcerative colitis.
5. Is there some blood in the stool? If so, consider *Salmonella, Campylobacter* and *Shigella* infection and inflammatory bowel disease.
6. Is there any blood in the stool? If not, consider traveller's diarrhoea, cholera, *C. difficile,* viral and protozoal causes.
7. Has the diarrhoeal episode been continuing for more than a week? If so, consider non-infectious causes, giardiasis and other protozoa, *Salmonella* infection and immunodeficiency (AIDS, hypogammaglobulinaemia).

Some infectious diarrhoeal illnesses are related to specific exposures. For example, *Cryptosporidium* diarrhoea is more frequently associated with visits to farms, haemorrhagic colitis with beef products, especially beefburgers, and *Campylobacter* infection with poultry. However, only in the context of an outbreak is it usually possible to ascertain the food or other source reliably.

Pain. Abdominal pain and tenesmus are particularly related to large bowel involvement found in *Campylobacter, Salmonella* and *Shigella* infections. Grumbling mild abdominal pain and chronic diarrhoea is typical of giardiasis.

Table 20 Distinguishing characteristics of the causes of acute intestinal infection

	Salmonella	*Shigella*	*Campylobacter*	Traveller's diarrhoea	Haemorrhagic colitis	*Clostridium difficile*	Viral infection including rotavirus	*Entamoeba histolytica*	Other protozoa*
Blood in stools	−/+	−/++	−/+	−	+++	−	−	++	−
Abdominal pain	++	+	+++	+	+	+	−	+	+/++*
Tenesmus	++	+++	+++	−	++	+	−	++	−
Fever	+++	++	+++	−/+	−	++	−/++	+	−/+
Vomiting	++	++	++	+	+	++	+++	+	+
Acquired in UK	++	++	++	+	++	++	++	−	+/++
White cells in stool	++	+++	+++	+	+	+++	−	−/+	−
Incubation period	12–48hr	12–48hr	2–5 days		3–9 days	N/A		5–14 days	
Requires antibiotic treatment	S	S	S	N	N	Y	N	Y	S

Y, yes; N, no; S, sometimes, depending on condition of patient and/or infecting species
Giardia lamblia, Cryptosporidium parvum, Cyclospora spp., *Isospora belli* and *Blastocystis hominis*

Physical signs. Signs of sodium and water depletion are described on page 170. Common physical signs in acute infectious diarrhoea vary with the organism and the patient:

- fever is typical of *Salmonella*, *Shigella*, *Campylobacter* and *C. difficile* infection (Table 21)
- dehydration (sodium and water depletion) is common if the diarrhoea is severe (e.g. > 10 stools daily) and particularly if associated with vomiting; elderly people are especially prone
- abdominal distension may be mild but if marked could indicate dilatation of the colon. This is seen particularly in *Salmonella*, *Campylobacter* and *C. difficile* infections.

Occasionally, patients are extremely unwell with features of sepsis (e.g. fever, tachycardia, renal impairment) and diarrhoea. They usually have invasive *Salmonella* infections caused by the more virulent species, such as *S. cholerasius* or *S. dublin*. Such patients often develop acute renal failure, shock and may die within 3 or 4 days of first symptoms.

Investigations

Stools should be sent to the laboratory in all cases for (standard) culture, which will yield evidence of infection with *Salmonella*, *Shigella* or *Campylobacter* spp.

- If the stool is bloody, culture for *E. coli* 0157
- if *C. difficile* is a possible diagnosis, request *C. difficile* toxin estimation
- if a viral diarrhoea is possible (no blood, other members of family affected) request virology
- if the stool is not bloody, request ova, cysts and parasites, particularly if the patient has been abroad
- if the stool is bloody and the patient has been abroad, then request a 'hot stool', meaning direct observation of the stool for amoebae, together with standard and *E. coli* cultures.

The white cell count may be elevated in bacterial diarrhoea. Urea, creatinine and electrolytes should be measured in all patients admitted to hospital, to guide intravenous therapy. Stool white cells are helpful in presumptive diagnosis (Table 21). A blood culture is essential in all patients admitted to hospital with diarrhoea, even if afebrile. Abdominal radiographs are not useful unless the abdomen is distended and an alternative (surgical) diagnosis or constipation with overflow is likely.

If stool cultures are negative and diarrhoea continues, sigmoidoscopy and rectal biopsy are indicated to diagnose inflammatory bowel disease (p. 118).

Management

All patients admitted to hospital with diarrhoea must be placed in a single room. The local infectious disease unit should be involved, especially for very ill patients and those from abroad, as the diagnostic capabilities of their laboratories are better and they have much clinical expertise in this area.

Fluid replacement. Dehydrated patients require sodium and water replacement (usually 3–4 litres daily) with either oral or i.v. rehydration solution. Potassium depletion is common and requires replacement. In the acute phase, patients should avoid milk products because of temporary lactase deficiency.

Antidiarrhoeal remedies. These are relatively ineffective and sometimes dangerous. Loperamide is the best, but should be used *only* in patients with traveller's diarrhoea who have no systemic features of illness (e.g. no fever or vomiting) and only for 1 to 2 days. Loperamide should *not* be prescribed for children, elderly people, anyone with either bloody diarrhoea, or a possible alternative diagnosis or moderate to severe diarrhoea (e.g. > six stools daily) as it may lead to toxic dilatation of the colon.

Antimicrobial therapy. Antibiotics are necessary for certain patients only. Table 21 indicates which are

Table 21 Antimicrobial treatment for intestinal infection

Organism/syndrome	Patients that should be treated	Preferred antibiotic
Salmonella spp. } *Campylobacter* spp.	Ill, immunocompromised, extremes of age	Ciprofloxacin
Shigella spp.	All symptomatic	Ciprofloxacin, cotrimoxazole
Escherichia coli 0157	None	–
Traveller's diarrhoea	If desired and therapy available	Ciprofloxacin, loperamide
Clostridium difficile	All symptomatic	Metronidazole (p.o./i.v.), vancomycin (p.o.)
Cholera	All	Tetracycline, ciprofloxacin
Viral	None	–
Entamoeba histolytica	All	Metronidazole, diloxanide furoate (for cyst carriage)
Giardia lamblia	All	Metronidazole, tinidazole
Cryptosporidium parvum	None	–

the preferred agents for which pathogen. Until the pathogen is known, the following groups require empiric antimicrobial therapy, usually with oral or intravenous quinolones (e.g. ciprofloxacin):

- immunocompromised patients
- very ill patients (high fever, frequent stools (e.g. > 10–20 per day), severe dehydration, renal impairment, etc.)
- patients over 60 yearse.

Overall, quinolones shorten diarrhoea by 24 hours. However, in patients with *Salmonella* infection, their use may not prevent longer-term carriage.

Notification

All patients with food poisoning and/or diarrhoea must be notified to the public health authorities even if the cause of the episode is not identified (p. 375).

Tumours

Resected appendixes may contain small carcinoid tumours, which are derived from neuroendocrine cells. Much more rare is the **carcinoid syndrome**, which occurs with extensive liver metastases from an ileal carcinoid tumour. Large amounts of 5-hydroxytryptamine (5-HT) are produced, together with other active substances. Common symptoms are flushing of the upper body, secretory diarrhoea, weight loss and wheezing. Fibrosis of the tricuspid and pulmonary valves may occur. Urinary 5-hydroxyindole acetic acid levels are markedly raised (breakdown product of 5-HT). Treatment is palliative, with the use of 5-HT antagonists and, occasionally, surgical resection/embolisation of metastases.

Inflammatory bowel disease

Crohn's disease is discussed on page 119.

3.5 The large intestine

Learning objectives

You should:
- be able to take an appropriate history from someone with possible bowel disease and construct a differential diagnosis
- be able to target investigations according to the probabilities in the differential diagnosis so as to narrow down or make a definitive diagnosis.

Normal structure and function

The large bowel starts at the caecum and consists of ascending, transverse, descending and sigmoid sections leading into the rectum. There is an inner circular layer

and an incomplete longitudinal layer of smooth muscle. The mucosa is flat, lacking crypts and has a large number of goblet cells.

The blood supply is important when considering sites of ischaemia and possible resection. The superior mesenteric artery supplies the colon to the splenic flexure and the inferior mesenteric artery supplies the descending colon and sigmoid section. The splenic flexure and the sigmoid are more vulnerable to ischaemic colitis (see below).

The prime action of the colon is to reduce the water content of the faeces from approximately 2 litres per day to 150 ml.

Normally the rectum is empty; passage of faeces into it produces the desire to defaecate. The internal sphincter and the puborectalis muscle relax, and the acute angle between the rectum and the anus decreases. Defaecation is produced by voluntary relaxation of the external sphincter and contraction of the abdominal muscles.

Diverticular disease

Diverticula are outpouchings of the colon through the muscle layer, usually at the point of entry of small arteries through the submucosa. The term **diverticulosis** implies no inflammation/infection, whereas **diverticulitis** implies their presence. It is probably better to talk about **diverticular disease**, unless there is definite evidence of an acute problem.

The diverticula are thought to be produced by the high intraluminal pressures forcing the mucosa through weaknesses in the bowel wall. They are more common in countries with a low fibre diet.

The prevalence of diverticular disease increases with age, with most patients over the age of 70 years having diverticula on barium examination. The most common site is the sigmoid colon, but they occur throughout the large bowel.

In most people, diverticular disease is asymptomatic. Some patients experience bouts of constipation and diarrhoea, with left-sided abdominal pain. The differential diagnosis is with colonic carcinoma, which must be actively excluded.

Occasionally, patients present with a infected inflamed diverticulum (abscess). The patient is ill, with left iliac fossa pain and tenderness together with fever and leucocytosis. The diverticulum may perforate, causing faeculent peritonitis, which has a high mortality. Sometimes a fistula is formed with the bladder or vagina.

In acute diverticulitis, blood cultures and an abdominal radiograph (for perforation) should be performed. The management is:

- i.v. broad-spectrum antibiotics. These should cover coliforms (e.g. cefotaxime) and *Bacteroides* spp. (metronidazole)
- i.v. fluids and pain relief
- inform the surgical team.

Sometimes, diverticular disease presents with rectal bleeding, leading to hypovolaemic shock. Mostly, the bleeding stops spontaneously and rarely is surgical resection necessary.

The main management of uncomplicated diverticular disease is reassurance as to the absence of more serious disease and advice on a high-fibre diet.

Irritable bowel syndrome

Functional bowel disorders, including non-ulcer dyspepsia and irritable bowel syndrome (IBS), are very common. There is no clear evidence as to the cause. In IBS, abnormal gut motility and sensitivity to distension may be present. Many patients also have considerable psychological morbidity.

Clinical presentation

In most patients, the history extends over many years. A significant number report recurrent abdominal pain in childhood. Enquire carefully about stresses and psychological disturbances. The story is often one of being relatively symptom-free for long periods interspersed with bouts of symptoms. The abdominal pain varies in site, with the commonest site being in the left iliac fossa, but it can be periumbilical or in the right hypochondrium. Alternating constipation and diarrhoea are common, with tenesmus and feelings of incomplete emptying. The stools are often described as ribbon-like or pellet. Mucus may be passed. There are no abnormal findings on examination other than some tenderness.

Investigation

You should resist ordering a series of investigations in patients whom you strongly suspect of having a functional bowel disorder. Investigate those patients where there are other important features, such as recent foreign travel or:

- onset of symptoms over the age of 40 years
- recent change in symptoms
- other symptoms not usually associated with IBS, such as rectal bleeding or weight loss.

Management

Management of irritable bowel disease is difficult, with symptoms persisting over many years. You should remember that most patients will respond to a placebo. You should be aware of psychological problems and treat depression. The mainstay of therapy has been a high-fibre diet, but many patients are made worse with the addition of bran, whilst only a minority improve. The use of antispasmodics such as mebeverine or peppermint oil may help.

Tumours

Benign tumours (polyps)

Polyps are very common in developed countries. There are different types:

- *metaplastic*: small, associated with regeneration, no malignant potential
- *hamartomatous*: developmental abnormalities. Seen in the **Peutz–Jeugher syndrome** (autosomal dominant inheritance). There is oral mucocutaneous pigmentation and extensive haematomas in the small and, to some extent, the large bowel. No malignant potential
- *adenoma*: malignant potential.

The malignant potential of adenomas rises with increasing size, and it is likely that most colonic carcinomas originate in polyps. Adenomas come in different forms: tubular or villous. The latter occasionally are associated with diarrhoea and loss of potassium. Rarely, multiple adenomas are seen, in familial **polyposis coli** (autosomal dominant).

Most polyps are asymptomatic and only come to light because of a barium enema or colonoscopy carried out for a different reason. Some large polyps may bleed and can cause a chronic iron-deficiency anaemia.

Management

Once identified, all polyps should be removed and sent for histological analysis. Removal can usually be achieved by snaring or diathermy via a colonoscope. Further polyp development is common and repeated surveillance is necessary. The management of polyposis coli is pancolectomy with ileoanal anastomosis.

Malignant tumours

Aetiology and epidemiology

Adenocarcinoma of the rectum/colon is the second commonest cause of cancer death in the UK. It is associated with inflammatory bowel disease, adenomas and polyposis coli (rare). It is thought to be linked to a diet high in animal fat, together with low vegetable fibre.

There is a genetic predisposition. The p53 gene is considered to be central to the development of many tumours. Its role is to prevent *entry* into the S phase of cell replication (DNA replication) until the genetic material has been checked and repaired. If abnormal, then the p53 gene permits the duplication of cells with abnormal genotypes. Very rare syndromes, such as Li–Fraumeni, lead to early development of a wide range of cancers. Much more common is somatic mutation, which is similarly associated with a range of tumours, including colonic carcinoma. Screening programmes for affected families are now in operation. Mutations of p53 protein and allelic loss of chromosome 18q are both associated with a poor prognosis.

Pathology and staging

Most tumours are adenocarcinomas and can be annular (apple core), ulcerative or polypoid (cauliflower) in appearance. The majority are located in the rectum or sigmoid colon. Histological staging according to **Duke's classification** is important for predicting survival:

> Stage A: involves mucosa or submucosa only; 95% 5-year survival
>
> Stage B: tumour has penetrated muscle; 50% 5-year survival
>
> Stage C: lymph node involvement; 25% 5-year survival
>
> Stage D: distant metastases (including liver): very few 5-year survivors.

Clinical presentation

You should consider colonic carcinoma in any person presenting over the age of 40 years with recent onset of symptoms referable to the large bowel. Change in bowel habit is a common symptom, or rectal bleeding with left-sided tumours. Caecal carcinomas are often asymptomatic until late in the disease. These may present with an iron-deficiency anaemia. Occasionally, patients present with a constant pain resulting from anal or sacral invasion; some have colicky pain because of bowel obstruction. If the tumour erodes into the vagina or bladder, then faecal material may be passed, or gas, per urethra. In advanced disease, the presentation may be cachexia, hepatomegaly or ascites.

In any patient suspected of having large bowel pathology, you must perform a rectal examination and arrange a sigmoidoscopy (preferably flexible).

Investigation

Patients may have an iron-deficiency anaemia. In those with hepatic metastases, alkaline phosphatase may be elevated. Your main aims of investigation are to image adequately the large bowel and, where necessary, have a tissue diagnosis. Other than an examination of the rectosigmoid bowel as indicated above, the first investigation is usually a double-contrast barium enema with careful bowel preparation. Where doubt remains, a colonoscopy should be arranged to visualise and biopsy lesions and remove polyps.

Management

The principal management is surgical resection, with preservation of the anus if possible. Sometimes, this is not feasible and a permanent colostomy is fashioned. Survival is related to Duke's staging. Where resection is not possible, a defunctioning colostomy may be indicated. Laser therapy can help in debulking large tumours and preventing/relieving obstruction. The tumours do not respond to radiotherapy. Adjuvant chemotherapy (e.g. 5-fluorouracil) prolongs survival.

Inflammatory bowel disease

Learning objectives

You should:
- know the important differences between ulcerative colitis and Crohn's disease, both in pathology and common clinical patterns/symptoms
- understand which investigations are best to make the diagnosis and assess extent and severity
- be able to discuss with a patient what the diagnosis means, including the long-term future, risks of complications and management
- understand the value of medical and surgical management.

Chronic inflammatory bowel disease can be divided into:

- Crohn's disease, which affects the GI tract anywhere from mouth to anus
- ulcerative colitis, which is confined to the large bowel.

Both are much more common in developed countries and have a peak incidence in young adult life but can occur at any age.

There are many theories about the causation of both conditions, but nothing proven. Environmental factors appear important and disease may be an unusual (immune) response to an infectious agent or some other trigger. There is increasing evidence that Crohn's disease is related to infection by cell wall-deficient mycobacteria.

Pathology

The two diseases are contrasted in Table 22. Crohn's disease characteristically 'skips' lengths of bowel and is patchy. It has a particular tendency to involve the terminal ileum. Ulcerative colitis affects the rectum, spreading up the colon.

Crohn's disease affects all the layers of the bowel, producing thickening and matting. There are deep fissures and ulcers in the mucosa: 'cobblestone' appearance. Apthous ulceration is an early feature. An increase in inflammatory cells and lymphoid hyperplasia are usual and most patients have non-caseating granulomata.

Ulcerative colitis remains confined to the mucosa and submucosa, which is reddened and bleeds readily. There is widespread ulceration with preservation of adjacent mucosa, which has the appearance of polyps (pseudo). In the lamina propria, an inflammatory cell infiltrate is found. Crypt abscesses and goblet cell depletion are usual.

Clinical presentation

The main symptoms are gastrointestinal. Non-GI manifestations are given in Table 23.

Table 22 Histopathological comparison between ulcerative colitis and Crohn's disease

Histological feature	Ulcerative colitis	Crohn's disease
Inflammatory process	Superficial, continuous	Transmural, skip lesions/patchy
Granulomas	Infrequent	Majority
Crypt abscesses	Frequent	Some
Goblet cells	Depleted	Preserved

Table 23 Non-GI complications of inflammatory bowel disease, together with their relative frequency and response to bowel therapy

System	Complication	Crohn's disease	Ulcerative colitis	Response to bowel therapy
Eyes	Uveitis	+	+	Yes
	Episcleritis	+	+	Yes
	Conjunctivitis	+	+	Yes
Skin	Erythema nodosum	++	+	Yes
	Pyoderma gangrenosum	+	+	Yes
Liver	Fatty infiltration	++	++	No
	Pericholangitis	++	++	No
	Sclerosing cholangitis	+	+++	No
	Cirrhosis	+	++	No
Locomotor	Sacroiliitis	+	+	No
	Ankylosing spondylitis	+	+	No
	Peripheral arthropathy	+	+	Yes

Crohn's disease

The main symptoms of Crohn's disease are:

- diarrhoea
- abdominal pain
- constitutional disturbance: weight loss.

The symptoms depend on the parts of the bowel affected. Some patients present with acute disease and others with a chronic problem. For example, anal disease may be the problem, with swelling, skin tags, fistulae or perianal abscesses.

Significant active disease is indicated by:

- weight loss
- general malaise
- loss of appetite
- low-grade fever.

The abdominal pain is variable, but is often colicky. Most patients have diarrhoea and, in colonic disease, this may contain blood. A significant proportion of patients simply have constitutional upset. Others may present with acute right iliac fossa pain, suggestive of appendicitis.

On examination, apart from extra-GI complications (see below) and low weight (always have patients weighed), very few signs may be present. In the mouth, apthous ulcers may be seen. There may be some discomfort on abdominal palpation and, occasionally, there is a right iliac fossa mass or fistulae. You must always examine the anal region.

Ulcerative colitis

In almost all patients, the dominant symptom is diarrhoea mixed with blood and mucus. In acute, severe disease, there is usually constitutional upset. In some patients, the disease is limited to a proctitis with diarrhoea, urgency and tenesmus. The frequency of defaecation, both night and day, can be very debilitating and socially very difficult.

The severity of an acute attack can be assessed by:

- constitutional upset
- stool frequency
- fever and tachycardia
- hypoalbuminaemia, anaemia and high ESR.

A severe attack always requires admission to hospital, given the potential development of toxic dilatation of the colon.

There are few signs in ulcerative colitis. Patients may have some abdominal distension or be tender to palpation. Rectal examination will show blood and mucus. Table 23 lists non-GI complications.

Investigation

The diseases can be distinguished clinically and radiologically to some extent, but histological differences seen on biopsy are important. In some cases, the conditions cannot be separated.

Blood

Using simple blood indices, a measure of disease activity and response to therapy can be achieved. In acute exacerbations, the ESR, plasma viscosity, CRP and other acute-phase reactants (e.g. ferritin) are raised.

Most patients have a normochromic normocytic anaemia, though iron and folate deficiencies should be identified and treated. Although Crohn's disease commonly affects the terminal ileum and vitamin B_{12} levels are low, a megaloblastic anaemia is unusual.

Hypoalbuminaemia is common. Abnormalities of liver enzymes should alert you to the presence of hepatobiliary involvement.

Imaging

Your aims are to:

- diagnose inflammatory bowel disease
- distinguish Crohn's from ulcerative colitis
- estimate the extent of the bowel involvement.

A plain abdominal radiograph may show fluid levels suggestive of bowel obstruction in Crohn's disease or colonic dilatation (toxic) in ulcerative colitis. A small bowel enema is useful in Crohn's disease, demonstrating strictures, proximal bowel dilatation, 'rose-thorn' ulcers and fistulae. The extent of colonic disease is assessed by a barium enema. In Crohn's disease, it will again show deep ulcers and skip areas. In ulcerative colitis, there are loss of haustrations, dilatation and superficial ulceration. The disease is contiguous from the anus. In longstanding disease, the colon is narrow and shortened ('pipestem'). In fistulae (Crohn's disease), contrast media can be used to delineate the tract. Ultrasound or CT scanning may be helpful in showing matted bowel, thickened wall, abscesses or hepatobiliary disease.

Endoscopy allows visualisation and biopsy of the abnormal bowel, particularly of any possibly malignant areas.

Other investigations

Stool cultures and microscopy should always be performed if the patient has diarrhoea. The major differential diagnoses of ulcerative colitis are amoebic and bacillary dysentery. Administration of steroids can be disastrous in these patients. Breath tests can be useful in those patients in whom, because of the damaged small bowel, bacterial overgrowth is suspected. In patients with possible liver disease, ERCP (endoscopic retrograde cholangiopancreatography) and liver biopsy may be helpful.

Management

You need to know about the drugs used in inflammatory bowel disease and have a grasp of the general approach to management, including the use of surgery.

5-Aminosalicylic acid drugs

Sulphasalazine is effective in inducing remission in inflammatory bowel disease and in preventing relapses in ulcerative colitis. The drug consists of sulphapyridine bound to 5-aminosalicylic acid by an azo bond. The linkage is broken in the large intestine and the prime effect is through the unabsorbed (i.e. topical) action of the 5-aminosalicylic acid.

Very little of the drug is absorbed. Toxicity can be severe, particularly in slow acetylators and results from the sulphapyridine moiety. The main side-effects are anorexia, vomiting, headaches and a low mood. A much smaller number develop haemolysis or agranulocytosis.

Newer drugs have been developed that do not contain the sulphonamide component and are probably less toxic. Mesalazine has a resin coat which is pH dependent and releases 5-aminosalicylic acid in the ileum and colon. Olsalazine is two molecules of 5-aminosalicylic acid bound by an azo bond which is cleaved by intestinal bacteria. Alternatively, in colonic disease, 5-aminosalicylic acid enemas may be used.

Corticosteroids

These are of major benefit in inflammatory bowel disease but have long-term side-effects, such as osteoporosis, skin atrophy and cataracts. Corticosteroids can be used orally, or as enemas when the disease is localised to the rectum and sigmoid colon.

Surgery

Surgery has an important role in the management of inflammatory bowel disease. Most patients with Crohn's disease will require bowel resection at some stage. For ulcerative colitis, a pancolectomy with an ileostomy is curative.

For Crohn's disease, the main indications for surgery are:

- failure of medical therapy, with severe ill health
- persistent bowel obstruction or enteric fistulae
- acute perforation/appendicitis
- chronic perirectal infection
- failure to grow in adolescence
- development of malignancy

Given the high probability of recurrence in Crohn's disease, the surgery undertaken should always be the minimum required.

For ulcerative colitis, surgery should be considered in:

- severe colitis that is not controlled by intensive medical therapy
- those with high risk for the development of carcinoma; longstanding (> 10 years) extensive disease
- acute megacolon, perforation or life-threatening bleeding
- unacceptable side-effects from therapy.

Approach to the management of Crohn's disease

You should have some understanding as to how to use the different therapies in Crohn's disease. In acute ileitis, steroids will usually induce a remission. For colitis, these are combined with sulphasalazine. There are *no* proven therapies for maintaining remission.

The bowel complications of Crohn's disease may need specific treatment. Metronidazole may help with fistulae or perianal disease, but some require surgical intervention. Broad-spectrum antibiotics are used in proven bacterial overgrowth.

After bowel resection, or in severe iliitis, the diarrhoea caused by colonic irritation by bile salts can be helped by cholestyramine. Extensive bowel resection may require nutritional supplements, including medium-chain triglycerides and parenteral vitamins (fat-soluble: A, D, E, K and B_{12}). Ultimately, a short-bowel syndrome may result, necessitating total parenteral nutrition.

Approach to the management of ulcerative colitis

In an acute attack, fluid balance must be maintained and the nutritional state monitored; steroids are prescribed. High-dose oral (i.v. in severe attacks) prednisolone and rectal hydrocortisone are used. In mild attacks, sulphasalazine may help. Be alert to the incipient development of perforation or toxic dilatation, which will require surgical intervention.

Maintenance therapy is with sulphasalazine or equivalent. Steroids are not used.

Prognosis

Crohn's disease

Most patients with Crohn's disease will run a relapsing and remitting course and will require surgery at some stage.

Ulcerative colitis

In patients with localised sigmoproctitis, the prognosis is good, with most going on to long-term remission. In fulminant pancolitis, there is a significant mortality and aggressive therapy is required. A minority of patients will require a colectomy.

In ulcerative colitis, extensive disease over several years (> 10 years) is a very high risk factor for the development of malignancy. Furthermore, there is a much higher risk of malignancy with Crohn's disease than indicated by previous estimates. Regular screening by colonoscopy for malignancy in *longstanding inflammatory bowel disease* should be advised.

Other inflammatory bowel disease

Non-specific colitis

In some patients, a local sigmoproctitis develops with troublesome diarrhoea. Sigmoidoscopic appearance is non-specific as is biopsy. An infective cause should always be excluded. Treatment is by steroid enemas.

Ischaemic colitis

In elderly people, colonic ischaemia can occur, particularly around the splenic flexure and the descending colon. The main features are bloody diarrhoea and abdominal pain. A barium enema classically will show 'thumb printing'— indentations of the bowel wall. In most patients, the symptoms resolve spontaneously. Management is to maintain fluid balance and prescribe analgesics.

Radiation colitis

Radiation damage can occur secondarily to therapy directed towards a pelvic tumour. In the acute phase, the patient experiences bloody diarrhoea, tenesmus and abdominal pain. The proctitis can be treated with local steroids. In the late phase, the proctitis may remain troublesome, with bleeding, ulceration and stricture formation.

Bleeding from the lower GI tract

Bleeding from the lower GI tract can be divided into:

- occult: major causes are caecal carcinoma and angiodysplasia (arteriovenous malformations which can be visualised on colonoscopy; this is a relatively common cause of iron-deficiency anaemia in elderly people)
- blood mixed with stool: left-sided colonic tumour, inflammatory bowel disease, diverticular disease, infective colitis and angiodysplasia
- fresh blood in small amounts: haemorrhoids, Crohn's disease of the anus, carcinoma of the rectum
- severe bleeding (rare): diverticular disease and ischaemic colitis.

You can usually narrow the possible diagnoses by a careful history and examination. Thus, carcinoma of the colon is extremely rare under the age of 40 years.

The management of chronic iron-deficiency anaemia is considered on p. 232. Faecal occult blood testing is of very limited benefit in reaching a diagnosis.

3.6 The liver

Learning objectives

You should:
- know the major metabolic functions of the liver and be able to predict the consequences of significant liver dysfunction
- know the anatomy of the liver and its relationship to other organs.

Normal anatomy and function

The liver lies immediately underneath the right diaphragm, with the left lobe of the liver lying underneath the heart and left diaphragm. Inflammatory lesions (such as abscesses) may lead to pulmonary or pericardial disease because of this close proximity.

The liver has two arterial supplies: the hepatic artery, which is a branch of the coeliac axis, and the portal vein, which is formed from the mesenteric vein and the splenic vein. The portal vein drains most of the blood from the GI tract. The venous drainage of the liver passes via a number of hepatic veins into the vena cava.

The liver has five distinct functions:

- it contains the components of the major excretory pathway for many large molecules, producing bilirubin, urea and others
- it synthesises a number of important specialised proteins, including albumin and all clotting factors
- it maintains stable levels of amino acids and glucose in the blood
- it supplies bile salts and bicarbonate to assist in digestion
- it detoxifies many potential toxins and drugs.

Major hepatic dysfunction leads to metabolic derangement and bleeding.

Symptoms of liver disease

Most symptoms of liver disease are indirect and do not immediately focus your attention on the liver. Typical symptoms are:

- anorexia
- fatigue.

Acute liver disease leads to:

- nausea and vomiting
- jaundice
- bleeding (especially nose bleeds and/or GI bleeding)
- encephalopathy (if severe, e.g. liver failure).

Chronic liver disease has a multitude of clinical manifestations, which are described in the relevant sections.

Signs of liver disease

Few signs in *acute* liver disease are specific to the liver. Important signs include:

- jaundice
- hepatomegaly or reduced liver size (as in hyperacute hepatic failure)
- right hypochondrial tenderness
- fever (sometimes).

There are usually no signs associated with mild chronic hepatitis. In contrast, there are a plethora of signs associated with severe chronic liver disease and cirrhosis.

Investigations

Blood tests

Specific tests for liver disease fall essentially into two groups:

- measuring synthetic function (albumin, clotting times, urea and glucose)
- measuring direct liver damage or excretory function (bilirubin, alkaline phosphatase and other hepatic enzymes).

A number of specific tests are used to diagnose particular liver diseases (see below).

You should consider abnormal liver function tests in two broad categories:

- cholestatic (raised alkaline phosphatase and bilirubin)
- hepatocellular (raised transaminases: alanine aminotransferase (ALT) and aspartate aminotransferase (AST), usually with elevated gamma-glutamyl transferase (GGT))

A cholestatic pattern suggests obstructive jaundice or cholangitis (such as sclerosing cholangitis). A hepatocellular pattern suggests direct liver cell damage, as in viral hepatitis, hepatotoxicity from drugs or ischaemia.

Abnormal liver function tests are extremely common in very sick patients. They are probably multifactorial in origin. Mostly, the abnormalities are mild and no action is required. There are five differential diagnoses that you should consider in very ill patients:

- cholestasis caused by sepsis
- ischaemic hepatitis
- acute hepatitis C (p. 127)
- total parenteral nutrition hepatitis
- drug-induced hepatitis (including halothane).

Sometimes, the abnormalities may be part of multiorgan failure, contributing to the patient's death or prolonged recovery.

Imaging

Ultrasound. This is extremely useful for:

- identifying gall stones and the diameter of the common bile duct
- assessing the approximate size of the liver and spleen
- detecting liver or splenic abscesses/masses
- detecting subpleural fluid
- targeting liver biopsy.

Ultrasound is quick, inexpensive and non-invasive. The sensitivity for gall stones or abscesses exceeds 90% but is not 100%; it is relatively poor at identifying pancreatic disease, especially in the body or tail of the pancreas.

CT scan. A CT scan is excellent for visualising liver texture and identifying small abscesses or collections of fluid and pus. It is better than ultrasound for visualising the pancreas and para-aortic nodes.

Biopsy. Often the only way to establish the diagnosis of liver disease is to do a biopsy and examine the tissue histologically. The main indication is chronic hepatitis, but it is also used for staging lymphomas and diagnosing tumours.

Acute liver disease

Learning objectives

You should:
- know the causes of acute liver disease and to be able to initiate appropriate investigations and outline a management plan for the important causes of acute liver disease
- be able to recognise acute liver failure and know the principles of management and determinants of outcome.

Paracetamol poisoning

Most cases of paracetamol poisoning are intentional and a suicide attempt. Normally, paracetamol is easily detoxified by the liver. Excessive doses overwhelm the normal hepatic detoxification system and so a highly reactive metabolite accumulates. This causes liver damage or failure, and occasionally renal failure.

Few symptoms accompany paracetamol poisoning itself. The history may not be forthcoming from the patient.

Investigations

Measurement of serum paracetamol and aspirin levels should be made as soon as possible. In addition, baseline biochemistry (liver function tests, prothrombin time, electrolytes, creatinine and glucose) is important. Consider whether any other drugs have been taken and if appropriate phone the local poisons unit for advice.

Management

If the patient presents to hospital within 4 hours of ingestion and has taken at least 15 tablets (7.5 g) then you should consider a gastric washout.

Three key pieces of information are needed to manage a patient with paracetamol overdose:

- the interval between taking the overdose and presentation
- the plasma concentration of paracetamol
- whether the patient is an alcoholic or taking P450 enzyme inducers (e.g. carbamazepine, phenytoin, rifampicin) as these all increase the amount of reactive metabolite produced.

The administration of i.v. acetylcysteine will reduce liver damage by increasing the amount of glutathione available to counteract the effects of the highly reactive metabolite. The decision to treat is based on the plasma concentration of paracetamol (Fig. 22). Treatment should be started as soon as possible. In patients who present

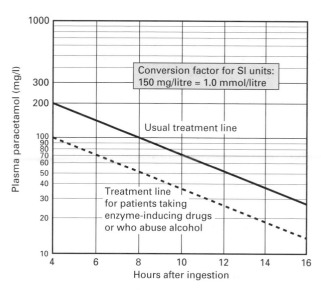

Fig. 22
Treatment graph for paracetamol overdose.

16 hours or more after poisoning, the serum concentration is not a useful guide to the need for treatment. The quantity of paracetamol ingested and whether the patient is developing hepatic encephalopathy are better indicators (see below). The assessment of liver damage can be made by:

- serial INR
- liver enzymes: aspartate transaminase
- plasma paracetamol concentration.

INR (International Normalised Ratio) is a standardised value for the prothrombin time. In severe liver dysfunction, lower levels of clotting proteins are produced and the INR prolonged. Patients who develop hepatic failure should be considered for transplantation.

Hepatotoxicity of other drugs

There are numerous drugs which, rarely, cause liver disease. For example, the antituberculous agents isoniazid and rifampicin may cause severe (fatal) liver damage weeks or months after starting treatment.

Early warning signs of liver toxicity include feeling tired, anorexia and abdominal tenderness (right upper quadrant). Jaundice is a late feature. Any of these features should prompt you to do liver function tests immediately. Drug-induced hepatotoxicity may be cholestatic or hepatocellular. Hepatocellular derangements are usually more life-threatening. If the liver function tests are significantly abnormal, the implicated drugs should be stopped immediately.

Gilbert's syndrome

This is a benign inherited disorder that causes jaundice with no other abnormality of liver function tests. The patient has a partial inability to conjugate bilirubin and so unconjugated hyperbilirubinaemia results, especially when the load is increased during infections, operations, following fasting, etc. The major differential diagnosis is haemolytic jaundice (p. 235).

Alcoholic hepatitis

In contrast to hepatic cirrhosis, alcoholic hepatitis is an acute illness associated with acute or chronic alcohol abuse. Patients present with:

- deep jaundice
- right upper quadrant abdominal pain
- tender hepatomegaly
- fever
- raised white cell count
- elevated prothrombin time.

Sometimes the patients have spider naevi and palmar erythema, suggesting chronic liver disease but they do not usually have cirrhosis. Liver function is somewhat deranged. You can make the diagnosis with a combination of history, physical findings and liver function test abnormalities. The differential diagnoses are:

- extrahepatic obstructive jaundice (e.g. gallstones or pancreatic tumour)
- liver abscess, cholangitis or other infection.

Investigations
Liver function, coagulation tests and full blood count are mandatory. Ultrasound will help exclude other differential diagnoses.

Management
Management is supportive (fluids, nutrition, etc.). Abstinence from alcohol, assuming the patient recovers, is key to long-term survival. Laparotomy and other invasive procedures may lead to early death. The mortality is 30–60%.

Pyogenic liver infection

The broad differential diagnosis of patients with fever and jaundice or substantially abnormal liver function tests (Table 24) other than in the intensive care unit (p. 122), is:

- cholecystitis (p. 134)
- bacterial liver abscess
- cholangitis (p. 135)
- amoebic liver abscess.

Bacterial liver abscess
Bacterial liver abscesses in the Western world are more common than amoebic liver abscesses, whereas the opposite is true in the developing world (Table 25). They are more common in elderly people and the presentation may be subtle. The aetiology is:

- associated with infection of the biliary tree, portal drainage area and local spread from, for example, a subphrenic abscess
- haematogenous spread from other sites, e.g. lungs
- trauma
- cryptogenic (20–30%).

Predisposing factors include diabetes, alcoholism, corticosteroid therapy, malignancy and immune deficiency.

Clinical presentation. The presentation is usually insidious over several weeks. There is usually low-grade fever, raised white cell count and ESR and, sometimes, tender hepatomegaly. Other common features include:

Table 24 Clues to the diagnosis of infections of the liver

	History	Signs	Investigations
Hepatitis A, B, C and E	Epidemiology (see text)	Absence of fever when jaundiced; enlarged diffusely tender liver	Very high AST/ALT, bilirubin normal (or low), white cell count and ESR
Leptospirosis	Water exposure (well, etc.); sewer worker	Cough; fever, bleeding tendency	Renal impairment; proteinuria; raised white cell count; moderately elevated liver function tests
Glandular fever	Typical age group (teenage, early 20s)	Non-tender lymphadenopathy; sore throat; fever	Atypical lymphocytes on blood film; positive Monospot and Paul Bunnell test
Bacterial liver abscess	Older age group; underlying pathology; subacute presentation	Fever (usually); right-sided chest signs	Raised white cell count and ESR; mildly abnormal liver function tests; low albumin; abscess on scan
Amoebic liver abscess	Travel abroad in preceding 3–18 months	Fever; point hepatic tenderness; right-sided chest signs	Raised white cell count and ESR; moderately abnormal liver function tests; large abscesses on scan
Hydatid cyst of liver	Residence in endemic area, e.g. Wales, developing world	Usually none, sometimes hepatomegaly	Normal liver function tests; normal white cell count; cyst on scan with septae and/or calcified rim; no useful serology

AST, aspartate aminotransferase; ALT, alanine aminotransferase; ESR, erythrocyte sedimentation rate.

- right-sided pleural effusion and/or crackles
- ascites
- splenomegaly
- mental confusion.

Jaundice and significant abnormalities of liver function are uncommon unless the disease is associated with another source of infection in the biliary tree.

Management. The number of organisms that cause liver abscesses is large, including anaerobes, *Streptococcus milleri*, and several Gram-negative bacilli. Abscesses are usually polymicrobial. Blood cultures are positive in about 50% of patients but may be so for only one of the organisms involved in the abscess. For this reason, percutaneous aspiration is appropriate to optimise antimicrobial therapy. As much pus as possible should be removed. If the abscess is small, no further action is required other than antibiotic therapy. If the abscess is large, percutaneous drainage may be appropriate. Empirical antibiotics should include:

- pencillin or ampicillin
- metronidazole
- an antibiotic active against Gram-negative bacteria.

Overall mortality is around 10–15%.

Amoebic liver abscess

The typical patient has travelled in the prior few months to an endemic area for *E. histolytica*. The clinical presentation is:

- acute fever
- right upper quadrant abdominal pain of < 10 days
- right shoulder, epigastric or pleuritic pain
- enlarged, painful liver (50% of patients)
- crackles at the right lung base.

Jaundice is *unusual* and indicates severe disease or, more likely, an alternative diagnosis.

Investigation. The key investigations are:

- ultrasound of the liver (which usually reveals one to three abscesses)
- antibody test to *E. histolytica* (positive in 95% of patients).

Other useful indicators of disease include leucocytosis, a high ESR (erythrocyte sedimentation rate) and mild anaemia. Increased levels of alkaline phosphatase and occasionally of the transaminases are found. Chest radiograph will often show elevation of the right diaphragm, sometimes with a pleural effusion. The stools are negative for *E. histolytica*.

Management. Aspiration of the contents of the liver abscess will establish whether it is or is not bacterial in origin. In patients with a positive amoebic serology and the appropriate epidemiologic indicators, you can give empirical therapy without aspiration. Metronidazole in high doses over 10 days is the treatment of choice. It can take 4–7 days for the fever to resolve.

Viral hepatitis

There are many causes of hepatitis, most of which cause jaundice but not all. Some are common (e.g. hepatitis A), others less so, but all are important for management reasons. Clues to the clinical diagnoses are shown in Tables 24 and 25.

Hepatitis A

Hepatitis A causes acute self-limiting hepatitis and is extremely common in all parts of the world except Northern Europe and North America. In developing countries, it typically presents in children. Most adults born in the UK have not been infected and are at risk.

Clinical features. Hepatitis A presents with nonspecific symptoms, such as malaise and weakness, followed by anorexia, which is usually profound, sometimes nausea and vomiting and a vague dull right upper quadrant pain. During this phase, there may be fever although typically there is not. The early symptoms last between 3 and 10 days prior to the onset of jaundice, which is associated with dark-coloured urine. The patient starts to feel better shortly after they become jaundiced, which usually lasts between 2 and 3 weeks, although sometimes less in mild cases. Most patients remain tired for some weeks.

Investigations. Liver function tests are extremely helpful as patients usually have marked elevations of

Table 25 Hepatitis viruses

	A	B	C	E
Transmission	F/O	I/V, vert, horiz, B/T, sexual	I/V, B/T, sexual	F/O
Incubation period (weeks)	3–6	5–26	2–3	4–20
Chronic carriage	N	Y	Y	N
Causes chronic hepatitis	N	Y	Y	N
Causes hepatocellular carcinoma	N	Y	Y	N(?)
Treatment with interferon beneficial	N	Y	Y	N

F/O, faecal/oral: I/V, intravenous drug abuse; vert, mother to child; horiz, sibling to sibling; B/T, blood transfusion; Y, yes; N, no.

aminotransferases and bilirubin, with slight increase in alkaline phosphatase and LDH (lactate dehydrogenase) (see Fig. 23). The white cell count is normal or low and the plasma viscosity or ESR is not elevated. Renal function is normal unless the patient goes into acute liver failure. The INR is typically prolonged, but usually only slightly. Monitoring of aminotransferases and INR is the most helpful guide to progress.

Management. Management consists of bedrest and maintenance of nutrition, if possible. Patients who exercise early after initial recovery are more likely to suffer a relapse of hepatitis. Patients with INRs greater than two should be admitted to hospital. Deteriorating hepatic function, which occurs in about 1 in 2000 patients, is an indication for transfer to a liver transplant unit.

Banning alcohol is only appropriate in alcoholic hepatitis or where alcohol withdrawal would carry other general health benefits for the patient. Once the liver function tests have returned to normal, alcohol may be consumed again.

Hepatitis B

Compared with hepatitis A (Table 25), the incubation period of hepatitis B is much longer. Gay patients and those sharing needles are most at risk. Occasionally the disease is acquired by heterosexual sex, in institutions for the mentally handicapped or during medical procedures.

Symptoms. The presentation is similar to that of hepatitis A, though less acute. There is a slightly greater likelihood of arthritis or rash (a form of serum sickness-like syndrome). The other major distinction between hepatitis A and B is the possibility of carriage and chronic liver disease in patients with hepatitis B (see below).

Investigations. You should do the same investigations you would do for hepatitis A. Also do hepatitis B tests (see Table 26). If there is doubt about the diagnosis, a liver ultrasound is helpful.

Hepatitis B surface antigen (HBsAg) is always positive during the acute phase of hepatitis B (Table 28). The problem can be confirmed as an acute episode of hepatitis B (rather than another form of hepatitis on top of a chronic hepatitis B carriage) using the hepatitis B core IgM test (anti-HBc IgM). This test is only useful in patients who are acutely ill with jaundice or just recovered. The anti-HBc IgG test is used to find out if a patient has ever had hepatitis B.

Management. The management of acute hepatitis B is very similar to that of hepatitis A. Patients with hepatitis B may develop fulminant liver failure as in hepatitis A.

Chronic infection. Patients with hepatitis B need to be followed up to establish whether they have become chronic carriers. The likelihood of a patient who develops jaundice becoming a chronic carrier is substantially

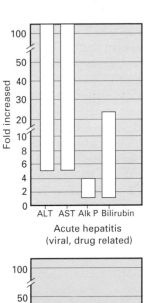

Acute hepatitis
(viral, drug related)

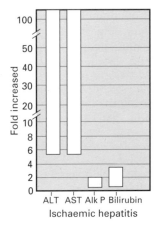

Chronic hepatitis
(viral, idiopathic)

Ischaemic hepatitis

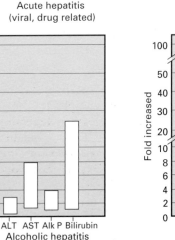

Alcoholic hepatitis

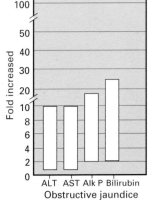

Obstructive jaundice

Fig. 23
Elevation of key serum enzymes and proteins in acute viral hepatitis and other common liver diseases. ALT, alanine aminotransferase; AST, aspartate aminotransferase; Alk P, alkaline phosphatase.

Table 26 Hepatitis B tests

	Interpretation of tests	
	If positive	**If negative**
Surface antigen tests		
Antigen itself (HBsAg)	Acute hepatitis B or carrier	Non-infectious, not acute hepatitis B
Antibody to surface antigen (anti-HBs)	Prior hepatitis B or prior immunisation	Not protected (if immunised)
Core tests		
IgM test (anti-HBc IgM)	Recent acute hepatitis B	No evidence of recent hepatitis B infection
IgG test (anti-HBc IgG)	Hepatitis B infection in past	Never had hepatitis B
e antigen tests		
e antigen itself (HBeAg)	Acute hepatitis B or highly infectious carrier	Not highly infectious
Antibody to e antigen (anti-HBe)	Prior hepatitis B but not highly infectious	Not useful

less than for patients who have 'silent' (anicteric) hepatitis B, which is quite common. If patients remain HBeAg positive they are termed 'supercarriers' because they are so infectious.

Hepatitis C

The presentation of hepatitis C is very similar to that of A and B. It essentially always follows a blood transfusion or sharing of needles. Sexual transmission is uncommon but does occur. Transmission of hepatitis C vertically to neonates is also uncommon (10%).

Symptoms and signs. These are similar to those of hepatitis A and B. Patients are frequently not jaundiced with acute hepatitis C.

Investigations. The same investigations as for hepatitis A and B are required, but serology in hepatitis C is not usually requested unless the patient is negative for A and B. Hepatitis C antibodies are positive during the acute phase and persist for a long time.

Management. The management of acute disease is the same as for hepatitis A and B. Patients may develop acute liver failure. Patients with acute hepatitis C must be followed up to establish whether they become chronic carriers or not (Fig. 24). This requires measurement of liver function tests and hepatitis C RNA in the blood. Patients with circulating hepatitis C RNA are much more likely to get chronic liver disease and are potentially infectious. Patients who are hepatitis C RNA positive or who have hepatitis C antibodies and abnormal liver function tests should be managed as if they have chronic hepatitis (see below).

Acute liver failure

Acute liver failure has three facets:

- encephalopathy
- jaundice
- markers of extreme hepatic malfunction (e.g. prolonged INR).

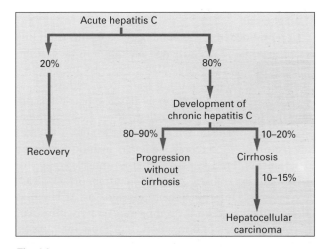

Fig. 24
The course of infection with hepatitis C.

The causes of acute liver failure in patients referred to a liver unit in the UK are:

- paracetamol overdose (55%)
- hepatitis A (5%)
- hepatitis B (10%)
- non-A, non-B hepatitis (20%)
- other causes (10%).

Clinical presentation

There are few physical signs of acute liver failure other than jaundice and encephalopathy. The liver may be so small that there is no overlying dullness to percussion.

Encephalopathy. Encephalopathy may be mild or profound. Conscious level varies from drowsy to unresponsive to pain. There are some distinctive features of hepatic encephalopathy:

- specific cognitive abnormalities
- liver flap
- hepatic foetor (sweet-smelling breath).

If the patient is not unconscious, test for liver flap and specific cognitive abnormalities. Spatial awareness is grossly impaired. Common tests include drawing a five-pointed star and putting the numbers and hands on a clockface. Patients tend to put all the numbers in one or two quadrants.

Investigations

Investigations will include:

- liver function tests (showing high transaminases and bilirubin)
- arterial blood gases (respiratory alkalosis caused by hyperventilation)
- INR (very prolonged)
- blood glucose (usually low)
- serum creatinine (usually elevated)
- blood cultures (Gram-negative sepsis, including cholangitis, is an important differential diagnosis).

Management

Cerebral oedema. Cerebral oedema results from loss of cell membrane integrity and alteration in the permeability of the blood–brain barrier. The very high intracerebral pressures produced lead to a reduction in cerebral perfusion, diffuse cerebral ischaemia and sometimes herniation of the brainstem. Rises in intracranial pressure are often sudden and unpredictable. The clinical features of cerebral oedema include systemic hypertension, bradycardia, increased muscle tone progressing to decerebrate posturing and abnormal pupillary reflexes. Unfortunately, these signs occur late and intervention based on their appearance rarely improves outcome. Intracerebral monitoring of intracranial pressure with a probe is used to guide treatment. Patients should be kept supine. If cerebral oedema is documented clinically or with a probe, mannitol (20%) is given rapidly. Other cerebral oedema-reducing measures such as dexamethasone are not effective.

Coagulopathy. Coagulopathy (as measured by a prolonged INR) results from the reduced synthesis of several clotting factors, though there are more complex events that contribute to bleeding, including reduced platelet function. Fresh frozen plasma should be given if there is bleeding. Vitamin K is of limited value.

Oliguric renal failure. Approximately 50% of patients develop oliguric renal failure, and this worsens the prognosis. This is sometimes called the hepatorenal syndrome. Renal failure may be directly caused by paracetamol overdose, poisoning by other toxins or by leptospirosis.

Hypoxaemia. Hypoxaemia is common and may necessitate ventilation. High inspired oxygen concentrations should be given. Prostacyclin improves peripheral oxygen delivery.

Hypoglycaemia. Hypoglycaemia is common and is related to defective gluconeogenesis as well as high circulating insulin levels resulting from inadequate hepatic uptake. Blood glucose levels should be monitored frequently and 10% glucose administered as appropriate. Hypokalaemia can occur as a result of this and sometimes large amounts of potassium are required to maintain normokalaemia.

Infection. Bacterial and candidal infections are common. Patients have faulty neutrophil function and impaired cell-mediated immunity. Frequent blood and other cultures, with appropriate antibiotic or antifungal therapy, are commonly required.

Outcome of liver failure and transplantation

Liver failure can be divided into three broad categories depending on the interval between the appearance of jaundice and encephalopathy (Table 27). The outcome depends on which group the patient falls into.

Transplantation (p. 342) is particularly indicated for those with acute and subacute liver failure as the prognosis is particularly poor.

Chronic hepatitis

Learning objectives

You must:
- know how chronic hepatitis presents
- know the main causes of chronic hepatitis
- know what to do when arranging a liver biopsy, the precautions to take and its complications
- have a broad framework of appropriate therapy for the various causes of chronic hepatitis
- be comfortable advising a patient with hepatitis B or C with regard to sexual practice, blood donation and dentistry.

Chronic hepatitis is essentially a histopathological diagnosis. Previously it was classified into chronic persistent

Table 27 Subgroups and outcome of acute liver failure

	Interval between jaundice and encephalopathy (days)	Outcome without transplantation (% survival)
Hyperacute liver failure	0–7	35
Acute liver failure	8–28	7
Subacute liver failure	More than 28	15

and chronic active (or chronic aggressive) hepatitis; but these classes have been abandoned. Chronic hepatitis is graded histologically into minimal, mild, moderate and severe activity, together with mild, moderate or severe fibrosis, also termed cirrhosis. Mild disease remains restricted to the portal tracts. The severity increases to include disease damaging the border between lobules (limiting plate) including bile duct proliferation, extensive inflammatory cell infiltrate and fibrosis.

Certain forms of chronic hepatitis have characteristic features that allow a specific aetiological diagnosis. Examples include alcoholism (fatty infiltration, Mallory's hyaline bodies and a central zonal type of liver damage), α_1-antitrypsin deficiency (intracellular PAS-positive material) and granulomatous hepatitis.

Clinical presentation

Chronic hepatitis presents in three ways:

- abnormal liver function tests
- hepatomegaly
- markers of active hepatitis B or hepatitis C infection.

Chronic hepatitis is often discovered accidentally when liver function test abnormalities are found. Some patients present with fatigue. Patients who are particularly ill may have a fever and other manifestations of disease, as in autoimmune chronic hepatitis and granulomatous hepatitis. Some patients with chronic hepatitis C, granulomatous hepatitis or haemachromatosis have normal liver function tests but have hepatomegaly.

Causes of chronic hepatitis

Deficiency of α_1-antitrypsin

Deficiency of α_1-antitrypsin is an uncommon inherited problem in which the enzyme produced by the patient is abnormal and unable to be exported out of the liver, where it is made. This leads to accumulation and chronic liver disease (usually in childhood). The systemic deficiency causes emphysema (p. 78). Variations in the degree of deficiency lead to differing levels of severity of disease. Because α_1-antitrypsin is an acute phase protein, tests for deficiency can only be done successfully when the patient does not have any degree of acute inflammation. There is no treatment, although smoking should be avoided.

Haemochromatosis

Haemochromatosis is an autosomal recessive condition leading to increased iron absorption from the gut and deposition in the body. The clinical manifestations are:

- diabetes mellitus
- bronzed appearance
- symmetrical arthritis (knees, MCP joints)
- gynaecomastia
- hypogonadism
- hepatomegaly, hepatic cirrhosis and hepatoma.

Liver function may be normal, but hepatomegaly is present. Serum iron ferritin is usually very high. Liver biopsy shows large liver stores of iron. It is best treated by venesection.

Wilson's disease

Wilson's disease is a disorder of copper metabolism inherited as an autosomal recessive. Heterozygotes have no clinical features. The biochemical stages in homozygotes are:

1. Defect in copper excretion from hepatic lysosymes to bile
2. Increased copper in liver
3. Reduced caeruloplasmin levels in blood (carries copper)
4. Increased free copper in blood
5. Increased urinary copper excretion
6. Deposition of copper in tissues (brain, kidney, etc.).

In Wilson's disease, many of the above indices overlap into the normal range. Chronic liver disease is often the first manifestation in childhood/young adulthood. In some, an acute hepatitis/fulminant hepatic failure may be the first presentation. As the copper starts to spill out of the liver, the patient may develop acute haemolysis, renal tubular acidosis and/or neurological features (extrapyramidal). In the early stages, response to D-penicillamine is good, with increased urinary copper excretion.

Autoimmune chronic hepatitis

Autoimmune chronic hepatitis occurs mostly in young or middle-aged women. It is associated with other autoimmune diseases such as ulcerative colitis, pericarditis, thyroiditis, migratory arthritis and fibrosing alveolitis. The diagnosis is suggested by abnormal liver function tests, positive antinuclear antibody (ANA) and smooth muscle antibodies. The onset is often insidious and may lead to cirrhosis relatively rapidly. Immunosuppressive therapy is usually successful.

Primary biliary cirrhosis

Primary biliary cirrhosis is a chronic obstructive cholangitis usually seen in middle-aged women. Patients present with marked pruritus, because of retention of bile salts, and abnormal liver function tests typical of cholestasis. The antimitochondrial antibodies are detectable in high titre in almost all patients. The patients also have a raised serum IgM. There is no proven treatment; many progress to cirrhosis.

Granulomatous hepatitis

Granulomatous hepatitis is a hotch-potch of around 30 diseases caused by both infectious and non-infectious agents. Around 10% of normal people have hepatic granulomata on biopsy. Therefore, granulomatous hepatitis implies hepatic dysfunction or generalised illness and the presence of granulomata. Causes include:

- classical causes of granulomata such as tuberculosis and sarcoidosis
- tropical parasitic diseases such as schistosomiasis
- Q fever
- chronic fungal disease (e.g. histoplasmosis).

Sometimes granulomatous hepatitis is the cause of PUO (pyrexia of unknown origin, p. 373). Treatment is directed towards the underlying cause, although sometimes none is required.

Investigation

The management of chronic hepatitis requires knowledge of the underlying cause and assessment of the extent of inflammation and fibrosis. Therefore, serological tests to identify the cause and a liver biopsy are essential.

Serological tests

Useful tests for the diagnosis of chronic hepatitis are shown in Table 28.

Liver biopsy

A liver biopsy is one of the most invasive 'medical' investigations and warrants detailed discussion with the patient. The primary risk is bleeding, which occurs, to a minor degree, following almost all liver biopsies. Occasionally, it is severe, unrelenting and ultimately fatal. The overall risk of death is 1 in 2000 liver biopsies, but there are some factors that make some biopsies more risky than others:

- abnormal clotting times
- cirrhosis
- abnormal platelet function.

If you are involved in organising a liver biopsy you need to:

- seek written consent

- ask about any recent drug ingestion, including aspirin, non-steroidal anti-inflammatory agents
- make a clinical assessment with regard to the likelihood of cirrhosis, e.g. spider naevi, evidence of oesophageal varices, radiological reports suggesting cirrhosis, etc.
- measure clotting times and platelet count
- group and save blood for cross-match.

Although liver biopsy may be done as a day case, the patient must be in a bed and spend a minimum of 4 hours resting after the biopsy. This is partly for observation for possible bleeding problems. Many patients complain of pain in the right lower chest or the right shoulder following liver biopsy. If the pain and pulse rate are increasing and they look unwell, you should summon senior colleagues immediately and arrange for cross-matching of at least 4 units of whole blood.

The information gained from a liver biopsy is vital to the diagnosis and management of patients with chronic hepatitis, as the liver function tests only give part of the picture. For patients on treatment, it may be necessary to repeat the liver biopsy at intervals of 6 or 12 months to ascertain whether there has been any response to treatment and whether it should be continued.

Management

Management is guided by the cause and extent of disease.

Hepatitis B and C are currently treated with α-interferon. Response rates are in the 30% range.

Immunosuppressive therapy is required for patients with autoimmune chronic hepatitis and primary biliary cirrhosis, copper chelation for Wilson's disease, abstention from alcohol for alcoholic liver disease and specific treatment for the underlying cause of granulomatous hepatitis. Progressive deterioration in younger patients may be an indication for transplantation.

Table 28 Investigations for chronic hepatitis

Cause	Abnormal liver function tests	Blood test useful for establishing aetiology
Hepatitis B	Yes	HBsAg
Hepatitis C	Yes or No	Anti-HCV, PCR for HCV
Haemochromatosis	Yes or No	Serum iron and iron-binding capacity
Deficiency of α_1-antitrypsin	Yes	Serum levels of AAT when no inflammation
Wilson's disease	Yes	Copper and caeruloplasmin levels
Chronic hepatitis of unknown aetiology	Yes	None
Primary biliary cirrhosis	Yes	Antimitochondrial antibodies
Autoimmune chronic hepatitis	Yes	ANA, smooth muscle antibodies
Alcoholic liver disease	Yes	Blood alcohol (sometimes)
Granulomatous hepatitis	Yes or No	Sometimes, e.g. Q fever, schistosomiasis, gammaglobulins

AAT, α_1-antitrypsin

Cirrhosis of the liver

Learning objectives

You should:
- understand cirrhosis in pathological terms
- know the main causes of liver cirrhosis
- know the clinical features and understand the metabolic derangements of liver cirrhosis
- be able to manage patients with cirrhosis.

Hepatic cirrhosis is the end-stage of many chronic inflammatory processes of the liver. It is characterised histologically by fibrosis and regenerating nodules. The most common cause is excess alcohol consumption, others include all the causes of chronic hepatitis. There is a parallel between the development of fibrosis in the liver and the clinical manifestations. Progressive fibrosis leading to cirrhosis can sometimes be arrested or slowed by correction of the underlying cause.

Clinical presentation

The clinical manifestations of cirrhosis include:

- palmar erythema
- more than five spider naevi on the face or upper trunk
- evidence of portal hypertension
- evidence of deranged hepatic synthetic function.

Numerous other associated clinical features may be present (Table 29). Some are not very specific. These include ankle oedema, which has multiple causes, and haemorrhoids, which are common in the normal population. However, when several of these features are present, the possibility of cirrhosis should rise in your mind.

Recognising alcohol abuse

There are some clues to the diagnosis of alcohol abuse:

- hypertension
- raised uric acid
- asymptomatic rib fractures found on chest X-ray.

Direct questions about alcohol intake sometimes are helpful (> 3–4 units/day in men, 2–3 in women). The CAGE questionnaire may be useful; a yes answer to

Table 29 Clinical findings in patients with cirrhosis

Cause	Clinical features
Cirrhosis itself	Spider naevi Gynaecomastia Testicular atrophy Palmar erythema (also rheumatoid arthritis, pregnancy, etc.) Dupuytren's contracture Low-grade PUO
Portal hypertension	Splenomegaly Ascites Oesophageal varices and/or GI haemorrhage Haemorrhoids
Hypoalbuminaemia	White nails (leuconychia) Ankle oedema Sacral oedema

Poor nutritional status
  Lack of adequate intake
  Lack of adequate caloric intake and utilisation
  Folate, iron, riboflavin, pyrodoxine deficiency
  Chronic thiamine deficiency
 	
  Acute thiamine and other nutritional deficiencies
	Proximal muscle wasting and myopathy
	Weight loss
	Glossitis/angular cheilitis
	Ankle oedema and ascites
	Global cardiac dysfunction
	Korsakoff's psychosis
	Wernicke's encephalopathy and retinal haemorrhage

Prolonged bleeding time
  Prolonged INR, reduced platelet function,
  vitamin C deficiency
	Bruising
	GI haemorrhage

Reduced immune function	Subacute bacterial peritonitis Pneumococcal pneumonia Bacteraemia Pulmonary tuberculosis Skin sepsis

Cerebral problems
  Directly caused by alcohol or chronic
  subdural haematomas
	Dementia
	Korsakoff's psychosis
	Wernicke's encephalopathy

three or four questions indicates problematic drinking. The questions are:

1. Have you ever felt you should cut (C) down your drinking?
2. Have you ever been annoyed (A) by criticism of your drinking?
3. Have you ever felt guilty (G) about your drinking?
4. Do you drink in the morning (eye (E) opener)?

Alcoholism is extremely destructive (Box 5).

Portal hypertension

Portal hypertension is caused by increased resistance to flow of the blood draining the GI system and spleen, leading to venous engorgement. As the resistance to flow increases so venous connections between the portal and systemic circulation open up:

- around the lower oesophagus: oesophageal and stomach varices
- around the rectum: haemorrhoids
- around the umbilicus: rare caput medusae and other dilated veins over the anterior abdominal wall
- dilated splenic vein: splenomegaly

Oesophageal varices

Bleeding of oesophageal varices is common and partially preventable by prophylactic sclerotherapy. After a provisional diagnosis of hepatic cirrhosis, an endoscopy should be arranged specifically to inject any varices present.

The control of bleeding varices can be difficult for three reasons:

- approximately 50% of patients with oesophageal varices bleed from another site within the GI tract, usually a gastric or duodenal ulcer
- the varices may be in the stomach and difficult to access
- clotting and platelet abnormalities.

The presence of large amounts of blood in the GI tract produces additional absorption of toxic compounds, such as ammonia and bilirubin, which the diseased liver cannot metabolise and this leads to encephalopathy.

The emergency management of GI bleeding is outlined in the box on this page. In varices, reduction of portal pressure can be achieved by infusion of somatostatin (octreotide) or vasopressin. Emergency sclerotherapy is of proven value. Only rarely is it necessary to use balloon tamponade (Sengstaken–Blakemore tube).

Ascites

The other major effect of portal hypertension is the development of ascites, which only occurs with sinusoidal obstruction *within* the liver, not in obstruction of the portal vein. The reason is that cirrhosis is associated

---

> **Box 5**
> **The effects of chronic excess alcohol consumption**
>
> **Physical effects**
>
> Hepatic
> fatty inflammation
> alcoholic hepatitis
> cirrhosis
> Pancreatitis
> Gastritis
> Peripheral neuropathy
> Korsakov's encephalopathy
> Wernicke's encephalopathy
> Chronic subdural haematomas
> Cardiomyopathy
>
> **Psychological effects**
>
> Suicide
> Withdrawal
> Depression
> Anxiety states
> Morbid jealousy
> Dementia
>
> **Social effects**
>
> Financial problems
> Employment problems
> Marital breakdown
> Violence
> Sexual dysfunction
> lack of libido
> impotence
> Legal problems
> drunk driving
> manslaughter
> theft

with alterations in sodium and water handling by the kidney because of increased activity of the renin–aldosterone system. Figure 25 shows the mechanisms leading to ascites. Without understanding these, it is difficult to treat appropriately.

Management. A graded approach is required depending on the severity of the ascites and the patient's compliance with diet and therapy. Excessive diuretic use will lead to hypovolaemia, electrolyte disturbance, significant prerenal impairment and sometimes renal failure. All treatment should be introduced gradually with careful observation in hospital, monitoring weight and salt and water balance. Bedrest is an important component of successful therapy of ascites. The steps in therapy are as follows:

1. Sodium-restricted diet only: 10% response
2. Sodium restriction plus spironolactone 100–200 mg daily: extra 50% response
3. Sodium restriction plus spironolactone 200 mg daily plus frusemide 40 mg daily: extra 25% response.

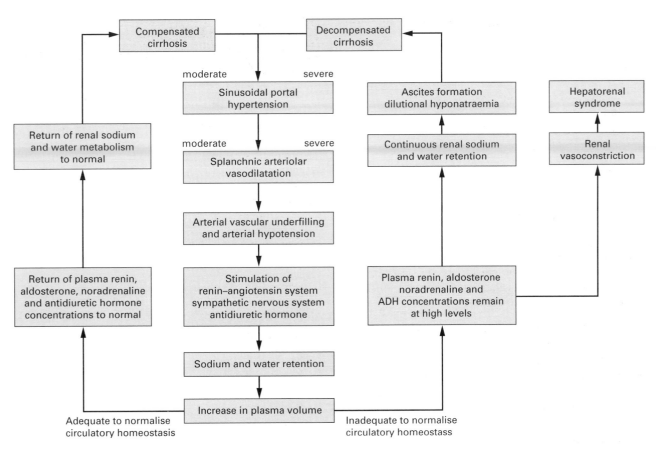

Fig. 25
The mechanisms leading to ascites. ADH, antidiuretic hormone.

During the time that these are introduced, renal function and urine output should be measured. Drug doses should be gradually increased.

Reformed alcoholics or patients with other reasons for cirrhosis may be candidates for liver transplantation.

Spontaneous bacterial peritonitis

Occasionally, ascites becomes infected from passage of gut bacteria into the intestinal lymph vessels and ascitic fluid. It occurs in about 10% of patients with ascites. It is almost always caused by Gram-negative bactaeria such as *Escherichia coli*. Risk factors include:

- GI haemorrhage
- raised serum bilirubin
- low ascitic fluid protein (low complement and immunoglobulin content)
- prior spontaneous bacterial peritonitis.

Patients present with abdominal pain and usually fever. On examination there are marked ascites with a very tender abdomen, often with rebound tenderness.

In suspected bacterial peritonitis, ascitic fluid should be taken for a white cell count and differential, protein, glucose, amylase, Gram-stain and culture.

Treatment is with a Gram-negative antibiotic such as cefotaxime. Mortality is 20–40%.

Tumours

Benign tumours

Both adenomas and haemangiomas are very rare. The former are associated with use of the oral contraceptive pill and anabolic steroids. They can present with shock caused by intraperitoneal rupture and haemorrhage.

Malignant tumours

Primary

Compared with metastatic disease, you will see very few primary hepatocellular carcinomas. It is associated with cirrhosis from any aetiology. In other parts of the world, the vast majority of patients with a hepatocellular carcinoma are hepatitis B antigen positive.

The presentation is usually non-specific with general deterioration in a patient with known cirrhosis. Some will complain of abdominal pain, others will have abdominal swelling caused by ascites. The possibility should be considered in any unwell patient with known chronic liver disease.

Liver function tests are usually unhelpful. *Serum α-fetoprotein* is often markedly increased. Ultrasound or CT scan imaging will show the tumour, which is usually solitary. A biopsy (under image guidance) should be done if possible to confirm the diagnosis; often it is not possible because of clotting abnormalities.

The outlook is bleak with only a few patients surviving beyond 3 months. If the tumour is confined to one lobe, it can be resected, but this is rare. Some patients gain temporary remission with chemotherapy, either systemically or direct into the hepatic artery.

Secondary

By far the most common liver tumour you will see is a metastasis, particularly from the GI tract, bronchus and breast. Often, it is the first presentation of the primary tumour. Patients may complain of geneal malaise, weight loss and non-specific abdominal pain. Most patients will have hepatomegaly (irregular edge), but not all.

A raised alkaline phosphatase is suggestive of the diagnosis, but imaging with ultrasound or CT is necessary. As with primary tumours, a biopsy may be required. Often, there is little active therapy that can be offered, though patients with (for example) breast disease may respond.

3.7 The biliary system

Learning objective

- You should know the different clinical patterns of biliary disease and understand how these affect management.

Normal form and function

The role of the biliary system is to collect the bile salts and bilirubin secreted by the hepatocytes and deliver these to the small intestine. The function of bile salts is to form micelles so that key lipid-soluble substances such as cholesterol and phospholipids can be absorbed.

Bile canaliculi channel bile salts from the hepatocytes to interlobular bile ductules in the portal tracts. These converge into the right and left hepatic duct, and then into the common hepatic duct. Outside the liver, the cystic duct joins the gall bladder where about 50 ml of bile can be stored. The common bile duct starts at the junction of the cystic duct with the common hepatic duct and runs to enter the second part of the duodenum with the pancreatic duct at the **ampulla of Vater**. The **sphincter of Oddi** prevents passage of bile into the small intestine in the absence of food.

Bile acids are synthesised from cholesterol in the hepatocytes. Conjugation (with taurine or glycine) increases the solubility. The bile acids are secreted in the bile, metabolised to some extent by bacteria in the small intestine and then almost all reabsorbed in the terminal ileum. Subsequently, they are resecreted by the liver. This recirculation takes place several times per day.

Failure of bile salt absorption (for example in Crohn's disease or after ileal resection) can cause colonic irritation and diarrhoea, which can be relieved by using cholestyramine to bind the bile salts. The ability of the drug to deplete the bile acid pool can help to alleviate the skin irritation and pruritus in prolonged obstructive jaundice.

The prime action of bile acids is to act as detergents. They aggregate into micelles so that there is a water-soluble envelope surrounding a hydrophobic (lipophilic) core, which allows the transport of cholesterol and phospolipids (particularly lethicin). Imbalance leads to aggregation and formation of gall stones.

Gall stones and cholecystitis

Gall stones are more common in women and become increasingly prevalent with age. The major factors leading to stones are:

- supersaturation of bile with cholesterol
- impaired gall bladder motility
- bile stasis.

Pigment stones are mostly seen when there is prolonged increased red cell turnover, for example in hereditary spherocytosis.

Clinical presentation

There are three presentations.

Asymptomatic. Most gall stones are asymptomatic and remain so. Often they are identified incidentally during ultrasound scanning

Symptomatic. Intermittent pain in the right upper quadrant, classically occurring after food and lasting several hours (biliary colic). The pain may be severe and require narcotic analgesics for relief. Once symptoms have occurred, they tend to recur and worsen, with increased risk of cholecystitis and pancreatitis.

Complicated. Most common complications are cholecystitis and duct obstruction together with cholangitis or pancreatitis. Acute cholecystitis with cystic duct obstruction can lead to abscess formation, gall bladder perforation or mucocoele. Finally, chronic cholecystitis causes a scarred, shrunken, non-functioning gall bladder. Carcinoma is an uncommon long-term problem.

Investigation

Pointers to gall stones may be the typical history described above, raised serum bilirubin and alkaline phosphatase. If you suspect gall stones, you should request an ultrasound examination, which has a sensitivity and specificity of over 90% for identification of stones. The gall bladder may be small and thick-walled. The width of the common bile duct is important (< 8 mm) as dilatation indicates extrahepatic biliary obstruction.

Acute cholecystitis is usually diagnosed on the history, physical examination and ultrasound findings.

Management

Management of gall stones can be either medical or surgical. The first decision is whether to do anything at all. Where stones are diagnosed by chance and the patient is asymptomatic, it is reasonable to do nothing.

Non-surgical treatment. This includes gall stone dissolution, extracorporeal shock wave lithotripsy and mechanical litholysis. However, these are suitable for only about 20% of patients and have a higher gall stone recurrence rate.

Surgery. The principal therapy is cholcystectomy; the aims are to remove the stones and avoid the risk of future recurrence. The operation can be done 'open' or using a laparoscope. The latter is associated with reduced pain, scarring, length of stay and convalesence.

Common bile duct stones. Stones in the common bile duct may be passed spontaneously or may have to be removed. They present with right hypochondriac pain, jaundice, and fever (caused by ascending cholangitis). Surgical exploration may be necessary, but many stones can be removed using endoscopic retrograde cholangiopancreatography (ERCP).

Ascending cholangitis

Infection of the biliary tree has high morbidity and significant mortality. It is usually associated with stones and can present with an unexplained pyrexia, or it may cause Gram-negative septicaemia with shock. A plain abdominal radiograph may show stones (10% radio-opaque) or gas in the biliary tree. The latter is an important sign as it signifies the presence of a gas-forming organism unless there has been no recent biliary operation.

Treatment is with i.v. fluids, high flow oxygen and antimicrobials. A reasonable choice is a combination of cefotaxime (a broad spectrum of activity against Gram-negative organisms) and metronidazole (anaerobes).

At some stage, subsequent to an ultrasound scan, ERCP is often performed, looking for stones in the common bile duct or a stricture.

Tumours

Cholangiocarcinoma is a rare tumour that is usually associated with gall stones in elderly people. It presents with obstructive jaundice, which may be painless. Most tumours are inoperable and the management is symptomatic, with the relief of biliary obstruction using a stent inserted via an ERCP.

The most common cause of obstructive jaundice in elderly people is gall stones. When the obstruction results from malignant disease this is usually a carcinoma at the head of the pancreas or metastatic disease in the lymph nodes at the porta hepatis.

3.8 The pancreas

Learning objectives

You need:
- to know about the normal structure and function of the pancreas and how derangement leads to the common presentations of pancreatic disease
- to be able to construct a plan of investigation and subsequent management of a patient with suspected pancreatic disease.

Normal structure and function

The pancreas is situated retroperitoneally with the second part of the duodenum wrapping around the head. The tail of the pancreas lies over the spleen. The exocrine secretion is drained by a branching system of ducts, draining into the main pancreatic duct. This usually enters the second part of the duodenum together with the common bile duct at the *ampulla of Vater*. There is considerable anatomical variation.

The vast majority of the pancreatic cells are concerned with its exocrine function. Release of **secretin** from acid stimulation of the duodenum causes the production of water, electrolytes and bicarbonate from the pancreas. Cholecystokinin is released when fat and amino acids enter the duodenum. As well as stimulating gall bladder contraction and relaxation of the sphincter of Oddi, it promotes pancreatic enzyme secretion and is trophic to the pancreas.

The main pancreatic enzymes act on:

- fat: lipase, phospholipase
- starch: amylase
- protein: chymotrypsin, trypsin. Importantly, these proteolytic enzymes are secreted in an inactive form. Activation within the gland is seen with acute pancreatitis.

The endocrine function of the pancreas is served by the **islets of Langerhans**. Within these, most cells are beta-cells secreting insulin. Others are alpha-cells, releasing glucagon, D-cells producing somatostatin and PP-cells secreting pancreatic polypeptide. Rarely, specific tumours of these cells produce symptoms through excess hormone production.

Pancreatitis

Inflammation of the pancreas can be acute or chronic; both can be relapsing.

Acute pancreatitis

You should always consider acute pancreatitis as a possible diagnosis in any patient with an acute abdomen. Most cases are associated either with gall stones or high alcohol intake. There are other much rarer associations, such as with hyperlipidaemia, hyperparathyroidism, hypothermia, AIDS and drugs (e.g. corticosteroids). The trigger for the attack may be an alcoholic binge or passing of a gall stone causing a temporary increase in the intraductal pressure. Activation of phospholipase and proteases set up an ongoing inflammatory response.

Clinical presentation

Abdominal pain is the dominant symptom, which is usually central/epigastric and may radiate through to the back. It is severe and the patient is often in great distress with pallor and sweating. Shock may develop with hypotension, poor peripheral perfusion and tachypnoea. Ask about possible triggers, as outlined above. On examination, other than the signs of shock, the patient will have tenderness, rigidity and guarding. Occasionally with severe haemorrhagic pancreatitis, there may be bruising in the flanks (**Grey–Turner's sign**) or around the umbilicus (**Cullen's sign**).

Investigations

The main differential diagnoses are:

* perforated peptic ulcer
* acute cholecystitis
* myocardial infarction.

Your investigations should exclude these and establish the diagnosis of acute pancreatitis as well as looking for evidence of complications. A rise in serum amylase more than five-fold above the upper limit of normal is highly specific for the diagnosis. Lower rises occur with the other conditions and results should be considered in conjunction with the clinical features.

Other biochemical features indicating severe disease are hypoalbuminaemia, hypocalcaemia (corrected), and a rise in urea and creatinine (which may progress to overt acute renal failure). The blood sugar may be elevated and sometimes needs control with insulin. Prolongation of the prothrombin time, elevated fibrin degradation products (FDPs) and thrombocytopenia indicates disseminated intravascular coagulation. Hypoxia resulting from ventilation/perfusion mismatching and a metabolic acidosis are commonly found on blood gas analysis.

An ultrasound scan will help to exclude acute cholecystitis and identify gall stones. The pancreas may be oedematous with evidence of necrosis. Ascites may be present or there may be collections of fluid around the pancreas. A plain abdominal radiograph helps to exclude a perforated viscus and may show the *sentinal* sign of a distended loop of small bowel surrounding the pancreas.

Management

There is no specific treatment of pancreatitis other than supportive management:

* pain relief with opiates: avoid morphine as it causes spasm in the sphincter of Oddi
* nil by mouth, i.v. fluids, and antibiotics (reduces mortality)
* regular aspiration through a nasogastric tube: nausea and vomiting are common
* high flow oxygen.

The pain usually subsides after a couple of days. In severe cases, the patient may need to be admitted to the intensive care unit. Mortality varies from 1% to almost 100%. It is important to have some knowledge of factors that predict a high mortality (Box 6).

Complications

Early complications: shock, disseminated intravascular coagulation (DIC), renal failure, hypoxia, ileus and hypo/hyperglycaemia.

Late complications: pseudocyst, ascites, pleural effusions (high amylase concentrations), abscess formation and candidaemia (p. 360).

A pseudocyst may be suspected because of continuing ileus, pain and a smooth epigastric swelling. It is diagnosed using ultrasound and may require drainage, though most resolve spontaneously.

Abscesses have a high morbidity and mortality. The responsible organism is often *Escherichia coli* and apart from broad-spectrum antibiotics (cefotaxime, metronidazole), drainage is required.

Box 6
Indicators of poor prognosis in acute pancreatitis

Clinical features

Age > 60 years
Associated with gall stones
Hypotension
Grey–Turner sign[a]: flank bruising
Cullen's sign[a]: periumbilical bruising
Ascites (particularly if haemorrhagic)

Investigation results

Low albumin
Low corrected calcium (NB hypercalcaemia is associated with pancreatitis)
Low haemoglobin, high white cell count
Increased blood glucose
Increased serum urea
Low PaO_2

[a](indicates haemorrhagic pancreatitis)

Chronic pancreatitis

Chronic pancreatitis is strongly associated with heavy, continuing alcohol intake. It is thought that protein plugs block the small ducts, leading to damage to the exocrine and endocrine cells. A large fibrotic response takes place, the ducts dilate and calcification occurs in the gland. The condition is non-reversible, but will arrest if the person stops drinking.

Clinical presentation

The dominant symptom is chronic pain. It is usually centred around the upper abdomen but may radiate through to the back. Some patients find relief by sitting forward. The condition may run a relapsing and remitting course, with episodes of severe pain and features of acute pancreatitis.

You can predict the other symptoms from the functions of the pancreas. Malabsorption causes weight loss. Reduction in lipase secretion causes steatorrhoea. The patient complains of bulky offensive faeces that are difficult to flush away. Damage to the endocrine function leads to diabetes mellitus, which may be non-insulin dependent or insulin dependent depending on the degree of beta-cell damage.

Investigation

The main differential diagnosis is with pancreatic carcinoma.

A plain radiograph may show intragland calcification. Ultrasound will demonstrate the small, shrunken fibrotic gland with ductal dilatation. Cysts may be present. An ERCP can show the disruption of the normal pancreatic anatomy. The amylase levels are not usually raised except where the condition runs a relapsing course. Biochemical and haematological investigations may show evidence of malabsorption. Faecal fat collections will show the large increase in fat excretion.

Management

The course of the condition is long. The main therapeutic aims are to stop alcohol intake and to treat the symptoms.

The pain from chronic pancreatitis is often severe and may lead to depression. It commonly requires narcotic analgesics and patients may need the expertise of a pain clinic.

Malabsorption may be helped by pancreatic enzyme supplements. An H_2-antagonist is used to prevent very low pH values occurring in the duodenum and limiting residual enzyme activity. Medium-chain triglycerides

(MCT) are given, as these do not require breakdown before absorption. Supplementation with fat-soluble vitamins (A, D, E, K) may be needed.

Tumours

Benign (endocrine activity) tumours

The pancreas can give rise to a number of rare tumours which are hormonally active, e.g. VIPoma, glucagonoma, insulinoma.

Malignant tumours

Adenocarcinoma of the pancreas is rising in incidence. It is more common in males and with increasing age. The tumour is associated with smoking, but there are no other proven strong aetiological links. Most tumours are in the head of the pancreas.

Clinical presentation

Most patients present late in the course of the disease. Pain, similar to that of chronic pancreatitis, is common, as is painless obstructive jaundice. Many people simply present with lethargy and weight loss. On examination, the patient may be jaundiced, often has hepatomegaly and/or an abdominal mass resulting from lymph node involvement. You may find ascites. A known association is thrombophlebitis, which may be superficial and migratory.

Investigation

Serum biochemistry may show a high alkaline phosphatase and bilirubin, but these are non-specific signs. Ultrasound can usually demonstrate the tumour or metastatic spread. It can also guide a biopsy for histopathological confirmation. Sometimes a CT scan is needed.

Management

Operative resection is usually not feasible and, where resection is undertaken, the perioperative mortality is high and the results poor. There are very few survivors at 5 years.

Surgery may help by creating biliary or intestinal bypass to alleviate the symptoms. ERCP can also be used to relieve jaundice by the insertion of stents. Early and regular use of appropriate narcotic analgesics should be used to prevent pain occurring rather than taking it away.

Self-assessment: questions

Multiple choice questions

1. In the small intestine:
   a. If there is bile salt deficiency, micellar formation is reduced
   b. Long-chain triglycerides are transported from the gut in the lymph as chylomicrons
   c. There is no lymphatic tissue
   d. The entire mucosa is turned over every 2–3 weeks
   e. Is the site of most nutrient absorption

2. Histological features more consistent with ulcerative colitis than Crohn's disease are:
   a. Depleted goblet cells
   b. Crypt abscesses
   c. Granulomata
   d. Diffuse lymphocytic infiltrate
   e. Mucosal involvement only

3. Colorectal cancer:
   a. May arise from a metaplastic polyp
   b. Most often occurs in the rectum and sigmoid
   c. There are further polyps in most cases
   d. Involvement of local lymph nodes does not affect prognosis
   e. Obstruction is more common in right compared with left-sided lesions

4. Angiodysplasia of the colon:
   a. Is more common in the caecum and ascending colon
   b. Is associated with a macrocytic anaemia
   c. Is best shown by barium enema
   d. Usually requires surgery
   e. Is a congenital lesion

5. Causes of acute pancreatitis include:
   a. Alcohol
   b. Hypocalcaemia
   c. Hyperlipidaemia
   d. Self poisoning with diazepam
   e. ERCP

6. Recognised side-effects of sulphasalazine include:
   a. Irreversible oligospermia
   b. Haemolysis
   c. Folate deficiency
   d. Teratogenicity
   e. Acute pancreatitis

7. Coeliac disease:
   a. The patient will almost always have had symptoms since childhood
   b. Is best diagnosed on colonic biopsy
   c. Is associated with HLA-B8
   d. The diagnosis is incorrect if a patient fails to respond to a gluten-free diet
   e. Requires a diet free from wheat, barley and rye

8. Features of non-ulcer dyspepsia include:
   a. Epigastric pain
   b. Abdominal fullness after meals
   c. Response to histamine H_2 antagonists
   d. Are more common in men than women
   e. Can be reliably separated from peptic ulcer clinically

9. Pseudomembranous colitis:
   a. Can only be diagnosed by sigmoidoscopy
   b. Is usually a relatively mild self-limited disease
   c. Can only be acquired in hospital
   d. Usually responds to treatment with oral metronidazole
   e. Has a >10% relapse rate after therapy

10. In a ward with several patients where one of the nurses has had vomiting and diarrhoea over a 48-hour period, you should:
    a. Send the patients home
    b. Culture stools (and vomitus) for viruses
    c. Treat everyone with metronidazole
    d. Exclude visitors from the ward
    e. Prevent the patients (affected or not) leaving the ward for investigations, physiotherapy, etc.

11. The differential diagnosis of acute bloody diarrhoea includes:
    a. Amoebic dysentery
    b. Campylobacter enteritis
    c. Haemorrhagic colitis caused by *E. coli*
    d. Traveller's diarrhoea
    e. Cholera

12. The following episodes of illness should be reported to the local consultant in communicable disease control (CCDC):
    a. Rotavirus infection of a family
    b. A couple both with acute diarrhoea and vomiting 3 days after an Indian meal
    c. A nursery nurse with *Salmonella* group D enteritis
    d. Three people admitted over 24 hours with acute vomiting who had attended a wedding reception 36 hours before
    e. A teenager admitted with acute bronchospasm and laryngeal oedema after eating a Chinese spring roll containing prawns

13. The following are correct:
    a. Hepatitis B can be acquired from serous fluid from a wound

b. Hepatitis C is not a cause of hepatocellular carcinoma
c. Hepatitis A is a cause of chronic liver disease
d. Hepatitis E can be acquired by sharing needles
e. A person with only a hepatitis B core IgG test positive is infectious for hepatitis B

14. Direct complications of acute viral hepatitis include:
   a. Aplastic anaemia
   b. Fulminant hepatic failure
   c. Chronic hepatitis
   d. Renal failure
   e. Fetal death during pregnancy

15. The following are causes of chronic hepatitis:
   a. Hepatitis C
   b. Deficiency of α_1-antitrypsin
   c. Gilbert's syndrome
   d. Sarcoidosis
   e. Isoniazid

16. A 'fatty liver' may represent:
   a. Simply an obese person
   b. Alcoholism
   c. Hepatitis C infection
   d. Acute vitamin A poisoning
   e. An ultrasound artefact

17. With regard to cirrhosis of the liver:
   a. Oesophageal varices are almost always present
   b. There is a > 60% likelihood of GI bleeding
   c. It may be caused by schistosomiasis
   d. If itching is a prominent symptom, the diagnosis is likely to be primary biliary cirrhosis
   e. It may cause low-grade fever, without apparent infection

18. Complications of acute liver failure include:
   a. Cerebral oedema
   b. Bleeding
   c. Drug hypersensitivity
   d. Candidaemia
   e. Hypoglycaemia

Case history questions

History 1

> You see a 79-year-old woman in the general medicine outpatient clinic because of poor mobility. It transpires that this results from marked osteo-arthrosis of both knees. A full blood count shows:
>
> Hb   10.8 g/dl
> MCV   70 µl.

1. What would you do now?

> A few days later, you are on call and she presents to the Accident and Emergency department with brisk rectal bleeding.

2. What should you do?

> Subsequently, a barium enema does not show any abnormalities other than severe diverticular disease. She is keen to go home and when you review her 4 weeks later, she still has a significant iron-deficient anaemia.

3. Outline a management plan.

History 2

> You are a house officer on call for medicine. A 69-year-old woman presents with severe, constant, low central chest pain of several hours' duration. The only medical history of note is that she is awaiting a cholecystectomy for gall stones. She also admits to drinking 'a couple of bottles of sherry a week'.

1. What are you going to do now?
2. A diagnosis of acute pancreatitis is made; how would you treat this?

> She is making a reasonable recovery, but when you examine her at 7 days, she has a smooth swelling in her epigastrium.

3. What do you think this is and what actions should you take?

History 3

> A 27-year-old i.v. drug abuser is admitted with cellulitis of his left groin. You treat him with cefuroxime and metronidazole and his skin improves. However, his liver function tests remain abnormal (normal range in parentheses) as follows:
>
> bilirubin 16 (1–20 IU/L)
> albumin 32 (35–50 IU/L)
> alkaline phosphatase 101 (30–130 IU/L)
> aspartate aminotransferase 123 (11–55 IU/L)
> gamma-glutamyl transpeptidase 63 (10–43 IU/L)

1. What is your initial differential diagnosis?
2. What other tests would you request?
3. What would you advise with respect to sexual practice?

History 4

You admit a verbose marketing executive, 39 years old, to hospital one evening because of a possible head injury. He weighs 95 kg and vital signs are temperature 36.8°C, pulse 95 regular, BP 130/95, respiratory rate 14/min. He has a 2 cm laceration on his left temple and his clothes are filthy, where he fell in the rain on his way home from work. He has no other signs of injury or abnormalities on neurological or general examination.

His plain skull X-rays are normal and so you arrange 2 hourly neurological observations and an overnight stay.

You are telephoned at 6:30 a.m. by the night sister because your patient tried to get up and leave but fell over and bruised his left thigh. He is being argumentative. He looks pale and sweaty and appears anxious and jittery. You try and examine him neurologically, but he is uncooperative. His pulse is 130/min and weak and his respiratory rate 24/min. His thigh has a large bruise on it. You try and examine him neurologically, but he is uncooperative. He insists on going home although he does not appear rational.

1. What are your diagnostic considerations?
2. What should you do?

An hour later he is calmer and willing to undergo further tests.

3. What additional history would you like?
4. How might you obtain a more complete history?
5. What further tests would you want to do?

History 5

You admit a 44-year-old Pakistani woman from casualty with a low-grade fever and bloody diarrhoea. She arrived from Lahore 2 days previously. The stool is offensive and contains blood and mucus. She has moderate left lower quadrant pain on deep palpation.

1. What are the three most likely pathogens?
2. What are three useful tests you can do that evening?

You admit her to hospital and treat her initially with intravenous fluids and oral rehydration solution (e.g. Diarolyte). The next morning she is more unwell and still has bloody diarrhoea.

3. What specific tests can the laboratory do on her stool to help you make a therapeutic decision?

History 6

You are called to a ward you are covering on a Sunday because two patients have developed diarrhoea. One is 76 years old and came in from a nursing home 3 days ago where she had not responded to oral cephalexin for a cough. She has been treated with intravenous and oral ampicillin since admission. The other patient is a 'long stay' patient who is bed- and chair-bound following a stroke 10 weeks ago. She has an indwelling urinary catheter.

The nurse in charge tells you that the diarrhoea is voluminous in both but not bloody. The fluid intake in both patients is suboptimal. She has started fluid charts on both.

1. What should you do now with respect to the management of each patient?
2. If you decide to treat one or other patient what should you use?
3. What action should the nurse in charge take with respect to the patients?

History 7

You see a 57-year-old man in the outpatient clinic complaining of a feeling of incomplete emptying when he goes to pass a motion. He has had some constipation over the last 4 months and has been taking regular senna. In the past, he has had some heartburn and investigations showed a mild iron-deficiency anaemia. He has been on regular iron therapy for 6 months. On examination, you find that his descending colon is full of faeces, but his rectum is empty on P.R.

1. What would be your initial management plan?
2. Figure 26 is one of the films from his barium enema:
   a. What are the abnormalities?
   b. What is the likely diagnosis?

Data interpretation

Table 30 gives the liver function test results for nine patients. Match the results to the patient for the following patient scenarios.

1. Vomiting patient 22 years old, referred by GP
2. A 47-year-old with fever and abdominal pain
3. A 19-year-old college student with sore throat
4. A 44-year-old hill walker admitted with fever

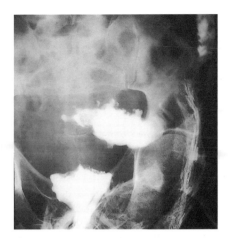

Fig. 26
Barium enema film for History 7 question.

5. A 52-year-old retailing executive investigated for ankle swelling

6. A intensive care unit patient (third week) with adult respiratory distress syndrome and renal impairment on haemofiltration

7. A 21-year-old 72 hours after acute admission with vague abdominal pain and unwell

8. A 'routine' blood test preoperation on a 49-year-old woman who had a major car accident 12 years ago

9. A 44-year-old male ex-prisoner, now a car mechanic with 2 cm hepatomegaly

Picture questions

1. Picture 3.1 is a CT scan of the liver in a 69-year-old woman with a PUO of 2 weeks' duration. She has mildly deranged liver function tests, a total white cell count of $12.8 \times 10^9/l$ with 80% neutrophils, mild normochromic normocytic anaemia, an ESR of 68 mm/hour and an albumin of 29 g/l. She has no abnormal physical findings.
   a. Describe the abnormality.
   b. What is the likely diagnosis?
   c. What investigations are now appropriate? (Give two.)
   d. How should she be managed?

2. Picture 3.2 is a chest radiograph taken preoperatively of a 78-year-old man, who was having peripheral vascular surgery.
   a. Give three abnormalities
   b. What action should be taken?

3. Picture 3.3 is of a barium enema in a 25-year-old woman with a 6-month history of general malaise, weight loss and bloody diarrhoea with mucus.
   a. Describe the abnormalities
   b. What is the diagnosis?
   c. What would be your initial management?

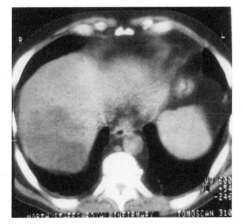

Picture 3.1

Table 30 Liver function test results for nine patients (normal range in parentheses) – see Data interpretation question opposite

Patient	1	2	3	4	5	6	7	8	9
Bilirubin (1–20)	123	145	45	48	16	22	75	11	9
Albumin (35–50)	34	31	38	29	21	23	19	39	43
Alkaline phosphatase (30–130)	165	470	135	210	95	220	350	75	92
Aspartate aminotransferase (11–55)	2365	227	550	350	65	195	750	110	27
Creatinine (blood 60–120)	92	75	80	225	125	470	225	75	95
INR (≤ 1.0)	1.2	1.1	1.1	1.9	2.5	1.5	4.8	1.0	1.1
White cell count (4–11)	4.3	17.1	9.3	15.3	7.4	13.4	12.5	8.5	6.3

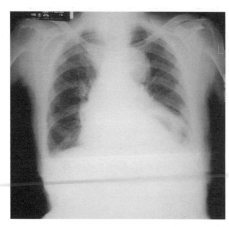

Picture 3.2

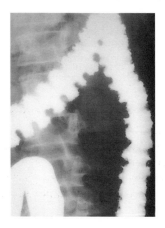

Picture 3.3

Short notes

1. A patient is admitted from Outpatients who is said to be malnourished and malabsorption is suspected. Outline your approach, including the investigations that you would initially request.
2. A 64-year-old man in the outpatient clinic was diagnosed as having a peptic ulcer 8 weeks previously at endoscopy. Unfortunately, he is still complaining of the same symptoms of upper abdominal pain. What should be done?
3. What is your management plan for a patient with jaundice and severe pain caused by a carcinoma of the pancreas which is inoperable?

Viva questions

1. You see a man of 48 years in clinic who is complaining of difficulty in swallowing. What are the key features that you will want to explore with him?
2. You have requested an ultrasound scan on a 75-year-old woman with a suspected aortic aneurysm. The report comes back 'aorta clearly seen, no aneurysm. Multiple stones seen in the gall bladder'. What are you going to do?
3. Discuss the different therapies used in inflammatory bowel disease. What would you use to maintain remission in a patient with ulcerative colitis? What side-effects would you discuss with the patient?

Self-assessment: answers

Multiple choice answers

1. a. **True.** Bile salts are essential for micelle formation.
   b. **False.** Fat is broken down to monoglycerides and fatty acids in the gut, absorbed across the cell and then reesterified to triglycerides for transport as chylomicrons.
   c. **False.** Lymphatic tissue is prominent in the gut, e.g. Peyer's patches.
   d. **False.** The gut turns over its mucosa every 2–3 days.
   e. **True.** The small intestine is the main area for the breakdown and absorption of nutrients.

2. a. **True.** Goblet cells are depleted in ulcerative colitis.
   b. **True.** Ulcerative colitis is a mucosal disease associated with crypt abscesses.
   c. **False.** Granulomas are uncommon.
   d. **False.** A polymorph infiltration occurs.
   e. **True.** Ulcerative colitis is a superficial inflammation which is continuous from the rectum.

3. a. **False.** Metaplastic polyps have no malignant potential.
   b. **True.**
   c. **False.** Additional polyps do occur but only in about one-third of cases.
   d. **False.** Prognosis is assessed by Duke's staging; lymph node involvement is stage 3 with 25% 5-year survival.
   e. **False.** Rectal bleeding and obstruction are more common with left-sided lesions.

4. a. **True.** It usually occurs in the right side of the colon.
   b. **False.** It causes iron-deficiency anaemia.
   c. **False.** It is visualised on colonoscopy.
   d. **False.** It is usually treated with diathermy.
   e. **False.** It is an acquired abnormality of the vascular system.

5. a. **True.** Most cases are associated with gall stones or high alcohol intake.
   b. **False.** Hypocalcaemia can occur during acute attacks, but *hypercalcaemia* is a cause of acute pancreatitis.
   c. **True.** There is an association with hyperlipid-aemia, but it is an uncommon cause.
   d. **False.**
   e. **True.** ERCP is used in the diagnosis of pancreatic disease, but can precipitate an acute attack.

6. a. **False.** Causes reversible oligospermia.
   b. **True.** In a small number of patients.
   c. **True.**
   d. **False.** It is safe in pregnancy.
   e. **True.**

7. a. **False.** Peaks of incidence occur in young children and in 20–40-year-olds.
   b. **False.** A jejunal biopsy is needed.
   c. **True.** It is associated with HLA-B8 and HLA-DRW3 antigens.
   d. **False.** Failure to respond to diet usually means poor compliance, but secondary lactose intolerance, associated infection and nutritional deficiencies should also be considered.
   e. **True.** All contain gluten.

8. a. **True.** Both ulcers and non-ulcer dyspepsia give epigastric pain.
   b. **True.**
   c. **True.** Patients do respond to H_2-antagonists and this cannot be used as a diagnostic test to separate non-ulcer dyspepsia from that caused by a peptic ulcer.
   d. **False.** Women are more often affected.
   e. **False.** There is no way of differentiating clinically.

9. a. **True.** It is a visual/pathological diagnosis. However, *Clostridium difficile*-related diarrhoea can be diagnosed by detecting cytotoxin in stool.
   b. **False.** It is often fatal in the elderly debilitated patient; it requires treatment.
   c. **False.** However, most cases are acquired in hospital.
   d. **True.** Over 90% response rate (but not 100%).
   e. **True.** However, they usually respond to retreatment with oral metronidazole or vancomycin.

10. a. **False.** Impracticable and would further spread the likely cause.
    b. **False.** The likely cause is Norwalk virus or another of the 'small structured round viruses' (SSRVs), which are diagnosed by electron microscopy and are not cultured.
    c. **False.** *C. difficile* diarrhoea is the most important differential but vomiting is less common with this and it rarely affects the staff, so a viral aetiology is more likely. You would send stools for detection of *C. difficile* toxin though.
    d. **True.** To prevent further spread, unless necessary for, say, a dying patient.
    e. **True.** Unless the investigation was absolutely vital.

11. a. **True.** This has much mucus and tenesmus.
    b. **True.** The amount of blood is usually small.
    c. **True.** The classic cause, with mostly blood and little stool and no fever.
    d. **False.** This is a watery diarrhoea caused by *E. coli*.
    e. **False.** Cholera has very watery diarrhoea in large volumes (rice-water stool).

12. a. **True.** Although rotaviruses can be transmitted via many routes only one of which is food and water.
    b. **True.** This is likely to be campylobacter because of the incubation period; the CCDCs will instruct the environmental health officers to inspect the restaurant. There may also be other cases you do not know about.
    c. **True.** *Salmonella* infection is notifiable, and given her work with small babies who are at risk of *Salmonella* meningitis, etc., she should not be allowed back to work until her stools are negative.
    d. **True.** Notify by phone as it may be a large outbreak with affected people spread all over the country. The caterers will need to be inspected. The investigation by the CCDCs may form the basis of a prosecution by the bride's family (also consider alcoholic gastritis!).
    e. **False.** Clearly the patient is allergic to something in the spring roll, possibly prawns. He needs to be referred to an allergist/immunologist for detailed advice on what foods to avoid, etc.

13. a. **True.** This is the likely mode of horizontal transmission among siblings in developing countries.
    b. **False.** Hepatitis C can lead to chronic liver disease and its sequelae.
    c. **False.** Hepatitis A causes an acute self-limiting disease.
    d. **False.** It is a waterborne disease.
    e. **False.** Only those HBsAg positive are infectious.

14. a. **True.** Generally rare but life-threatening and common in Asia.
    b. **True.** It only occurs in about 1 in 2000 cases of jaundiced hepatitis A patients.
    c. **True.** If hepatitis B and C viruses are involved.
    d. **False.** Unless the patient first has fulminant hepatic failure. If renal impairment or failure are present, consider leptospirosis, haemolytic uraemic syndrome or acute poisoning, e.g. paracetamol.
    e. **True.** But only in hepatitis E which also is often severe and life-threatening in pregnancy.

15. a. **True.** About 20% of hepatitis C infections lead to cirrhosis.
    b. **True.** This is rare and untreatable.

   c. **False.** Gilbert's syndrome involves a rise in unconjugated bilirubin only.
   d. **True.** Granulomatous hepatitis, usually evidence of disease in other organs.
   e. **False.** Emphatically wrong. A cause of acute hepatitis. It is vital to stop isoniazid or seek immediate expert help if abnormal liver function tests are found in patients taking isoniazid or rifampicin or both.

16. a. **False.**
    b. **True.** A common 'early' abnormality.
    c. **True.**
    d. **False.** Vitamin A poisoning is caused by eating fish or polar bear liver and causes severe headache, cerebral oedema, flushing of the face and skin, peeling of the nose and, in severe cases, death. Chronic vitamin A ingestion may lead to cirrhosis.
    e. **False.** But is often found on ultrasound.

17. a. **True.** As a result of portal hypertension.
    b. **False.** About one-third of patients have bleeding varices but sometimes they have gastric ulcers or other causes of bleeding.
    c. **True.** In Asia and Africa: *S. japonicum* and *S. mansoni*.
    d. **True.**
    e. **True.** But beware subacute bacterial peritonitis, tuberculosis and other occult infections.

18. a. **True.** The most likely cause of death.
    b. **True.** Especially nose bleeds and/or GI bleeding.
    c. **False.** Although toxicity is a problem because of failure to metabolise many drugs.
    d. **True.** However, it usually follows serious bacterial infection.
    e. **True.** Blood glucose requires constant monitoring and treatment.

Case history answers

History 1

1. She has a mild, microcytic anaemia. You should look carefully at the blood count report to see what other information is given. There may be a low MCHC and an increased red cell distribution width. The reticulocyte count may be increased and, if actively bleeding, there may be a raised platelet count. A blood film would confirm the presence of small cells together with hypochromia. At this stage, you should confirm the iron-deficiency anaemia with serum ferritin, or serum iron and total iron-binding capacity. You should also ask why she is anaemic. The temptation is to treat simply with iron supplements on the basis that the anaemia is only mild.

In an elderly person, there may be an element of poor nutrition, but more likely she has organic disease. You should enquire carefully about upper GI symptoms and also whether she is, or has recently been, taking NSAIDs because of her arthritis. The other main concern is that she has an occult large bowel carcinoma.

2. You should establish i.v. access; if she is hypovolaemic, you should use a plasma expander such as Gelofusin whilst waiting for cross-matched blood. Renal function should be measured. In significant GI bleeding, you should inform the on-call surgical team so that, if intervention is needed, it does not come too late.

   Assuming that the bleeding stops and that a transfusion has been given, the next step is to decide on investigations to determine the cause. Occasionally, anal disease can haemorrhage, but the most likely problem is a large bowel carcinoma, diverticular disease or angiodysplasia. It is reasonable to request a barium enema, but in this case no cause for the bleeding is found.

3. You need to consider whether the patient has been complying with therapy; iron supplements can produce GI upset. You need to consider the value of the barium enema. Was the examination a complete one or was there considerable faecal loading? You need to decide whether to accept that the probable cause was diverticular disease, whether a carcinoma was missed or whether you should look for angiodysplasia. If you wish to pursue one of these, you need to request a colonoscopy. Occasionally, despite intensive and repeated investigation, no cause for GI bleeding is found, in which case management is by iron supplements and transfusion.

History 2

1. The differential diagnoses are myocardial ischaemia, aortic dissection (but no history of pain through to the back or arterial insufficiency), and an intra-abdominal catastrophe (biliary colic, perforated peptic ulcer or acute pancreatitis). Your next step would be a focused examination looking for supportive evidence of one of the possibilities. There may also be signs which help to exclude a diagnosis. For example, absence of abdominal tenderness would be strongly against the diagnosis of a perforated peptic ulcer. In addition, you should look for signs of shock, such as hypotension and tachypnoea.

   Investigations are again targeted towards your differential diagnosis. In all patients with chest pain, you should request an urgent ECG and chest radiograph. A serum amylase should also be checked. It may be mildly elevated in the other conditions, but gross elevation is diagnostic of acute pancreatitis. In any patients who are shocked, you

should also perform blood gas analysis, urea and electrolytes and measure urine output. If you suspect a perforated peptic ulcer , then a plain upright abdominal radiograph is indicated.

2. You are told that the patient has acute pancreatitis. Clues to this in the history are the heavy alcohol intake (you should also consider why — this may be associated with depression) and gall stones. Management is supportive (p. 136). Remember fluids, oxygen, antibiotics and pain relief.

3. She almost certainly has a pancreatic pseudocyst. Ascites can also occur in severe cases, but this would cause generalised swelling. You should request an ultrasound scan to confirm the diagnosis. Many small collections of fluid resolve spontaneously, but some need drainage. Remember the other complications of pancreatitis (p. 136).

History 3

1. The initial differential diagnosis is:
   - chronic hepatitis: hepatitis B or C, drug-induced hepatotoxicity or alcohol abuse
   - granulomatous hepatitis
   - cirrhosis of liver (low albumin is more consistent with acute illness).

2. Tests that should be requested are:
   - hepatitis B surface antigen and anti-HBc IgG
   - hepatitis C antibody
   - HIV (if he gives consent)
   - ultrasound of the liver
   - smooth muscle and antimitochondrial antibodies
   - clotting screen.

3. If hepatitis B surface antigen or hepatitis C RNA positive, then safe sex and immunisation of any partners for hepatitis if they are not already positive should be undertaken.

History 4

1. Delirium tremens (alcohol withdrawal) is by far the most likely diagnosis although it is usually manifest 24–36 hours after admission. However, hypo-glycaemia, serious sepsis and intracranial bleeding must be excluded. Disorientation may also be caused by concussion.

2. Steps that should be undertaken are:
   a. BM stix immediately
   b. blood culture and white cell count
   c. sedation with chlormethiazole infusion if BM stix normal, with close monitoring of respiratory rate and blood pressure
   d. re-examine him carefully when he is quieter, seeking neurological signs and signs of hepatic cirrhosis
   e. CT scan of brain (when sedated)
   f. if febrile or with features of pneumonia or sepsis investigate as you would any pneumonia (chest

radiograph, blood gases, etc.) and treat empirically with antibiotics, e.g. cefotaxime.

3. Additional history:
   - is he a drinker (use CAGE questionnaire, p. 132)?
   - has he travelled anywhere (malaria, typhoid)?
   - does he have any past medical history of note?
   - has his behaviour changed lately (? manic/ depressive, hyperthyroidism, intracranial pathology, such as encephalitis, meningioma).
4. Speak to a close relative or work colleague in confidence later that day.
5. Further tests:
   - assess his liver function status (? cirrhosis): albumin, clotting, endoscopy for oesophageal varices
   - assess him neurologically: CT scan (?), lumbar puncture
   - assess his endocrine status, especially thyroid function
   - assess him psychiatrically (refer).

History 5

1. *Shigella, Entamoeba histolytica, Salmonella* infections.
2. Useful tests:
   - send stool for culture
   - urea and electrolytes
   - blood culture
   - full blood count and differential.
3. Stool microscopy on a 'hot stool' for amoebae, red and white cells and parasites. (The bedpan should be taken directly to the laboratory (or a generous portion of stool without urine) immediately.)

History 6

1. Examine each patient with respect to fluid state and any intra-abdominal pathology. It is easy to assume that they have the same problem, but it may be coincidental. Do urea and electrolytes and send stool for culture and *Clostridium difficile* toxin. Use i.v. fluids if oral rehydration solution is not adequate.
2. If *C. difficile* is implicated use oral metronidazole, for salmonella or other bacterial diarrhoea use ciprofloxacin. If diarrhoea is severe, it is appropriate to start therapy before the results are available.
3. Put each patient in a separate cubicle. Inform the infection control sister as soon as possible so that the area around each patient's bed can be cleaned to reduce dispersal of clostridial spores.

History 7

1. The patient is complaining of a change in bowel habit, which must be taken seriously. Iron therapy can cause constipation, but you should not assume that this is the cause. The empty rectum with a full descending colon suggests an obstructive lesion. A common error is for an iron-deficiency anaemia to be ascribed to 'reflux oesophagitis'; many of these patients have lower bowel disease and, unless a barium meal or gastroscopy shows a definite cause, a barium enema or colonoscopy should be carried out.

You need to repeat the blood count and check the iron status. As the patient may have a large bowel carcinoma, you should request liver function tests and ultrasound. A high alkaline phosphatase would suggest liver metastases. You need to examine the lower bowel; a flexible or rigid sigmoidoscope will visualise the rectum and lower sigmoid colon. If a barium enema is inconclusive, colonoscopy would be indicated.

2. a. With barium studies, always try to orientate yourself. This is a lateral film showing the rectum and lower sigmoid colon. The hip, pelvis and sacroiliac joint are visible. There is a gross filling defect, with a thin line of barium in communication with the sigmoid colon. Even if you cannot see the thin column, you can deduce that there is not total obstruction by the filling of the sigmoid colon. The appearances are described as an 'apple core'.

   b. A rectal carcinoma. The tumour must have been just beyond the tip of the finger on rectal examination.

Data interpretation answers

1. Typical hepatic liver function test abnormalities, with normal white cell count and typical clinical presentation: acute hepatitis, probably A but could be B, C or E or possibly Epstein–Barr virus (EBV).
2. Typical cholestatic liver function test abnormalities, with fever and a raised white cell count: cholecystitis, cholangitis, liver abscess.
3. Consistent with viral hepatitis but not very high aspartate aminotransferase (AST). Must account for the sore throat: glandular fever, could be hepatitis A (but why sore throat) or primary HIV.
4. Mixed cholestatic/hepatitic picture with fever and impaired renal function. Leptospirosis (p. 000), haemorrhagic fever with renal syndrome (Hautaan virus), severe sepsis including liver abscess or cholangitis, alcoholic hepatitis.
5. Note the low albumin and raised INR, typical of acute or chronic liver failure: alcoholic cirrhosis (consider heart failure, thiamine deficiency). Impaired renal function occurs with severe cirrhosis because of poor renal perfusion and diuretic therapy.
6. Note the typically low albumin of patients in the intensive care unit (ICU) (non-specific). Raised white cell count alerts you to infection: sepsis including candidaemia, TPN-induced hepatitis (mild), drug-induced hepatitis.

7. Typical biochemical features of acute liver failure with renal impairment: for example caused by paracetamol poisoning, hepatitis A, B or C, drugs. Look for liver flap and encephalopathy.

8. Isolated raised AST typical of chronic hepatitis, most likely C but consider B and autoimmune disease. Consider primary sclerosing cholangitis (but alkaline phosphatase normal).

9. Hepatitis C, haemachromatosis, alcoholic liver disease, emphysema (caused by downward displacement of the liver without enlargement).

Picture answers

1. a. Low attenuation irregular area posteriorly in the right lobe of the liver.
   b. Bacterial liver abscess. Usually amoebic abscesses are more clearly circumscribed and found in younger people; metastases or liver tumours are virtually always more clearly outlined and often higher attenuation.
   c. (i) Direct aspiration of abscess contents for Gram stain and aerobic and anaerobic culture, (ii) amoebic serology and/or (iii) blood culture
   d. Intravenous antibiotics to cover the likely organisms and to penetrate into a large abscess cavity, e.g. ampicillin (*Streptococcus milleri*), third-generation cephalosporin (Gram-negatives) and metronidazole (anaerobes).

2. a. He has cardiomegaly (cardiothoracic ratio >0.5), an unfolded aorta (prominent aortic knuckle) and a hiatus hernia (gas bubble behind the left heart border).
   b. You would probably do nothing. The anaesthetist may want to assess his cardiovascular function in more depth. You may want to question him about any symptoms of reflux oesophagitis. Patients with 'rolling' (portion of stomach rolling alongside the oesophagus) rather than the very common 'sliding' hiatus hernia are more at risk of complications such as gastric volvulus. However, if the patient is asymptomatic, you would do nothing.

3. a. The barium enema visualises the transverse and descending colon. There are fine spiculating superficial ulcers throughout, giving a fuzzy contour. There are also examples of 'collarstud' ulcers and 'pseudopolyps' — luminal filling defects that are inflamed mucosal islands between ulcer craters. The colon in the lower left of the picture has lost its haustration pattern and is featureless ('hosepipe').
   b. The history points to inflammatory bowel disease and the barium enema confirms ulcerative colitis.
   c. Given the severity of the disease, the patient needs admission. Initial management would be oral and rectal corticosteroids.

Short note answers

1. There is very little information about the patient (which is often the case for a house-officer; patients will 'turn up' on the ward). An initial step would be to recap the history and examination findings. There are two interdependent problems. The first is whether the patient is malnourished. Find out about the length of the history and try and quantify any weight loss. Arrange for the patient to be weighed and *you* should record this in the patient's notes. Ideally, the height of the patient should be measured to calculate the **body mass index** (weight/height^2). Are there any are other pointers towards nutritional deficiency? Is there marked oedema, possible ascites, indicating protein malnutrition? Is there evidence of folate or B_{12} deficiency, e.g. a peripheral neuropathy (p. 211)?

   Having decided that the patient is malnourished, the second question is then why? Is it because of a poor diet? This can be difficult to assess and a dietary assessment by a nutritionist might help. Is there a previous history of bowel problems? The patient may have had a gastrectomy years ago, extensive gut resection or surgery that has created a blind loop. The patient may have a disease such as scleroderma which, because of the interference with gut motility, has permitted bacterial overgrowth. Are there pointers from the history, or examination findings suggestive of inflammatory bowel disease?

   It may then be decided that the patient is malnourished and that GI disease is suspected. The investigations take the same logical approach:
   - document the degree of malnourishment: iron, total iron-binding capacity, B_{12}, folate, calcium, alkaline phosphatase and plasma albumin should all be measured
   - what is the underlying disease: in coeliac disease, a small bowel enema and a jejunal biopsy may be requested. For bacterial overgrowth, a hydrogen breath test may be required.

2. The first task is to look back at the records from 8 weeks ago and check the details. Was the ulcer in the stomach? If a gastric ulcer, then were biopsies taken and are the results in the notes? Even if the biopsies were negative, he needs a repeat endoscopy to assess healing, as there are false-negative biopsies with gastric carcinoma.

   Assuming that he has a proven duodenal ulcer, why have the symptoms persisted? Is the ulcer a coincidental finding with another cause for his symptoms, e.g. myocardial ischaemia? If the dyspepsia is caused by a duodenal ulcer, what therapy was he prescribed (if any!) and has he been complying with it? If he was given a proton pump inhibitor, almost all ulcers should have healed by 8 weeks. If an H_2-antagonist was prescribed, the healing rate is less and is slower. It may be worth continuing with the therapy, changing to a proton pump inhibitor or repeating an endoscopy. This last option should include reculture for *H. pylori* (p. 109).

3. In dealing with a patient who has a terminal carcinoma, it is important not to focus on physical symptoms to the detriment of the psychological care. Involvement of the MacMillan nurses or a palliative care team should be strongly considered. There is also a high probability of a reactive depression. In this patient there are two goals: relief of jaundice and pain control.

The jaundice may be managed by insertion of a stent using ERCP. Alternatively, surgical bypass may be used. If the jaundice cannot be relieved, the pruritus may be helped by antihistamines and/or cholestyramine to bind the bile salts. Pancreatic insufficiency may also be a problem, with steatorrhoea (p. 112).

Pain relief should start with simple analgesics such as paracetamol, stepping up through codeine, dihydrocodeine to morphine. Bone pain may be helped by the use of NSAIDs or radiotherapy, though adenocarcinomas tend not to be very radiosensitive. If morphine is used, it should be rationally prescribed. Initially, the patient is placed on regular oral morphine (4 hourly), with supplementation for breakthrough pain. A pain chart will indicate the degree of control obtained. The dose of morphine is adjusted according to the amount of PRN dosing being used. Finally, the 4 hourly dosing is converted to sustained release morphine. Always prescribe a PRN dose for ready access to pain relief. A prophylactic laxative should be prescribed whenever using narcotic analgesics.

Viva questions

1. You must allow the patient to describe his difficulty. Is it dysphagia, nasal regurgitation or aspiration (violent coughing on eating)? The main differential diagnoses are neurological or oesophageal disease. What is the context of the symptoms? Does the patient have a history suggestive of neurological disease or does he give a story of longstanding heartburn? Is the problem more with liquids (neurological) or solids (obstructive)? If we assume that the pointer is towards GI disease, then the main differential diagnoses are a benign stricture and carcinoma. Even with a long history of reflux and heartburn, it cannot be assumed that the problem is benign. A barium swallow may help, but oesophagoscopy will allow direct visualisation (after an oesphageal toilet to clear out the debris) and biopsy.

2. Given that she has gall stones, you need to know whether these are asymptomatic. If so, then the correct course of action would be to do nothing. If she gives a history of recurrent right upper quadrant pain and the gall bladder is shrunken and scarred on ultrasound scan, you may discuss the possible need for surgery and that you would like to send her for a surgical opinion. Remember that abdominal pain may have other causes and do not assume that it is necessarily caused by the gall stones.

3. The question is 'open', asking you to state your knowledge on drug therapy in inflammatory bowel disease. It then closes down onto maintenance and potential side-effects (see p. 120).

Renal disease, fluid/electrolyte and acid/base balance

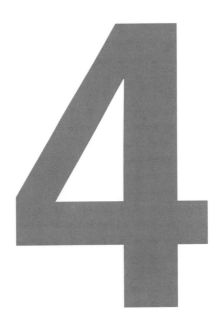

4.1 Background

Learning objectives

You need:

- to feel confident about diagnosing renal failure on the basis of abnormal biochemistry
- to understand those aspects of renal physiology which explain renal failure and its treatment
- to understand how the kidneys, heart and circulation form a functional unit in the regulation of fluid and electrolyte balance
- to understand how abnormalities of renal perfusion can affect renal function
- to understand how renal function is affected by urinary outflow.

You may regard the topics of this chapter as very difficult to understand, and feel that you have had little experience of renal failure. However, about one patient in three on any acute medical ward has abnormal renal function. The difficulty arises because most of the symptoms and signs of renal disease are non-specific and the diagnosis is usually based on abnormal 'Us and Es' (urea and electrolytes) or proteinuria. You may feel uncomfortable about making a really important diagnosis like renal failure from a mere laboratory report.

Another problem arises because practising clinicians are all too often shaky on the assessment of fluid/electrolyte balance. Many a patient with heart failure is wrongly given saline because he 'looks dry'. A reader who comes to the end of this chapter able to distinguish a volume-depleted patient from one who is volume overloaded and able to look with interest and understanding at biochemistry results has the basic skills to recognise and manage renal disease.

This chapter will show that renal function and fluid/electrolyte homeostasis are inextricably linked and that the kidneys form a functional unit with the heart and circulation. The emphasis is more towards physiological concepts than structural pathology, which is covered in pathology and reference textbooks. However, the traditional anatomical framework makes it easier to remember the causes of renal disease.

Prerenal factors:

- something wrong with the circulation
  - volume depletion/shock, e.g. blood loss, excess GI losses, burns
  - fall in peripheral vascular resistance, e.g. caused by sepsis
  - heart failure
  - hypertension
- something wrong with the renal vasculature
  - renal arterial disease
  - renal venous disease
  - drug-induced shutdown of renal perfusion, e.g. ACE inhibitors, NSAIDs
- something wrong with the blood

- hypoxia
- infection
- toxin.

Renal factors:

- glomerular disease
- tubular disease
- parenchymal/interstitial disease.

Postrenal factors:

- diseases of the renal papillae, renal pelvis, ureters, bladder or urethra.

Renal anatomy

The kidneys are approximately 12 cm in length and situated retroperitoneally at the level of T12–L3, the right being 1–2 cm lower than the left. Each has one or more main renal arteries entering at the hilum, dividing into interlobular arteries which run radially out to the cortico-medullary junction and then into the arcuate arteries and ultimately into the glomerular capillaries. The functional unit is the nephron (Fig. 27).

The glomerulus can be thought of as an epithelial pouch invaginated by a tuft of capillaries running from

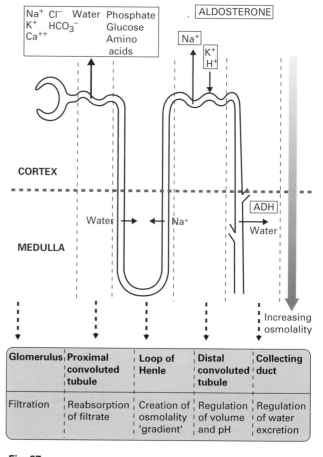

Glomerulus	Proximal convoluted tubule	Loop of Henle	Distal convoluted tubule	Collecting duct
Filtration	Reabsorption of filtrate	Creation of osmolality 'gradient'	Regulation of volume and pH	Regulation of water excretion

Fig. 27
The anatomy and physiology of the nephron. The site of action of the two principal hormones controlling water and electrolyte levels are shown. (Modified from Textbook of Medicine, ed. Souhami and Moxham, Churchill Livingstone, Edinburgh.)

the afferent to the efferent arteriole. The endothelial and epithelial cell junctions and basement membrane constitute a semi-permeable filter. The other cellular element of the glomerulus is the mesangium. The mesangial cells are contractile and can alter bloodflow and the glomerular filtration rate (GFR). They are commonly involved in glomerular disease. The juxtaglomerular apparatus is formed by the afferent arteriole and distal tubule of the same nephron.

Renal physiology

Filtration and flow

The kidneys receive 25% of cardiac output. About 20% of the blood volume which enters the glomeruli passes through the glomerular filter, which is permeable to every component of blood except cells and large protein molecules. The glomerular basement membrane is negatively charged and this charge barrier retains anionic proteins such as albumin which are small enough to pass through the pores. Damage to the glomerular basement membrane disrupts the charge barrier before it disrupts pore size, making albumin an exquisitely sensitive marker of glomerular damage.

Filtration is a passive process determined by the pressure balance across the capillary wall. Haemostatic pressure in the glomerular capillaries causes filtration. It is opposed by the hydrostatic pressure in the urinary space and the oncotic pressure exerted by proteins in glomerular capillary blood.

In order to understand renal disease, a crucial concept is the distinction between **filtration** and **flow**. Nitrogenous waste can only reach the urine by filtration since it is not actively secreted into the tubule. Maintenance of filtration is therefore crucial to homeostasis. It is maintained by renal autoregulation over a wide range of perfusion pressures (80–200 mmHg). Filtration only fails if there are insufficient functioning nephrons or the perfusion pressure falls below the lower limit of autoregulation. The latter can be caused by one of the prerenal processes listed in the anatomical classification on p. 150 or if there is 'back pressure' from the tubule, as in ureteric obstruction.

Within the physiological range of perfusion pressures, there is a vastly different rate of urine flow after celebrating your exam results from when you play squash on a hot summer afternoon. In both situations, a glomerular filtrate amounting to 180 1/24 hour is needed to clear nitrogenous waste and about 90% of the fluid is obligatorily reabsorbed to prevent circulatory collapse. It is in the handling of the remaining 10% of filtrate that the controlling mechanisms operate; they can alter flow between a minimum of 0.5 and a maximum of over 20 1/24 hour. There are two controlling mechanisms.

Sodium reabsorption. This is the main factor which determines extracellular fluid **volume**: it is controlled primarily by the renin–angiotensin–aldosterone system and the recently discovered natriuretic peptides.

Water reabsorption. This controls extracellular fluid **osmolality**: it is controlled by antidiuretic hormone (ADH, p. 167).

Filtration should be regarded as the 'waste disposal' function and flow the regulator of volume and osmolality.

Tubular 'processing' of the glomerular filtrate

Urine reaches the proximal convoluted tubule as a cell-free ultrafiltrate of plasma. Two-thirds is reabsorbed in this segment as a consequence of active sodium reabsorption. Water in the renal tubule diffuses passively down the concentration gradient created by sodium reabsorption and there is little change in urine osmolality from one end of the proximal tubule to the other. Chloride, potassium, calcium, phosphate, glucose and amino acids are also reabsorbed in this segment.

Another tubular function is acidification of the urine. Water and carbon dioxide combine in the tubular cells to form carbonic acid, catalysed by the enzyme carbonic anhydrase. Dissociation into hydrogen and bicarbonate ions yields free hydrogen ions, which are pumped into tubular fluid in exchange for sodium. The hydrogen ions are buffered by recombination with bicarbonate to yield water and diffusible carbon dioxide, and by combination with phosphate buffers and ammonia. The net effect is absorption of bicarbonate and increase in the acidity of urine.

The function of the loop of Henle can be summarised as a mechanism which progressively increases the osmolality of the renal interstitium from cortex to medulla by 'countercurrent multiplication' (summarised in any physiology textbook) and removes a further 15% of filtrate. It is in the distal convoluted tubule and collecting duct that the mechanisms which control the non-obligatory handling of sodium and water operate. **Aldosterone** increases sodium reabsorption in exchange for potassium. About 15% of glomerular filtrate enters the collecting ducts and passes through an increasingly hyperosmolar interstitium. **Antidiuretic hormone,** secreted primarily in response to changes in plasma osmolality, regulates the permeability of the collecting ducts to water and, together with aldosterone, controls urine flow.

Endocrine function

The endocrine functions of the kidney can be summarised as:

- secretion of renin by the juxtaglomerular apparatus; this controls angiotensin and aldosterone secretion in response to volume depletion and hyponatraemia
- erythropoietin synthesis in response to anaemia and hypoxia
- the 1α-hydroxylation of vitamin D, controlled by parathyroid hormone.

Urea and creatinine as markers of renal disease

The renal handling of urea and creatinine deserves special mention, not just because these are important nitrogenous waste products but because they are measured in almost every 'medical' patient and are a key to understanding fluid and electrolyte biochemistry.

Creatinine. In health, there is a steady rate of creatinine synthesis from the turnover of muscle protein. Creatinine is freely filtered and is not actively secreted; only a small proportion is reabsorbed. Plasma creatinine concentration is thus primarily determined by glomerular filtration rate (GFR). Unless there is accelerated muscle catabolism, an increase in plasma creatinine signifies a sign of a fall in GFR.

Urea. General protein catabolism produces urea, synthesis of which is dependent on intact liver function. Urea production is, therefore, more labile than creatinine production, rising in catabolic states (and after eating a large protein meal) and falling in liver failure. More important still, between 10 and 70% of tubular urea is reabsorbed depending on the rate of urine flow. Thus plasma urea concentration can be increased by both reduced **filtration** and reduced **flow**. The relationship between plasma urea and creatinine concentrations can be used to distinguish between these two very different physiological conditions. If urea alone is raised, the cause is reduced flow (e.g. caused by reduced renal perfusion within the range which can be compensated for by autoregulation). If both are raised, there is hypofiltration ('renal failure'). Remember that a small increase in urea may result from protein catabolism after large protein meals or GI bleeding.

Summary of renal physiology

When considering renal disease and its management, it is useful to have the following simple framework of renal function in your mind:

- clearance of nitrogenous waste
- regulation of sodium, potassium and water balance
- retention of essential proteins
- regulation of blood pressure
- regulation of acid–base homeostasis
- endocrine function: erythropoietin synthesis and 1-hydroxylation of vitamin D.

Renal pathology

Glomerular disease

The nephrons are vulnerable to abnormal oxygenation, abnormal perfusion and to toxins in the incoming blood. The glomeruli can also be damaged by immunological processes, notably autoantibodies to glomerular structures (e.g. antiglomerular basement membrane in Goodpasture's syndrome) and circulating immune complexes. Glomerulonephritis may follow infection or complicate connective disease or malignancy. Metabolic processes also cause diffuse glomerular damage. Diabetes is the commonest example. The effects of glomerular disease are proteinuria and renal failure.

Tubular disease

This may be congenital (e.g. Fanconi syndrome) or acquired (e.g. multiple myeloma). It causes abnormal water/electrolyte handling and acidosis, as discussed on page 160.

Postrenal disease

Obstruction to the urinary tract is an important cause of renal dysfunction; remember, however, that there is so much reserve capacity in the two kidneys that both must be obstructed for there to be significant renal failure. Infection and stones often present with their own symptoms long before they cause renal failure.

Symptoms and signs

These can be separated into those of any underlying disease and those of renal failure itself.

The symptoms of renal disease can be elusive. Urinary frequency and dysuria suggest lower urinary tract disease. Polyuria and nocturia, the most specific symptoms of renal failure, are caused by failure of renal tubular sodium reabsorption and/or collecting duct disease. Renal failure is only one cause of polyuria and polydipsia. Others include:

Common causes:

- anxiety or habit
- diabetes mellitus.

Uncommon causes:

- diabetes insipidus
  — nephrogenic
  — cranial
- hypokalaemia
- hypercalcaemia.

Table 31 lists the symptoms and signs of renal disease. You should remember that the symptoms and signs of **uraemia** do not occur until the GFR is severely impaired (< 20 ml/min).

No assessment of a patient with renal disease is complete without an assessment of blood volume (as described on p. 169). This is because:

- volume depletion (shock, 'dehydration') impairs renal perfusion and can cause or worsen renal failure
- renal failure impairs salt and water excretion and can cause volume overload
- heart failure impairs renal perfusion and can ultimately cause renal failure.

These points emphasise a crucial concept: the heart and kidneys are a functioning unit in terms of fluid balance. At the bedside, the haemodynamic effects of 'heart failure' (p. 22) and 'renal failure' can be indistinguishable. Another important relationship is between renal disease and hypertension. Fluid retention and renin oversecretion both cause hypertension and both can exacerbate and be caused by renal disease. You must measure blood pres-

Table 31 Symptoms and signs of renal disease

Symptoms	Signs
Renal failure	
Failure to excrete nitrogenous waste	
Pruritis	Uraemic foetor
Nausea, anorexia, vomiting, dyspepsia	Pale, sallow skin
Lethargy	Scratch marks
Chest pain	Pericardial or pleural rub
Mental dullness	Cognitive impairment, twitching, fits and/or coma
Paraesthesiae	Sensori-motor neuropathy
Hiccoughs	
Protein loss and failure to regulate fluid/electrolyte balance and blood pressure	
Thirst	Oedema
Polyuria	Signs of left ± right heart failure
Nocturia	Hypertension or hypotension
Oliguria or anuria	
Weakness (hypo- or hyperkalaemia)	
Breathlessness	
Acidosis	
Breathlessness	Kussmaul respiration
	Cognitive impairment
Failure of endocrine function	
Anaemia	Pallor
Lethargy	
Dyspnoea	
Impaired hydroxylation of vitamin D	
Bone pain	Signs of osteomalacia or rickets
Underlying disease	
Urinary tract disease	
Haematuria	Loin tenderness
Loin pain	Palpable kidneys and/or bladder
Dysuria	
Systemic disease	
E.g. symptoms of diabetes and its complications in collagen vascular disease	e.g. Vasculitic skin rash in collagen vascular disease

sure carefully (p. 41) and assess your patient carefully for the complications of hypertension (p. 42).

4.2 Investigation of renal disease

Learning objectives

You should:
- know the range of investigations for renal disease and understand their use in different clinical situations
- appreciate that proteinuria is easy to detect with a dipstick, usually indicative of renal/urinary tract disease and all too often overlooked at an early stage when referral, investigation and treatment could preserve renal function.

Urine analysis

Stick testing

Dipsticks can accurately measure pH and detect the presence of blood, protein and white cells. Urine test-

ing for albumin is an essential adjunct to physical examination since healthy people do not have proteinuria except during intercurrent illness or menstruation and, in some cases, in the upright posture ('benign orthostatic proteinuria'). Proteinuria needs further investigation. Its causes (with the most common in bold) are:

- General
  — **fever**
  — benign orthostatic proteinuria
  — Pre-eclampsia
- abnormal plasma protein
  — myeloma (p. 243)
- glomerular disease
  — hypertension
  — **diabetes**
  — **acute or chronic glomerulonephritis**
- tubular disease
  — acute tubular necrosis
- other renal diseases
  — renal tumours or cysts
  — **chronic pyelonephritis**
  — renal tuberculosis
  — interstitial nephropathy

- lower urinary tract disease
  — **urinary tract infection**
  — tumour.

Microscopy and culture

Both microscopy and culture can give valuable information. The presence of red and/or white cells signifies infection or structural pathology at any level from the glomerulus to the bladder. The presence of casts must be taken seriously. Red cell casts are pathognomonic of glomerular disease. Hyaline or granular casts may be caused by disease of the glomeruli or tubules.

Culture should be performed on a fresh, midstream urine sample. Infection is distinguished from contamination by the presence of white cells and growth of pathogenic rather than commensal organisms.

Urine biochemistry

Unlike plasma biochemistry, there are no clearly defined normal ranges for any urinary solute except protein (less than 150 mg/24 hours). In health, the urinary excretion of sodium and potassium reflect intake and are determined by food preferences rather than physiology. In disease, measurement of urinary sodium or potassium can tell you whether or not depletion or overload of these solutes is caused by abnormal renal handling.

Similarly, creatinine excretion varies widely between individuals with different muscle bulks, but measurement of its clearance in a 24 hour urine sample (excretion in relation to plasma concentration) gives an estimate of GFR. In acute renal failure, measurement of the ratio of urine to plasma urea concentration can help you decide whether the problem is impaired renal perfusion with intact glomerular function (ratio > 8)or whether the capacity to concentrate urea is lost (ratio < 8).

Plasma biochemistry

Plasma creatinine concentration is a useful proxy for GFR provided you remember that the steady-state serum creatinine concentration is determined also by muscle bulk. Therefore, a wasted elderly patient may have significant renal failure at a creatinine concentration which is normal for a muscular rugby player. This is reflected in the wide 'normal' range for serum creatinine. Changes in serum creatinine within an individual can be a sensitive guide to changes in renal function, although serum creatinine rises in a near-exponential relationship to GFR. Therefore, a rise in creatinine from 130 to 140 μmol/l may signify the same proportional loss of renal function as a rise from 400 to 600 μmol/l. Plasma creatinine does not rise above normal until over 50% of glomerular filtration is lost. Plasma urea is usually measured together with creatinine for reasons discussed on page 152.

Measurement of potassium is important because renal failure impairs its excretion and that may be exacerbated by drugs (see p. 159). Hyperkalaemia is a potentially fatal complication of renal disease. Renal failure may also cause acidosis by failure of the tubular processes described on page 151.

Measurement of GFR

This can be measured isotopically (^{51}CrEDTA) or chemically (inulin clearance). These measurements are usually confined to specialist nephrological practice.

Imaging

Plain X-ray and i.v. pyelography

High-quality ultrasound has made these investigations all but obsolete. A plain radiograph can show calculi and the renal outlines but provides little other useful information. Pyelography gives good definition of the kidneys and indicates whether they are functional, but opacification is poor in renal failure. Moreover, even modern 'non-ionic' contrast media present a considerable osmotic load which can cause heart failure and precipitate acute renal failure, particularly in patients with myeloma or diabetes. You must ensure that such patients are not volume depleted at the time of contrast radiology or the risk is increased further still.

Ultrasound

In the hands of a skilled radiologist, this gives detailed information about the structure of the kidneys and urinary tract. It cannot, however, assess function. Because ultrasound is non-invasive and very informative, it is usually the first and often the only form of imaging in renal disease.

Computerised tomography

CT gives detailed information about abnormalities within the renal parenchyma and the relationship of organs of the urinary tract to surrounding structures.

Antegrade and retrograde pyelography

The renal pelvis and ureters can be cannulated endoscopically and imaged following contrast injection. These techniques are used in obstructive uropathy, in which cannulation may relieve obstruction as well as demonstrating its anatomical level and cause.

Cystography

Cystography is used primarily in paediatric practice. It is performed by instilling contrast into the bladder to demonstrate ureteric reflux during micturition.

Angiography

Digital i.v. angiography allows detailed non-invasive imaging of the renal arterial circulation and is used to investigate renovascular disease. Direct intra-arterial cannulation is more invasive but is the 'gold standard' to detect stenosis. Renal venography is used to investigate suspected renal vein thrombosis.

Isotope renography

Isotope studies are used not just to image the kidneys but also to measure renal function. For example, asymmetrical uptake between the two kidneys supports a diagnosis of unilateral renal artery stenosis. Delayed clearance of isotope suggests obstruction. Renography is the screening technique of choice for renovascular disease, especially when used in conjunction with captopril, which amplifies the haemodynamic effects of renal artery stenosis (p. 161).

Biopsy

Biopsy is performed by placing a biopsy needle into the kidney substance through a posterior loin approach under ultrasound guidance in a conscious patient. Cooperation is needed because the kidneys move several centimetres with respiration and the patient must stop breathing when the biopsy is taken. It can precipitate renal failure or be complicated by haemorrhage. Renal biopsy is indicated for the investigation of acute or chronic renal failure of unknown cause, or unexplained persistent proteinuria and haematuria. It is primarily indicated to diagnose diffuse disease of the glomeruli, tubules and interstitium. The biopsy sample is analysed by light microscopy, electron microscopy and immunohistochemistry.

4.3 Clinical presentations of renal disease

Learning objectives

You need to understand:
• the common presentations of renal disease
• their causes and management.

Table 32 shows a 'matrix' correlating pathologies with clinical presentations. This chapter first discusses the clinical presentations and then fills in details about specific pathologies.

Renal failure

Renal failure may be acute, chronic or 'acute-on-chronic'. There are three potentially **reversible** factors which can cause or exacerbate renal failure:

• impaired perfusion
• urinary obstruction
• infection.

Impaired perfusion not only causes renal failure but can be made worse by it since uraemic anorexia and vomiting cause volume depletion. You should approach a patient with renal failure with the following questions in mind:

• what is the patient's blood volume?
• have obstruction and infection been excluded?

In addition, the size of the kidneys (easily measured by ultrasound; p. 154) gives you important information about the chronicity of the problem.

Acute renal failure

Epidemiology
Acute renal failure requiring dialysis has an annual incidence of approximately 70 cases per million. Of these:

• 60% are caused by prerenal disease, usually acute tubular necrosis (see p. 150)
• 10% are caused by urinary obstruction
• 10–15% result from vasculitides and rapidly progressive glomerulonephritis
• 10% are caused by drugs and interstitial nephropathies.

Pathology
The diseases which cause acute renal failure are rapid in their onset and usually prerenal. There are few pathologies which will simultaneously occlude both ureters, so 'postrenal' disease rarely causes truly **acute** (as opposed to acute-on-chronic; p. 159) renal failure. The exception is in patients with a congenital absence of or pre-existing disease in one kidney. Likewise, there are few renal parenchymal diseases which cause simultaneous acute failure of 1.3 million nephrons: glomerular vasculitis

Table 32 Clinical presentation of renal/urological disease

Pathology	Acute nephritis	Acute renal failure	Chronic renal failure	Nephrotic syndrome	Tubular disease	Haematuria	Pain	Symptomless mass
Glomerulonephritis	+	+	+	+		+		
Renovascular disease		+	+					
Renal involvement in systemic disease	+	+	+	+	+	+	+	
Congenital nephropathies			+	+	+			
Renal tumours						+	+	+
Stone			+			+	+	
Infection	±		+			+	+	

and rapidly progressive glomerulonephritis are striking exceptions.

Since each kidney has a separate arterial supply, the same logic might apply to vascular causes, except that aortic disease may involve both renal arteries simultaneously. Prerenal changes are the most common cause of acute renal failure and are most often seen in the context of severe illness *exogenous* to the kidneys. The causes include:

Prerenal factors leading to renal hypoperfusion and acute tubular necrosis (ATN) (listed on page 150).

Other causes:

- rhabdomyolysis with urinary excretion of myoglobin
- drugs — e.g. gentamicin
- structural abnormalities of renal vasculature:
  — large vessel occlusion (renovascular disease)
  — small vessel occlusion
     accelerated hypertension, DIC (p. 248), haemolytic/uraemic syndrome, thrombotic thrombocytopenic purpura, systemic sclerosis, pre-eclampsia
  — acute cortical necrosis
- acute glomerulonephritis and vasculitis
- interstitial nephritis
- myeloma
- urinary tract obstruction.

The most important concept in the understanding of acute renal failure is that *failure of renal perfusion can progress from a functional abnormality (reversible if perfusion is restored) to established renal damage (acute tubular or cortical necrosis).*

Clinical features

As often as not, renal failure is diagnosed in an already 'ill' patient. The diagnosis may be made biochemically or from the development of oliguria or anuria. Oliguria is defined as a urine flow less than the obligatory minimum for nitrogen excretion (0.5 litres/24 hours). Oliguria/anuria are not *necessary* conditions for the diagnosis of acute renal failure, since flow may be maintained or even exaggerated despite hypofiltration. Progression from oliguria/anuria to polyuria is common during recovery from acute tubular necrosis. Patients with polyuric acute renal failure have an impaired ability to control *flow* and are extremely vulnerable to volume depletion, which can secondarily exacerbate their renal failure. Other symptoms of renal failure are as shown in Table 31. The symptoms in any individual patient depend on the severity and duration of their disease but do not usually include the effects of renal endocrine failure since these take time to develop.

The clinical assessment of patients with acute renal failure should concentrate on:

- duration of symptoms: is the disease truly acute?
- symptoms and signs of causative diseases, either specifically renal or multisystem

- assessment of blood volume (p. 168)
- assessment of cardiac function
- exclusion of obstruction: rectal and vaginal examinations are essential in all patients
- assessment for the other features listed in Table 31.

Investigations

Biochemistry. You should measure plasma sodium, potassium, urea and creatinine and venous bicarbonate. Arterial blood gas sampling is not necessary to diagnose metabolic acidosis but may be indicated for other reasons. Measurement of urea and sodium in a 'spot' urine sample helps to distinguish between failure of perfusion and 'established' renal failure; in the former, urinary sodium is low (< 20 mmol/l) and the ratio of urinary to plasma urea > 8.

Urinalysis. Culture and microscopy of fresh urine for cells and casts is essential in all cases.

Imaging. *Immediate* ultrasound is indicated to assess renal size and exclude bladder outflow obstruction, hydronephrosis and other lower urinary tract disease. A chest radiograph is needed to assess heart size and look for signs of pulmonary oedema.

Haematology. Normochromic anaemia is suggestive of **chronic** renal failure. Other haematological changes such as thrombocytopenia, fragmentation of red cells, etc. may give clues to underlying microvascular disease (e.g. DIC).

ECG.

Renal biopsy. The procedure and indications are described on page 155.

Other investigations. These are indicated by your suspected cause of renal failure. Immunological tests should include antineutrophil cytoplasmic antibody, glomerular basement membrane antibody and antinuclear factor.

Management

Fluid therapy. Just as assessment of blood volume is crucial to the diagnosis of acute renal failure, fluid therapy is central to its management. In many cases, the need for fluid can be determined by clinical signs (see Fig. 32, below). If in doubt, a central venous pressure line or pulmonary arterial flow catheter should be used. Management is guided not just by the initial assessment but by frequent bedside reassessment of blood volume and close observation of fluid balance and weight. A urinary catheter can introduce infection and is best avoided in any patient who is able to cooperate, but it may be needed for accurate hour-to-hour monitoring of output. It is mandatory to weigh the patient daily to assess net gains and losses. More precise and hour-to-hour weighing needs a 'weighing bed'. The aim of fluid therapy is to achieve adequate but not excessive volume replacement. The choice of fluid depends on the context. Blood loss is treated by blood transfusion. Massive protein loss, as in burns, is treated by 'colloid' infusions. In other cases, saline is the fluid of choice because volume-depleted patients need volume expansion with salt and water, sometimes with dextrose to correct imbalances in the plasma sodium concentration.

Management of fluid overload. If the patient is in heart failure, cardiac function should be optimised by treating arrhythmias and, if necessary, giving inotropic agents. Low-dose dopamine specifically improves glomerular perfusion and may be given conjointly with dobutamine for maximum inotropic effect. There are two indications for diuretics in acute renal failure: to treat volume overload and, as a therapeutic trial, to re-establish urine flow in a volume-depleted patient. A loop diuretic (frusemide or bumetanide) should be given i.v. in high dose and repeated as necessary. Fluid overload which does not respond to these measures is an indication for dialysis (see below).

Obstruction. If present, this must be relieved. In the case of bladder outflow obstruction, a urethral or suprapubic catheter should be passed. In ureteric obstruction, a drainage catheter can be positioned in one or both renal pelvices percutaneously (nephrostomy).

Hyperkalaemia. Failure of tubular potassium excretion is potentially the most serious metabolic complication of acute renal failure since it can cause fatal ventricular fibrillation. A serum potassium concentration > 7 mmol/l is a medical emergency and should be managed as described on page 172.

Diet and fluid intake. The fluid and sodium intake should be adjusted to maintain a normal blood volume, allowing for insensible loss (500 mg/24 hours, higher if pyrexial). Patients who are volume overloaded should be salt and water restricted; those who are volume depleted should drink freely and may need salt supplements. Potassium intake should be restricted. Nutrition is important, particularly in patients whose renal failure is secondary to some other severe illness, because catabolism increases urea production. Carbohydrate must be the predominant source of calories and patients should take as high a calorie intake as is commensurate with their fluid and potassium allowances. A protein intake of 1 g/kg body weight is often recommended. If oral feeding is impracticable, enteral or parenteral nutrition is needed.

Dialysis for acute renal failure. This is indicated for:

- nitrogen retention (uraemic symptoms or 'high' blood urea: threshold individualised to the patient)
- pericarditis or neurological complications of uraemia
- intractable fluid retention; even if primarily caused by cardiac failure
- intractable hyperkalaemia, acidosis or other electrolyte disturbance.

Haemodialysis is used in preference to peritoneal dialysis for acute renal failure.

Prognosis

Partly because it often develops in the context of multiorgan failure and partly because it causes severe catabolism and widespread tissue damage, ac[u] has an overall mortality around 50% in the stage of needing dialysis. If the patient su[r] most of the prerenal causes of acute renal failure have an excellent renal prognosis.

Chronic renal failure

Epidemiology
The annual incidence of end-stage renal failure in the UK is approximately 80 cases per million. The causes are:

- chronic glomerulonephritis: 30%
- chronic reflux nephropathy: 25%
- polycystic kidney disease: 10%
- diabetic nephropathy: 15% (higher incidence in Asians and Afro-Caribbeans)
- obstructive uropathy: 10%
- renovascular disease: 10%.

Pathology
Figure 28 shows causes of chronic renal failure. An important point to understand is that it can become self-perpetuating because loss of functioning nephrons causes glomerular hypertension which leads to further nephron loss. For this reason, treatment rarely reverses established chronic renal failure and renal function may deteriorate progressively despite correction of an underlying disease.

Clinical features
The presentation varies from a chance biochemical finding to the most florid and fully developed uraemia. A typical presentation is with non-specific lethargy and anaemia with or without urinary symptoms. Unlike acute renal failure, the symptoms of bone disease may be prominent. Clinical assessment follows exactly the same steps as described under acute renal failure (p. 156) including exclusion of reversible factors.

Investigation
This follows the same principles as acute renal failure except that there are some investigations, for example micturating cystography, which are specific to diseases causing chronic renal failure. Renal biopsy is indicated if no diagnosis has been made, 'macroscopic' causes have been excluded and renal failure is not too far advanced.

Management
Management consists of:

- treating underlying causes
- optimising fluid/electrolyte balance and nutrition
- retarding the progression of chronic renal failure
- treating complications
- renal replacement for end-stage renal failure (ESRF).

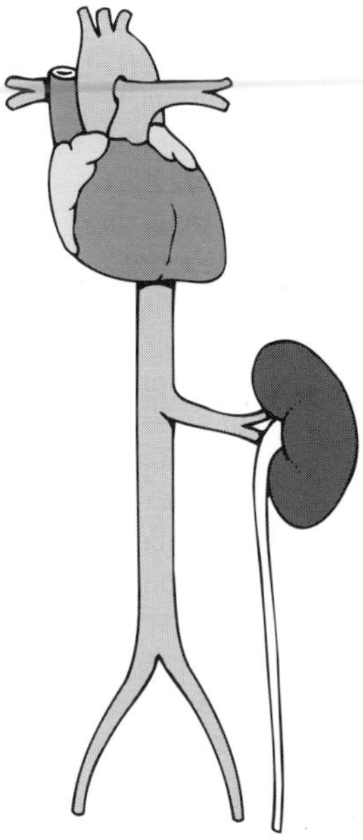

Pre-renal:
- Cardiogenic
  Severe cardiac failure

- Vascular
  Renal artery stenosis; bilateral or
    complicated by ACE-I therapy
  Intra-renal atherosclerosis
  Hypertension

Renal:
- Immunological /vasculitis:
  Glomerulonephritis–primary or
    secondar to systemic disease
  Microscopic polyarteritis
  Wegener's granulomatosis
  Systemic sclerosis
- Other microvascular disease:
  Diabetes
- Neoplastic
  Multiple myeloma
- Toxic
  Gold, penicillamine, cyclosporine
- Tubulo–interstitial nephropathy
- Infection and/or reflux
  Chronic pyelonephritis
  Renal TB
- Cystic diseases
  Polycystic kidneys

Post-renal:
- Disease of the renal pelvis
  Stone
  Pelvi-ureteric obstruction
- Bilateral ureteric obstruction
  Retroperitoneal tumour or fibrosis
  Pelvic or bladder tumour or fibrosis
- Obstruction of solitary kidney
- Bladder outflow obstruction
  Urethral stenosis
  Prostate hypertrophy

Fig. 28
Causes of chronic renal failure.

Fluid/electrolyte management. Patients with chronic failure may be fluid overloaded or fluid depleted. Their fluid and salt intake should be adjusted to achieve euvolaemia. Dietary potassium restriction is usually necessary. When diuretics are needed, care must be taken not to cause volume depletion and prerenal uraemia. Potassium-conserving diuretics are contraindicated.

Acid/base management. In some cases, chronic treatment with oral bicarbonate is needed to correct acidosis.

Diet. There is evidence that restriction of dietary protein below 1 g/kg body weight daily can improve hydrostatic pressures within the glomeruli and attenuate the self-perpetuating renal deterioration. As the patient approaches end-stage renal failure, dietary protein restriction may delay the need for dialysis. Together with salt, potassium and water restriction, this can make an extremely bland and unpalatable diet, so advice should be tailored to the patient's willingness to comply.

Antihypertensive therapy. There is strong evidence that, for at least some causes of chronic renal failure, antihypertensive therapy can halt or attenuate renal deterioration. ACE inhibitors are particularly beneficial but can be harmful if the patient has renal artery stenosis or is volume depleted. Close monitoring of renal function after starting ACE inhibitors is essential and 'arteriopaths' may need renography or angiography to exclude renal artery stenosis before starting them.

Hyperlipidaemia. Most patients with chronic renal failure are hyperlipidaemic and this is one factor contributing to the formidably high cardiovascular morbidity and mortality. Fasting lipids should be checked periodically and treated (as described on p. 273). This is not without difficulty, because fat restriction is yet another imposition on the renal patient's diet, and lipid-lowering drugs may cause a myalgic syndrome in patients with renal failure.

Renal replacement. This is indicated for patients with advanced renal failure whose general state of health, psychosocial wellbeing and support are such that it is likely to improve the quality as well as the quantity of life. Renal replacement should be planned and discussed with patients well in advance of end-stage. It is started when uraemia seriously affects their wellbeing or any of the complications discussed on page 157 develop. Transplantation, where possible, achieves a higher level of rehabilitation than maintenance (home or hospital) haemodialysis or continuous ambulatory peritoneal dialysis.

Prescribing in renal disease

At its simplest, this can be covered in five words: 'refer to British National Formulary'. This should be carried in every doctor's pocket or briefcase and gives detailed information about drugs which affect or are affected by renal disease. The ways in which renal disease affects the action of drugs and how drugs can damage the kidneys are summarised in Table 33.

Renal bone disease

Pathophysiology

The pathogenetic mechanisms, summarised in Figure 29, are relatively specific to chronic renal failure. Renal tubular phosphate retention and failure to 1α-hydroxylate vitamin D lead to osteomalacia and secondary hyperparathyroidism, with failure of mineralisation and increased osteoclastic bone resorption. There may also be osteosclerosis, which causes the 'rugger jersey spine' appearance on plain radiographs.

Clinical and biochemical features

There may be weakness, bone pain, deformity and fractures. Plasma calcium is usually normal or low. Plasma phosphate is high. Alkaline phosphatase is high if there is significant bone disease. Serum parathyroid hormone is usually raised.

Management

Phosphate-binding agents should be given to all patients with established chronic renal failure. Calcium

Table 33 Important drug effects in renal failure

	Drug	Effect	Action
Accumulation	Digoxin	Potential toxicity	Reduce dose, monitor drug level
	Aminoglycosides	Ototoxicity	Use prescribing nomogram, monitor levels
	Sulphonylureas	Hypoglycaemia	Use non-renally excreted drugs, e.g. gliclazide
Nephrotoxicity	Aminoglycosides	Tubular toxicity in acute renal failure	Use prescribing nomogram, monitor levels
	Radiographic contrast media	Acute-on-chronic renal failure	Ensure patients are adequately hydrated before radiographic procedures
May have side effects	NSAIDs	Fluid retention Worsened GFR	Use with caution Monitor serum creatinine
	ACE inhibitors	Worsened renal function in renal artery stenosis Hyperkalaemia	Avoid in renal artery stenosis, monitor creatinine Monitor serum K$^+$ and creatinine
	Dopamine	May cause renal vasoconstriction	Use at low dose
Less effective in renal failure	Diuretics		Increase effectiveness by: using loop diuretics, giving i.v., using high dose
Contraindicated	Potassium-sparing diuretics	Hyperkalaemia	
	Nitrofurantoin	Renal tubular necrosis, peripheral neuropathy	
	Tetracycline	Worsened uraemia	
	Metformin	Lactic acidosis	

carbonate is a good choice because it provides supplemental calcium as well. Hypocalcaemia is treated with 1,25-dihydroxycholecalciferol or an analogue. Tertiary hyperparathyroidism is treated by parathyroidectomy.

Acute-on-chronic renal failure

Patients with chronic renal failure are vulnerable to the prerenal and postrenal diseases summarised on page 000 and the effects of intercurrent illness and urinary infection, all of which can acutely exacerbate chronic renal failure. The clinical features, investigation and management are as for acute renal failure. The search for exacerbating factors, volume depletion in particular, is paramount. With prompt and effective treatment, it is usually possible to reverse the functional deterioration.

Nephrotic syndrome

Nephrotic syndrome is a chronic condition defined by the triad of:

* proteinuria (> 3 g/24 hour)
* hypoproteinaemia (serum albumin < 30 g/l)
* oedema.

It is to be distinguished from acute nephritis (p. 160), although both syndromes may be caused by glomerulonephritis. Proteinuria is the primary abnormality; hypoproteinaemia ensues and this lowers plasma oncotic pressure so that salt and water leak from capillaries into the interstitial fluid. Plasma volume is reduced and there is compensatory hyperaldosteronism, which increases total body sodium content. Nephrotic syndrome signifies increased permeability of the glomerular filter caused by glomerular disease.

Causes
The most classical cause of nephrotic syndrome is **minimal change nephropathy** in children. A more complete list includes:
* glomerulonephritis
  — primary: minimal change glomerulonephritis, other glomerulonephritides
  — secondary to autoimmune disease such as SLE
* other immunological disease: amyloid
* metabolic: diabetes mellitus
* neoplasia: carcinoma, lymphoma, leukaemia, myeloma
* infection: subacute bacterial endocarditis, malaria, hepatitis B
* drugs/toxins: gold, other heavy metals, penicillamine, intravenous drug abuse
* vascular: renal vein thrombosis.

The most common causes are glomerulonephritis, diabetes and drugs.

Complications and management
Apart from salt retention (oedema, pleural and pericardial effusions, ascites), patients may suffer from malnutrition and increased susceptibility to infection as an effect of protein loss. Hypercholesterolaemia and hypercoagulability predispose to coronary artery disease. Nephrotic syndrome predisposes to one quite specific complication, renal vein thrombosis, which should be suspected in any nephrotic patient whose protein-

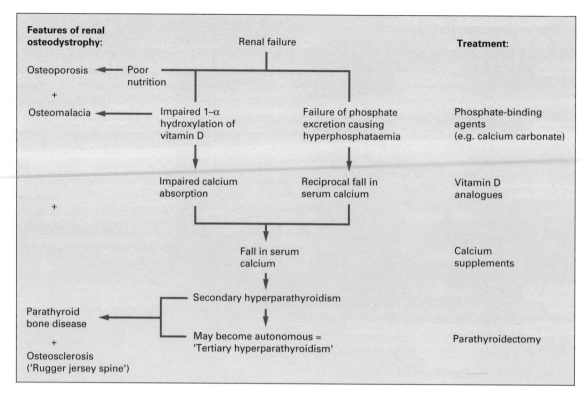

Fig. 29
Mechanisms of renal bone disease.

uria or renal function worsens abruptly. It is diagnosed by renal venography or Doppler ultrasound and treated with anticoagulants both to preserve renal function and prevent pulmonary embolism.

Diuretics are prescribed for oedema but their use is problematic because they may further contract an already reduced plasma volume and worsen renal perfusion. If plasma volume contraction prevents effective diuretic therapy, colloid may be infused to increase plasma colloid oncotic pressure and provide a temporary 'bridge' between the interstitial fluid and glomeruli. Minimal-change disease can be treated with corticosteroids or other immunosuppressives; many other causes of nephrotic syndrome are unremitting, even with treatment.

Acute nephritis

At its most florid, the acute nephritic syndrome consists of oliguria and oedema of the face, hands and legs. The urine is 'smoky' because of glomerular haematuria, proteinuria and urinary casts. Historically, the most common cause was streptococcal infection, but post-streptococcal nephritis is now rare in the developed world. The acute nephritic syndrome is more commonly caused by rapidly progressive glomerulonephritis, sometimes associated with collagen vascular disease. It may also follow a range of non-streptococcal infections. It may be benign and self-limiting or lead to acute renal failure. Management is as described for other causes of acute renal failure, with specific treatment aimed at any underlying cause.

Renal tubular acidosis

This name strikes terror into the heart of all but the nephrologist or the physician who has recently passed MRCP. In fact, the principles are simple and follow exactly from the description of tubular function (p. 151).

- there is failure of bicarbonate reabsorption (type 2, proximal tubular) or hydrogen ion secretion (type 1, distal tubular) leading to reduced serum bicarbonate and metabolic acidosis
- the urine is inappropriately alkaline
- there is a compensatory rise in serum chloride to maintain electrical neutrality, a 'hyperchloraemic acidosis'
- there may be other tubular dysfunctions, such as increased leakage of sodium, potassium, glucose, calcium, amino acids and phosphate
- the disease may be congenital or acquired
- there may be calcification of the kidneys, particularly at the cortico-medullary junction (nephrocalcinosis)
- the tubular phosphate leak may cause a vitamin D-resistant form of rickets (renal rickets).

The best recognised form of renal tubular acidosis is **Fanconi syndrome**. This inherited disorder is caused by proximal tubular dysfunction and comprises glycosuria, aminoaciduria, 'renal rickets' and renal tubular acidosis. Acquired renal tubular disease may result from multiple myeloma, collagen vascular disease, heavy metal poisoning, acquired aldosterone deficiency and chronic parenchymal kidney disease. Treatment is with alkali, phosphate, sodium and potassium and the synthetic analogue of aldosterone, fludrocortisone.

4.4 Specific renal and urinary tract diseases

The clinical presentations described so far are core knowledge. Many individual renal diseases, including the glomerulonephritides, are 'non-core'. A description of them can be found in a reference textbook.

The ways in which individual **systemic diseases** affect the kidneys is best learned when learning about the diseases themselves.

Parenchymal and vascular diseases

Interstitial nephropathy

Glomerulopathy is one renal response to injury; another is interstitial or 'tubulo-interstitial' nephropathy, where the tubules and interstitium bear the brunt of disease. The classical stereotype is analgesic nephropathy, but this is now uncommon. Important causes include:

- vesico-ureteric reflux
- reflux nephropathy (formerly known as chronic pyelonephritis)
- chronic urinary obstruction
- idiopathic.
  Less common causes include:
- collagen vascular disease
- neoplasia
- metabolic causes: hypercalcaemia, hypokalaemia, gout.

Interstitial nephropathy presents with moderate proteinuria, acute or chronic renal failure or renal tubular dysfunction. Diagnosis rests on clinical suspicion and, where appropriate, renal biopsy. Treatment is by correction of underlying causes; in some patients, steroids are effective. The disease may progress to end-stage renal failure.

Renal papillary necrosis

Renal papillary necrosis is caused by ischaemic necrosis and sloughing of renal papillae. It is characterised by:

- loin pain (sometimes of a colicky nature)
- haematuria
- variable degrees of renal impairment.

It is an acute and extreme variant of interstitial nephropathy, most commonly caused by drugs/toxins and acute infections, particularly in diabetes mellitus.

Renovascular disease

Narrowing of the renal artery or its tributaries proximal to the glomeruli reduces glomerular pressure and increases renin secretion, irrespective of systemic pressure. This may result from a single narrowing of a main renal artery or diffuse intrarenal arterial disease. Renal artery stenosis causes hypertension and, if bilateral, renal failure. Renal arterial disease is suggested by otherwise unexplained renal failure or hypertension in a patient with peripheral vascular and/or generalised arterial disease; renal bruits are the only clinical sign and are present only in a minority. It should also be suspected in a patient whose renal function worsens when given an ACE inhibitor, because they adversely affect the compensatory haemodynamic response to renal arterial disease. Because of this risk, renal function should be measured frequently after initiation of ACE inhibitor therapy in arteriopaths or elderly patients.

Ultrasound may show a small kidney on the side of unilateral renal artery stenosis; isotope renography and angiography are the definitive investigations. Renal artery stenosis can be treated by:

- angioplasty
- stenting
- surgery.

Renal vein thrombosis has been mentioned under nephrotic syndrome.

Cystic disease

There are three main forms of cystic disease:

- solitary benign cysts
- cysts associated with renal cell carcinoma
- polycystic disease.

A solitary cyst may be found by chance on abdominal examination or ultrasound or in the investigation of loin pain and/or haematuria. Most are benign. If in doubt, cyst fluid may be aspirated percutaneously for cytological examination.

Adult polycystic disease is an important diagnosis because it accounts for about 10% of cases of end-stage renal failure, typically presenting between 40 and 50 years of age. Patients may also present with:

- loin pain
- haematuria
- symptoms and signs related to the massively enlarged kidneys.

In established disease, the appearances on ultrasound or CT are pathognomonic and the diagnosis can even be made by abdominal examination (large, irregular masses in both loins). The disease follows an autosomal dominant pattern of inheritance and progresses slowly but inexorably towards end-stage renal failure. Treatment is with:

- good control of blood pressure
- general management of chronic renal failure
- dialysis when end stage is reached.

There are liver cysts in 70% of patients and 25% have berry aneurysms which may lead to subarachnoid haemorrhage. A chromosomal marker has been identified and genetic counselling must be offered in all cases.

Neoplasia

Neoplasia can be classified into:

- urothelial tumours
- renal cell carcinoma
- exogenous or secondary tumours directly or indirectly affecting the urinary tract, the renal parenchyma, the renal circulation, the glomeruli and/or the tubules.

Haematuria and pain are the main symptoms: the exact distribution and nature of the pain depends on the site, size and invasiveness of the tumour. Renal adenocarcinoma is a tumour notorious for its systemic effects. In addition to its local effects, it may present with:

- pyrexia of unknown origin
- weight loss and systemic malaise
- bony or pulmonary metastases
- hypercalcaemia.

Relevant investigations are urinalysis, ultrasound, CT, intravenous pyelography and cystoscopy. Table 34 summarises key facts about tumours of the kidneys and urinary tract.

Urinary stone

Stones may present with:

- pain and/or haematuria
- symptoms of infection
- renal failure in patients with a solitary kidney or chronic disease.

They may be a chance radiographic finding. Most stones are radio-opaque. Those which are not can be detected with pyelography or ultrasound. The management is with analgesics, a high fluid intake and, occasionally, lithotrypsy or surgery for large stones or acute obstruction.

The 'medical' approach to stones is to consider underlying causes which predispose to stone formation. These are:

- chronic infection
- hypercalcaemia
- hyperuricaemia
- cystinuria.

A small minority of patients with stones will have one of these diseases. The majority have hypercalciuria or hyperoxaluria, for which the management is a high fluid intake and avoidance of foods with high calcium or urate contents. Hypercalciuria can be treated with thiazide diuretics. The treatment of hypercalcaemia is discussed on page 317. Hyperuricaemia is treated with allopurinol. Cystinuria is managed by alkalinisation of the urine and with penicillamine.

Urinary tract infection

Learning objectives

You should:
- be able to distinguish acute cystitis from the urethral syndrome in young women
- be able to distinguish upper tract infection (pyelonephritis) from lower tract infection (cystitis)
- be conversant with the concept of a complicated urinary tract infection and how it is distinguished from a simple urinary infection
- be able to interpret a urine microscopy and culture report.

Clinical syndromes
Several different bacterial diseases of adults come under the heading of 'urinary tract infection'. They can be grouped as follows:

- cystitis and acute urethral syndrome in young women
- acute uncomplicated pyelonephritis in women
- urinary tract infection in young men
- catheter-associated urinary tract infection
- asymptomatic bacteriuria in the elderly
- complicated urinary tract infection.

Table 34 Tumours of kidney and urinary tract

Type	Demography	Clinical features	Management
Renal adenocarcinoma	Male > female, Adults	PUO, malaise, loin pain, haematuria, mass, effects of local invasion, metastases, hypercalcaemia, polycythaemia	Surgery, embolisation (chemotherapy, radiotherapy)
Nephroblastoma (Wilms' tumour)	Infants or children	Mass, haematuria, pain	Surgery, chemotherapy, radiotherapy
Transitional cell carcinoma			
Kidney and ureters	Adults	Haematuria, mass, hydronephrosis	Surgery
Bladder	Adults	Haematuria, urinary symptoms	Superficial: regular cystoscopic surveillance, diathermy, intravesical chemotherapy Invasive: cystectomy, radiotherapy, chemotherapy

Infection can also be caused by *Mycobacterium tuberculosis*, fungi and parasites. Many viruses are excreted in the urine but only adenoviruses cause infection.

Diagnosing urinary tract infection

Diagnosis rests on microscopy and culture of an appropriately collected specimen (Table 35). Rapid tests include the detection of nitrates, dehydrogenase activity and proteinuria.

Occasionally, pyuria occurs without a positive culture ('sterile pyuria'). This may occur in elderly people and is rarely significant unless symptoms are also present. Causes are:

- a partially treated urinary tract infection
- fastidious bacteria, e.g. *Lactobacilli*, *Corynebacteria*, *streptococci*
- urinary tract tuberculosis
- papillary necrosis.

In symptomatic patients with sterile pyuria, it is important to culture urine for *M. tuberculosis* and fastidious organisms.

Cystitis

Cystitis in young women

Cystitis is common, affecting about 1 million women annually in the UK. Typically, they present acutely ill with frequency, urgency and dysuria. Physical signs are few and fever is usually absent. There are several risk factors, including:

- sexual intercourse
- the use of a contraceptive diaphragm and spermicide
- failure to micturate after intercourse
- a history of prior cystitis.

Over 85% of cases are caused by *Escherichia coli* and *Staphylococcus saprophyticus*, the remainder being caused by other Gram-negative rods. A midstream urine specimen will usually contain more than 10^5 organisms/ml and > 10 white cells/mm^3.

Treatment regimens include single doses or short courses of amoxycillin, trimethoprim, cotrimoxazole or a quinolone, depending on the local prevalence of resistance. Women should be advised to drink plenty of fluids and urinate immediately after intercourse.

Recurrent cystitis

A significant number of women suffer from recurrent cystitis. Risk factors include:

- the Lewis blood group secretor phenotype
- increased vaginal colonisation with *E. coli* or other Gram-negative rods, sometimes related to diaphragm use
- upper urinary tract abnormalities, present in < 5% and easily excluded by renal ultrasound.

Antibiotic prophylaxis may be administered continuously, after intercourse or on first symptoms.

Recurrent infection in older women

Older, particularly multiparous, women may have a cystocoele preventing complete bladder emptying during micturition. Postmenopausal loss of urethral elasticity and increased *E. coli* colonisation of the vagina may also contribute. Oestrogen pessaries often substantially reduce the frequency of urinary infection in post menopausal women.

Acute urethral syndrome

This term refers to a clinical syndrome in young women akin to cystitis but with negaitive urine culture and microscopy. Symptoms are generally milder but more chronic than in cystitis. Like cystitis, this problem is common. Sexually transmitted infections such as chlamydia need to be excluded (p. 368). A large percentage of these women, particularly if the infection is chronic, appear to have bacterial infection and inflammation of the periurethral tissues of the distal ureter. The causative organisms are frequently unusual and missed in routine urine cultures. A urethral swab and/or the first portion of urine during micturition from such patients is usually positive. Antibiotic management should be directed at the pathogen isolated

Table 35 Laboratory diagnosis of urinary infection in various clinical settings

	Cystitis	Acute urethral syndrome	Pyelonephritis	Catheterised patient[a]	Complicated UTI	Elderly nursing home patient[a]
White cell count	+++	–/+	+/++	–/++	–/+++	+/++
Significant bacterial count	> 10^5/ml	?	> 10^4/ml	>10^2/ml	Variable	>10^4/ml
Common pathogens	*E. coli*, *Staphylococcus saprophyticusans*	Negative[b]	*E. coli*	Any	*Proteus* spp., *M. tuberculosis*, *Candida* spp., *Pseudomonas* spp.,	*E. coli*

*UTI, urinary tract infection.
[a]Clinical assessment essential as asymptomatic bacteriuria common, which does not require therapy.
[b]Special cultures required (see text).

and continued for longer than the standard urinary tract infection course (e.g. 10–14 days).

Pyelonephritis in women

The spectrum of illness is wide. Clinical features include:

- fever (common)
- back or loin pain (common)
- chills and rigors (common)
- nausea and vomiting
- hypotension and features of the sepsis syndrome (p. 356) (occasional).

Severe pain and radiation of the pain into the groin is rare but if present suggests a renal calculus. Pyelonephritis is proportionally more common in pregnancy, partly because of dilatation of the ureters and decreased ureteral peristalsis, and may lead to premature labour. Asymptomatic pyelonephritis sometimes accompanies cystitis.

Diagnosis

Over 80% of cases of pyelonephritis in young women are caused by invasive E. coli that have specific virulence mechanisms. Blood cultures are often positive, especially in the more severely ill patients. The urine usually shows pyuria and is culture positive. The 10^5/ml cut-off for bacteriuria used for cystitis does not apply to pyelonephritis, as at least 20% of patients with pyelonephritis have less than this number of bacteria in their urine.

Pyelonephritis in older patients or with other organisms is most likely to represent a complicated urinary tract infection, even though the presentation is very similar (see below).

Investigation

Investigations for abnormalities of the urinary tract are unrevealing in most young women with pyelonephritis. Indications for investigation include:

- slow resolution of infection
- more than one episode
- prior urinary infection in childhood
- unusual features, e.g. haematuria, impaired renal function, colicky pain, etc.

Treatment

The vast majority of patients with pyelonephritis require admission to hospital. Intravenous antibiotics are appropriate for all but the mildest cases. Aminoglycosides, quinolones or third-generation cephalosporins are most appropriate. Patients should have a repeat urine culture and renal ultrasound to seek a perinephric abscess if they have not responded after 3

days. Second- or third-generation cephalosporins are the preferred agents in pregnancy.

Urinary tract infections in men

Urinary tract infections are rare in men up to the age of 60. The same uropathogenic E. coli strains that cause pyelonephritis in young women cause cystitis and occasionally pyelonephritis in men. Risk factors include anal intercourse, lack of circumcision and a female sexual partner with vaginal colonisation by uropathogenic E. coli. Occasionally urinary infections are complicated by epididymitis and/or prostatitis. Oral antibiotics are usually appropriate. Investigations for a structural urological abnormality are usually negative but should be undertaken if the organism isolated is unusual or the patient has more than one episode. Likewise, chronic prostatitis should be excluded.

Epididymitis

Epididymitis is a common infection that varies in aetiology depending on the age of the patient. Over 35 years of age it is usually caused by Gram-negative rods, sometimes Gram-positive cocci. Under the age of 35 years, Neisseria gonorrhoeae and Chlamydia trachomatis are the most common causes. Patients present with painful swelling of the scrotum over 1–2 days. It is often asymmetrical and appears to involve the testis. Fever, dysuria and frequency of micturition are common. In younger patients, urethritis is common and should be sought clinically. A gratifying response to antibiotics is usual.

Catheter-associated urinary tract infection

Urinary catheters may be placed for short- or long-term use. Ascending infection from the use of short-term catheters in hospital is the most common cause of Gram-negative bacteraemia, sometimes with fatal consequences. Therefore, early removal of a catheter is appropriate, if possible. However, in the incontinent patient, catheterisation may prevent skin breakdown and bed sores so, as in all aspects of medicine, a reasonable balance between two opposing risks is necessary. Careful, aseptic changing and draining of catheter bags and the use of a closed collecting system reduce infection rates.

Diagnosis and management

Bacteriuria of only 10^2/ml drained through a catheter is significant when the patient is symptomatic. Asymptomatic pyuria and bacteriuria is common and does not require therapy. The organisms causing catheter-associated urinary tract infection are much more varied and are more likely to be resistant to antibiotics than those causing cystitis in healthy women. Therefore, broader-spectrum antibiotics, such as quinolones, may be appropriate for treatment. As the infecting bacteria often produce biofilms on catheters, treatment failure or relapse is common and a catheter change or removal is important for eradication.

With respect to long-term catheterisation, intermittent self-catheterisation (as for example in paraplegic patients after spinal injury) is far less likely to lead to infectious problems than continuous long-term indwelling urinary catheters. Long-term indwelling silastic catheters should be changed, 3-monthly.

Asymptomatic bacteriuria in elderly people

Bacteriuria is relatively common (up to 40%) in immobile elderly patients, especially in nursing homes, and may or may not reflect disease. Surprisingly, symptomatic infections, including pyelonephritis and/or sepsis, are uncommon. Therefore, screening and treatment of those found to be positive is unjustified. Furthermore, routine cultures of urine in elderly people on admission to hospital are wasteful as asymptomatic bacteriuria and pyuria are more common than urinary infections. Elderly patients with a new confusional state and/or symptoms suggestive of a urinary infection (e.g. frequency, nocturia, etc.) should, however, be treated promptly after cultures have been obtained. Pyuria may be present but is a less useful guide to symptomatic infection in elderly people.

Complicated urinary tract infection

A complicated urinary tract infection is defined as an infection that either occurs in patients with a functionally or anatomically abnormal urinary tract, or is caused by pathogens resistant to standard antibiotics (e.g. *M. tuberculosis*, *Pseudomonas* spp., etc.) or both.

However, these factors are not necessarily discernible when the patient first presents. There is a wide spectrum of presentation, from mild cystitis to life-threatening sepsis syndrome. Clues to the diagnosis of a complicated urinary tract infection include:

- history of renal tract disease, such as stones, surgery, haematuria, etc.
- prior urinary tract infection or bacteriuria
- prior antibiotic therapy (possibly for other problems)
- prior hospitalisation, especially if catheterised
- abnormal renal function on presentation.

All patients with complicated urinary tract infections need referral to a specialist physician and/or a urologist as surgery may be necessary. Unusual antibiotic regimens are also usually necessary and so obtaining a culture before antibiotic treatment is fundamental to good management.

Fungal urinary tract infection

Candida is found in the urine of 5–10% of hospitalised patients. In the intensive care unit it is almost synonymous with life-threatening candidaemia and patients should be treated for systemic candidiasis (p. 360). In other patients, it carries little significance unless accompanied by symptoms or white cells. *C. albicans* is the most common species. *C. glabrata* is also common.

Tuberculosis of the urinary tract

Urinary tract disease is a relatively unusual manifestation of tuberculosis. Patients complain of frequency and urgency, with little dysuria. Tuberculosis is a classic cause of sterile pyuria and should be suspected in symptomatic patients in whom straightforward bacterial infection has been excluded and the patient is from the Indian subcontinent. Heaf or Mantoux tests are usually strongly positive in these patients.

Early morning urine samples for *M. tuberculosis* culture are frequently requested for 'generally ill patients in whom tuberculosis is a possibility'. Their utility is, however, very poor as they have a low yield and the results take 4–8 weeks to come back. If the diagnosis of urinary tract tuberculosis is a serious possibility, cystoscopy and biopsy of the bladder wall is a quicker way to reach the diagnosis.

Treatment is as for pulmonary disease (p. 73), for at least 6 months.

Antibiotic management of urinary tract infections

Useful antibiotics for uncomplicated urinary tract infection include trimethoprim (about 80% of infecting organisms are sensitive) and quinolones (about 90%). The duration of therapy for cystitis should not exceed 5 days and 3 days is often sufficient. Longer treatment (e.g. 10 days) is required for the acute urethral syndrome.

For ill patients with pyelonephritis, cephalosporins such as cefuroxime or cefotaxime, or quinolones are appropriate. Aminoglycosides are also very useful and effective. For patients with other complicated urinary tract infections, empirical therapy with the above is appropriate but coverage for *Pseudomonas* spp. with ciprofloxacin or gentamicin is superior.

4.5 Fluid and electrolyte balance

For the tissues to function effectively, they have to be perfused with oxygenated blood of the correct electrolyte composition. Perfusion depends upon:

- cardiac pumping
- vascular tone
- maintenance of vascular volume.

This section primarily concerns vascular volume and the electrolyte composition of plasma. Cardiac pumping and vascular tone are discussed in Chapter 1 (p. 9). Remember, however, that renal function, fluid/electrolyte homeostasis and cardiovascular function are intimately related physiologically, biochemically and in terms of symptoms and signs.

The underpinning physiology may be a distant memory but the moment you collect your bleep for the first time you assume responsibility for interpreting the physical signs and biochemistry of fluid/electrolyte and acid/base balance and maintaining the volume and composition of your patients' fluid compartments. This section will 'lock together' simple physiological concepts with the everyday measurements made by clinicians and show how they relate to disease states. The approach is deliberately simplistic because it is by failure to apply simple physiological concepts that clinical errors are made.

Learning objectives

You need to:
- understand the concept of fluid 'compartments'
- know the composition of 'barriers' which divide the compartments
- understand the mechanisms which control vascular volume and electrolyte homeostasis
- be able to assess vascular volume reliably at the bedside
- be able to interpret abnormalities of plasma sodium, potassium, urea, creatinine, bicarbonate and albumin concentrations and know how to use physical signs to help interpret them
- understand how to manage common fluid/electrolyte disorders.

Physiology of fluid and electrolyte balance

Compartments

A 70 kg man has a total fluid content of approximately 42 litres. Figure 30 shows how this divides between a large intracellular and a smaller extracellular compartment. The cell membrane acts as a barrier which maintains the different electrolyte composition of the two compartments by active electrolyte transport. The predominant intracellular cation is potassium and the predominant anions are proteins and phosphate. Sodium and chloride are the predominant extracellular anion and cation, respectively. The extracellular fluid (ECF) is subdivided into a larger interstitial and smaller vascular compartment. The barrier between them is the capillary wall, which acts as a semi-permeable membrane. The vascular and interstitial fluids have the same electrolyte composition but protein cannot pass across the capillary wall.

Osmolality and filtration

Osmotically active substances, predominantly electrolytes, attract water. The degree of dilution of these

Compartments:	Intracellular fluid (ICF)	Extracellular fluid (ECF)	
		Interstitial	Vascular
Volumes in a 70 kg man	28L	10L	5.5L

Composition:

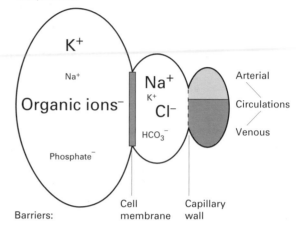

Fig. 30
Fluid compartments.

solutes is regulated by homeostatic mechanisms and measured as osmolality. Water diffuses freely between the intracellular and extracellular compartments and their osmolality is, therefore, identical. In the ECF, sodium is the most abundant low-molecular-weight solute and, therefore (as discussed on p. 170), the sodium content of the extracellular fluid determines its volume. Plasma is protein-rich compared with the interstitial fluid. Plasma proteins exert an osmotic force termed the **colloid osmotic pressure** which maintains **vascular** volume.

The capillaries have a higher hydrostatic pressure than the interstitial compartment, with a gradient between the arterial (high pressure) and venous (low pressure) ends. Capillary pressure forces an ultrafiltrate into the interstitial fluid. This process of filtration leaves an increasingly protein-rich fluid in the capillary which, at its low pressure venous end, osmotically draws sodium and water back into the vascular compartment. Excessive accumulation of interstitial fluid (oedema) occurs if the colloid osmotic pressure is low (hypoproteinaemia), the capillary wall leaks protein or there is increased venous pressure, which opposes the colloid osmotic 'draw' of fluid back into the capillary (as occurs in venous obstruction or the raised central venous pressure of heart failure).

Volume

The vascular compartment is the 'central player' in fluid and electrolyte physiology because it is the vehicle by which solutes and oxygen reach the tissues and waste is removed. Its composition determines the composition of the interstitial compartment and, indirectly, the intracellular compartment. It is small, about 5.5 litres, two-thirds of which is in the venous circulation and one-third in the arterial circulation. The all-important part of the system is the arterial circulation because it maintains oxygen delivery. Even transient disruption of arterial oxygen supply can have catastrophic consequences.

Since the circulation is a closed system, cardiac function depends upon venous return as well as on an intact myocardium. The veins are the 'capacitance' vessels, which can absorb extra fluid volume or 'top up' the circulation in states of volume depletion. The single most important term in understanding fluid balance is *volume*, and this can be subdivided conceptually into venous and arterial volume. The terms **volume depletion** and **volume overload** will be used here to discuss disease and clinical management in preference to 'dehydration' and 'overhydration', because disease usually affects sodium and water homeostasis rather than water alone. Figure 31 illustrates the vascular system schematically and shows how it changes in different pathological conditions.

Homeostatic mechanisms

Haemorrhagic shock is the most extreme example of volume depletion. Arterial baroreceptors activate the sympathetic system leading to:

- vasoconstriction to divert blood away from skin, intestine and kidneys and maintain arterial volume (pale, clammy, oliguric)
- venoconstriction to maintain venous return from the reserve volume in the capacitance vessels
- tachycardia to maximise cardiac output.

In health, homeostatic mechanisms have to compensate for variations in the intake of fluid and dietary sodium and loss through the kidneys, skin, intestinal tract and lungs. Two mechanisms operate: thirst, which regulates water intake, and the endocrine system, which regulates renal water and electrolyte handling. The sensation of thirst is controlled by hypothalamic osmoreceptors. There are several endocrine mechanisms.

Arginine vasopressin. AVP (or antidiuretic hormone, ADH) is primarily secreted in response to changes in plasma osmolality sensed by the hypothalamic osmoreceptors; in states of volume depletion, the arterial baroreceptors increase AVP secretion, irrespective of osmolality, to 'preserve volume at all costs'. AVP increases water absorption in the collecting duct (p. 151).

Aldosterone. This is the end-product of the renin–angiotensin–aldosterone system (p. 268). Aldosterone secretion is determined by renal perfusion (i.e. afferent arteriolar bloodflow) as sensed by the juxtaglomerular apparatus; it increases sodium/water reabsorption (in exchange for potassium) in the distal tubule.

Atrial natriuretic peptide (ANP). This is controlled by atrial stretch receptors and increases renal sodium/water loss; ANP and aldosterone have opposing effects.

Measurement of fluid/electrolyte balance

Having described the various compartments, it is now possible to discuss the clinical assessment which must always be done before attempting to interpret abnormal electrolyte biochemistry. Three compartments can be independently assessed at the bedside.

The interstitial compartment. An increase in **interstitial fluid** causes **oedema**. If the increase is caused by raised venous pressure (heart failure), the oedema is in dependent parts. If caused by venous obstruction, it is in the affected venous territory. If caused by increased capillary permeability or hypoproteinaemia, it is generalised. Remember that lymphatic obstruction also causes oedema, by preventing drainage from the interstitial compartment.

The venous compartment. The 'window' into the **venous compartment** is the jugular venous system. Significant volume overload increases jugular venous pressure and volume depletion reduces it. Dogmatic rules taught about cardiovascular examination ('2 cm above the sternal angle at 45°') obscure the simple fact that bedside examination allows an estimate of central venous pressure by relating the height of the jugular venous pulse to the surface anatomy of the right atrium. If the pulse cannot be seen with the patient lying at 45°, it can be made visible by lying the patient flat. Likewise, a very high venous pressure can best be assessed by sitting the patient upright. This is illustrated in Figure 32.

The arterial compartment. This is affected by cardiac disease and degrees of volume depletion or overload which cannot be compensated for by venous capacitance. Arterial overload is rare because there are powerful homeostatic mechanisms to prevent it. Likewise, depletion of the arterial circulation only occurs when the capacitance vessels are empty. It causes hypotension and tachycardia, initially only on standing. The way to assess the arterial compartment is to measure the lying and standing pulse and blood pressure.

Volume depletion. Reduced urine output is a sign of volume depletion which begins as the homeostatic mechanisms operate at the stage of venous volume depletion. It proceeds to oliguria/anuria when there is significant arterial volume depletion.

One of the greatest disservices done to medical students by conventional teaching is the concept of 'dehydration' and its physical signs of increased skin turgor, sunken eyes and dry mouth. These are indeed signs of reduced total body water, but more often mislead than help because:

- they are insensitive: body water rarely changes in isolation from sodium, so changes in vascular volume occur long before there is a detectable reduction of interstitial fluid volume
- they are not specific: skin turgor is affected by ageing, and dryness of the mouth by the respiratory rate.
- they are notoriously difficult to assess accurately.

Unusually, this discussion has focussed upon physical signs before symptoms. That is because careful physical

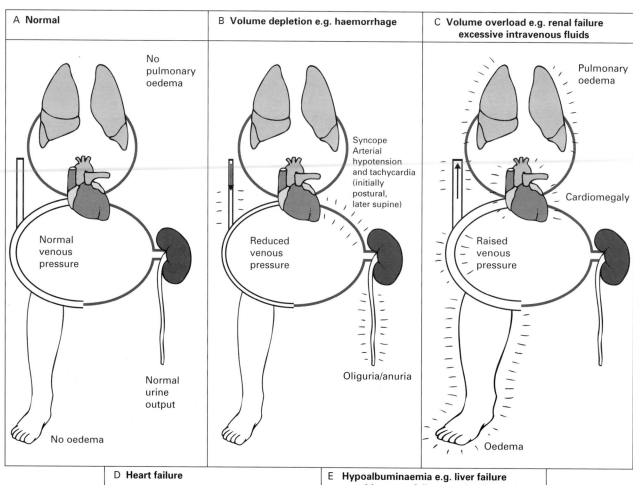

A **Normal**

No pulmonary oedema

Normal venous pressure

Normal urine output

No oedema

B **Volume depletion e.g. haemorrhage**

Syncope Arterial hypotension and tachycardia (initially postural, later supine)

Reduced venous pressure

Oliguria/anuria

C **Volume overload e.g. renal failure excessive intravenous fluids**

Pulmonary oedema

Cardiomegaly

Raised venous pressure

Oedema

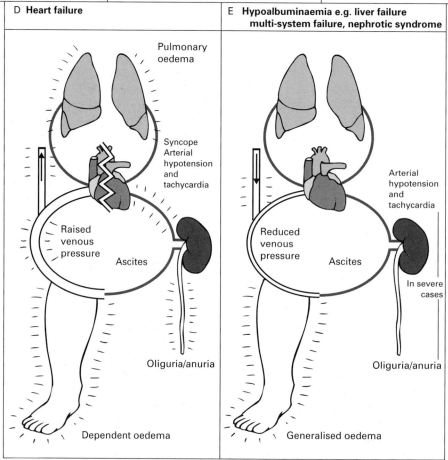

D **Heart failure**

Pulmonary oedema

Syncope Arterial hypotension and tachycardia

Raised venous pressure

Ascites

Oliguria/anuria

Dependent oedema

E **Hypoalbuminaemia e.g. liver failure multi-system failure, nephrotic syndrome**

Arterial hypotension and tachycardia

Reduced venous pressure

Ascites

In severe cases

Oliguria/anuria

Generalised oedema

Fig. 31
Fluid physiology in health and disease.

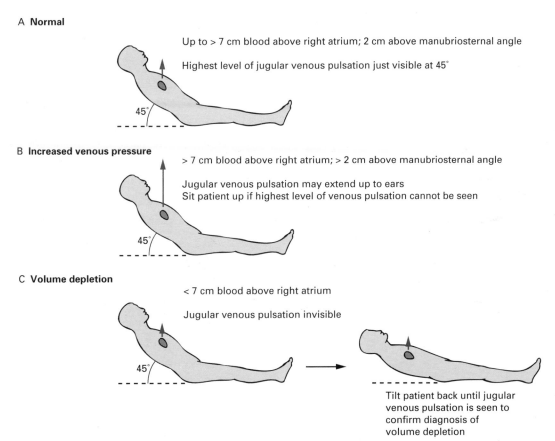

A **Normal**

Up to > 7 cm blood above right atrium; 2 cm above manubriosternal angle

Highest level of jugular venous pulsation just visible at 45°

45°

B **Increased venous pressure**

> 7 cm blood above right atrium; > 2 cm above manubriosternal angle

Jugular venous pulsation may extend up to ears
Sit patient up if highest level of venous pulsation cannot be seen

45°

C **Volume depletion**

< 7 cm blood above right atrium

Jugular venous pulsation invisible

45°

Tilt patient back until jugular
venous pulsation is seen to
confirm diagnosis of
volume depletion

Fig. 32
Assessing venous pressure.

examination is the key to clinical management. Headache is an early symptom of volume depletion. Others do not occur until the *arterial* circulation is depleted: they are fatigue, lightheadedness, dizziness and syncope (particularly on standing), and oliguria. Symptoms of volume overload arise from the systemic and pulmonary *venous* circulation: they are breathlessness and oedema.

Fluid physiology in disease

Figure 33 relates the physiological principles discussed above to common disease states. Table 36 lists the causes of volume depletion and overload. Heart failure and hypoproteinaemia are two disease states which deserve special mention because they present with mixtures of volume depletion and overload and can be understood by applying exactly the same principles.

Heart failure
Cardiac disease causes *effective* arterial volume depletion. There is reduced renal perfusion to which the homeostatic response is increased aldosterone secretion causing salt and water retention. The combination of pump failure and fluid retention increases venous volume. Heart failure is, therefore, a combination of effective arterial volume depletion and venous volume overload.

Hypoproteinaemia
This occurs in nephrotic syndrome and hepatocellular disease and may also be seen in severe illness when increased capillary leakage acts together with hypoproteinaemia to reduce the osmotic pressure difference between plasma and the interstitial fluid. The vascular colloid osmotic pressure is reduced and the interstitial fluid volume expanded at the expense of the vascular compartment. Patients may have symptoms and signs of volume depletion together with oedema.

Table 36 Causes of volume depletion and overload

Volume depletion	Volume overload
Excessive loss	**Insufficient loss**
Skin: sweating, as in fever, burns	Renal failure
Lungs: tachypnoea, as in asthma	Heart failure
GI tract: vomiting, diarrhoea, fistulae	Steroid excess
Kidneys: salt-losing kidney, diabetes	Conn's syndrome
mellitus and other causes of osmotic	Cushing's syndrome
diuresis, hypoadrenalism	Steroid therapy
Inadequate intake	**Excessive intake**
Severe illness, anorexia, neglect	Excessive saline therapy

Diabetes insipidus, psychogenic polydipsia and the syndrome of inappropriate antidiuresis are not listed because they are pure abnormalities of water balance and affect total body water, not extracellular volume (p. 166).

The treatment of volume depletion and overload

Extracellular volume is primarily determined by the total body content of sodium, which itself determines water content. Volume depletion is treated by replacing salt and water (orally or intravenously). Volume overload is treated by removing salt and water. This is done with dietary restriction, diuretics and — in extreme cases — dialysis or haemofiltration.

The treatment of heart failure is more difficult and consists of

- optimising cardiac function (e.g. correction of dysrhythmias), inotropic therapy, reducing cardiac work and increasing efficiency by reducing ventricular overload and 'stretch' with arterial and venous vasodilators
- removing salt and water with diuretics.

The physiological principles discussed above explain the major limitation of the treatment of heart failure: effective arterial volume is already reduced so diuretics and vasodilators which reduce it further can cause syncope and impair renal perfusion. The treatment of severe heart failure consists of 'tight-rope walking' between the effects of treatment on the different compartments.

The management of hypoproteinaemia has been discussed under Nephrotic syndrome (p. 159).

Disorders of sodium and osmolality

The biochemistry laboratory can only measure *concentrations* and *osmolalities*, which are uninterpretable unless *volume* in the compartments has been estimated at the bedside. So, for example, a patient with severe burns can have massive salt and water loss and circulatory collapse without any immediate effect on the plasma urea and electrolytes; only as the homeostatic mechanisms and reduced urine flow have their effects will the biochemistry become abnormal.

Since sodium is the main determinant of plasma osmolality and 'water follows sodium', the plasma concentration is not a reliable marker of total body sodium content. It can only reflect the relative amounts of sodium and water in the extracellular fluid. Therefore, a low serum sodium concentration is caused by an excess of water relative to sodium; total body sodium might be normal or low. Likewise, a high serum sodium is caused by *relative* water depletion, usually in the context of a low total body sodium.

Hyponatraemia

Hyponatraemia has a number of causes (Box 7). **Water overload** may be caused by:

- excessive water drinking or i.v. dextrose treatment (e.g. postoperative)
- a primary abnormality (syndrome of inappropriate

antidiuresis or SIAD — see below) in which there is excessive AVP secretion and impaired water excretion.

In both cases, total body water is increased and total body sodium normal. In excessive water drinking, the urine is very dilute but the capacity of the kidneys to excrete water is overwhelmed. In SIAD, the urine is very concentrated. Thus, measurement of urine osmolality distinguishes between them.

Hyponatraemia may also be caused by **volume depletion** (e.g. from diuretic therapy) **with continued water drinking**: hyponatraemia is caused by homeostatic AVP secretion in response to volume depletion. In this case, total body sodium is low.

The distinction between SIAD and hyponatraemia associated with volume depletion is made by assessing venous and arterial volume, measuring urea (a biochemical marker of volume depletion) and considering the patient's history. A fuller list of causes of hyponatraemia is shown in Box 7. In severe heart failure, it is caused by increased AVP secretion and thirst, caused by effective arterial volume depletion and often made worse by diuretic therapy.

SIAD

Box 7 lists causes of SIAD; it may be idiopathic, drug-related, caused by ectopic AVP secretion or caused by disease of the chest or hypothalamus. It may be the presentation of hypothyroidism or hypoadrenalism. Water retention lowers plasma osmolality and causes non-specific malaise and neurological problems including confusion, personality change and fits/coma owing to cerebral oedema (particularly likely at a serum solution < 125 mmol/l). Apart from a low serum sodium and normal or low urea, plasma osmolality is low and uri-

---

Box 7
Causes of hyponatraemia

Water overload
Psychogenic polydipsia
Excesive i.v. dextrose

SIAD
    Carcinoma of the bronchus
    Inflammatory lung diseases
    Hypothyroidism
    Hypoadrenalism
    Idiopathic
    Drugs: chlorpropamide, carbamazepine, syntocinon, phenothiazines, tricyclics
    Hypothalamic disease: meningitis, encephalitis, tumour or granuloma

Homeostatic response to volume depletion
Any cause of volume depletion, if patient has access to water

Heart failure

nary osmolality high (because excess AVP prevents the formation of a dilute urine). In mild cases, the management consists of water restriction, allowing loss through the lungs, skin and bowel to clear excess water. If the problem is prolonged, demeclocycline may be given to induce nephrogenic diabetes insipidus. In emergencies (e.g. uncontrolled fitting) hypertonic saline is given with a loop diuretic (to prevent volume overload and increase free water clearance). Correcting hyponatraemia too quickly can cause neurological complications so this should only be done under expert supervision.

Hypernatraemia

Because 'water follows salt' and the osmoreceptors trigger thirst and AVP secretion when osmolality rises, hypernatraemia is unusual and can really only occur if the patient

- is elderly or neurologically disabled and has lost perception of thirst
- is too ill to drink
- has an osmotic diuresis and loses water disproportionately to sodium.

'Hyperosmolar dehydration' may arise with severe and prolonged hyperglycaemia (hyperosmolar non-ketotic diabetic coma) or other causes of osmotic diuresis. It may also be caused by diabetes insipidus, in which there is uncontrolled renal water loss. Since water is lost from both the ECF and ICF, patients rarely become hypernatraemic in this disease because they develop life-threatening water depletion with florid thirst before there is a major change in plasma sodium.

Investigations are directed towards the underlying cause and treatment consists of volume repletion, sometimes with judicious use of hypotonic saline or 5% dextrose.

Disorders of potassium

Since potassium is predominantly intracellular, major changes in total body potassium can occur with only minor changes in the plasma concentration. An important factor affecting plasma potassium concentration is pH, since potassium and hydrogen ions exchange with one another between the intracellular and extracellular compartments. So, for example, **acidosis** can *increase* plasma potassium by displacing it from the intracellular compartment and **alkalosis** can *lower it* without any change in total body content. Likewise hydrogen ion takes the place of potassium lost from cells, so hypokalaemia is accompanied by alkalosis. Catecholamines shift potassium into cells, as does insulin and any drug/disorder with a sympathomimetic effect.

Hypokalaemia

This is the most common electrolyte disorder. It causes nerve and muscle dysfunction (particularly at a concentration <2.5 mmol/l) so its effects are:

- weakness
- ileus
- cardiac dysrhythmias.

Chronic hypokalaemia can also induce nephrogenic diabetes insipidus (p. 266) and cause thirst and polyuria.

The most common cause of hypokalaemia is renal loss through diuretic therapy. Table 37 lists others. Measurement of potassium excretion in a 24-hour urine sample is the main investigation. It is increased if the primary problem is renal loss and reduced in all other cases.

Table 37 Causes of hypokalaemia and hyperkalaemia

Hypokalaemia	Hyperkalaemia
Excessive loss	**Insufficient loss**
Renal: potassium-wasting diuretics	Renal: potassium-conserving diuretics, ACE inhibitor therapy
Steroid excess: steroid therapy, Conn's syndrome	Steroid deficiency: Addison's disease, congenital adrenal hyperplasia
Osmotic diuresis: diabetes mellitus	
Potassium-losing kidney	Renal failure
Liquorice addiction	
GI tract: persistent vomiting, diarrhoea, villous adenoma of the rectum, enterostomies, purgative abuse	
Inadequate intake	**Excessive intake**
Malnutrition	
Prolonged intravenous therapy without added potassium	Excessive intravenous potassium
Shifts	**Shifts**
Metabolic alkalosis	Metabolic acidosis
Insulin therapy	Insulin deficiency (diabetic ketoacidosis)
Severe illness (e.g. myocardial infarction)	Cellular injury: burns, rhabdomyolysis, cytotoxic therapy
Theophylline and sympathomimetic therapy	
Poisoning: aspirin, theophylline	

Management consists of correcting the cause of loss and replenishing the pool. Remember that potassium has to pass through the small extracellular pool to reach the intracellular fluid, so overrapid potassium replacement can cause potentially fatal hyperkalaemia. Highly concentrated potassium solutions should never be given intravenously. The rate of replacement should not exceed 30 mmol/hour, even in severe hypokalaemia. Potassium replacement is best done orally.

Hyperkalaemia

The causes, effects and treatments of hyperkalaemia are the mirror image of hypokalaemia. Renal failure and potassium-conserving drugs are the most common causes, and these are potentially lethal in combination. Hyperkalaemia may be asymptomatic or may present with muscle weakness. A serum potassium over 7 mmol/l is a medical emergency because it can cause cardiac arrest. Cardiographic signs of hyperkalaemia are 'tented' T waves, loss of P waves and widening of the QRS complex progressing to a 'sine wave' pattern. Management is shown in the emergency box.

Emergency treatment: management of severe hyperkalaemia

- Give 50% dextrose 50 ml and soluble insulin 10 units: **this shifts potassium from the ECF into cells**
- Do an ECG
- Give 10–20 ml 10% calcium gluconate if there are signs of severe hyperkalaemia: tented T waves, loss of P waves and widening of the QRS complex: **this antagonises the effects of hyperkalaemia on the myocardium**
- Call for senior help
- Repeat plasma potassium and bicarbonate
- Prescribe calcium resonium orally or rectally: **this increases potassium excretion**
- Assess the patient's fluid status: give intravenous fluids if volume depleted to increase potassium excretion; consider giving isotonic bicarbonate if volume depleted *and* acidotic: bicarbonate shifts potassium into cells
- Resistant hyperkalaemia may be an indication for dialysis in renal failure or unresponsive cases

---

4.6 Acid/base disorders

If fluid/electrolyte physiology seems complex, acid/base homeostasis and its disorders can seem even more so. However, you will encounter a limited range of these disorders as a newly qualified doctor and an even more limited range without senior supervision, so this discussion picks out only salient points relevant to management.

Learning objectives

At the very least, you should:
- understand the terms *respiratory* and *metabolic acidosis* and *alkalosis*
- understand that these changes may be primary or compensatory
- be able to interpret arterial blood gas measurements in those terms
- know the common diseases which affect acid/base balance
- understand the main principles of management.

Mechanisms and terminology

Respiration affects acid/base balance because excess carbon dioxide combines with water to form carbonic acid. This is termed **respiratory acidosis** and may be an effect of respiratory disease or a homeostatic mechanism to maintain a normal pH in the face of **metabolic alkalosis**. Likewise, a reduced partial pressure of carbon dioxide (pCO_2) causes **respiratory alkalosis** which may be primary (caused, for example, by hyperventilation) or to compensate for **metabolic acidosis**. The biochemical marker of respiratory acidosis and alkalosis is a change in pCO_2.

Metabolic acidosis may be caused by:

- increased intake of hydrogen ions, as in salicylate overdosage
- increased production of hydrogen ions, as in lactic acidosis or ketoacidosis (p. 283)
- decreased renal excretion of hydrogen ions
- a shift of hydrogen ions out of cells, as in hyperkalaemia.

The biochemical marker of metabolic acidosis is a fall in plasma bicarbonate. Normally there is a difference of about 10–15 mmol/l between the sum of plasma sodium plus potassium (the main cations) and bicarbonate plus chloride (the main anions). This is termed the **anion gap** and is 'filled' by unmeasured organic anions. If acidosis is caused by excess lactate, ketoacids or other unmeasured anions (particularly drugs), the anion gap is increased.

The marker of metabolic alkalosis is a rise in plasma bicarbonate. It is caused by either excess intake of alkali or excess loss of hydrogen ions through the kidneys or into the ICF.

Investigations

To obtain a true measurement of acid/base and blood gas status, pH, pO_2 and pCO_2 must be measured in arterial blood; venous blood cannot be used because it is affected by local tissue metabolism. Bicarbonate is ideally measured in arterial blood but venous bicarbonate approximates closely enough to arterial bicarbonate to be used for the diagnosis of metabolic alkalosis and acidosis. Chloride can be measured in venous or arterial blood.

Table 38 Interpretation of acid/base biochemistry

	Metabolic acidosis	Respiratory acidosis	Respiratory alkalosis	Metabolic alkalosis
pH	$\downarrow$	$\downarrow$	$\uparrow$	$\uparrow$
pCO_2	($\downarrow$)	$\uparrow$	$\downarrow$	($\uparrow$)
Bicarbonate	$\downarrow$	($\uparrow$)	($\downarrow$)	$\uparrow$
Chloride	$\uparrow$[a]	($\downarrow$)	($\uparrow$)	$\downarrow$

$\downarrow$, fall; $\uparrow$, rise; () indicates compensatory as opposed to primary changes.
[a] Except where there is an excess anion such as lactate or ketoacids, in which case chloride is normal or low.

Causes and differential diagnosis

Table 38 shows the four main patterns of abnormality described above. Note how the patterns of pH, pCO_2 and bicarbonate differ between the four disorders. Box 8 lists their causes.

Clinical presentation

The symptoms and signs are usually those of an underlying disease, except that patients with metabolic acidosis characteristically have deep, sighing (Kussmaul) respiration.

Treatment

The treatment of respiratory acidosis and alkalosis is directed at the underlying respiratory disease. Metabolic alkalosis rarely needs treatment in its own right. The treatment of acidosis is directed primarily at the underlying disease. Intravenous sodium bicarbonate is used to correct severe metabolic acidosis but must be given judiciously for several reasons:

- it is a solute load and contraindicated if the patient is already volume overloaded
- hypertonic bicarbonate solutions are extremely damaging to peripheral veins
- abrupt correction of acidosis can cause acute, severe and potentially fatal hypokalaemia as potassium shifts into cells
- it can temporarily worsen cerebral acidosis because it immediately corrects plasma acidosis and reduces the compensatory respiratory alkalosis but takes time to diffuse into the CNS.

Oral bicarbonate is occasionally given to compensate for chronic bicarbonate loss, as in renal tubular acidosis.

Box 8
Causes of disordered acid/base biochemistry

Respiratory acidosis
Respiratory failure:
  Airway obstruction
  Mechanical problems
    of ventilation
  Neuromuscular disease

Respiratory alkalosis
Hyperventilation:
  Primary
  Secondary to:
    Alveolar disease
    Right-left shunting
    Salicylate poisoning

Metabolic acidosis
Normal anion gap:
  Renal tubular acidosis
  Bicarbonate loss from
    GI fistula

Increased anion gap:
  Lactic acidosis:
    Septic shock
    Tissue anoxia
    Liver disease
    Drugs: eg metformin
  Ketoacidosis:
    Diabetes
  Poisoning:
    Salicylate
  Renal failure

Metabolic alkalosis
Ingestion of alkali
Hypokalaemia
  Gastric acid loss
  (pyloric stenosis)

Self-assessment: questions

Multiple choice questions

1. Acute renal failure is a likely complication of the following:
   a. Septicaemia
   b. Polycystic kidney disease
   c. Major arterial surgery
   d. Retroperitoneal tumours
   e. Cardiogenic shock

2. In patients with acute renal failure:
   a. Sodium bicarbonate should be given routinely
   b. Diuretics have no place in acute management
   c. Skin turgor is a reliable guide to the need for intravenous fluid therapy
   d. Urinary catheterisation is sometimes needed to monitor the response to therapy
   e. Intravenous pyelography is the investigation of choice to exclude urinary obstruction

3. The following are true:
   a. Serum urea is a more reliable measure than creatinine for the diagnosis of renal failure
   b. Diuretic therapy of heart failure can increase serum urea
   c. Serum creatinine may be misleadingly low in wasted patients with renal failure
   d. Plasma creatinine is primarily influenced by glomerular filtration not urine flow
   e. The urinary urea concentration provides useful information in the investigation of suspected renal failure

4. The following are causes of chronic renal failure:
   a. Gout
   b. Atherosclerosis
   c. Analgesic abuse
   d. Non-insulin-dependent diabetes
   e. Hypothyroidism

5. The following are true of renal dialysis and transplantation:

   a. Maintenance haemodialysis gives a better long-term quality of life than renal transplantation
   b. Transplantation is the best treatment for elderly patients with renal failure
   c. Pericarditis is an indication for dialysis in acute renal failure
   d. Acute dialysis can correct metabolic acidosis
   e. Maintenance dialysis gives people with chronic renal failure a normal life expectancy

6. The following may cause the nephrotic syndrome:
   a. Minimal change nephropathy
   b. Treatment with beta-blockers
   c. Rheumatoid arthritis
   d. Diabetes mellitus
   e. Renal cell carcinoma

7. The following are true of the investigation of renal disease:
   a. No patient should go onto dialysis without having had a renal biopsy
   b. Intravenous pyelography may worsen renal failure
   c. Urine microscopy can give valuable information as to the cause of renal failure
   d. Renal venography may be indicated in the investigation of nephrotic syndrome
   e. Retrograde pyelography is usually needed to diagnose urinary obstruction

8. The following are features of urinary infections in elderly people:
   a. Patients usually complain of dysuria
   b. They may present with falls
   c. They may present with constipation
   d. Sterile pyuria is most likely caused by tuberculosis
   e. Oestrogen supplements may reduce their frequency in postmenopausal women

9. Renal cell carcinoma
   a. May be bilateral
   b. May present as a PUO
   c. May present with pulmonary metastases
   d. Commonly causes hypertension
   e. Is extremely radiosensitive

10. Renal artery stenosis:
    a. Is invariably caused by atherosclerosis
    b. May cause renal failure in patients given ACE inhibitor therapy
    c. Can be reliably diagnosed by auscultating for renal bruits
    d. May be seen on ultrasound as a unilateral small kidney
    e. Is a cause of hypertension

Case history questions

History 1

A 74-year-old man who has always had excellent health has been increasingly lethargic and short of breath for 3 months before he is admitted to hospital. He is found to have a serum urea of 58 mmol/l and a creatinine of 900 µmol/l.

1. In seeking a cause of his renal failure, name three particularly important points to be sought in his clinical history and examination.
2. What single investigation would you request first to elucidate the cause?

He is found to have an enlarged bladder with bilateral hydronephrosis.

---

3. How should he be managed?

Despite relief of his hydronephrosis, his serum urea and creatinine remain high.

---

4. What other treatable factors might be contributing to his renal failure?

History 2

A 23-year-old single female shop assistant presents to you as her GP complaining of frequent micturition and a 'burning sensation' when she passes water. She has never had this problem before. She is otherwise fit and well and you last saw her 9 months previously.

---

1. Which of the following are appropriate courses of action:
   a. Refer her to a urologist
   b. Send her urine for culture and microscopy
   c. Empirically treat her with a broad-spectrum oral antibiotic.
   d. Examine her, particularly looking for genital herpes
   e. Enquire about a new sexual partner and/or recent sexual activity.

In the event you prescribe amoxycillin for 5 days and tell her to return if it is not better. She returns with the same symptoms 5 days later.

---

2. What should your course of action be now:
   a. Refer her to a urologist
   b. Send her urine for culture and microscopy
   c. Re-treat her with another oral antibiotic
   d. Examine her, particularly looking for genital herpes
   e. Refer her to a genitourinary medicine department.

This time you take urine for culture and microscopy and then prescribe oral trimethoprim. She is advised to drink plenty of fluids and to urinate immediately after intercourse. She reports back in 7 days with improved symptoms but now complaining of 'irritating itchiness down below' and increased vaginal discharge. The urine result showed > 100 white cells per high power field and a culture of 10^6/ml of *E. coli* resistant to ampicillin and cephradine but sensitive to trimethoprim and gentamicin and norfloxacin.

---

3. Your course of action now is to:
   a. Refer her to a urologist
   b. Examine her and take a vaginal sample for *Candida* and *Trichomonas* and a cervical sample for *Chlamydia* and *Neisseria gonorrhoea*
   c. Empirically treat her with a third oral antibiotic
   d. Empirically treat her for vaginal candidosis
   e. Refer her to a genitourinary medicine department.

Data interpretation

1. Table 39 has biochemical findings for five patients. Suggest an interpretation.

Table 39 Biochemical data for patients 1–5

	1	2	3	4	5
Na$^+$ (mmol/l)	138	130	160	114	124
K$^+$ (mmol/l)	6.8	2.8	4.9	3.8	7.2
Urea (mmol/l)	43.0	16	58	2.1	8.8
Creatinine (µmol/l)	780	118	400	86	120
HCO$_3^-$ (mmol/l)	15	32	24	26	19

2. Comment on the following biochemical findings in a patient with chronic renal failure. What management would be appropriate? Calcium 1.90, phosphate 2.1, alkaline phosphatase 450.
3. Comment on the biochemical findings in Table 40

Table 40 Arterial blood data for patients 1–4

	1	2	3	4
pCO$_2$ (mmHg)	60	24	52	28
pH	7.2	6.9	7.6	7.5
HCO$_3^-$	32	5	36	18

4. Patients 1–6 in Table 41 had dysuria and/or frequency. Classify their disease appropriately and suggest a single course of action (e.g. treat with antibiotics, renal ultrasound, etc.).

Table 41 Microbiological and clinical data for patients 1–6

	1	2	3	4	5	6
Urine (white cells per high power field)	> 100	30	80	50	10	80
Culture result (cells/ml)	$\times 10^4$ Mixed flora	$< 10^2$	$> 10^5$ Proteus mirrabili	$< 10^4$ Mixed flora	10^4 E. coli	$< 10^2$
Age	78	82	22	26	79	43
Sex	F	M	M	F	M	M

Picture question

The ultrasound scan in Picture 4.1 is of the the left kidney of a 50-year-old woman with advanced ovarian cancer. She has recently lost over 1 stone in weight and complained of back pain. She is admitted vomiting, with a serum urea of 50 mmol/l, creatinine 1020 µmol/l.

1. What does the scan show?
2. What is the likely cause of this appearance?
3. How should she be managed?

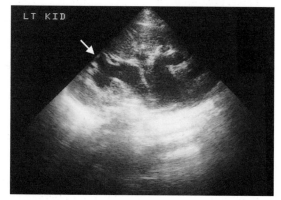

Picture 4.1

Self-assessment: answers

Multiple choice answers

1. a. **True.** Commonly caused by prerenal factors such as septicaemia.
   b. **False.** Polycystic kidneys cause chronic rather than acute renal failure.
   c. **True.** Major arterial surgery can cause renal ischaemia and acute tubular necrosis.
   d. **False.** Postrenal disease uncommonly causes *acute* renal failure, and retroperitoneal pathology is particularly unlikely to do so because it would need to involve both ureters simultaneously.
   e. **True.** Cardiac disease can critically impair renal perfusion.

2. a. **False.** Patients may be fluid overloaded in which case it would be unsafe to give any intravenous fluid. Not all patients have severe enough metabolic acidosis to need bicarbonate, and bicarbonate therapy could critically lower serum potassium if the patient were not hyperkalaemic. Bicarbonate therapy is used only in selected cases (p. 172).
   b. **False.** Patients who are fluid overloaded may respond to high-dose loop diuretics and this may avert the need for acute dialysis.
   c. **False.** Skin turgor, like eyeball pressure and the moistness of the tongue, is a poor guide to blood *volume*. (See p. 167 for reliable signs of volume depletion and overload.)
   d. **True.** It is important to measure urine flow in the fluid management of acute renal failure.
   e. **False.** Urinary obstruction should be excluded in all cases but pyelography is a poor method because visualisation of the kidneys depends on renal function to excrete the dye. The dye is nephrotoxic and may worsen renal failure. Ultrasonography is non-invasive, sensitive and specific for urinary obstruction.

3. a. **False.** Serum urea may be increased by protein catabolism and reduced urine flow as well as by renal failure. Serum creatinine is the more reliable marker.
   b. **True.** Poor cardiac output may increase serum urea by decreasing urine flow. Diuretic therapy can exacerbate the situation, in which case serum urea rises disproportionately to creatinine.
   c. **True.** Patients with reduced muscle bulk may have a normal serum creatinine even in the presence of renal failure because muscle bulk determines creatinine production.
   d. **True.** Creatinine is a marker of glomerular filtration.
   e. **True.** In renal failure, the kidneys are unable to excrete urea so the urinary urea concentration is low. This distinguishes renal failure from, for example, volume depletion, in which plasma urea is high but the kidneys retain the capacity to concentrate urinary urea.

4. a. **True.**
   b. **True.** As a result of extrarenal or intrarenal obstruction to the renal arterial circulation.
   c. **True.**
   d. **True.** Both insulin-dependent and non-insulin-dependent diabetes cause renal failure.
   e. **False.**

5. a. **False.** A successful transplant gives the best quality of life.
   b. **False.** The elderly tolerate immunosuppression poorly and are particularly susceptible to cardiovascular disease; they are treated with haemodialysis or peritoneal dialysis.
   c. **True.** Pericarditis is an indication for dialysis in acute renal failure.
   d. **True.**
   e. **False.** Even if treated with renal replacement, there is increased mortality from cardiovascular disease in patients with renal failure.

6. a. **True.** This is the characteristic form of nephropathy associated with nephrotic syndrome, particularly in children.
   b. **False.**
   c. **True.** It may be caused by amyloid associated with rheumatoid arthritis or by drugs used to treat the disease (gold or penicillamine). Rarely it is caused by a glomerulonephritis associated with the disease itself.
   d. **True.** Although the full-blown nephrotic syndrome is a relatively uncommon presentation of diabetic nephropathy.
   e. **False.**

7. a. **False.** There are limited indications for renal biopsy; usually in patients with mild to moderate parenchymal renal disease of uncertain aetiology.
   b. **True.** Particularly in elderly patients, those with diabetes or myeloma and particularly if they are volume depleted.
   c. **True.**
   d. **True.** Renal vein thrombosis may cause or exacerbate nephrotic syndrome.
   e. **False.** Renal ultrasound is far more commonly used than retrograde pyelography.

8. a. **False.** Many urinary tract infections in the elderly are subtle in their presentation and may be relatively asymptomatic. Typically, the patient presents with 'going off their feet', confusion,

anorexia or nocturia/incontinence. Fever is uncommon. Urine culture is an essential investigation in unwell elderly people.

b. **True.** See above.

c. **True.** Or it may be coexistent, perhaps reflecting anorexia and dehydration.

d. **False.** It could be caused by tuberculosis, but there are more likely causes such as incompletely treated infection, urinary tract disease, etc.

e. **True.** Elasticity of the urethra is reduced postmenopausally and this can lead to infection. Local oestrogen therapy helps.

9. a. **True.**
   b. **True.** Renal cell carcinoma is prone to cause systemic symptoms.
   c. **True.** Both bony and pulmonary metastases occur.
   d. **False.**
   e. **False.**

10. a. **False.** Fibromuscular hyperplasia and radiation fibrosis are two other pathologies which can cause renal artery stenosis, although atherosclerosis is the most common pathology.
    b. **True.**
    c. **False.** A renal bruit may be present but absence of a bruit is an unreliable way of excluding renal artery stenosis.
    d. **True.** Hypoperfusion causes reduction in renal size.
    e. **True.**

Case history answers

History 1

1. A common cause of renal failure in elderly men is prostatic disease. The history should concentrate on symptoms of prostatism and he should have a rectal examination and abdominal examination for bladder enlargement. Arterial disease is another likely cause. Symptoms and signs of cardiac and peripheral vascular disease should be sought. A full drug history should be taken. Ask for symptoms of urinary or systemic infection.

2. Immediate abdominal ultrasound to exclude urinary obstruction and assess renal size.

3. Urethral catheterisation. It is normal practice to clamp the catheter after 1–1.5 litre of urine has been drained because abrupt relief of pressure may precipitate severe polyuria and volume depletion.

4. He may be volume depleted or overloaded and should be treated accordingly. His urine should be cultured because stasis predisposes to urinary infection and this may worsen renal function.

History 2

1. a. **False.** She has the classical symptoms of acute uncomplicated cystitis. Referral is unnecessary.

b. **True.** However, over 80% of cystitis infections are caused by *E. coli* and most respond to antibiotics if treated empirically.

c. **True.**

d. **False.** The symptoms are so suggestive of a urinary infection that examination is probably unnecessary.

e. **True.** Cystitis in young women often follows sexual activity and these are sensible questions.

2. a. **False.** This is unnecessary.
   b. **True.** Now it is imperative to send a culture as she has failed therapy. If one had already been sent, a result to guide treatment would be available.
   c. **True.** She has the same symptoms and failed therapy with the first-line antibiotic. In fact, amoxycillin and ampicillin are poor empirical choices for urine infections as only about 40% of *E. coli* are susceptible in the UK. Trimethoprim or ofloxacin would be better.
   d. **True.** More justification now, to exclude vulval disease, but it is still very likely to be cystitis.
   e. **False.** Unnecessary for uncomplicated cystitis.

3. a. **False.** Urinary symptoms have improved.
   b. **True.** The symptoms are typical of vaginal candidosis and she has a good precipitating cause: two courses of antibiotics. However, if she has got (or had) a new partner (or an unfaithful regular partner) she could well have a sexually transmitted disease and examination and culture are important.
   c. **False.** New symptom complex not suggestive of cystitis.
   d. **True.** See (b) above.
   e. **True.** Now an appropriate course of action, particularly if you are not equipped to take appropriate cultures for sexually transmitted diseases *and* she has had a new partner.

Data interpretation answers

1. Patients with data in Table 39.

   Patient 1. Typical biochemistry of severe renal failure with very high creatinine and urea, hyperkalaemia and metabolic acidosis.

   Patient 2. There are multiple abnormalities. Plasma urea is high but creatinine is normal, suggesting volume depletion or impaired renal perfusion resulting in reduced urine flow. Plasma sodium is slightly low implying water retention as a result of increased AVP secretion. There is also a hypokalaemic alkalosis. These abnormalities could best be explained by heart failure, the hypokalaemic alkalosis being caused by treatment with a loop diuretic. Volume depletion from vomiting is another possibility.

   Patient 3. Hypernatraemia is uncommon because it usually causes extreme thirst; this patient has an extremely high plasma urea and moderately high creatinine. This suggests volume depletion with secondary renal failure. This picture is seen in diabetic non-ketotic hyperosmolar coma; note the *absence* of acidosis. The patient is drowsy and either unaware of the hyperosmolality or too ill to drink. Plasma glucose in this case was 76 mmol/l.

Patient 4. Plasma sodium is low. This may be because of excessive water retention or water retention in compensation for severe volume depletion. The latter is unlikely because urea is low–normal. This picture is seen in severe water intoxication resulting from psychogenic polydipsia or the syndrome of inappropriate antidiuresis.

Patient 5. The most striking abnormality here is the high serum potassium. Serum sodium is low and urea high, suggesting volume depletion with compensatory AVP secretion and water retention. This is characteristic of hypoaldosteronism as seen in Addison's disease. Note the mild acidosis. Serum chloride, in this case, will be increased in compensation for the reduced bicarbonate.

2. This is a typical picture of renal bone disease; serum phosphate is high because of renal phosphate retention and calcium is low. Alkaline phosphatase is high suggesting secondary hyperparathyroidism with bone disease. The patient may have bone pain, weakness and malaise. Management is with phosphate-binding agents by mouth (calcium carbonate) and a vitamin D analogue.

3. Patients with data in Table 40.

Patient 1. Acidosis (low pH) with a raised pCO_2 is a **respiratory acidosis**; there is a compensatory metabolic alkalosis. This picture is seen in, for example, an exacerbation of chronic obstructive pulmonary disease.

Patient 2. The acidosis here is **metabolic** because bicarbonate is low; there is compensatory hyperventilation and a reduced pCO_2.

Patient 3. This alkalosis (raised pH) is **metabolic** because bicarbonate is high; there is a compensatory respiratory acidosis (hypoventilation).

Patient 4. Again, alkalosis (high pH); in this case it is **respiratory** because pCO_2 is low; there is a compensatory metabolic acidosis.

4. Patients with data in Table 41.

Patient 1. A 'sterile pyuria' in an improperly collected sample contaminated from the vulva with some faecal contents. Repeat sample in a few days.

Patient 2. Also mild 'sterile pyuria'. Consider fastidious organisms, tuberculosis, antibiotic treatment, etc. If no prior antibiotics, consider tuberculosis, especially if Asian. However, mild pyuria is common in elderly people and this patient could have benign prostatic hypertrophy and no other urinary tract pathology.

Patient 3. A complicated urinary tract infection in a young man; possibly related to a stone. Needs a renal ultrasound in first instance.

Patient 4. Acute urethral syndrome. Urine findings similar to those of bacterial vaginosis but symptom complex different. Treat with prolonged (e.g. 14 days) antibiotics.

Patient 5. Normal urine in an elderly patient: consider prostatic hypertrophy or cancer. Rectal examination and acid phosphatase.

Patient 6. Sterile pyuria. Take early morning urine for mycobacterial culture and microscopy.

Picture answer

1. Pelvi-calyceal dilatation.
2. The ultrasound appearance could result from distal ureteric obstruction or from vesico-ureteric reflux. The patient is in renal failure and has an intra-abdominal malignancy. Hypercalcaemia is one possible explanation for her renal failure, and back pain might indicate bone involvement, but in this case the renal ultrasound appearance would be normal. The ultrasound appearance, in this context, suggests obstruction. For her to be in this degree of renal failure, the obstruction is likely to be bilateral. She might have bladder outflow obstruction but the most likely explanation is retroperitoneal spread of malignancy with bilateral ureteric obstruction. Her back pain fits that diagnosis.
3. She needs further investigation by ultrasound and/or CT to assess the state of her pelvic tumour and retroperitoneum. Her obstruction must be relieved. If the problem were bladder outflow obstruction, the treatment would be bladder catheterisation. If she has ureteric obstruction, she needs a percutaneous nephrostomy, which can be sited under ultrasound/fluoroscopic guidance, or a ureteric stent, which is a longer-term solution.

Neurological disease

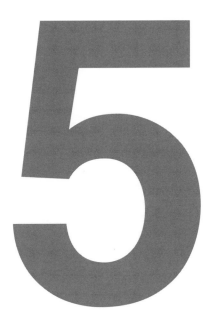

5.1 **Clinical aspects**

Introduction

Learning objectives

You should:
- understand the importance of neuroanatomy in neurological problem solving
- know enough about the major diseases affecting the nervous system to place them appropriately in your differential diagnoses
- be aware of other, less common, neurological diseases
- understand the principles of investigation and management of the major neurological diseases.

One of the keys in dealing with a neurological problem is using your knowledge of the anatomy of both the central and peripheral nervous system. In this chapter, neuroanatomy and physiology are linked with the clinical problems.

Terminology

In neurology there are many different terms which are easy to confuse and can distract you from understanding of a clinical problem. One common difficulty is the use of the prefixes 'a' and 'dys'. In precise terms, the former means the complete absence of the function (i.e. aphasia), whereas the latter simply implies impairment (i.e. dysphasia). In practice they can be used interchangeably. Similarly hemiparesis (weakness) and hemiplegia (complete paralysis) are used without distinction. Here is a list of definitions/explanations for terms which are particularly difficult.

Dyspraxia. This is the inability to carry out voluntary purposeful movement correctly despite apparently normal motor, sensory and coordinative functions. It is usually seen in left cerebral hemisphere damage.

Agnosia. This is a failure to recognise some object when the sense by which it is normally recognised remains intact (e.g. visual agnosia, sensory agnosia). This is different from nominal dysphasia where an object is recognised but cannot be named. Agnosias occur with either left or right hemisphere damage.

Neglect/inattention/denial. These usually occur (but not exclusively) in right hemisphere damage. The person shows less attention to one side of their body or space. Mild degrees need bilateral stimulation to be apparent (visual/sensory extinction). In severe forms, patients deny that one side of the body belongs to them.

Dysphasia. This is a problem with *language*, not simply speech. One important aspect is that if a patient has a marked expressive dysphasia then some receptive problems will be present. A common misconception is that the patient 'understands everything that is said to them'.

Dominance. Another common misunderstanding is the term **dominant hemisphere**; this refers to dominance for language and is almost always the left hemisphere (including 80% of left-handed people). Dominance does not mean the most important.

Impairment, disability and handicap. It is important to know the definitions and relationship between impairment, disability and handicap. If you think of a person with a stroke:

Impairment. Impairments are the direct neuropathophysiological consequences of the underlying pathology. You can think of them in terms of the 'symptoms and signs' you use to diagnose a stroke. Examples are dysphasia, hemiparesis and hemianopia.

Disability. A stroke causing impairment will usually affect a person's behaviour or function. Examples of disabilities include difficulty in walking, dressing or cooking. The relationships between impairments and disabilities are complex, with other influences such as the local environment (ward, house, work) and the person's psychological state (dependency, depression). In stroke, difficulty in dressing might be caused by impairment of movement (hemiparesis), coordination (limb ataxia), sensation (hemisensory loss) or planning movement (dyspraxia).

Handicap. Even more complex are the relationships between handicap and impairment/disability. Handicap refers to the social and societal consequences of pathology (i.e. a stroke) which arise at the level of the person's own roles and activities. Examples of handicap include loss of a job or breakdown of a relationship. One important aspect is that handicap can arise as a consequence of an impairment without any disability. An example would be the loss of an HGV licence as a consequence of a hemianopia (impairment, no disability).

Other disease. Impairment/disability/handicap can also be considered in terms of diseases in other systems. Examples would be the social stigma (handicap) attached to a positive test for HIV, or the change in working practice for a surgeon who is found to be hepatitis B antigen positive. These illustrate that handicap can result from a disease process without any impairment.

Common symptoms

In neurological practice, there are certain symptoms which you must be able to evaluate and either link to particular disease processes *or* discount so that the patient is reassured that there is no serious problem. One important pitfall to avoid is dismissing something you do not understand as being 'hysterical, psychosomatic, supratentorial' or some other demeaning label. As in all branches of medicine, someone with more experience may be able to make sense of the clinical picture. When in doubt — ask!

There are a number of crucial questions that you should ask yourself when taking a history from someone with possible neurological disease.

What is the age of the patient? An old person is unlikely to have multiple sclerosis. A young person is unlikely to have Parkinson's disease.

What is the time course of the symptoms? Abrupt onset is likely to be vascular or epileptic but could result from hypoglycaemia. Onset over a few hours may be infective, though occasionally viral meningitis has an abrupt onset. Progression over several weeks may point to a tumour. Years of gradual decline is likely to be degenerative.

What is the pattern of the symptoms with time? If it is a constant decline then a degenerative condition is probable. If the pattern is relapsing and remitting then an inflammatory condition such as multiple sclerosis may be responsible.

Is the problem a global one such as loss of consciousness or confusion? If so, then causes outside the brain may be responsible, such as hypoglycaemia or arrhythmia.

Are there focal neurological symptoms or signs? If yes, can they be placed at one level or do they cover more than one level?

Is there any relevant family history for vascular or degenerative disease? Not simply asking what the patient's parents died from, but in great detail — such as whether there is a 'family peculiar walk' or foot deformity suggestive of a spinocerebellar syndrome. You need to be able to construct a family tree.

Headache

Everybody gets a headache from time to time. The aim is firstly to separate out headache caused by underlying disease from the remainder. If you use headache as a model for the questions above, a template for sorting out the problem starts to develop. If a headache has an abrupt onset, particularly if it is severe with neck stiffness, then subarachnoid haemorrhage should be suspected. A headache that has been present for years ('never free from it') is unlikely to be caused by neurological disease. One that comes and goes and is associated with flashing lights/visual disturbance is likely to be migraine, but recent onset in an older person might suggest temporal arteritis. If the headache is global ('like a band round the head'), this suggests a tension headache, whereas an intense retro-orbital pain might suggest periodic migraine/cluster headache. If the headache is associated with focal neurological signs, a more sinister cause is likely, possibly a tumour. You should also consider other head and neck problems such as sinusitis. Remember most headaches are not indicative of serious disease, but you need to be able to identify the small number that are.

Blackouts/funny turns

Many patients will present with a 'funny turn'. The causes can be thought of as brain (e.g. fits) or non-brain (e.g. cardiac arrhythmia).

The first question is whether the person did, or did not, lose consciousness. This can be difficult to be sure of as patients may fill in gaps in their memory ('I must have tripped'). One clue may be the extensive facial bruising suggesting a fall without any protective out-stretching of the hands.

What was the person doing immediately before? A blackout in a hot crowded room whilst standing up suggests a simple vasovagal attack. Were there any prodomal features or, if they did not lose consciousness, how did they feel during the episode? Palpitations would suggest a disturbance in cardiac rhythm (**Stoke Adams attack**). An odd feeling prior to the event might be caused by the **aura** of epilepsy.

For any patient presenting with a blackout, you should seek out a witness to the event. They can describe what happened, which is important for the diagnosis of epilepsy.

A key feature is how the person felt following the attack. If it was caused by cardiac dysrhythmia, recovery is characteristically quick. Similarly, recovery following a vasovagal event (a 'faint') is rapid once they have laid down (never hold them up). In contrast, a person is commonly confused and drowsy after a fit, wishing to sleep for several hours.

Unfortunately, the aetiology of the blackouts may not be clear, and your examination (neurological and general) may not be helpful. Investigations may then be appropriate.

Cardiac causes. A 12-lead ECG is most useful for revealing stable abnormalities, e.g. left axis deviation with right bundle branch block (bifascicular block), which predispose to bradyarrhythmias. A 24-hour ECG recording is often requested, but the yield from these is *small* and should only be done if frequent attacks are present.

Neurological causes. An EEG is frequently ordered but is of limited value. It may show a potential epileptic focus with spike activity. A normal EEG does *not* rule out epilepsy. A CT scan is another common investigation, but seldom adds much.

The message is that careful histories from the person *and* witnesses are the most important steps to take in the diagnostic process.

Confusion

Chronic confusion is discussed under Dementia (p. 202). Acute confusional states occur at all ages, not just in elderly people. The features include a disturbance of conscious level (**delirium**), with disorientation in place and time. Patients may be agitated or withdrawn. As with any organic brain syndrome, *visual* hallucinations are common. The symptoms may vary over time. The causes are legion and you should think of them in broad categories:

- brain problems: stroke, infection, trauma
- metabolic and electrolyte disturbance, e.g. hypoglycaemia, hyponatraemia
- toxins: alcohol, drugs
- infections: pneumonia, urinary tract infection
- others, e.g myocardial infarction (brain perfusion).

Focal neurology

The key diagnostic questions you need to address in a patient with a focal deficit are:

- can the deficit result from a single lesion or must there be more than one site involved?
- at what level is the lesion: cerebral hemispheres, brainstem, spinal cord, peripheral nerve, motor endplate or muscle?
- What is the time course, e.g. sudden (vascular/fit) or gradual deterioration (degenerative)?

The clinical diagnosis can often be made from the answers to these questions. For example, a rapid deterioration in visual acuity with a previous history of ataxia and urinary difficulties in a young person suggests multiple sclerosis (multiple sites, affected at different times). In contrast, an episode of fleeting loss of vision in one eye in an older person (**amaurosis fugax**) is suggestive of a platelet embolus from the carotid artery (single site).

A further guiding rule is to try to place the lesion as peripherally as possible. Thus sensory loss should be considered first as a peripheral nerve problem. If this does not fit the clinical picture, then move through the spinal cord centrally towards the integrating centres in the parietal lobe until all the features can be accounted for. In another example, a hemiparesis could be anywhere from the high cervical cord upwards, but with an exaggerated jaw jerk would place the damage above the level of the pons; dysphasia would place it in the cerebral hemispheres. Without these other signs, little precision can be achieved.

Cranial nerve abnormalities

Damage to the cranial nerves must be diagnosed on the basis of the common symptoms and examination findings.

Optic nerve/visual disturbance. A common presenting symptom is visual difficulty. The important elements of the visual pathway must be known in trying to determine the cause and pathophysiological process involved (Fig. 33). Lesions along this pathway cause particular visual disturbances (Table 42).

You must also know the path involved in the light reflex (Fig. 34). The other pupillary reflex is **accommodation**, in which the pupils constrict, the eyes converge and ptosis occurs on looking at an object close-up. In an **Argyll–Robertson** pupil, the light reflex is lost, but accommodation is preserved. Characteristically, the pupils are small, irregular and unequal. In the past, the most common cause was neurosyphilis, but now diabetes mellitus is a common cause of pupillary abnormalities. The **Holmes–Adie pupil** is typically seen in young women, in which the pupil is large and responds to light sluggishly. There is an association with limb areflexia.

Horner's syndrome. In a Horner's syndrome there is damage to the *sympathetic* supply to the orbit. The pathway involved has a long course, starting in the hypothalamus, running down through the brainstem and flowing out through T1 in the spinal cord. Fibres

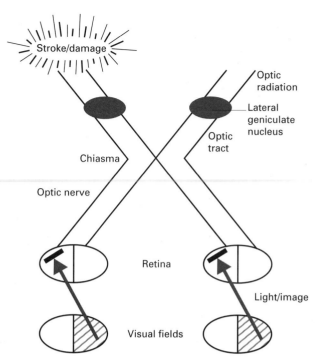

Fig. 33
The visual pathway. Damage on one side of the brain (e.g. stroke) causes a homonymous hemianopia on the opposite side.

then run back into the skull as a plexus round the carotid artery and into the orbit. Damage anywhere along this route can cause a Horner's syndrome. Commonest causes are cerebrovascular disease and tumours growing in the apex of the lung damaging the brachial plexus (**Pancoast's tumour**), though most cases are idiopathic. There are four cardinal signs of the syndrome:

- meiosis (constricted pupil)
- partial ptosis
- enophthalmos (eye shrunken into socket)
- anhydrosis (lack of sweating on ipsilateral side of face).

Oculomotor nerves. The third, fourth and sixth cranial nerves act together to produce smooth visual fixation and tracking. You must know the direction of the prime action of the muscles involved (Fig. 35). In trying to unravel diplopia it is useful to remember three simple rules:

- diplopia is maximal on looking in the direction of the prime action of the muscle
- the false image is always displaced furthest in the direction of action of the muscle affected
- The false image is always the least distinct.

Third cranial nerve palsy. This is commonly caused by either an aneurysm or diabetes (see p. 200 and p. 281) and it results in:

- complete ptosis
- the eye turned down (unopposed action of superior oblique muscle) and out (lateral rectus)
- an usually large pupil that is non-reactive to light (see Fig. 34).

Table 42 Visual symptoms arising from damage to the visual pathway, site of damage and common pathological processes.

Visual symptom	Site of damage	Common pathologies[a]
Fleeting loss of vision in one eye (amaurosis fugax): 'Like a curtain coming up/down'	Central retinal artery	Microemboli, often from carotid artery
Monocular blindness: 'Can't see at all out of one eye'	Optic nerve, eye	Trauma, infection, bleeding (diabetes), central retinal artery thrombosis, temporal arteritis
Field defects in one eye (scotomas) 'I seem to have a blind spot'	Retina, branch of retinal arteries, part of optic nerve	Glaucoma (arcuate scotoma), retinal artery thrombosis, MS, CMV retinitis in AIDS
Bitemporal hemianopia: 'Can't see things to the side'	Chiasma; if upper part, lower fields lost, and vice versa	Tumour: pituitary, craniopharyngioma (child)
Homonymous hemianopia: 'Can't see to the left (right)'	Optic tract Optic radiation Occipital cortex	Tumours, vascular damage: stroke
Sudden bilateral visual loss: 'Struck blind'	Occipital cortex: Anton's syndrome, patient may not complain of blindness	Vascular
Flashing lights/zigzag lights (fortification spectra) loss of part of visual field	Occipital cortex	Migraine

MS, Multiple sclerosis; CMV, cytomegalovirus.
[a]In the UK the most common causes of blindness are diabetes mellitus, glaucoma and senile macular degeneration.

Fourth nerve palsy. This is very rare in isolation. It causes diplopia when looking down and away from the affected side (eye adducted).

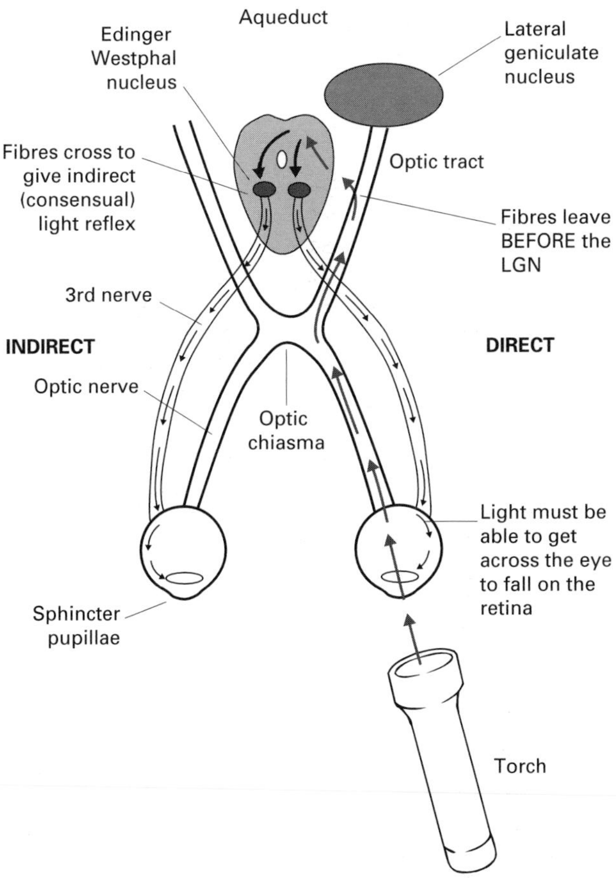

Sixth nerve palsies. These are relatively common, either from vascular lesions or as a false localising sign in raised intracranial pressure where the nerve is trapped as it crosses the falx cerebri.

Visual movements. Other problems with visual movements are described on page 197.

Fifth nerve. The fifth nerve supplies sensation to the face, including the cornea, through the ophthalmic branch. The mandibular division supplies the muscles of mastication (temporalis, masseter and pterygoids). An important element in examining trigeminal function is the corneal reflex (efferent arc: facial nerve). An absent or diminished corneal reflex may be an early

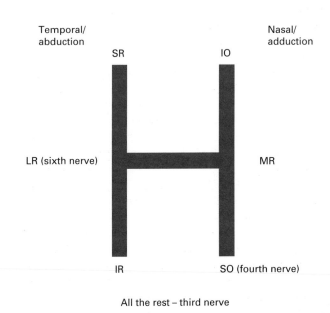

Fig. 34
Pathway for light reflex.

Fig. 35
Primary action of extrinsic ocular muscles and their innervation.

sign of an **acoustic neuroma** (pressure on the fifth nerve in the cerebello–pontine angle). Divisions of the fifth nerve are commonly affected by herpes zoster.

Trigeminal neuralgia. This is an important clinical problem affecting the fifth nerve. It is a condition of unknown aetiology which runs a relapsing and remitting course. It is sometimes bilateral. Patients describe *lancinating* pain, which may be precipitated by stimulating a *trigger zone* or by activities such as yawning or brushing teeth. On examination there are *no* physical signs. The main treatment is **carbamazepine**.

Seventh nerve. The most common cranial nerve lesion you will see in practice is a facial nerve palsy. You must know the diagram in Figure 36 in order to understand how facial nerve damage manifests. An important additional detail is that the upper part of the face is *bilaterally innervated*. What this means is that the each motor cortex (left and right precentral gyrus) sends fibres to the facial nucleus on both sides. Consequently:

- an upper motor neurone lesion (e.g. caused by a stroke), affecting the pathway from only one cortex, will spare the upper part of the face
- a lower motor neurone lesion (damage to the nucleus or the nerve) will cause complete paralysis of one half of the face.

Facial weakness often results from damage to the facial nerve. In trying to pinpoint where the damage is located, you need to know the information in Figure 36.

For example, an acoustic neuroma (VIIIth nerve) may compress the facial nerve as it runs towards the internal auditory meatus and all function may be lost. Whereas damage in the facial canal, for example in **Bell's palsy**, will spare the greater superficial petrosal nerve and hence lacrimation.

Ramsay–Hunt syndrome. A complete facial palsy may be caused by geniculate herpes zoster. Some vesiculation may be observed around the ear canal. Prognosis for recovery is much worse than in Bell's palsy.

Eighth nerve. In neurological practice, the most important diagnosis is the rare acoustic neuroma, which is discussed on page 194.

Ninth and tenth nerve. The ninth nerve is mainly sensory to the palate, with branches to the carotid sinus (monitoring blood pressure) and carotid body (monitoring arterial oxygen partial pressure). The vagus nerve is mainly motor to the palate including the pharyngeal constrictors. The principal effect of damage to the nerves/nuclei, e.g. in the medulla (vascular, motor neurone disease) or around the jugular foramen, is **dysphagia**. Swallowing is a complex act requiring coordination between a number of different centres. Three stages are recognised:

- oral/preparatory: lip closure (seventh nerve), mastication (fifth nerve), manipulation by the tongue (twelfth nerve) and presentation of the bolus to the pharynx.

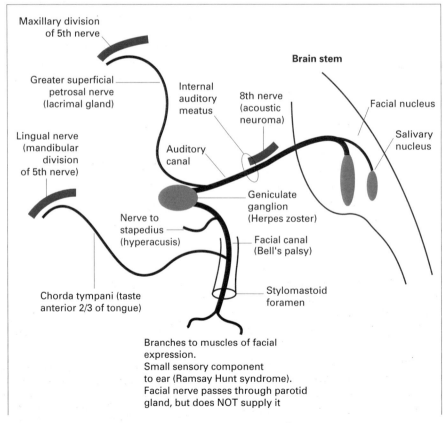

Fig. 36
Pathway of facial nerve, including branches and important relationships.

- pharyngeal (ninth and tenth nerve): the soft palate lifts together with the larynx, and the pharyngeal constrictors assist the bolus through to the upper end of the oesphagus
- oesophageal (discussed on p. 102).

You must be aware that presence or absence of the gag reflex (sensory ninth nerve, motor tenth nerve) is of no use in predicting aspiration. All patients who are drowsy should be considered at risk and a Glasgow Coma Score (see Table 47) of ≤ 6 is an indication for endotracheal intubation in an acutely ill patient. Main features to look for are a 'wet' voice and coughing on taking a small amount of fluid. In neurological dysphagia, unlike obstructive dysphagia, the greater difficulty is with thin liquids rather than solids because of difficulty in controlling the former.

Twelfth nerve. Tongue function can be affected by bulbar (i.e. medullary) damage or pseudobulbar damage. In a unilateral lesion, the tongue will point *towards* the affected side. Bulbar weakness, caused by ischaemia, encephalitis, motor neurone disease or **syringobulbia** (very rare, cavity in the middle of the brainstem), will cause wasting of the tongue with fasciculation, dysphagia and dysarthria.

Pseudobulbar palsy. This is caused by *bilateral* damage of the pyramidal tract system (e.g. stroke, motor neurone disease). It causes dysphagia, *emotionalism* (inability to control emotions with crying at inappropriate times or excessively) and a tongue which appears small and 'stuck' to the floor of the mouth. The dysarthria is likened to talking with a mouthful of marbles.

Basic investigations

Examination of cerebrospinal fluid

The brain is covered by the meninges, which consist of the thick dura mater externally, the arachnoid lining the dura and the pia mater adherent to the brain and spinal cord. The arachnoid and the pia bound the subarachnoid space, which is filled by the cerebrospinal fluid (CSF). The CSF is produced at a constant rate of about 450 ml/day by the **choroid plexuses** of the lateral (most important), third and fourth ventricles. Flow is from the lateral ventricles into the third ventricle and then the fourth ventricle by way of the aqueduct. Foramina allow drainage from the fourth ventricle into the pontine cistern and cisterna magna. Blockage along this route may cause a **non-communicating hydrocephalus.** Causes include tumour or blood within the ventricular system.

The CSF flows through the cisternal spaces and over the cerebral hemispheres. Absorption into the dural venous sinuses is through the **arachnoid villi**. Block here, e.g. by blood from a subarachnoid haemorrhage, may cause a **communicating hydrocephalus.**

Rarely a **normal pressure hydrocephalus** occurs in elderly people. In this, slow pressure waves can be demonstrated by continous monitoring (these gradually dilate the ventricles), but isolated pressure readings are normal. Patients have a triad of dementia, gait dyspraxia and urinary incontinence. It is important because around half of patients will respond to insertion of a ventricular shunt.

Another rare condition is **benign intracranial hypertension**, where there is an overproduction of CSF. The disease is most common in young women and is associated with the oral contraceptive pill, pregnancy and obesity. Presentation is with headaches, an enlarging blind spot and progressive visual failure. Papilloedema is found on examination. A CT, or MR, scan will show slit-like ventricles and effacement (compression) of the sulci of the cerebral hemispheres. A lumbar puncture reveals a greatly elevated CSF pressure (≥ 20 cm H_2O) and repeated lumbar punctures may improve the symptoms. It is important to make the diagnosis, as patients can respond to corticosteroids. Sometimes neurosurgical intervention is needed to decompress the brain.

The CSF volume is around 80–200 ml, with a recumbent pressure of 80–180 ml H_2O. It is important to know the approximate normal values for CSF constituents as this is essential to make decisions on the results of an urgent CSF specimen. Key values are given in Table 43.

The indications for a lumbar puncture are suspected:

- meningitis
- encephalitis
- subarachnoid haemorrhage (if CT scan negative)
- benign intracranial hypertension.

The main contraindications to lumbar puncture are focal signs, evidence of raised intracranial pressure, a space-occupying lesion on CT scan or a significant bleeding tendency. Papilloedema takes several hours to develop, you have to acquire the skill of assessing whether retinal venous pulsation is present; absence of which is a reliable indicator of raised pressure. If in doubt — request a CT scan. The patterns of abnormalities found in the CSF with different disease processes are the keys to synthesising the information into a differential diagnosis (Table 44).

Imaging techniques

CT and MR imaging techniques have revolutionised neurological practice. When looking at a CT or MR scan, go through a set routine:

Table 43 Normal values for CSF constituents

Protein	0.25–0.50 g/l
Glucose[a]	2.5–5.5 mmol/l
White cells	< 5 cells (lymphocytes)/mm³
Red cells[b]	0

[a]This is dependent on the blood glucose value (should be 50–70% of the blood value: N.B. diabetes mellitus).
[b]Should be zero. However a 'bloody tap' may contaminate the fluid. If some red cells are present in all specimen samples, this suggests subarachnoid haemorrhage. If decreasing values in successful samples, this suggests a 'bloody tap'. One white cell is allowed for every 1000 red cells.

Table 44 Relevant tests and abnormalities in CSF with disease processes

Disease process	Pressure	Cells	Glucose	Protein	Microbiology	Special notes
Bacterial meningitis	May be increased	High, neutrophils (95–100%)	Very low or undetectable	High or very high	Gram stain or culture positive	Partially treated: may be culture negative
Viral meningitis	Usually normal	High lymphocytes (10–100%); early disease: neutrophils	Low	Normal or slightly high	PCR useful	Common
Viral encephalitis		Mild increase lymphocytes	Low	Normal or slightly raised	PCR for herpes simplex useful	May be red cells in herpes simplex
Brain abscess/ parameningeal focus	May be increased	High, neutrophils (60–100%)	Normal or low	High	Culture and Gram stain negative	Check CT scan carefully
Fungal meningitis	May be increased	High lymphocytes	Low or normal	Normal or raised	India ink stain (75%); culture positive, cryptococcal antigen positive (95%)	Usually AIDS or other immunoccompromised patient
Tuberculous meningitis	May be increased	Lymphocytes, usually 100%	Low	High or very high	ZN stain (10–20%) and culture (30%)	Uncommon
Malignancy	Variable	Malignant cells on cytology	Low	Some increase	Negative	Rare
Guillain–Barré syndrome	Normal	Slight increase in lymphocytes in early stages	Normal	Raised after first week	Negative	
Multiple sclerosis	Normal	Slight increase in lymphocytes in relapse	Normal	Mild rise	Negative	May have oligoclonal protein bands
Subarachnoid haemorrhage	May be raised	Red cells increased	Normal	High	Negative	Xanthochromia (red cell pigment) present

PCR, polymerase chain reaction; ZN, Ziehl–Neelsen.

- orientate yourself: left/right; anterior/posterior
- was contrast given? If not, then on a CT scan any dense white areas in the brain are either blood or (less common) calcium
- describe any obvious abnormality in terms of its position, size, shape and any effects on surrounding brain tissue (compression: midline shift)
- look for other abnormalities which may be more subtle and present in other areas of the brain.

The use of CT/MR scanning is discussed within the common neurological problems described below.

Electroencephalography

Though now regarded as an 'old' investigation, electroencephalography (EEG) is still useful as a tool for unravelling a neurological problem but it has its limitations. Approximately 5% of the population have an 'abnormal' EEG; particularly young people. Therefore, it cannot be used to 'diagnose' epilepsy; it is there as an adjunct to careful history and examination. In certain cases, 24-hour recordings of events or telemetry can be useful.

There are certain conditions in which an EEG can yield characteristic findings (Table 45). In most other conditions in which abnormalities are seen, for example drug toxicity or cerebral oedema, the findings are non-specific, for example generalised or localised slow waves.

Nerve conduction tests and electromyography

You do not need to know the detail of the specialised nerve conduction tests and electromyography (EMG). What you must know are the clinical problems for which you should request these investigations and understand what the results will tell you.

Nerve conduction studies determine the *conduction velocities* within the nerves and will be impaired if the

Table 45 Characteristic EEG abnormalities with disease processes

Disease processes	Notes on EEG abnormality
Petit mal epilepsy	3/s spike and wave activity
Partial epilepsy	May be no abnormality; may have 'focus' with spike activity
Hepatic encephalopathy	Triphasic waves
Herpes simplex encephalitis	Temporal lobe abnormality (30–50%)
Creutzfeldt–Jakob disease (prion disease)	Slow background repetitive spikes

myelin sheath is damaged. Therefore, conditions such as **Guillain–Barré syndrome** show marked slowing of conduction. Diseases that attack the axons or nerve bodies, such as **motor neurone disease**, will show minimal impairment of conduction but reduced number of motor units (amplitude of signal). Nerve conduction studies can show localised areas of demyelination resulting from pressure, such as in the carpal tunnel syndrome (wrist) or ulnar nerve palsies (elbow).

EMG is useful for showing changes in the innervation of muscles or disorders of muscles themselves. Therefore, acute/subacute denervation, such as in motor neurone disease, will show fibrillating potentials. Problems at the motor endplate, such as in **myasthenia gravis** or **Eaton–Lambert syndrome** will produce characteristic changes, as can inflammation in the muscles (**myositis**) or an intrinsic abnormality such as **dystrophia myotonica**.

Common drugs

The most common drugs used in neurological practice are antiepileptic (p. 206) and antiparkinsonian. These are dealt with below. The use of hypnotics and neuroleptics are outside the scope of this book. Analgesia is dealt with elsewhere (p. 303). Occasional use of corticosteroids and immunosuppressives are discussed in the context of the target disease.

5.2 Infection

Bacterial meningitis

Learning objectives

You should:
- be able to recognise rapidly the symptoms of meningitis and be clear about the immediate management plan once this diagnosis is suspected
- be able to distinguish, using clinical features and the CSF results, bacterial meningitis from viral meningitis and encephalitis
- understand the role and priority of CT scanning in the evaluation of possible CNS infection.

Pathogenesis and epidemiology

Bacteria enter the meningeal space either directly because of a hole in the dura or via the bloodstream. The two most common organisms causing meningitis in adults are *Neisseria meningitidis* and *Streptococcus pneumoniae*. Both of these enter the body through the nasopharynx. Why *S. pneumoniae* causes pneumonia in some individuals and meningitis in others is unclear. Likewise why *N. meningitidis* causes meningococcal septicaemia (see p. 358) or meningitis is not understood.

N. meningitidis infection is more common in young adults and teenagers; the incidence of *S. pneumoniae* meningitis increases with age.

Clinical features

The onset of bacterial meningitis is usually abrupt and rapidly progressive. The time from first symptom to death is frequently as short as 48 hours and sometimes as little as 24 hours. Therefore bacterial meningitis *must* be treated as a medical emergency. The symptoms that should lead to suspicion of meningitis are:

- headache
- vomiting
- fever
- impaired consciousness.

Patients may also complain of photophobia, chills, sore throat, rash and painful or stiff neck.

Clinical evaluation and emergency management

Your evaluation of the patient with possible meningitis should be rapid and focused, so as not to delay therapy. Apart from the above symptoms, seek information about immunocompromising factors and allergies. Your examination should look for neck stiffness, papilloedema/absence of pulsation in retinal veins, focal neurological signs, ear disease, rash, signs of pneumonia and ventilatory status. If neck stiffness is present, together with the above symptoms (especially if consciousness is impaired) you should make a presumptive diagnosis of meningitis.

At this stage in hospital practice the emergency treatment outlined in the box should be initiated. You should endeavour to ensure that all patients with meningitis receive antibiotics within 30 minutes of arriving in the hospital. Delay will worsen outcome.

Differential diagnosis

If the patient is hospitalized or immunocompromised, other causes of meningitis should be considered. Examples include *Listeria monocytogenes*, Gram-negative organisms or the fungus *Cryptococcus neoformans*. The lumbar puncture is *critical* for these patients otherwise treatment is likely to be wrong. In addition, penicillin resistance in pneumococci is an increasing problem and optimum therapy for these patients can only be decided if the organism is cultured. The lumbar puncture also distinguishes viral from bacterial meningitis and allows herpes simplex encephalitis to be diagnosed with confidence (see p. 192). If the patient is young and acutely ill with the typical purpuric rash of meningococcal disease, a lumbar puncture adds little in addition to a blood culture and need not be done.

Management

Steroids are definitely indicated for meningitis in children. Studies in adults have not been done satisfactorily, but the data show an improved outcome in unconscious patients with pneumococcal meningitis.

1. Prescribe cefotaxime 2 g or ceftriaxone 4 g i.v. (if none available use penicillin 5 mega units) and ask nurses or colleague to prepare drugs immediately
2. Take blood for blood culture, serology, full blood count, creatinine, urea, electrolytes and glucose
3. Set up an intravenous infusion
4. Give antibiotics
5. If patient unconscious give dexamethasone 4 mg i.v.
6. If focal signs or papilloedema or lack of retinal venous pulsation, arrange an urgent CT scan, with contrast. Lumbar puncture with a focal lesion in the posterior fossa or causing mass effect could lead to coning of the brainstem: often a fatal complication. The CT scan will usually be normal in meningitis (and encephalitis) and so it is used primarily in this setting to exclude a brain tumour or abscess
7. If no focal features or signs of raised intracranial pressure, do a lumbar puncture before CT scan; if CT scan normal, do LP; if CT shows focal disease seek senior guidance
8. Do blood gases and administer oxygen if necessary
9. Take complete history and do full physical examination
10. Speak to consultant microbiologist or infectious disease physician about case and decide empirical antibiotic regimen
11. Transfer to single room or intensive care.

They should be given for only 3–5 days. Antibiotics are usually given for 7–10 days. Avoid giving too much fluid: keep patients slightly sodium and water depleted to reduce cerebral oedema.

Outcome and complications
The mortality of meningococcal meningitis is 10% and of pneumococcal meningitis is 25%, rising to 60% in elderly people, even if treated appropriately. Bacterial meningitis, especially pneumococcal, carries a high rate of neurological sequelae if the patient survives. Deafness is the most common deficit. Memory deficits, motor disability and more complex problems are quite common, perhaps affecting a third of survivors. This is probably because of cerebral venous infarction as the major veins run on the surface of the brain, adjacent to the meninges.

Prevention
All forms of meningitis are notifiable diseases. Household contacts or those who have given mouth-to-mouth resuscitation to patients with meningococcal meningitis or septicaemia require antibiotic prophylaxis (see p. 358).

Brain abscess

Pathogenesis and epidemiology

Most abscesses are related to chronic ear disease, but dental, sinus, pulmonary and cyanotic congenital heart disease are also predisposing factors. In many patients, no underlying cause is found. An increasing number of cerebral abscesses occur in immunocompromised patients. In these patients, opportunistic pathogens such as *Nocardia*, *Aspergillus* or *Toxoplasma* are more frequent than bacteria. For this reason, you should always try and ascertain the immune status of the patient. About half the cases occur in young adults.

Clinical features

Typically patients have symptoms for 1–2 weeks before admission and diagnosis. Chronic ear infection is found in 40%. Nausea and vomiting with drowsiness are common. However, the clinical findings are not distinctive:

- headache is the most common symptom (75%)
- only 10% of patients are unconscious
- fever is only present in 30%
- focal signs are found in 70%
- neck stiffness is found in only 15%.

Investigations

Radiological findings
The typical CT appearance (with contrast) is an area of central necrosis, with ring enhancement surrounded by oedema. Frequently there is midline shift. The appearances are usually sufficiently distinctive to distinguish a brain abscess from tumour. Abscesses are found throughout the brain and are multiple in about 25% of patients.

Management

If the patient has AIDS, empiric therapy for toxoplasmosis is given without confirmation of the diagnosis. In all other patients, needle aspiration of the lesion through a burr hole is the next step. As anaerobic organisms are common, rapid transport of the specimen to the laboratory is crucial. In over one-third of patients, four or more organisms are grown from the abscess. Antibiotic management is then directed against the appropriate pathogens. Empirical therapy of brain abscess always includes metronidazole and should include an antistreptococcal agent (such as penicillin or ampicillin) and a broad-spectrum Gram-negative agent (such as cefotaxime), all in large doses.

Outcome

If managed appropriately, the overall mortality from brain abscess should be < 10%, with all deaths occurring in patients presenting unconscious. The mortality from brain abscess in immunocompromised patients is much higher, especially with *Aspergillus*, when virtually all patients die.

Tuberculous meningitis

You must be able to distinguish the common treatable forms of lymphocytic meningitis (e.g. tuberculous meningitis) from viral meningitis, using primarily the CSF results (see Table 44).

Epidemiology

Tuberculous meningitis is an uncommon cause of meningitis in the UK but is the most common cause worldwide of subacute meningitis in non-AIDS patients. About 3–10% of all patients with tuberculosis have meningitis.

Clinical features

Symptoms increase in severity over 2–6 weeks prior to presentation. In the UK, most cases occur in patients from the Indian subcontinent. Vomiting, headache and anorexia are the most common features (50–75%). Drowsiness is seen in a third of patients. More severely affected patients, usually those who present late, may be unconscious, have cranial nerve palsies, hemiparesis or other localising features. Fever is not common. Examination shows

- neck stiffness (90%)
- papilloedema (30%)
- focal neurological signs (25%, in more severe cases).

In the UK, a previously well Asian patient with a 2 week history of vomiting and headache is likely to have tuberculous meningitis. If he also has neck stiffness, the diagnosis is highly likely.

Investigations

Key investigations are:

- chest radiograph: to seek evidence of concurrent, prior pulmonary or miliary tuberculosis
- Mantoux/Heaf test
- CT scan of brain (to visualise tuberculomata and rule out other brain abscess or tumour)
- CSF examination (see below and Table 44).

The typical CSF shows many white cells — usually 100–400/mm^3 — which are predominantly or exclusively lymphocytes, a very high protein (e.g. >1.0 g/l) and a low glucose content. This picture is characteristic and clinically useful, as acid-fast bacilli are seen in the CSF in only a minority and culture is positive in only 25–50% of patients. Therefore, confirmation of the diagnosis is difficult. The usual problem is that the CSF is consistent with tuberculous meningitis but no confirmatory data (such as a strongly positive Mantoux test) are available. In these circumstances, you should seek expert advice.

Management

Treatment for tuberculous meningitis is similar to that for other forms of tuberculosis with two exceptions:

1. Four drugs should be given initially rather than three, as this disease has such a poor outlook if undertreated; resistance is an increasing problem
2. Dexamethasone should be used.

Outcome

The mortality of tuberculous meningitis is about 15–50% depending on how delayed treatment is. Neurological sequelae, such as diplopia, deafness, hemiparesis and mental retardation, are common in survivors (20–25%). A significant proportion of patients (10–20%) develop hydrocephalus (headache or declining mental status) and require a ventricular shunt.

Fungal meningitis

Cryptococcal meningitis

The most common cause of fungal meningitis is *Cryptococcus neoformans*. In the UK, there are about 150 cases each year, mostly in AIDS and other immunocompromised patients.

Cryptococcus is acquired through inhalation and can cause pneumonia or lung nodules. However 85% of patients have meningitis. It presents subacutely, rather like tuberculous meningitis. CSF examination will show yeasts (by India ink examination) in 75% of cases and cryptococcal antigen is usually positive, as is culture.

Treatment is with amphotericin B and flucytosine followed by fluconazole. If treatment is initiated promptly the outcome is good, especially in AIDS.

Viral meningitis

Learning objectives

You should:
- know how to distinguish viral meningitis from encephalitis and other forms of meningitis
- know the main causes of viral meningitis and encephalitis
- know the few indications for therapy.

Epidemiology

Overall, viral meningitis is more common than bacterial meningitis. The widespread use of mumps vaccine has reduced the number of cases substantially. There are many causes of nonbacterial meningitis, some of which require specific therapy. To make things easier for you, Table 46 includes all major infectious causes of a lymphocytosis in the CSF.

Clinical features

Viral meningitis presents with headache and neck stiffness, without impairment of consciousness (see section on viral encephalitis). The headache is often severe, coming on gradually over 1–6 hours. Occasionally it has a sudden onset, but you should think first of subarachnoid haemorrhage. Occasionally, there are associated features such as parotitis or orchitis in mumps or cranial nerve herpes zoster, or other features of primary HIV infection (see p. 337). Headache is a common feature of influenza and atypical pneumonia, so consider these diagnoses. Often, there are no useful clinical features to make an aetiological diagnosis.

Investigations

Lumbar puncture is useful. The total cell count is elevated with a neutrophil predominance (up to 90%) in most patients in the first 2 days or so with a lymphocyte predominance thereafter. The glucose is usually normal, but in about 10% of patients it can be slightly low but is never extremely low. The protein may be mildly elevated (up to about 0.8 g/l) but is rarely above 1.0 g/l (Table 44). Virus is grown from the CSF in only about 10–20%. PCR tests are increasingly useful.

The most useful tests for the enteroviruses (the commonest cause) are throat and stool viral cultures. Mumps virus can be grown in the urine. HIV is best identified by the HIV p24 antigen or viral load tests, as seroconversion can be delayed. If HIV is identified, this would be an indication to treat early with antiretroviral therapy (see p. 338). All forms of meningitis are notifiable diseases.

Management

Viral meningitis is a benign illness which is self-limiting in normal people. Bed rest and symptomatic relief for headache is all that is required. If deterioration in the level of consciousness occurs, then the diagnosis is

Table 46 Infectious causes of lymphocytic CSF

	Treatment required
Viral causes	
Enteroviruses[a]	No
Mumps virus	No
Adenovirus	No
Lymphocytic choriomeningitis virus	No
Varicella zoster virus	No
Herpes simplex virus	Yes
Human immunodeficiency virus	Yes
Other causes	
M. tuberculosis[a]	Yes
Lyme disease	Yes
Leptospirosis	Yes
Syphilis	Yes
Mycoplasma pneumoniae[a]	Yes
Cryptococcus sp.	Yes
Coccidioidomycosis	Yes
Brucellosis	Yes

[a] Most common in UK.

probably a meningoencephalitis (or other non-viral disease) with implications for management (see below).

Viral encephalitis

Epidemiology

Around 1000 documented (and many more undocumented) cases of viral encephalitis occur in the UK each year. There are several causes of viral encephalitis, which generally present in the same way. Most cases of encephalitis in the UK are caused by common viruses present worldwide. These include Coxsackie and echoviruses (enteroviruses), adenovirus, mumps, measles, varicella zoster, Epstein–Barr virus and others.

Clinical presentation

Encephalitis is characterised by the acute onset of a febrile illness, with mental status abnormalities. Any or all of the following features can occur:

- headache
- altered level of consciousness
- behavioural and speech disturbance
- neurologic signs
- seizures which may be focal or generalised.

Many patients with viral encephalitis have neck stiffness and cells in the CSF, and the term meningoencephalitis is often used. The cardinal features distinguishing viral encephalitis from meningitis are alterations in consciousness and behavioural changes.

Differential diagnosis

The differential diagnosis of viral encephalitis is broad. It includes bacterial infections of the CNS (including *Listeria* and tuberculosis), cryptococcal meningitis, Lyme disease, drug overdoses, vascular disease and others. It also includes carbon monoxide poisoning and systemic lupus erythematosus. The diagnosis can be established with reasonable certainty by excluding structural lesions on CT and MR scanning, lumbar puncture, serology and repeated careful observation. In addition, stool, urine and throat swabs may grow the virus.

Investigations

The lumbar puncture is of value provided the CSF findings are interpreted correctly (Table 44). Rarely, if ever, is the CSF entirely normal in encephalitis. Typically, white cells are increased but may be only just abnormal, e.g. 7 cells/mm^3. Red cells are often increased in herpes simplex encephalitis. The glucose is normal, except in a few cases of mumps meningoencephalitis, when it is slightly low. The protein may be normal, or more commonly slightly elevated. A virus may be grown from the CSF, although this is uncommon. Molecular diagnosis of herpes simplex encephalitis using PCR or CSF is now routinely available. Other conditions including tuberculosis, neurosyphilis and *Listeria*, etc. can usually be excluded by lumbar puncture.

The EEG is not specific enough to establish with certainty the aetiology of encephalitis, although a temporal focus suggests herpes simplex encephalitis (Table 45).

CT and MR scans are principally of use in excluding other diseases. Occasionally a focus of haemorrhagic necrosis or inflammation is identified, but the specificity of such findings is poor.

Management

The treatment of encephalitis is mostly supportive but may include admission to the intensive care unit if the Glasgow coma score is low (Table 47). Treatable causes are:

- herpes simplex encephalitis, which is treated with acyclovir i.v. for 10 days
- mycoplasma meningoencephalitis, treated with erythromycin or tetracycline
- primary infection with HIV, which should be treated with zidovudine and didanosine.

Outcome

Encephalitis is an extremely unpredictable disease. Some patients are ill for only a few days and make a complete recovery. Most are unwell for 2–6 weeks and then make a slow recovery. Many never regain their full mental faculties and short- or long-term memory loss is common. In the UK, the mortality is low. Encephalitis is notifiable disease.

Post-infective encephalitis

Encephalitis may appear after a generalised viral infection (most commonly measles, varicella, influenza and mumps) has resolved. The onset is often abrupt with

seizures and reduced consciousness or memory change, but the prognosis usually good.

Rabies

A 'rabies scare' following a dog bite among travellers in rabies endemic areas is not rare (2% of all UK travellers), hence the need for you as a practising doctor to have some knowledge of the disease and immunisation.

Pathogenesis and clinical features

Rabies is an RNA virus that is transmitted to humans by an animal bite, almost always a dog. The virus is present in the saliva of the animal. A break in the skin is necessary to transmit the virus. The virus then enters unmyelinated nerves and travels gradually up the axon until it reaches the spinal cord. It disseminates rapidly through the CNS causing an illness with characteristic stages, ending in death. The incubation period is very variable, from 2 weeks to 11 years. The earliest symptoms are pain or paraesthesia at the wound site together with malaise, fever and anorexia. CNS disease is manifest as intermittent hyperactivity, hallucinations, bizarre behaviour and convulsions. Later pharyngeal spasms occur on swallowing.

Management of a bite

Following a dog bite in a rabies endemic country, three actions are appropriate if the skin was broken:

- wash the wound with soap and water
- instillation of rabies immunoglobulin locally around the wound and systemically
- active immunisation (five injections over a month).

Immunoglobulin and vaccine should be administered within 48 hours if possible, but certainly within 5 days. If followed, this regimen has been 100% effective. Rabies is a notifiable disease.

Prion disease

Human prion disease causes dementia is known as Creutzfeldt–Jakob disease (CJD). It has been transmitted from human tissue to human via

- corneal transplantation
- human growth hormone injections derived from pituitary glands collected from cadavers.

Fortunately there are only about 50 cases in the UK annually. Most occur in middle age and are sporadic. In 1996 a variant of CJD was described in younger people, possibly related to consumption of meat products, contaminated with the prion responsible for bovine spongiform encephalopathy (BSE).

Table 47 Glasgow Coma Scale: the scores are summed to give an overall rating between 3–14; minimum score is 3

Category	Score
Eye opening	
Spontaneous	4
To speech	3
To pain	2
None	1
Best verbal response	
Orientated	5
Confused	4
Inappropriate	3
Incomprehensible	2
None	1
Best motor response	
Obeying commands	5
Localising	4
Flexing	3
Extending	2
None	1

Clinical features

Memory loss, diminished intellect and poor judgement are typical presenting features of CJD. Florid psychiatric symptoms including visual and auditory hallucinations are frequent. Myoclonus and/or muscle fasciculation and wasting are common but may not be present initially. Cerebellar forms also occur with ataxia and incoordination, followed later by dementia and myoclonus. EEG is helpful late in the disease (Table 45). CT scan and other imaging contributes little to the diagnosis, which is essentially clinical. Cerebral biopsy and/or autopsy is required for precise diagnosis. If cerebral biopsy is undertaken, all surgical instruments have to be discarded afterwards as there is no known way to 'sterilise' them.

Outcome

All patients with CJD die, usually over a period of 1 to 3 years. No treatment is known.

Tetanus

Although only 5–15 cases of tetanus occur annually in the UK, hundreds of cases occur in most developing countries. Tetanus is almost completely preventable by immunisation but as *Clostridium tetani* is a soil organism, all immunisation programmes will have to continue indefinitely.

Clinical features

The cardinal features of tetanus are:

- trismus: involuntary clenching of the jaw (100%)
- muscle spasms
- dysphagia.

Common presenting features include back pain and an infected wound.

Management

Management must be in an intensive care unit, with specific treatment including wound excision, metronidazole, antitetanus immunoglobulin intramuscularly and intrathecally and, in severe cases, tracheostomy and paralysis.

Outcome

The mortality is about 10% in the UK, but much higher abroad. Tetanus is a notifiable disease.

5.3 Tumours

Learning objectives

You should:
- know the natural history of tumours
- know how they are diagnosed

- understand how the different pathological types influence natural history and diagnosis.

Epidemiology and presentation

Cerebral tumours (25% are metastatic) account for approximately 10% of all tumours. Three modes of presentation predominate:

- focal neurological deficit as the tumour invades and compresses surrounding tissue
- focal epilepsy, which may become generalised from the outset
- signs of raised intracranial pressure: somnolence, headache, vomiting.

Headache on its own is a *very rare* presentation of a brain tumour.

Benign tumours

Meningioma

Meningiomas arise commonly in the parasagittal region around the falx, or over the cerebral hemispheres, the wing of the sphenoid bone or the olfactory groove. They are slow growing vascular tumours which often calcify. The overlying bone commonly either erodes or becomes hyperostotic. A CT scan shows a homogeneous, space-occupying lesion which densely enhances after contrast media. Surgical removal can be curative, but is often difficult and the tumour may regrow.

Cerebello–pontine angle tumour

Acoustic neuromas (**schwannomas**) arise from the eighth cranial nerve (vestibulo-cochlear). They slowly grow and may invade the surrounding tissue. As they enlarge, progressive deafness occurs as well as damage to the other nerves in the cerebello–pontine angle. Therefore, patients may have facial sensory loss (fifth nerve: particularly loss of corneal reflex), facial weakness (seventh nerve: lower motor neurone), together with ipsilateral cerebellar signs. Eventually, hydrocephalus develops. Plain skull radiographs may show erosion of the internal auditory meatus, but an MR scan is the investigation of choice, showing a mass that enhances with contrast media. A CT scan is also useful, but bone may interfere with the image. If the tumour is not invasive, surgical removal is feasible.

Malignant tumours

Pathology

Primary tumours arise from glial cells (hence glioma) with most originating from astrocytes. There is a spectrum of malignancy amongst astrocytomas (graded

I–IV). Grade I is very slow growing with patients surviving many years with little deficit as the brain has time to adapt and deform as the tumour increases in size. At the other extreme is **glioblastoma multiforme** (grade IV) which are rapidly growing with patients rarely surviving more than 1 year. The tumour invades surrounding tissue and may cross the corpus callosum to the contralateral hemisphere. Gliomas rarely metastasize.

Brain metastases from distant tumours are common, particularly from bronchus, breast and kidney. In some patients, the location of the primary tumour remains unknown. Lymphomas may also affect the CNS, including the spinal cord. This is particularly common in AIDS (see p. 341).

Clinical presentation

The most common presentation is an insidious progressive neurological deficit over weeks or months. Some patients present with fits (focal or generalised). Later symptoms and signs of raised intracranial pressure supervene with headache, vomiting and somnolence. When you see a person with a focal deficit such as a hemi/monoparesis, hemisensory loss or limb ataxia, your main differential diagnosis will be with a stroke. The main questions to ask are the length of the history and the onset. A stroke happens quickly, then, in most cases, there is some recovery. In tumour, the progression is relentless. Occasionally, bleeding takes place into the tumour with a sudden deterioration in the neurological deficit. In these cases, differentiation from a stroke is difficult.

Investigations

Neuroimaging (either CT or MR) is the key to diagnosis. On plain CT scanning, an irregular, heterogeneous mass may be seen compressing the surrounding brain with a mass effect giving:

- effacement of cerebral sulci
- obliteration of the ipsilateral ventricle
- midline shift
- dilatation of the contralateral ventricle.

Slow growing, grade I, astrocytomas may show small areas of calcification. Rapidly growing tumours often have large areas of surrounding oedema, which appear on a CT scan as very low-density (black) regions. Irregular enhancement is seen after contrast. It may be very difficult to distinguish a solitary metastasis from a primary brain tumour, although metastases are often multiple.

Management

In malignant brain tumours, the treatment is predominantly palliative. Surgical removal is usually not feasible. Lymphomas may temporarily respond to chemotherapy. For palliation of metastatic disease, radiotherapy may be of help. A significant proportion of patients may obtain benefit lasting several weeks to months from high-dose dexamethasone, which reduces the surrounding oedema. Side-effects from the high steroid dose are common, with myopathy, hyperglycaemia and hypokalaemia.

5.4 **Cerebrovascular disease**

Strokes are common and, as a house physician, you will be dealing with one or two new strokes per week.

Learning objective

You should be able to:
- establish the diagnosis and describe the neurological impairment
- advise people on the prognosis for survival and disability
- assess risk factors for stroke
- understand the principles of rehabilitation, including the importance of multidisciplinary teamwork.

Vascular and neuroanatomy

The brain is supplied by four arteries (two carotid and two vertebral). It is important to realise that, although these feed the circle of Willis, sudden occlusion of a major vessel *cannot* be compensated for by collateral flow because the circle is usually incompletely formed. If the reduction in blood flow takes place over several weeks or more, then there can be some compensation.

The circulation should be considered in terms of the **carotid** (anterior) and the **vertebrobasilar** (posterior) circulation. The common carotid bifurcates into the external and internal carotid arteries. The bifurcation is one of the most common sites for atheroma. The main branches of the internal carotid artery (none outside the cranium) are:

- the **ophthalmic artery**, which is important because platelet emboli originating in the carotid bifurcation cause **amaurosis fugax** (see Table 42)
- the **middle cerebral artery**, which supplies most of the parietal, temporal and some of the lateral surface of the frontal lobe: occlusion causes massive damage, i.e. hemiparesis (arm > leg), dysphasia (left hemisphere), neglect (right hemisphere) and hemianopia
- the **anterior cerebral artery**, which supplies the anterior pole of the frontal lobe and the medial surface: occlusion causes hemiparesis (leg > arm), dysphasia (left hemisphere), urinary incontinence and personality changes
- the arteries on either side are joined by the **anterior communicating artery**, which is one of the sites for berry aneurysm (see Subarachnoid haemorrhage below)

- The **posterior communicating artery** is another major site for a berry aneurysm. Expansion of this causes a painful third nerve palsy with a large pupil owing to compression of the parasympathetic fibres running on the outside of the nerve. Berry aneurysms cause approximately one-third of third nerve palsies (the other major cause being diabetes mellitus). The artery joins the posterior cerebral artery.

The vertebrobasilar system is formed by the two vertebral arteries (one may be rudimentary or absent) joining to form the basilar artery. The vertebrobasilar system supplies the brainstem and midbrain. After giving off several branches, including the **posterior inferior cerebellar artery** (PICA; see Lateral medullary syndrome, p. 197), it terminates in the posterior cerebral artery, which supplies the occipital lobe. This is predominantly concerned with vision. Unilateral damage causes a hemianopia, in which the macula may be spared (see Table 50) and bilateral damage can result in cortical blindness.

Stroke

Stroke is the preferred term rather than cerebrovascular accident or CVA. You should take care in diagnosing and describing a stroke. In describing the stroke, you should refer to the side of the brain affected. Thus a left stroke would describe a left cerebral hemisphere infarct leading to a right hemiparesis and dysphasia. Ask the patient (or a witness) the following questions.

How quickly did it happen? Sudden onset is classically seen in an embolic stroke, but thrombotic occlusion or haemorrhage may progress over a few hours. A longer time course (> 24 hours) would be against the diagnosis of stroke.

Are there focal neurological symptoms or signs? Many strokes lead to impaired consciousness, but lack of focal signs is against the diagnosis.

Have the symptoms persisted for longer than 24 hours? By definition *complete* recovery within 24 hours is diagnostic of a **transient ischaemic attack** (TIA) and is not a stroke.

Epidemiology

Cerebrovascular disease is the third most common cause of death in the UK. It consumes approximately 6% of the NHS budget mainly in long-term care/nursing costs. The incidence rises exponentially with age. In an average health district population of 250 000, the incidence is 200–300 new strokes each year with a prevalence of 600–700 people disabled by stroke.

Pathology

Strokes can be divided into two main pathophysiological types:

- **infarction** is caused by sudden occlusion of an artery either by thrombosis or embolus from a distant source; damage to the neurones occurs as a result of ischaemia with subsequent disruption of function and death
- **haemorrhage** is caused by bleeding, often originating from penetrating vessels deep within the brain substance. Damage occurs as the blood tracks between neurones and fibres causing pressure and occlusion of supplying and draining vessels. Small aneurysms (**Charcot–Bouchard**) associated with hypertension are one source of this bleeding. Another is from vessels weakened by amyloid deposition, which is associated with age.

It is useful to know the relative frequencies of the different pathologies. In every 100 strokes, approximately 80 will be caused by infarction secondary to thromboembolism. It is now thought that an embolus is the most common cause rather than thrombosis in situ, because atheroma is relatively uncommon in the intracerebral vessels. The common sources of emboli are shown in Figure 37.

Clinical presentation

A stroke can affect any part of the brain and may be very small or very large. There is a huge number of possible permutations of symptoms and signs. You do not need to know all of these; what you must be able to do is assess a patient and document accurately the neurological impairment at the time you see them — the picture will change over time.

Strokes may be silent, that is no symptoms were noticed yet on a CT or MR scan there is evidence of old damage. In these patients, close questioning may elicit an 'odd' episode.

Once you have diagnosed that the patient has had a stroke, the next question is what is the nature of the stroke? As stated above, infarction is the commonest pathology. It is *not* possible to differentiate reliably at the bedside between haemorrhage and infarction; a CT or MR scan is needed.

The third stage is to decide on the site and extent of the stroke. Many patients present with a hemiparesis, but remember that the path of the pyramidal tract starts in the precentral gyrus then runs down through the cerebral peduncles and the midbrain, before decussating low down in the brainstem. Consequently, unilateral weakness tells very little about the site of the stroke and you need to ask about other symptoms and seek out other signs. The main divisions in stroke are between:

- cerebral hemisphere
- lacunar
- brainstem.

The location of major functions are shown in Figure 38. Dysphasia, dyspraxia and neglect have been described and can be used to locate the site of a stroke. For anterior circulation (carotid) ischaemia, it is useful to think of **total anterior circulation infarcts** (TACI) and **partial anterior circulation infarcts** (PACI).

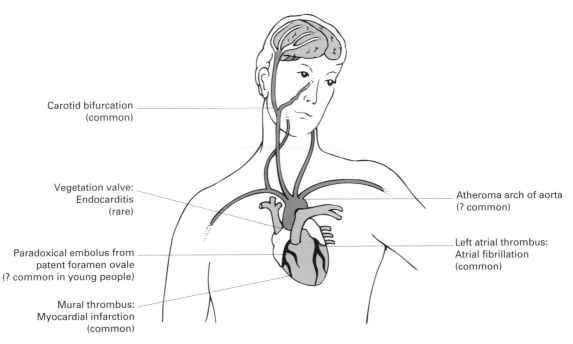

Carotid bifurcation
(common)

Vegetation valve:
Endocarditis
(rare)

Paradoxical embolus from
patent foramen ovale
(? common in young people)

Mural thrombus:
Myocardial infarction
(common)

Atheroma arch of aorta
(? common)

Left atrial thrombus:
Atrial fibrillation
(common)

Fig. 37
Possible sources of emboli to the brain.

TACI. A TACI is a huge stroke, either caused by occlusion of the internal carotid or the middle cerebral artery on one side. Virtually all of one hemisphere is damaged, so the picture is:

- drowsiness/unconsciousness
- complete hemiparesis
- hemisensory loss
- dysphasia (left) or neglect (right)
- incontinence
- hemianopia and forced deviation of the eyes towards the side of the lesion.

In summary, this stroke causes gross brain damage and a poor prospect for survival or good recovery.

PACI. A PACI is a smaller event, with a wedge-shaped infarct caused by blockage of one of the small arteries supplying the cerebral hemispheres. The symptoms and signs will vary according to where the lesion is but may simply be, for example, an expressive dysphasia. Patients have a good probability of recovery, but have a significant risk of a further stroke.

Lacunar strokes. These are small discrete infarcts (occlusion of small penetrating arteries) around the internal capsule, thalamus and basal ganglia. They are often multiple. Patients present with one of the following:

- isolated hemiparesis
- hemisensory loss
- hemiparesis with limb ataxia (clumsy).

Prognosis for survival and recovery is very good. There is a strong association with hypertension.

Posterior circulation (vertebrobasilar) infarction (POCI). Patients present with symptoms and signs of brainstem damage. Features include:

- severe truncal ataxia (midline vermis lesion)
- limb clumsiness (signs ipsilateral to cerebellar hemisphere damage)
- gaze palsies
  — *conjugate* (involuntary, '*forced*', parallel deviation of the eyes away from the site of the lesion)
  — *dysconjugate* (where the eyes do not act together)
- respiratory rhythm disturbance
- hemiparesis (contralateral).

Mortality is high because of damage to vital centres, but, if the patient survives, prospects for functional recovery are good with a low probability of recurrence.

Lateral medullary syndrome. This is caused by an infarction in the territory of the posterior inferior cerebellar artery. Classical symptoms are ipsilateral facial paraesthesia or pain (spinal nucleus of fifth nerve), severe vertigo and vomiting, dysphagia, dysphonia, ataxia and contralateral limb sensory impairment. On examination, a Horner's syndrome may be present, with ipsilateral facial loss of pain and temperature and contralateral limb spinothalamic sensory impairment.

Investigations

In casualty, one of the main decisions is choosing the investigations that will make a difference to the immediate management. These vary according to the presentation and your assessment of the patient. Table 48 (p. 199) summarises the important ones to consider both as urgent and non-urgent. In general, patients who are very unlikely to survive (e.g. deeply unconsciousness: Glasgow coma scale 3) should not be subjected to investigations.

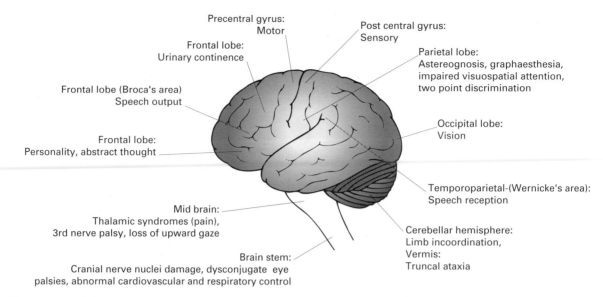

Precentral gyrus:
Motor

Post central gyrus:
Sensory

Frontal lobe:
Urinary continence

Parietal lobe:
Astereognosis, graphaesthesia,
impaired visuospatial attention,
two point discrimination

Frontal lobe (Broca's area)
Speech output

Occipital lobe:
Vision

Frontal lobe:
Personality, abstract thought

Temporoparietal-(Wernicke's area):
Speech reception

Mid brain:
Thalamic syndromes (pain),
3rd nerve palsy, loss of upward gaze

Cerebellar hemisphere:
Limb incoordination,
Vermis:
Truncal ataxia

Brain stem:
Cranial nerve nuclei damage, dysconjugate eye
palsies, abnormal cardiovascular and respiratory control

Fig. 38
Anatomical localisation of important brain functions.

Prognosis

It is important that you are aware of the prognosis following a stroke in terms of survival, recovery and risks of further events, so that you can advise patients and carers appropriately. Almost half of all patients who are admitted will die in hospital. Early deaths result from compression/damage to major structures, for example the respiratory centre in the brainstem. Subsequent brain swelling leads to further deterioration, with coning of the hemispheres into the posterior fossa and the brainstem through the foramen magnum. Unlike myocardial infarction, those stroke patients who die do so within a few days rather than the first few minutes.

Deaths in the next few weeks are often caused by pulmonary emboli or pneumonia. Late deaths are commonly caused by further stroke or myocardial ischaemia.

On admission, the single most unfavourable prognostic sign is a reduced conscious level. If the patient has a Glasgow Coma scale of 3 (see Table 47) then the chances of survival and good recovery are very slim. Other bad prognostic signs are complete hemiparesis, urinary incontinence and forced deviation of the eyes.

Of the 50% who survive, half will make a very good recovery. The remainder will be left with significant disability and handicap. In relation to stroke type:

- TACI: poor prognosis (survival or disability)
- PACI: recover well, but have a high chance of recurrence
- LACI: do reasonably well and have a low risk of recurrence
- POCI: high mortality but may do well if they survive.

Management

The management of stroke patients can be divided into early and late phases.

Early stages

In the immediate aftermath of a stroke, there is no direct treatment that will affect outcome. Management is directed at preventing complications. Dysphagia is common and carries a risk of aspiration pneumonia. In almost all patients, the problem is transient and can be dealt with by giving nothing by mouth and providing hydration by some other means (i.v., s.c. or n.g.) until swallowing recovers. Patients are at risk of deep vein thrombosis and pulmonary emboli. Heparin therapy may be needed, but care should be taken beforehand to exclude haemorrhage as a cause of the stroke. Pressure sores may develop, unless the patient is assessed as being at risk and correctly nursed.

High blood pressure may be noted in the first few hours following a stroke. This should not be treated unless **hypertensive encephalopathy** is diagnosed (very rare, see p. 44). Otherwise lowering blood pressure is more likely to do harm as **autoregulation** of cerebral bloodflow is lost.

In a insulin-dependent diabetic patient, any major event may precipitate ketoacidosis. This should be managed in the standard way, avoiding hypoglycaemia.

Late stages

The late management of stroke is based on active rehabilitation and reducing the risk of further events. Of the survivors, approximately one quarter will make a rapid recovery and one quarter will make a very poor recovery requiring long-term care. The remainder (half) benefit from referral to a specialist stroke rehabilitation service. This is associated with:

- lower death rate
- shorter hospital stay
- less disability on discharge
- greater chance of going home.

Table 48 Main investigations in stroke, with indications for urgency

Investigation	When to perform	Reason
Blood sugar (BM stix)	All patients, on admission	Hypoglycaemia can cause focal signs; missing it can cause irreversible damage
Chest radiograph	Some patients, on admission	Semiconscious, may have or at risk of aspiration pneumonia
	All patients, non-urgent	Exclude neoplasia
Full blood count	All patients, non-urgent	To exclude erythrocytosis, thrombocythaemia
Urea and electrolytes	Some patients on admission	May be or at serious risk of water depletion; if electrolyte disturbance suspected
	All patients, non-urgent	To exclude renal impairment and to help to manage fluids
CT brain scan	Some patients on admission	1. Those on anticoagulants 2. Suspected **cerebellar haematoma**: only indication for surgical intervention 3. Suspicion of abscess, meningitis or subarachnoid haemorrhage
	Most patients within 7 days	1. Considering anticoagulants, aspirin 2. Still uncertain of diagnosis 3. Determine nature of stroke
ESR	On admission	If suspect temporal arteritis
	Non-urgent	To exclude vasculitis
Electrocardiogram	Some patients, on admission,	If suspect recent myocardial infarction
	All patients, non-urgent	For rhythm, LVH, old infarction
Duplex colour flow Doppler studies of carotid artery	Non-urgent	Candidate for carotid endarterectomy
Echocardiography	Non-urgent	Suspicion of a cardiac source of emboli (e.g. valve lesions, replacements)
Other tests, e.g. blood culture	Some patients, on admission	If suspected septicaemia/meningitis/endocarditis
Other tests: cholesterol, TPHA. RF, ANF, etc	Some patients, non-urgent	1. Young, strong family history of vascular disease 2. Suspected neurosyphilis 3. Suspected vasculitis

Most recovery will take place in the first few months; by about 6 months the patient may have *plateaued*. Patients with significant *right* (non-dominant) hemisphere damage tend to have a worse prognosis. However, most patients will walk again, possibly using aids, though many of these will be severely restricted (disability and handicap). Recovery of hand function is often poor, particularly if there is no movement at all by 7 days. Speech can go on improving for more than a year.

Prevention

In patients who have made a good or reasonable recovery, the risk of further stroke should be assessed. For the UK, the 'Health of the Nation' has set the target of a reduction in the death rate from stroke of **40%** by the year 2000 in both those under 65 years and those 65–74 years. What can be done to achieve this? Since the turn of the century, the incidence of both cerebral haemorrhage and infarction has been declining. This *predated* any medical advances, for example antihypertensives, but the continuing decline *may* be influenced by medical intervention.

For the decline in stroke incidence to continue, the **target population** and the major factors causing

stroke need to be known, together with any means whereby these can be altered. Schemes can be implemented to reduce stroke by targeting either *whole populations* or *individuals*. The approach can be further refined by aiming at **primary** prevention for the person who has had no previous episodes (including TIAs) and **secondary** prevention for the person who has had an event.

A key concept in prevention is the *risk* of something happening. This can be divided into:

- **absolute** risk: applies to an individual without any external reference, e.g. a 70-year-old man has a 12% absolute stroke risk over 10 years (1 in 8 chance).
- **relative** risk refers to the chances of an event occurring relative to something else, e.g. in a woman taking the oral contraceptive pill, the *relative* risk of stroke is increased several fold, but the *absolute* risk remains extremely small.

In relation to stroke and specific treatments:

- if a person has a TIA or stroke, the absolute risk of a future stroke is approximately 8%/year

- a person following a stroke also has an *absolute* risk of 8%/year of having a myocardial infarction; this is the most common cause of death
- the biggest risk factor is hypertension: this accounts for at least half of all strokes. The ideal blood pressure is < 150/90
- carotid disease is an important risk factor (emboli); if a patient has had a TIA and has > 70% stenosis on the relevant side, then a carotid endarterectomy is beneficial (*secondary* prevention).
- aspirin (low dose) is beneficial in *secondary* prevention; it reduces the risk of a stroke by 30% and vascular death by 15% (*relative* reduction)
- in a person with atrial fibrillation, particularly with valvular heart disease, *anticoagulation* will reduce the relative risk of a stroke by two-thirds (the change in absolute risk, if the person had a stroke/TIA, is from 12%/year to 4%/year)
- treating elderly hypertensive people (up to the age of 80 years), because of their high *absolute* risk, is more beneficial than in younger people (more strokes prevented).

Subarachnoid haemorrhage

The pathophysiology and presentation of subarachnoid haemorrhage (SAH) are different to those of stroke. Most are caused by bleeding from **berry aneurysms** around the circle of Willis. These classically occur at the bifurcations, commonly at the origins of the middle cerebral, anterior cerebral and the anterior and posterior communicating arteries. SAH occurs in young people, but the risk increases with age. There is also an association with polycystic kidneys. Most aneurysms are in the anterior circulation (75%) and a small proportion are multiple (20%). A minority of SAH (10%) is caused by bleeding from an arteriovenous malformation. In some patients (10%) a site is never identified.

Clinical presentation

The classical presentation of SAH is with a severe headache. The person may say that they thought that 'someone had hit them on the head with a hammer'. They may remember a severe headache a few days/weeks earlier (**herald bleed**). There is a very high risk (20–40%) of rebleeding within the first 3 weeks. If bleeding extends into the brain, there may be focal signs, rapid loss of consciousness and death. An aneurysm on the posterior communicating artery may cause a third nerve palsy. Blood in the CSF causes meningeal irritation (neck stiffness, headache, photophobia). Another problem is vascular spasm, which particularly affects the artery where the aneurysm is situated. Large bleeds promote spasm which, in turn, may cause widespread brain infarction.

Investigations

Because of the high mortality and risk of rebleeding, it is vital that the diagnosis is established early and a referral made to a neurosurgical centre. The investigation of choice is a CT scan to demonstrate the blood within the sub-arachnoid space. If the scan is negative (10% of SAHs) and there is no evidence of raised intracranial pressure, a lumbar puncture should be done. Blood-stained fluid will be obtained and, after 24 hours, xanthochromia develops because of breakdown of haemoglobin. For patients in whom surgery would be considered (< 65 years, not deeply unconscious), angiography should be performed.

Management

All patients should be given **nimodipine** (a calcium antagonist) to reduce the risk of spasm. In those patients fit enough, early surgery to clip accessible aneuryms is advised, given the high risk of early rebleeding. In a patient who deteriorates, you should consider rebleeding, spasm and hydrocephalus. A CT scan can help to distinguish between these.

Prognosis

The mortality from SAH is high, with as many as a third dying within a few hours and a further third dying in the first month.

Arteriovenous malformations

Bleeding is often less pronounced compared with berry aneurysms, with episodes over a number of years producing mild neurological deficits. Epilepsy is common. An enhanced CT scan may be abnormal and an MR scan may be diagnostic, though the definitive investigation is angiography. Surgery or embolisation of feeding vessels is sometimes undertaken but may be technically difficult with a very high risk.

Subdural haematoma

Acute extra and subdural bleeds usually occur as a result of trauma. Chronic subdural haematoma is a problem of elderly people and alcoholics. In the history, there may be a story of a minor head injury. The patient presents with a fluctuating level of consciousness with or without focal signs (e.g. hemiparesis) over several weeks/months. The condition is caused by oozing from damaged subdural veins. Osmotic changes in the haematoma causes it to expand and contract. A CT scan will usually show a characteristic abnormality of a localised rim of hypodensity between the brain and the skull (sometimes bilateral). The patient should be referred to a neurosurgical unit.

5.5 Degenerative conditions

Learning objective

- You should have a framework for describing degenerative conditions of the nervous system and know about examples in each category.

The central and peripheral nervous system is affected by many different degenerative conditions. You will find it useful to divide them into inherited and acquired conditions.

Inherited conditions

Spinocerebellar ataxias

The spinocerebellar ataxias are a complex set of disorders. They range from very rare cerebellar disorders seen in childhood through to **spastic paraparesis** (autosomal dominant) affecting the corticospinal tracts, which usually is diagnosed in middle age.

Friedreich's ataxia

The typical disorder is Friedreich's ataxia, which is inherited as an autosomal recessive. In this, three systems are affected in the CNS:

- cerebellum
- spinocerebellar tracts
- corticospinal tracts.

In addition, there is degeneration in the axons of the dorsal root ganglia, resulting in loss of joint position sense (posterior columns) and a sensory neuropathy.

Patients usually present in late childhood/early adulthood with nystagmus, ataxia, dysarthria, spastic paraparesis and extensor plantars with *absent* reflexes. Other features include a cardiomyopathy, diabetes mellitus and low intelligence. Life expectancy is reduced, with death from cardiac failure/arrhythmias around the fourth decade. **Forme frustes** are seen, that is affected family members may be only slightly affected, e.g. 'funny' walks or being bad at games.

Huntington's chorea

Huntington's chorea is a rare autosomally dominant inherited condition. It typically presents in the fifth or sixth decade of life with a progressive basal ganglia movement disorder (chorea, parkinsonism) and dementia. Because of the late onset, there are major family implications as the patient has usually had children. Specialist counselling services are available and, as with most inherited conditions, gene probes are now providing information for affected families, with the possibility of diagnosis prior to the onset of symptoms and of carrier states in autosomal recessive conditions.

Wilson's disease

Wilson's disease arises as a disorder of copper metabolism inherited as an autosomal recessive (see p. 129). Heterozygotes have no clinical features. In the CNS, copper deposition in the basal ganglia and elsewhere cause dyskinesias (chorea, athetosis) and parkinsonism together with a progressive dementia. In the eye, copper deposition at the margin of the cornea causes a **Kayser–Fleischer** ring best seen on slit lamp examination. Onset is often insidious. The condition needs to be diagnosed early and treated with **D-penicillamine** for any chance of remission.

Benign essential tremor

This is seen either as a sporadic disorder or running in families (50% of cases) with an autosomal dominant inheritance. It may present at any time in adult life and worsens over the years. It is a positional tremor, often mild and worsened by emotion. The tremor is helped by alcohol and responds to **propranolol.**

Acquired degenerative disorders

Parkinson's disease

Learning objectives

You should:
- know the difference between Parkinson's disease and parkinsonism
- be able to describe the features of Parkinson's disease
- understand the principles of its management.

Aetiology

The most important concept you need to understand is that **Parkinson's disease** refers to degeneration of the neurones of the substantia nigra of unknown aetiology which causes progressive akinesia, rigidity and a tremor, whereas **parkinsonism** refers to the same symptoms and signs, but occurring secondary to some other condition. The most common causes of parkinsonism are anti-dopaminergic drugs (metoclopropamide, neuroleptics) and cerebrovascular disease (see Vascular dementia, p. 204). Other rare causes include carbon monoxide poisoning, exposure to a 'designer' drug MTPP and, with other signs, Huntington's chorea and Wilson's disease.

Epidemiology and pathophysiology

The prevalence of Parkinson's disease increases with age, affecting around 1 in 200 people over the age of 65 years. The aetiology is not clear but may involve exposure to some environmental toxin. The symptoms start to appear after the loss of at least 80% of the neurones of the substantia nigra, which show depigmentation. These dopaminergic neurones project to the basal ganglia where other neurotransmitter abnormalities and receptor changes are found. Microscopically, **Lewy bodies** are found and the more widespread and dense the distribution of these, the greater the cognitive impairment (see below).

Clinical features

You need to consider the following:

- tremor
- bradykinesia
- rigidity (cogwheel/lead pipe)
- flexed posture.

Symptoms commonly start in the sixth decade of life, but there is a wide variation. Even with treatment, the life expectancy is reduced, with the disease taking approximately 10 years to run its course. The symptoms and signs are often asymmetrical. You will find that diagnosing Parkinson's disease in the early stages is difficult. The symptoms are vague, and signs minimal.

Tremor. Initially, the patient may complain only of *tremor*. This is coarse (4–6 Hz) and starts in the thumb and fingers; as the disease progresses it may worsen to affect the hand, arm and trunk. It disappears during complete relaxation/sleep and is made worse by holding a posture and by anxiety.

Bradykinesia and rigidity. Reduction in movement may be noticed by people close to the patient. Gradually, there is a slowness and difficulty in initiating and changing any voluntary movement. Accompanying the bradykinesia is an increase in tone. This rigidity is present throughout passive movement of a limb and is described as **lead pipe** (cf. the 'clasp knife' increase in tone seen in pyramidal tract disorders). The superimposition of the tremor on the hypertonia leads to **cogwheel rigidity.**

Posture. Observing the patient you will notice a **flexed posture** with a shuffling gait (**festinant**) and loss of arm swing. Falls are frequent because of loss of postural control. Other features are loss of facial expression, dysphagia and dribbling of saliva. The voice is reduced in amplitude (**dysphonia**) with little intonation and a tendency to peter out. As the disease progresses, the dopamine transmission starts to become inconsistent, with sudden freezing of movement (**on–off phenomena**), gross difficulty in starting movement and stopping walking.

Other symptoms. Parkinson's disease is also associated with marked cognitive slowness and impairment. In some of these people, *Lewy bodies*, which are usually confined to damaged neurones in the basal ganglia, are found much more widely in the cerebral cortex (**Lewy body dementia**). Alzheimer's disease is also more common in patients with Parkinson's disease.

Overall management

Your role in the management of Parkinson's disease involves much more than simply prescribing drugs. One important aspect is counselling patients and their families/carers about the effects of a progressive neurological condition leading to a premature death. You must recognised that anxiety and depression go with this, which may be amenable to therapy. Other disciplines may help: physiotherapy with mobility, occupational therapy with activities of daily living, speech therapy with communication and swallowing and social work with financial worries and social support.

Drug treatment

The main defect is failing dopamine transmission in the basal ganglia. Therapy is aimed at preserving transmission for as long as possible. Dopamine cannot cross the blood–brain barrier so the precursor **L-dopa** is used, which is then converted to dopamine within the substantia nigra. An alternative approach is to use a direct dopamine agonist like **bromocriptine.**

For many years, prior to the introduction of L-dopa, anticholinergic drugs such as **benztropine** were used. Their main action is on tremor rather than bradykinesia and rigidity. They are often used in patients with parkinsonism secondary to neuroleptic drugs, in whom dopamine receptor stimulation must be avoided to prevent exacerbating the mental disturbance.

The main aims of currently available therapy are:

- to preserve independence for as long as possible
- to achieve smooth duration of effect
- to create minimum side-effects.

Achievement of these is dependent on tailoring therapy to individual patients and involving them in decision making. As the disease progresses, a combination of treatments is often employed, but, like epilepsy, therapy should be kept simple.

Various phenomena may be observed with disease progression:

- *peak dose effect:* choreiform movements are observed approximately 30 minutes after taking L-dopa and result from excessive stimulation of dopamine receptors
- *on–off phenomena* are caused by fluctuations in dopamine concentrations within the basal ganglia
- *end of dose effect* is because of the effect of L-dopa wearing off prior to the next dose being due.

The main approach to limiting these effects is to employ small frequent doses of L-dopa; this reduces the peaks and troughs found with larger, less-frequent doses. The different modes of action of the drugs used and the common side-effects are summarised in Table 49.

Dementias

Dementia is a chronic failure of cognitive function. It must be differentiated from an acute or sub-acute confusional state, though it predisposes to the development of these.

Learning objectives

You should:

- know the features of Alzheimer's and multi-infarct dementia and understand how these conditions differ
- understand the principles of the management of dementia and the value of multidisciplinary teamwork.

Epidemiology

The prevalence of dementia increases rapidly with advancing age; 20% of those aged 85 years have at least a mild form; 5% are severely affected. The vast majority of these result from Alzheimer's disease. This is predominantly seen in old people, but it can occur before the age of 65 years.

The other major cause of dementia is cerebrovascular disease, but this is less common than Alzheimer's disease. The prevalence of vascular dementia increases exponentially with age and is related to the known risk factors for vascular disease, such as hypertension.

In clinical practice, you will find it useful to keep in mind the relative frequencies of the different causes of dementia (see Fig. 39).

Alzheimer's disease

Pathophysiology

The histological hallmarks of Alzheimer's disease are **neuronal plaques** and **neurofibrillary tangles**, with widespread cortical loss of neurones. Some of these features are found in the brains of elderly people without dementia, but not to the same extent.

Within the cortex and the subcortical connections/projections, there are abnormalities in most transmitter systems, but a deficit in acetylcholine transmission is most closely linked to clinical features. Genetic factors are important; the dementia is inherited as an autosomal dominant in a small number of families. Furthermore, patients with Down's syndrome have a very similar dementia, but it develops much earlier. Most research is now focused on abnormal expression of β-amyloid protein.

Clinical presentation

Typically, patients present with an insidious decline. There is increasing disruption of cortical function with fragmentation of language, disorientation in time, difficulty with intellectual tasks such as money matters, personality changes including disinhibition, wandering and fragmentation of language. The memory loss is marked with failure to retain or recall important information. Over a period of months and years, cortical function becomes progressively disrupted until the patient is aphasic, incontinent (in the early stages urination/defaecation may occur inappropriately because of disinhibition), immobile and fails to recognise even close relatives. Weight loss can be marked.

Diagnosis. When faced with a patient with possible Alzheimer's disease you must understand two things:

- *There is no diagnostic test.* A CT scan may show 'cerebral atrophy', but it does so in many normal elderly people. The diagnosis is based mainly on the clinical history outlined above with use of psychological tests in some patients. There are no focal neurological signs.
- *It is difficult to differentiate between Alzheimer's disease and vascular dementia.* Important features to look for in the latter are hypertension, previous strokes (or CT scan evidence), stepwise deterioration with some improvement/plateau after each event and focal neurological signs.

Management

Effective treatments for Alzheimer's disease are starting to appear. Some anticholinesterases such as donepezil seem to produce an improvement in cortical function by improving the deficit in acetylcholine transmission in patients with mild to moderate disease. However, managing patients involves much more than offering specific treatment. The key is working as part of a multidisciplinary team looking at all aspects of support, including that of the carer. Many house-officers find it difficult to find their own role within this team. Your main responsibilities are:

- the diagnosis and management of any medical problems: acute illness (e.g. infection, myocardial infarction) and its treatment can cause an **acute on chronic confusional state.** Diagnosis of an acute illness may be difficult because of the lack of a clear history from a demented patient, but correct and

Table 49 Major drugs used in Parkinson's disease, mode of action and side-effects

Drug	Action	Side-effects	Notes
L-Dopa	Indirect agonist: supports dopamine transmission	Postural hypotension, nausea, confusion High doses: chorea (peak dose effect)	Need a peripheral decarboxylase inhibitor: prevents peripheral breakdown Short half life: give frequent doses (> 4/day)
Bromocriptine, pergolide	Dopamine agonist	Side-effects +++: nausea, postural hypotension, confusion, psychosis	Given 3 times/day
Apomorphine	Dopamine agonist	Nausea, postural hypotension	High efficacy, used in end-stage disease; has to be given subcutaneously
Selegiline	Monoamine oxidase type B inhibitor		Give once a day; well tolerated; mild antiparkinsonian and mood-uplifting effect; need to reduce l-dopa dosage (blocks metabolism)
Benztropine	Cholinergic antagonist	Blurred vision, urinary retention, dry mouth, confusion	Main effect is on tremor; not very effective

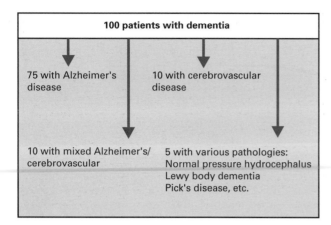

100 patients with dementia

75 with Alzheimer's disease

10 with cerebrovascular disease

10 with mixed Alzheimer's/ cerebrovascular

5 with various pathologies:
Normal pressure hydrocephalus
Lewy body dementia
Pick's disease, etc.

Fig. 39
The prevalence of dementia from different pathological causes. Lewy body dementia may account for some cases of apparent Alzheimer's disease and may be a more important cause than indicated here.

prompt treatment may make a large difference in functional outcome
- the judicious use of drugs such as neuroleptics (promazine, thioridazine) in patients who are very agitated, aggressive or have a gross disturbance of sleep pattern
- adopting a behavioural approach to management: caring for patients in a familiar environment with familiar people using a consistent approach
- coordinating the plans of the different agencies involved after an acute illness so as to ensure smooth discharge
- making time available for talking with the carers.

Prognosis. Alzheimer's disease progresses at different rates, usually with death after several years.

Vascular dementia

Pathophysiology
The mechanisms involved in vascular dementia are different to those of Alzheimer's disease. It can be conceptualised as the summative effects of lots of small strokes causing a stepwise deterioration in overall brain function. Occasionally, though, a single stroke in the deep structures around the basal ganglia can cause a permanent confusional state. In other patients, chronic ischaemia damages the white matter (axonal connections) at the junction with the cerebral hemispheres. (**Biswanger's disease**).

Clinical presentation
Typically, the patient will have a history of several strokes: some minor and some major. The progression is in steps, with acute deterioration caused by the stroke being followed by a period of partial recovery and a new (lower) functional plateau. There is commonly a history of hypertension or other vascular risk factors such as atrial fibrillation or diabetes.

On examination, as well as impaired cognition, there will be focal signs, for example brisk reflexes and an upgoing plantar response.

Investigations. The investigation of vascular dementia is similar to that of stroke (see Table 51). A CT scan may show multiple areas of infarction. An ECG may confirm the presence of atrial fibrillation.

Management
The general management of vascular dementia is the same as that for Alzhemier's disease. Although there is no firm evidence that it influences the course of the disease, the consensus is that the known vascular risk factors should be treated and the patient prescribed aspirin.

Motor neurone disease

Learning objectives

You should:
- know the features of motor neurone disease
- understand the importance of excluding other (potentially treatable) causes of the patient's problem.

Epidemiology

Motor neurone disease (amyotrophic lateral sclerosis) affects males much more than females and commonly presents in middle age, but it occurs over a wide age range.

Clinical presentation

The diagnosis should be considered in any patient with progressive motor symptoms and signs. An important aspect is to exclude other, potentially treatable problems, such as cervical spondylosis. *Any* sensory signs rule out the diagnosis of motor neurone disease.

The disease affects both upper and lower motor neurones, so the symptoms and signs depend on the relative involvement of different neuronal groups. Segments C8 and T1 may be affected with weakness, wasting and fasiculation of the small muscles of the hand (particularly 1st dorsal interossei). Another pattern is involvement of the pyramidal tract neurones innervating the lower limbs, causing weakness, spasticity and hyper-reflexia. As the disease progesses, a mixture of signs are seen, e.g. arreflexia in the lower limb with extensor plantar responses. Impact on the bulbar musculature is frequently severe, with dysphagia, aspiration and dysarthria. The oculomotor neurones are usually spared as are those controlling bladder and bowel function.

Investigations

Diagnosis is clinical, supported by electrophysiological studies. EMG will show a sub-acute denervation pattern. Nerve conduction studies show only minimal slowing.

Management

As with dementia, there is no effective treatment and the principles of management, including multidisciplinary teamwork, are similar. Unlike dementia, the patient is not cognitively impaired, even though communication may be difficult. A major challenge is to give support through the illness. You must always bear in mind the possibility of depression, which is amenable to treatment. Management often involves speech and language therapists, physiotherapists, occupational therapists, social workers and nurses, as well as referral to specialist clinics such as for seating/wheelchairs.

Prognosis

As with many degenerative conditions, the time course can vary, but death usually occurs within 1–2 years.

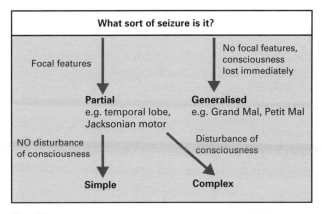

Fig. 40
Categorisation of epilepsy. Partial fits may generalise, causing a grand mal seizure.

5.6 Epilepsy

Learning objectives

You should
- understand how to make a diagnosis of epilepsy
- know how to classify seizures
- know the appropriate investigations to request and how to interpret these
- to be able to outline a management plan, including the advantages and disadvantages of the drug options, taking into account lifestyle and occupation.

A fit (seizure) is a symptom. It may be the first symptom of a brain tumour, cerebrovascular disease or encephalitis. Sometimes it is a manifestation of a metabolic disturbance or a reduced seizure threshold (e.g. caused by alcohol or malaria prophylaxis with chloroquine). Epilepsy is a continuing liability to seizures.

Epidemiology

Seizures are common, with a lifetime probability of approximately 1:20 of having a fit at some time. In adult life, the prevalence of epilepsy increases with age. The prognosis, though, is much better than is generally perceived. On treatment, two-thirds of people with epilepsy become fit free and, eventually, two-thirds do not require any medication.

Diagnosis

You must evaluate the diagnosis of a fit on clinical grounds using the patient's account and, most important of all, the account of a witness. There are two main questions that you should consider:

- is it a fit? Differentiation from other causes of blackouts and funny turns (p. 183)
- what type of fit is it? Seizures are classified into two large categories: *generalised* and *partial* (Fig. 40).

Examples of generalised fits are **grand mal** and **petit mal** (predominantly in childhood). In a grand mal seizure, there is no aura, consciousness is lost from the outset and tonic clonic movements are observed for a short time. An important point is that if someone has *bilateral* shaking and is fully conscious then it is *not* epilepsy. Tongue biting and urinary incontinence may be observed. Following the fit, in the **post-ictal** stage, the patient is drowsy.

In partial epilepsy, there is a focus which discharges periodically. Consequently, there are focal symptoms or signs depending on the location of the focus. In the temporal lobe, this may manifest as an aura (e.g. an odd feeling starting in the stomach, washing over the patient), new surroundings being intensely familiar (déja vu), failure to recognise familiar surroundings (jamais vu), or odd smells can be experienced (burning rubber). If the focus is in another part of the brain, there may be shaking of a limb (Jacksonian epilepsy).

Partial epilepsy can be divided into **simple partial epilepsy** with no disturbance of consciousness at any stage and **complex partial epilepsy** where consciousness is disturbed.

Many patients with epilepsy are referred to casualty after a seizure. In your assessment, you should be considering whether the patient is a known epileptic and if this represents a typical event or whether it is a manifestation of another disease process.

A careful examination should be carried out looking for focal signs and meningism. Fits can cause a fever and abnormalities in the CSF (raised white cells) so, at times, the picture can be confusing.

Status epilepticus

Status epilepticus is defined as a series of fits without regaining consciousness. Continued epileptic activity leads to exhaustion and cerebral damage, so you must take urgent action. The mortality is 10–30%. Intravenous (or rectal) diazepam and a loading dose of phenytoin are used. If the seizures continue, senior colleagues must be consulted.

Investigations

The diagnosis of epilepsy is based on the history *not* on EEG findings (see p. 188). The use of an EEG (Table 45) is both in identifying a focus and in showing the characteristic abnormalities of certain types of epilepsy.

A CT scan looking for a structural brain lesion is indicated in anyone either with focal signs on examination or partial epilepsy. It is *no* use in diagnosing epilepsy. A CT scan is indicated in late onset (>60 years) epilepsy, but you should note that most cases are *not* caused by a tumour but by a cerebrovascular disease.

Management

You must manage the patient in the context of their life. Does the diagnosis of epilepsy have major consequences for employment or recreational activities such as driving a car? The most common difficulty is with driving. Patients must let the DVLC and their insurance company know about *any* change in their health status which may affect their ability to drive. Your obligation is to inform patients of this requirement and to advise any driver who regard as a danger to themselves or other road users not to drive (and note your advice in the medical records).

For a person with epilepsy who holds a *standard* driving licence, they cannot drive until seizure-free for 1 year, on *or* off treatment. After this time, they can resume driving providing there is 'no ongoing liability to have seizures', e.g. an astrocytoma. An exception to this regulation is a person who only has nocturnal (during sleep) seizures. They can drive even though they are still having fits, providing the pattern has been established for 3 years. The law for those holding an LGV or a PSV licence is more stringent. The person can only drive if free from seizures for 10 years, on no antiepileptic drugs for 10 years and has been examined by a specialist.

Drug treatment

When talking to patients about their future, one important point is that 80% (less with partial epilepsy) will obtain acceptable control by use of a single drug. Recommended drugs are:

- sodium valproate for generalised epilepsy (carbamazepine and phenytoin are equally effective, but have greater toxicity)
- sodium valproate and carbamazepine for partial epilepsy (phenytoin effective but toxic).

Monitoring of drugs. Plasma level monitoring of drugs is generally not used apart from checking on compliance in patients whose seizures are not controlled. When starting, the dose is increased gradually until either toxic effects supervene or seizure control is obtained. The only exception to this approach is for phenytoin (see below).

Continuing therapy. Once seizure control is obtained, an important question is when to stop treatment? In 60% of adults who have had no fits for 2 years, it is usually possible to withdraw drugs over 2–3 months without a recurrence. However, there are other considerations, such as occupation and driving.

Specific drugs.

Sodium valproate. Used in generalised or partial seizures. It acts through increasing GABA activity (inhibitory). Its biological half-life (i.e. prevention of seizures) is longer than its physical half-life. Major side-effects in adults are weight gain (appetite stimulant), hair thinning, and tremor (high doses).

Carbamazepine. You must increase the dose of carbamazepine gradually to allow it to induce its own metabolism. Major side-effects are dizziness, nausea, headache, drowsiness, and a rash (5–10%). Toxic effects include hyponatraemia. As an enzyme inducer, carbamazepine reduces the efficacy of phenobarbitone, valproate, lamotrigine, theophylline and warfarin.

Phenytoin. Above a certain level, the metabolism of phenytoin becomes saturated. Consequently, a small increase in dose can cause markedly different changes in plasma levels, dependent on which part of the curve the patient lies (Fig. 41). There is also the potential for dangerous drug interactions, e.g. cimetidine (an enzyme inhibitor). Phenytoin has a long half-life and should be given once per day. Side-effects include gum hypertrophy, hirsutism and facial coarsening. Toxicity includes sedation, ataxia and nystagmus.

Vigabatrin. Vigabatrin is a new drug which inhibits GABA metabolism. It is used in resistant partial seizures. Side-effects are drowsiness, fatigue, irritability, weight gain and psychosis.

Lamotrigine. Lamotrigine inhibits glutaminergic excitation, thereby increasing the seizure threshold.

Gabapentin. Like vigabatrin and sodium valproate, gabapentin acts through the GABA system. It is excreted unchanged in urine and the dose should be reduced in renal impairment. Major problems are somnolence, dizziness and ataxia.

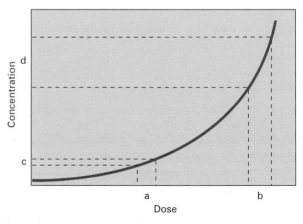

Fig. 41
Relationship between phenytoin dosage and plasma concentration, showing that the same increase in dose (a,b) can produce markedly different changes in plasma concentrations (c,d) dependent on saturation of the metabolic pathway.

Epilepsy and pregnancy

If any of your patients are pregnant or are considering starting a family it is important for them to know about the likely risks. Even without drug therapy, the relative risk of fetal malformation or fetal loss in an epileptic patient is increased by 25%; taking drugs doubles this. Abnormalities occur with *all* the main drugs; most are minor anomalies, such as odd facial appearance.

The main abnormalities are shown in Table 50. The risk increases with number and dosage of antiepileptic drugs used. The principle is to treat with a single drug.

After delivery, most drugs are excreted in breast milk, but concentrations are low, so breast feeding is acceptable.

Seizure control. In pregnancy, drug levels may fall leading to loss of control. This is mainly because of increased clearance by the maternal liver and reduced protein binding because of a fall in albumin concentration.

Contraception. Carbamazepine and phenytoin induce hepatic microsomal enzymes, so the combined or progesterone-only pill are unreliable as contraceptives (a way round this is to increase the dose of the pill). Valproate and the newer drugs, gabapentin, lamotrigine and vigabatrin, do *not* induce enzymes.

Prognosis

A single seizure has a much better prognosis for future recurrence compared with a series of fits. A different 'population' of newly diagnosed epileptics is seen within specialist clinics compared with primary care; most patients have already had a series of fits and the prognosis is one of definite epilepsy.

5.7 Inflammatory conditions

There are a number of conditions affecting the nervous system which have, as a central feature, evidence of a disordered defence/immune mechanism. One example of an acute problem is Guillain–Barré syndrome. An important example of a chronic problem is multiple sclerosis.

Learning objectives

You should:
- recognise Guillain–Barré syndrome in a patient presenting with progressive paralysis
- be able to assess the possibility of multiple sclerosis in a young person with neurological symptoms
- know the principles of management of multiple sclerosis.

Guillain–Barré syndrome

It is important that you consider this diagnosis in any patient with an acute progressive paralysis as survival and recovery depend on appropriate management. The condition occurs at all ages. In at least half, a minor illness ('viral') precedes the onset.

Table 50 Teratogenetic effects of anti-epileptic drugs

Drug	Effect
Carbamazepine	Spina bifida (1%), hypospadias
Sodium valproate	Spina bifida (1.5%), hypospadias and craniofacial and skeletal anomalies
Phenytoin	Congenital heart disease, cleft palate

Pathology

There is intense demyelination of the peripheral nerves. The brunt of the damage is to the most heavily myelinated and longest fibres.

Clinical presentation

The first symptom may be back pain or altered sensation in the feet, followed by progressive, ascending paralysis. Other patterns occur with involvement of the bulbar musculature and, importantly, the respiratory muscles. The natural history is progression over a few weeks to a nadir (it may be faster), then slow recovery as remyelination takes place.

Investigation

If the diagnosis is suspected, urgent nerve conduction studies may confirm the gross slowing consistent with demyelination. CSF examination will show evidence of disordered immune response with a mild pleocytosis in the first week followed by a rise in protein (see Table 44).

Management

When assessing a patient, the main concern is to identify the need for respiratory support by monitoring peak flow rate and arterial blood gases. A rising pCO_2 is an indication for ventilation. Repeated plasmapharesis modifies the disease process, with fewer patients requiring ventilation, and it also improves the outcome.

A major cause of death is the gross autonomic disturbance in patients with complete paralysis, who experience large swings in blood pressure together with dysrhythmias.

Multiple sclerosis

Multiple sclerosis is more common in young people and is very rare after the age of 60 years. It is a disease of temperate climates and, in the UK, increases in frequency from south to north. The risk is associated with a childhood spent within these zones. These clues point to a continuing disordered immune reaction initially triggered by an infection acquired as a child.

Pathology

The pathological process produces plaques of demyelination in the CNS (myelin produced by oligodendrocytes rather than Schwann cells). These plaques are disseminated in time and site but do have a predilection for certain areas, such as the visual pathway and the cervical posterior columns. In the initial demyelination, there is surrounding oedema and reactive changes, with subsequent shrinkage and maturation of the plaque. Hence, the clinical picture is a focal neurological impairment with subsequent (partial) recovery as involution takes place.

Clinical presentation

It is often difficult to make the diagnosis in the early stages. Hallmarks are disturbance of visual acuity and micturition. By the time the disease is established, over 90% will have urinary frequency, urge incontinence, urinary retention, etc. As with motor neurone disease, the pattern of symptoms and signs depends on where the lesions are. Patients may have, for example, cerebellar signs, proproceptive loss, spasticity or weakness.

Factors associated with a poor outcome (disability and survival) are:

- male gender
- onset at a later age
- predominant motor signs
- frequent relapses
- constant decline with no remission.

When talking to patients, you should remember that one-third:

- do well with no/few further attacks
- slowly deteriorate over 5–25 years but remain active and not grossly disabled for much of this time
- deteriorate rapidly and die (< 5 years).

Investigations

The clinical diagnosis is made on the basis of acute neurological deficits separated not only neuroanatomically but also over time, with no other clear cause (e.g. cerebral toxoplasmosis in AIDS). Investigations, up to relatively recently, were focused on supporting this, e.g. disordered **visual evoked potentials** (VEP) in patients with spinal cord symptoms and signs. Other investigations provided evidence of disturbance of CNS immunology, with oligoclonal immunoglobulin bands in the CSF indicating intrathecal production. Unfortunately, these investigations have limited sensitivity in a person with early, rather than established, multiple sclerosis.

The principal investigation now is **MRI**, which shows the distribution of the plaques of demyelination, both recent and old.

When considering the possibility of multiple sclerosis, you must bear in mind treatable diseases. One important example would be spinal cord compression in a patient presenting with a paraparesis.

Management

A team approach to the management is very important. Patients may need help and advice with their urinary difficulties; some will practise intermittent self-catheterisation. They may have to be registered partially sighted (through an ophthalmologist).

High-dose corticosteroids reduce the duration of relapse but do not have any effect on the ultimate outcome. More recently there is interest in the use of β-interferon, which decreases the number and severity of the relapses and may modify the course of the disease.

5.8 Coma

In the evaluation of a patient with impaired consciousness, you must know and use the Glasgow coma scale: (Table 47). Always contact senior colleagues. The principles of management are:

1. resuscitation with checks of airway (A), breathing (B) and circulation (C), then
2. consideration of cause and treatment.

A history is crucial and should be sought out from any witness; it will help to determine the cause as the list of possible aetiologies is huge (Box 9, p. 209). One important differentiating factor is the presence of focal neurological signs. A major consideration is identifying treatable factors. The management is dependent on the accurate diagnosis and, for specific disorders, is described elsewhere.

5.9 Diseases of the spinal cord

Anatomy

You will find it useful to be able to visualise the cross-sectional layout of the spinal cord (Fig. 42). Certain key points should be noted:

- sensory fibres enter the spinal cord through the **posterior (dorsal)** roots, motor fibres leave through the **anterior (ventral)** roots
- the cell bodies for the posterior column lie in the **dorsal root ganglia.** Their axons synapse in the cuneate and gracilis nucleus. From here, the fibres decussate and ascend in the **medial lemniscus** through to the thalamus and then the post-central gyrus
- in the posterior column, fibres from the lowest segments of the spinal cord lie *medially* and hence will be damaged by an expanding central cord lesion
- the fibres joining the **spinothalamic tracts** ascend the cord for a few segments before crossing; a central lesion, by interrupting this decussation, can cause a

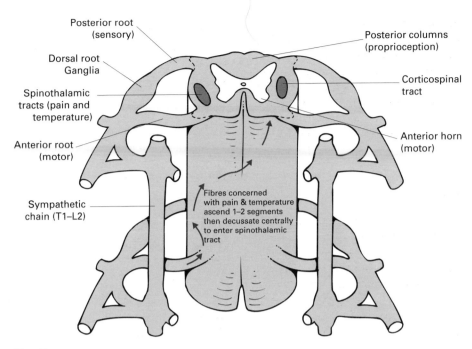

Fig. 42
Cross-sectional layout of the spinal cord.

suspended (normal sensation above and below) loss of pain and temperature over part of the trunk
- the **corticospinal tracts** decussate in the pyramids and run in the lateral part of the cord.

Common patterns of abnormal sensation

Unilateral loss of all modalities. Usually results from a lesion in the thalamus or the posterior part of the internal capsule.

Loss of pain/temperature on one side of face and opposite side of body. Usually caused by a lateral medullary syndrome (p. 197).

Bilateral loss of all forms of sensation below a definite level ('sensory' level). Caused by compression of the cord (or transverse myelitis). Upper part may be indicated by zone of hyperaesthesia. Note that the bony level does not correspond to cord segment level (i.e. the cord ends at the L1/L2 vertebra).

Hemisection (Brown–Séquard) of the cord. This results in paralysis and loss of proprioception/vibration on the same side of the body with loss of pain/temperature on the contralateral side, apart from a thin band of analgesia at the level of the damage (Fig. 42). It is more common to get incomplete forms.

Impairment of pain/temperature sensation over several segments. Indicates an intrinsic lesion of the cord, near the centre involving crossing fibres. Common in syringomyelia (cavity in the centre of the cord) and intrinsic cord tumours.

Loss of sensation of 'saddle' type. Impairment of all sensory modalities over the lowest sacral segments. Often accompanied by loss of leg reflexes and sphincter control. It is caused by a **cauda equina** lesion.

Sacral 'sparing'. This can occur with extrinsic cord compression caused by the fibres from the lower cord segments lying medially in the posterior column away from the pressure. This pattern is often seen with extradural tumours, with sparing of the saddle area.

Box 9
Causes of coma/disturbed conscious level

Without focal signs (mostly non-CNS pathology)

Hypoglycaemia

Subarachnoid haemorrhage (may be focal signs)

Electrolyte disturbance, e.g. hyponatraemia

Meningitis or encephalitis

Drugs: particularly taken in overdose. May be specific antagonists or therapies (e.g. narcotics, benzodiazepines, lithium)

Epilepsy

Trauma (extradural, subdural, concussion)

Encephalopathy: hepatic

Respiratory failure: acute rise in carbon dioxide

Carbon monoxide poisoning

Hypothermia (< 35°C)

With focal signs (mostly intracranial pathology)

Hypoglycaemia (check blood sugar in *all* unconscious patients immediately)

Stroke

Tumour: very late

Brain abscess: look for other evidence

Epilepsy

Trauma

Blood supply of the cord

Anterior spinal artery syndrome

The cord has a poor blood supply relying on penetrating arteries at multiple levels. The anterior spinal artery supplies all of the spinal cord *except* the posterior column. The anterior artery is heavily dependent on a branch of the aorta entering at around the 12th thoracic vertebra (**Giant artery of Adamkiewicz**). When blocked by atheroma or during repair of an aortic aneurysm, an anterior spinal artery syndrome occurs, with weakness below T10–T12 and loss of pain/temperature sensation but *not* light touch.

Spinal strokes

Spinal strokes can occur; because of the poor collateral supply, these often affect the cord in a patchy manner, with several segments being affected in an asymmetrical fashion.

Sub-acute combined degeneration of the spinal cord

Sub-acute combined degeneration of the spinal cord (SACD) is now a rare condition caused by vitamin B_{12} deficiency. There are usually concomitant haematological changes (p. 233). The main features in an established case are a combination of:

- posterior column loss: impairment of proprioception
- corticospinal damage: weakness in lower limbs
- peripheral neuropathy: loss of reflexes, stocking loss of sensation.

It was commonly seen in patients with pernicious anaemia and is treated with vitamin B_{12} injections, which will prevent further damage.

5.10 Peripheral nervous system

Dermatomes and myotomes

In order to identify precisely neurological impairment, you need a detailed knowledge of dermatomes. When examining the patient, place them in the anatomical position (palms facing anteriorly). Important points are:

- C2 supplies the back of the scalp up to the vertex
- C3 and C4 include the neck and upper part of the shoulder
- C5–C8: C5 area is the outer aspect of the shoulder and upper limb; C6 the lateral aspect of the forearm to the thumb and index; C7 a strip down the centre of the forearm to the middle finger; C8 the inner side of the forearm and the ring and little fingers; T1 the medial aspect of the upper arm to the axilla
- on the chest wall, C4 and T2 are adjacent; the nipple is at T5, the rib margin at T8, umbilicus at T10 and symphysis pubis at T12

- the anterior aspect of the thigh is supplied by L1–L3, the medial aspect of the calf by L4, and the lateral aspect and dorsum of the foot by L5; The sole and little toe are supplied by S1
- the perineum is supplied by concentric rings of S3–S5.

Similarly a knowledge of myotomes is essential.

diaphragm: C4
shoulder muscles and flexors of elbow: C5, 6
triceps and extensors of wrist and fingers: C7
flexors of wrist and fingers: C7, 8
hand muscles: C8, T1
intercostals and lumbar/abdominal muscles: T2–L3
quadriceps and adductors: L3, 4
Ilio-psoas: L1–L5
glutei: L4, 5
hamstrings: L4–S1
muscles controlling ankle: L5, S1
foot muscles: S1, 2
bladder, anal sphincter: S2–S4.

There are a few key points that you must know about the brachial plexus:

- it is the C5 and C6 roots which are most likely to be affected by cervical spondylosis (loss of biceps and supinator jerks)
- the medial cord (T1 and C8) is vulnerable to pressure from a cervical rib or infiltration from a bronchial carcinoma (**Pancoast's syndrome**).

Medial cord damage causes weakness and wasting of the intrinsic muscles of the hand (T1). A **Horner's syndrome** is also likely to be seen (T1 sympathetic outflow). Appropriate initial investigations would be chest and cervical spine radiographs.

Peripheral nerves

Examination of the arm should enable diagnosis of damage to the radial, ulnar and median nerves. The important muscles supplied and sensory distribution are summarised in Table 51.

Upper limb
Radial nerve. The radial nerve can be damaged at two main places:

- if pressure is applied in the axilla, for example by using a crutch, this will cause weakness of the triceps; neoplastic infiltration of the axilla may cause a similar problem
- a *Saturday night palsy* is caused by pressure on the radial nerve in the spiral groove of the humerus. Examination shows normal triceps power with weakness of the wrist and finger extensors; this causes the typical **wrist drop.**

In radial nerve palsies there is very little sensory loss.

Ulnar nerve. Commonly the ulnar nerve is damaged at the elbow as it passes behind the medial epi-

Table 51 Important (not all) muscles supplied by the three main nerves of the upper limb and the sensory distribution

Radial nerve	Ulnar nerve	Median nerve
Motor		
Triceps	Interossei (finger ab/adduction)	Abductor policis brevis
Wrist extensors	Medial lumbricals (3 and 4) (flex MCP joints)	Opponens pollicis
Finger extensors	Hypothenar eminence: little finger	Lateral lumbricals (1 and 2)
	Adductor pollicis: only muscle in thenar eminence supplied by ulnar nerve	
Sensory		
Back of hand *only* between thumb and index finger	Little finger and medial ½ ring finger	Thumb, index, middle and lateral ½ ring finger

condyle, resulting in weakness of the intrinsic muscles of the hand. Wasting and guttering will be seen, affecting the interossei and the hypothenar eminence. A key diagnostic feature is the deformity of the hand. If the lumbricals are paralysed, then the long extensors of the metacarpophalangeal (MCP) joints can pull these joints into hyperextension; because of this, the proximal interphalangeal (PIP) and the distal interphalangeal (DIP go into flexion and a **claw hand** is produced. For an ulnar nerve lesion, this affects the little and ring fingers (sparing the lateral two lumbricals: median nerve) with only a slight deformity of the middle and index fingers (**ulnar claw hand**). However, if the damage is at T1 then all the lumbricals are affected causing a **true claw hand.**

Median nerve. The median nerve is commonly damaged at the wrist in a **carpal tunnel syndrome.** Often the condition is idiopathic, but there are many specific causes, for example obesity, pregnancy, hypothyroidism and rheumatoid arthritis. The characteristic symptom of a carpal tunnel syndrome is pain in the sensory distribution of the nerve, though this may spread up the forearm. The pain is worse at night and the patient may relieve the pain by shaking the hand. On examination, other than detecting any sensory loss, the main focus should be looking for wasting of the thenar eminence and weakness of *abductor pollicis brevis* and *opponens pollicis.*

Investigation and management. For all nerve lesions, your clinical assessment will form the basis of diagnosis. Confirmation can be sought through nerve conduction studies (p. 188).

Radial nerve palsies (Saturday night or crutch). Relief of pressure will usually lead to recovery. A wrist splint should be used to support the hand in the neutral position whilst this takes place.

Ulnar nerve entrapment/damage at the elbow. Surgical freeing of the nerve is sometimes required.

Carpal tunnel syndrome. Treatment of the underlying condition may help as can local injection of corticosteroids. Commonly, surgical release is needed.

Lower limb

Femoral nerve. Damage to the the femoral nerve will result in weakness of knee extension and consequent difficulty in getting up from a chair or climbing stairs. Quadriceps wasting will be seen with loss of the knee jerk. **Femoral amyotrophy** is seen in poorly controlled diabetics and is often associated with pain, depression and weight loss. It is treated by improving diabetic control (converting to insulin).

Lateral popliteal nerve. The other important nerve lesion in the lower limb is damage to the lateral popliteal nerve as it winds round the head of the fibula. A foot drop occurs because of weakness of dorsiflexion. Again, a mononeuritis from diabetes may be the cause, but it is also seen following prolonged pressure, such as by a plaster cast or in an unconscious patient.

Peripheral nerve disease

Mononeuritis and mononeuritis multiplex

Mononeuritis and mononeuritis multiplex have complex aetiologies with a common factor being a vasculitic process affecting the vasa nervorum. Patients present with either a single nerve (often cranial nerve) or a mixture of nerve lesions. It may be painful. Mononeuritis occurs in, amongst other conditions, aggressive rheumatoid disease, SLE and polyarteritis nodosa. Treatment is directed towards the underlying problem.

Peripheral neuropathy

The hallmark of a peripheral neuropathy is a *symmetrical glove and stocking loss*, which is unlike the asymmetry seen in mononeuritis multiplex or other local nerve damage. There are hereditary sensorimotor neuropathies such as **peroneal muscular atrophy** (Charcot–Marie Tooth syndrome: autosomal dominant). Among acquired causes diabetes mellitus is the commonest; others include AIDS, drugs (amiodarone, nitrofurantoin) and pellegra (pyridoxime deficiency) and neoplasia. Most cases are idiopathic.

Early features are of dys/paraesthesiae in the feet ('like walking on cotton wool'), although many patients have no symptoms at all. On examination, the ankle jerks are lost and some distal wasting and weakness may be found, but the dominant feature is often symmetrical sensory impairment with a zone of impaired sensation giving way to numbness more distally. Occasionally, the neuropathy can be painful.

Investigation

Diagnosis is made on clinical grounds, supported by nerve conduction studies. If the pathological process is damaging myelin, the nerve conduction pattern will be different to one causing axonal/neuronal loss (p. 189). You should target investigations to the probable/possible cause(s) identified in the history and examination. The tests may include blood sugar (diabetes), rheumatoid factor (rheumatoid disease/amyloid), antinuclear factor (SLE), chest radiograph (neoplasia), full blood count (vitamin B$_{12}$, folate deficiency), ESR/plasma viscosity (inflammatory disease), biochemical profile (uraemia) and possibly HIV status (AIDS).

Management

Management is aimed at the underlying cause. Care must be taken about footwear and chiropody to prevent any ulceration/infection, which may result in gangrene particularly if vascular supply is affected.

Non-metastatic manifestation of malignancy

A peripheral neuropathy can be seen as a **paraneoplastic syndrome**. Non-neurological manifestations are discussed elsewhere (see p. 76), but malignancy may present or be associated with a primary cerebellar degeneration, a myasthenic-like syndrome (see below), a primary motor neuropathy or a myositis. Malignancy should always be considered in any patient with an odd neurological syndrome.

5.11 Muscle disease

Learning objectives

You should:
- know the commmon causes of muscle disease
- kow the common clinical presentations
- understand how to investigate a patient with possible muscle disease

Structure of muscle

The functional unit of muscle is the motor unit, which comprises a single motor neurone innervating, via its axon, a variable number of muscle fibres. Muscle fibres are divided using histology and biochemistry into:

- type I fibres: smaller than type II, larger numbers of oxidative enzymes and mitochondria; they contract and relax relatively slowly, being important in postural control

- type II fibres: a higher content of glycogen and are geared for anaerobic metabolism; these are **fast twitch** fibres.

Clinical presentation

The major features of muscle disease are weakness and fatigability. An inflammatory myopathy (and some metabolic syndromes) may be painful. Wasting is sometimes apparent and it is important that you document its distribution as it may help in diagnosis. The reflexes are usually preserved, unlike in a peripheral neuropathy.

Muscle disease can be divided into inherited disease (you should take a careful family history) and acquired disease.

Investigations

Initial investigations of suspected muscle disease should include a chest radiograph (malignancy, thymic tumour), full blood count, ESR (inflammatory/connective tissue process), rheumatoid factor, antinuclear factor creatine phosphokinase (muscle enzyme: may need skeletal muscle isoenzyme MM). Electromyography may show evidence of disordered muscle function. A muscle biopsy is sometimes indicated, with enzymatic assays, histological stains and electron microscopy.

Inherited disease

Many inherited diseases are rare conditions seen only in specialist clinics or in paediatric practice.

Dystrophia myotonica

Dystrophia myotonica is a rare, but important, muscle disease. It is inherited as an autosomal dominant, with the gene located on chromosome 19. Males, particularly born to affected females, are more severely affected and the severity is linked to increasing numbers of **repeat sequences** within the abnormal gene.

Myotonia (delayed relaxation) is the characteristic feature, which worsens in the cold. Wasting of temporalis and masseter muscles are observed, together with some distal muscle atrophy. Ptosis occurs. Dystrophia myotonia is a multisystem disorder associated with cataracts, frontal balding, diabetes, cardiomyopathy and gonadal atrophy. Sleep apnoea is common.

The condition presents in the third or fourth decade and life expectancy is reduced. The myotonia may be helped by procainamide and phenytoin.

Acquired disease

Myasthenia gravis

Myasthenia gravis occurs in adults of all ages, being slightly more common in females. It is more often associated with a thymoma in older people. The symptoms and signs result from failure of neuromuscular transmission because of blockade of the acetylcholine receptor on the muscle end-plate by receptor antibodies. Characteristic symptoms are:

- diplopia
- fatigability: increasing weakness with repetitive tasks (e.g. brushing hair, using screwdriver) or at the end of a day.

On examination, you may bring out the weakness when using repeated movements. Ptosis is often present and the patient may complain of diplopia in all directions. Unlike peripheral nerve damage, reflexes are preserved.

Investigations

A chest radiograph (PA and lateral) and a thoracic CT scan should be performed looking for a thymic tumour. Blood should be taken for receptor antibodies. If there are none, it is unlikely that the patient has the disease. An EMG will show diagnostic features and can be used to differentiate true myasthenia gravis from the much rarer **Eaton–Lambert syndrome**. The latter is a paraneoplastic syndrome with many of the features of myasthenia except the weakness *improves* on repetition.

Injection with the short-acting anticholinesterase edrophonium can confirm the diagnosis by showing immediate and dramatic improvement. The PEFR can be used to demonstrate the change objectively.

Management

For many years, the only treatment available for myasthenia was an anticholinesterase such as **neostigmine** or **pyridostigmine**. These have to be given frequently because of their short half-lives (3–4 hour dose interval) and can produce excessive cholinergic stimulation, but do not modify the underlying disease process. More recently, the aim has been towards disease modification. Thymectomy has been shown to be a safe procedure that will produce a remission over several months and will last a long time in those patients *without* a thymoma. Corticosteroids can also be beneficial; these have to be introduced in a low dose as they can temporarily produce a worsening of the condition. Sometimes other immunosuppressives (e.g. **azathioprine**) are used.

As a medical house officer, you need to be able to recognise a crisis in a patient with known myasthenia. If the person is receiving anticholinesterases, then the differential diagnosis lies between a **myasthenic crisis** and a **cholinergic crisis**. There may be clues to the correct diagnosis in the history, for example poor compliance with medication or treatment with amino-glycoside antibiotics, which have a curare-like (competitive antagonism) effect. Usually, it is very difficult to differentiate between the two different crises. Much more importantly, you should assess ventilation with PEFR, vitalograph and blood gases. A specialist opinion should be sought with a view to ventilation. An edrophonium test has been used to diagnose a myasthenic crisis, but this may cause respiratory paralysis if given to a patient who is overtreated with anticholinesterases. The test should *only* be done in an intensive care unit.

Myopathies

A number of conditions result in a myopathy. Almost always this affects the **proximal musculature**, resulting in difficulties with e.g. rising from a chair or lifting the arms high. Wasting may occur, but it may not be obvious.

Conditions causing a proximal myopathy include endocrine disease such as Cushing's disease, acromegaly and thyrotoxicosis. Toxins such as alcohol may be important, and binge drinking may cause acute muscle necrosis. A myopathy may be seen as part of a non-metastatic manifestation of malignancy (paraneoplastic syndrome). One of the most important causes of a proximal myopathy is treatment with corticosteroid at doses above 10 mg of prednisolone per day.

Myositis

Particularly in connective tissue disease (see Chapter 8), the skeletal musculature may be affected by vasculitis and inflammation. When chronic and mild, pain may not be a feature and the presentation is that of a proximal myopathy. The hallmark is a raised creatine phosphokinase.

In a small percentage of patients, a characteristic skin rash with a heliotrope (red-purple) discoloration of the skin over the dorsum of the metacarpophalangeal joints and around the eyelids may be apparent: **dermatomyositis**.

As with many neurological syndromes, myositis may be a marker for a malignant process. This is now known to be less common than previously thought. Management is of the underlying condition, but high-dose steroids are often used to suppress the inflammatory process.

Self-assessment: questions

Multiple choice questions

1. The following are true:
   a. There is weakness of elbow extension in a crutch palsy
   b. Wasting of the hypothenar eminence occurs in the carpal tunnel syndrome
   c. Abduction of the thumb is impaired in an ulnar nerve lesion
   d. The index finger is hyperextended at the MCP joint in an ulnar nerve lesion
   e. Sensation is lost over the whole of the back of the hand in radial nerve damage

2. In a patient treated for epilepsy the following are true:
   a. Drug levels of cabamazepine are useful in the management
   b. Sodium valproate is useful and safe during pregnancy
   c. A patient with epilepsy who has been fit-free for 4 years and who stops his medication must not drive for a further 2 year
   d. Respiratory depression is associated with chlormethiozole infusions for status epilepticus
   e. The use of sodium valproate makes the combined oral contraceptive pill unreliable

3. The following are true:
   a. A cerebellar vermis lesion will result in a marked intention tremor
   b. Macular sparing is a characteristic of lesions affecting the optic tract
   c. In a patient with marked visuo-spatial inattention, the lesion is most likely in the left cerebral hemisphere
   d. Agnosia means inability to plan and execute motor tasks
   e. Dyscalculia is a feature of Alzheimer's disease

4. The following are true of stroke risk:
   a. Following a transient ischaemic attack, most patients will have a stroke within 3 years
   b. Carotid endarterectomy is of proven value in preventing strokes in patients with severe stenosis and who have had recent events (TIA, minor stroke) in that territory
   c. Treating hypertension is of proven value in patients up to the age of 80 years
   d. Anticoagulation will reduce the risk of a stroke in patients in sinus rhythm
   e. The benefit of an intervention for a patient depends on the absolute risk

5. Features of a right sixth nerve palsy include:
   a. Convergent strabismus
   b. Diplopia worse on looking to the right
   c. False image parallel to the true image
   d. False image occurs further to the left than the true image
   e. Images become increasingly separated on looking to the left

6. Pressure on the facial nerve at the internal auditory meatus by an acoustic neuroma may cause:
   a. Loss of taste
   b. Loss of ability to blink
   c. Loss of supply to the parotid gland
   d. Loss of sensation to the cheek
   e. Loss of sweating over the cheek

7. Parkinson's disease is associated with:
   a. Loss of dopamine transmission
   b. Cogwheel rigidity
   c. Tardive dyskinesia
   d. Intention tremor
   e. Festinant gait

8. The following are true of myasthenia gravis:
   a. An equal sex incidence
   b. Diplopia and papilloedema are the main ocular signs
   c. Usually a loss of tendon reflexes
   d. A deficiency of acetyl cholinesterase
   e. Fasciculation often occurs

9. In a young female with paraplegia, which of the following would suggest a diagnosis of multiple sclerosis:
   a. Periventricular lesions on CT or MR scanning
   b. Raised CSF protein
   c. Raised CSF globulin
   d. Denervation of the muscles of the leg
   e. Episode of visual disturbance

10. A 19-year-old girl presents with a 12-month history of repeated falls. A diagnosis of epilepsy is supported by the fact that:
    a. There are abnormal sensations prior to the attack
    b. They only occur in the presence of the mother
    c. They only occur when watching television
    d. There have been feelings of increased anxiety over the last year when on a bus or in shops
    e. They only occur when standing upright

11. The following are more suggestive of dementia than of depression:
    a. Several episodes of antisocial behaviour
    b. Mutism
    c. Duration of symptoms less than one month
    d. Worsening of symptoms during the early morning
    e. Marked impairment of concentration

12. The following are causes of predominantly lymphocytic meningitis:
    a. Enteroviruses
    b. Sarcoidosis
    c. *Cryptococcus neoformans*
    d. Tuberculosis
    e. Herpes simplex virus

13. With respect to lumbar puncture:
    a. Coagulopathy is a contraindication
    b. Papilloedema is an absolute contraindication
    c. The procedure may cause meningitis
    d. The less CSF is removed, the less likely coning is to occur
    e. Postlumbar puncture headache is related to the size of the needle used

14. The following diagnoses should be considered when a patient presents with a combination of fever and impaired conscious level:
    a. Pneumonia
    b. Tuberculous meningitis
    c. Bacterial meningitis
    d. Viral meningitis
    e. Pontine haemorrhage

15. Outcome from bacterial meningitis relates to:
    a. Age of patient
    b. Time to first administration of antibiotic
    c. CSF concentration of antibiotic
    d. Development of antibiotic resistance during therapy
    e. The causative organism

Case history questions

History 1

A 57-year-old man with known diabetes presents to his general practitioner following an episode lasting a few minutes during which 'a curtain had descended down over my left eye'. Following this he had been fine. He had one similar episode 2 weeks previously when his speech had been 'garbled' as well as his vision 'going funny'. This had lasted a few minutes.

1. What are the diagnoses and where are the lesions?
2. What tests, if any, would you request?
3. How would you treat him?

Unfortunately, 2 weeks later he developed sudden onset of right-sided weakness, started to talk 'rubbish' and was noticed to be looking constantly to his left. He was admitted to hospital where his conscious level deteriorated over the next 8 hours. He developed constant urinary incontinence.

4. What tests would you do as an emergency?
5. What is the likely diagnosis and prognosis?
6. Assuming he survives, how should he be managed?

History 2

A 27-year-old woman felt unwell and feverish. She had vague urinary symptoms and was given trimethoprim. Ten days later she developed unsteadiness in walking and tingling in her feet. She complained of stiffness in her legs and ill-defined low back pain. Over the next few days she noticed increasing leg weakness.

1. Discuss the differential diagnosis

History 3

A 55-year-old man presented with a 1-year history of progressive dysarthria and trouble swallowing, with recurrent chest infections. Some wasting of the muscles of his hands was apparent. Nerve conduction studies in the legs showed a conduction velocity of 42 m/s (normal 50 m/s) and EMG showed some fibrillatory potentials and giant motor units. The creatine phosphokinase was normal.

1. What is the diagnosis?
2. If the patient had sensory disturbance how would this change the diagnostic possibilities?
3. Outline a management plan

History 4

A 19-year-old male Asian student is brought in to Casualty drowsy but communicating. He is accompanied by his flatmate. Staff nurse tells you he has a fever of 38.5°C, blood pressure of 100/60 and a pulse of 110/minute. He complains of headache and vomiting of about 36 hours' duration. He looks ill.

1. The following actions are appropriate immediately:
   a. Check his travel history in detail
   b. Do an urgent blood count
   c. Send him to a ward where you will see him very soon
   d. Arrange an urgent chest X-ray immediately
   e. Examine his skin while completing the history

> You learn that he was previously well and never admitted to hospital before. He was born in the UK, has not travelled anywhere for 2 months and is not allergic to any antibiotics that he knows of. He has marked neck stiffness, no skin rash and no focal neurological signs on examination of his cranial nerves, limbs or cerebellum. His chest is clear to auscultation and he has not coughed during the examination.

2. The following actions are appropriate:
   a. Administer i.v. antibiotics
   b. Do a lumbar puncture immediately after taking blood and inserting i.v. line
   c. Do a lumbar puncture after getting his platelet count
   d. Do a CT scan first (there is an on-call emergency CT scan service in the hospital)
   e. Give loading doses of phenytoin to prevent fits

> Two hours later, the patient has had a lumbar puncture, CT scan and his first dose of antibiotic and he has been admitted to the ward. The microbiologist on call says that the CSF was consistent with bacterial meningitis and Gram-negative cocci were seen intracellularly, consistent with *N. meningitidis* in the CSF.

3. Now you should:
   a. Put the patient in a side room
   b. Wear a mask when visiting him
   c. Administer rifampicin prophylaxis to his flatmate, the staff nurse in casualty, the ambulancemen and yourself
   d. Inform the consultant responsible for Communicable Disease Control now, by telephone, that the patient has been admitted
   e. Reassure his parents that he is likely to make a full recovery

Data interpretation

1. In a patient with a presumed diagnosis of Guillain–Barré syndrome, comment on the following sequences of spirometry and blood gases:

	Monday a.m	Monday p.m.
FEV$_1$ (l)	1.7	1.1
FVC (l)	2.5	1.7
pH	7.32	7.30
PaO_2 (mmHg)	80	70
$PaCO_2$ (mmHg)	43	47
HCO$_3^-$ (mmol/l)	27	29

2. Table 52 gives information for CSF in a patient with fever, impaired mental status or headache, or a mixture of these. Give the most likely diagnosis for cases A to F.

Table 52 Data obtained for CSF (data interpretation question 2)

	A	B	C	D	E	F
RCC/hpf	150	20	23,000	22	12	20
WCC/hpf	9	8	14	1,700	450	180
Polymorphs (%)	20	0	50	99	70	10
Protein (g/l)	0.58	0.69	0.9	1.2	0.51	0.9
Glucose (CSF) (mmol/l)	3.2	4.2	3.8	0.2	3.4	1.1
Serum glucose (mmol/l)	5.6	6.4	5.9	6.2	5.8	4.8

hpf, high power field: mm3 = ×10⁶/L

Picture questions

1. You see a 46-year-old-man is seen in Casualty. He has a 4-week history of left-sided weakness. A CT scan is done the following day (Picture 5.1). During examination, the patient is asked to draw a clock face (picture 5.2).

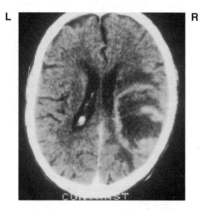

Picture 5.1

   a. What do you want to know about the history of the weakness?
   b. List three abnormalities shown on the scan
   c. What is the differential diagnosis?
   d. Why has he drawn the clock (Picture 5.2) this way?
   e. What day-to-day problems might he have because of this problem?

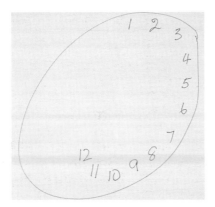

Picture 5.2

2. A 54-year-old woman is admitted through Casualty complaining of a severe headache. A CT scan is performed within 24 hours (Picture 5.3). A second scan is done at 2 weeks because of concerns (subsequently proved unfounded) about the diagnosis (Picture 5.4).
   a. Describe the abnormalities on the scan shown in Picture 5.4
   b. Why are these not present in Picture 5.3 given that her condition has not changed?
   c. What symptoms would she be complaining of other that her headache?
   d. What artery supplies the area of abnormality?

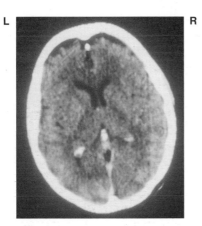

Picture 5.3

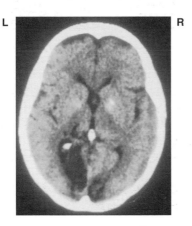

Picture 5.4

3. A 73-year-old man is brought to Casualty. He is drowsy. The history from his wife is that he is on long-term anticoagulants because of atrial fibrillation and a previous stroke. He suddenly deteriorated on the day of admission. Picture 5.5 is a CT scan of the patient.
   a. Why should you request an urgent CT scan requested?
   b. What does the scan (Picture 5.5) show?
   c. What should you do now?

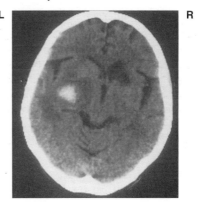

Picture 5.5

4. You are asked to see a 33-year-old woman in Casualty; she is drowsy and unable to give a history. Her temperature is 37.5°C and she has neck rigidity. An urgent CT scan is carried out (Picture 5.6).
   a. Describe two abnormalities on the scan
   b. What should you do now?
   c. If she survives, what neurological problems might she develop?

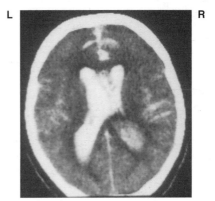

Picture 5.6

5. You are looking after a 34-year-old woman with Friedreich's ataxia who is confined to a wheelchair and is complaining of left-hand weakness.
   a. What does Picture 5.7 show?
   b. What particular features would you look for on examination?
   c. Why has she developed this problem?

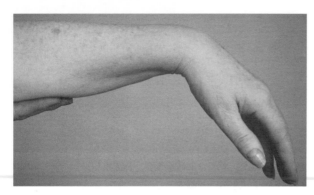

Picture 5.7

6. A 63-year-old man in the outpatient department complains of right-hand weakness which has developed over 5 months (Picture 5.8).
   a. Describe the abnormality
   b. Where is the neuroanatomical lesion likely to be?
   c. Name one possible cause

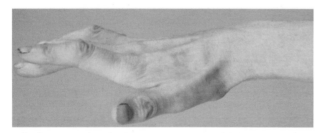

Picture 5.8

Short notes

1. The daughter of a patient who has been diagnosed clinically as having Alzheimer's disease wants to ask what tests you are doing, what treatment can be offered and what will happen in the future. Consider what you would do if the daughter became angry and aggressive (would be a suitable question for a viva).

2. What would be your immediate management, including pertinent questions in the history, examination findings, investigations and treatment in:
   a. A patient with three seizures over 30 minutes with no recovery of consciousness in between
   b. A patient with known myasthenia who is generally weak and drowsy.

3. In a patient with one of the following symptoms, where is the lesion likely to be and name a common pathological process:
   a. reduction in visual acuity over several hours with impaired colour vision (blurred and colours 'washed out')
   b. Loss of the left visual field with macular sparing
   c. Loss of both temporal fields starting with the lower fields
   d. Loss of left temporal vision in one eye in a 35-year-old man with progressive weight loss.

4. A 59-year-old man enters outpatients complaining of dizziness and almost immediately has a grand mal seizure. Moments after recovery from this, his pulse rate is 38/min. Discuss your management of him both diagnostic and therapeutic, from this moment.

Viva questions

1. How would you examine a patient whom you suspected had a space-occupying lesion in the right cerebral hemisphere.
2. Discuss the drugs used in Parkinson's disease with specific reference to control of symptoms and side-effects.
3. An ambulance team brings a comatose middle-aged woman into the casualty department. How would you assess her level of consciousness and what causes of her condition would you consider?

Self-assessment: answers

Multiple choice answers

1. a. **True**. The triceps is affected in a crutch palsy.
   b. **False**. It is the median nerve (**thenar** eminence) that is commonly damaged.
   c. **False**. The little and ring fingers are affected.
   d. **False**. There is deformity of the index finger (lumbrical supplied by median nerve).
   e. **False**. There is little sensory loss.

2. a. **False**. Drug levels are used simply to assess gross compliance.
   b. **False**. All the main drugs are associated with some teratogenicity.
   c. **False**. You must know the medico-legal position about epilepsy (p. 206): for an ordinary car licence in the UK, it is the fit-free period that counts (1 year), not withdrawal of treatment.
   d. **True**. It should only be used in high dependency.
   e. **False**. Sodium valproate is *not* an enzyme inducer (unlike carbamazepine and phenytoin).

3. a. **False**. A vermis lesion will result in gross *truncal* ataxia.
   b. **False**. Macular sparing is a feature of occipital pole damage.
   c. **False**. Visuo-spatial inattention can occur with left-sided lesions, but it is more common with *right* hemisphere problems.
   d. **False**. Agnosia is a problem with interpretation of sensory information (see p. 182 and Dyspraxia, p. 182).
   e. **True**. Rememer other higher cortical functionals, e.g. dysphasia, dyslexia.

4. a. **False**. After a TIA, the absolute risk of stroke is 8% per year.
   b. **True**. In symptomatic patients with 70–99% stenosis (not occluded) endartectomy is beneficial.
   c. **True**. Treating elderly hypertensive people is cost effective because of their high absolute risk.
   d. **False**. Anticoagulation is of proven benefit for those in *atrial fibrillation*.
   e. **True**. If the patient's absolute risk of something happening is extremely small, he/she is not going to get much benefit from an intervention.

5. a. **True.** Complete paralysis of the lateral rectus leaves the medial rectus unopposed hence producing a convergent strabismus, though mostly the paralysis is only brought out when the eye is abducted.

b. **True**. Diplopia is maximal on looking in the direction of the primary action of the muscle.
   c. **True**. Unlike a superior oblique palsy.
   d. **False**. False image is always displaced furthest in the direction of action of the muscle, in this case looking to the right.
   e. **False**. Images become increasingly separated looking to the right.

6. a. **True**. The chorda tympani runs along the facial nerve.
   b. **True**. An absent or diminished corneal reflex may be an early sign of an acoustic neuroma.
   c. **False**. Logical though it might be, the facial nerve does *not* supply the parotid gland, the glossopharyngeal nerve does.
   d. **False**. Many patients with a facial nerve palsy will say that their face feels 'funny', but on examination there will not be any sensory signs.
   e. **False**. Sweating is controlled through sympathetic fibres (impaired in Horner's syndrome).

7. a. **True**. Although the mechanism is unclear, it does involve loss of dopaminergic neurons.
   b. **True**. Cogwheel rigidity is a superimposed tremor on the 'lead pipe' increase in tone.
   c. **False**. Patients with tardive dyskinesia have slow stereotypic movements such as 'tromboning' of the tongue. It is associated with neuroleptic (e.g. haloperidol) treatment causing a blockade of dopamine receptors, which become supersensitive (up-regulated).
   d. **False**. Intention tremor is a sign of cerebellar disease.
   e. **True**. To festinate means to hurry/accelerate — always trying to catch up with the centre of gravity.

8. a. **False**. It is slightly more common in females.
   b. **False**. Papilloedema and loss of pupillary reflexes are *not* features, but over 90% have ocular involvement (diplopia).
   c. **False**. In muscle or neuromuscular disease tendon reflexes are usually preserved, unlike in a peripheral neuropathy.
   d. **False**. There is blockade of the acetylcholine receptor on the muscle end-plate by antibodies.
   e. **False**. Fasciculation is brief spontaneous contraction of muscle fibres causing a flicker of movement under the skin; it is often associated with motor neurone disease. In myasthenia gravis, fasiculation would imply overtreatment with anticholinesterases.

9. a. **True**. Periventricular plaques would imply disease remote from the spinal cord. MR scanning is the preferred imaging technique.
    b. **False**. The danger here is that you will diagnose MS, for which there is no very effective treatment, and miss spinal cord compression from a treatable condition.
    c. **True**. CNS immunology is disturbed in MS.
    d. **False**. Denervation suggests peripheral nerve damage.
    e. **True**. Disturbances of visual acuity are an early sign.

10. a. **True**. An aura would suggest partial epilepsy.
    b. **False**. This suggest attention-seeking behaviour.
    c. **True**. A stroboscopic effect is known to occur when watching TV or video games, and in clubs.
    d. **False**. This is indicative of agoraphobia, although this is unusual in a young person.
    e. **False**. This suggests a vasovagal attack.

11. a. **True**. Antisocial behaviour is more in keeping with the personality change of dementia.
    b. **False**. Mutism can occur in depression.
    c. **False**. Short duration of symptoms suggests depression.
    d. **False**. Diurnal variation suggests depression.
    e. **False**. Poor concentration can occur also in depression.

12. a. **True**. Polio, coxsackie and enterovirus all cause viral meningitis.
    b. **True**. Although it is a rare cause and virtually always associated with other (e.g. pulmonary, skin) manifestations of disease and cerebral lesions on CT scan.
    c. **True**. It is relatively common in AIDS, lymphoma and transplant patients; also occasionally occurs in non-immunocompromised patients.
    d. **True**. The most common cause worldwide of *chronic* lymphocytic meningitis; early in disease neutrophils may predominate in CSF.
    e. **True**. However, it usually causes viral encephalitis with few cells in the CSF. Impaired consciousness is a hallmark of encephalitis.

13. a. **True**. However, if correctable (e.g. haemophiliac) and the indication for lumbar puncture is strong enough then it should be corrected and lumbar puncture done.
    b. **False**. It is the presence of a mass lesion and displacement of the ventricular system which leads to papilloedema that is the contraindication. It is essential to do a lumbar puncture in certain events, for example in benign intracranial hypertension for diagnostic and therapeutic reasons, despite papilloedema.

    c. **False**. Given the number of lumbar punctures done for myelograms and other investigations, the incidence of meningitis following lumbar puncture is exceptionally rare.
    d. **False**. Coning (the brainstem being forced down into the foramen magnum) is *not* related to the amount of CSF removed. It is related to a mass lesion *and* high intracranial pressure. In fact after a lumbar puncture is done, much more CSF leaks out from the dural hole than is removed during the procedure. So you should try and take at least 5 ml of CSF for diagnostic purposes.
    e. **False**. Most postlumbar puncture headache is not related to anything other than entering the epidural space. A small minority of cases are related to continued leakage of CSF through the dura. A blood patch procedure is helpful if postlumbar puncture headache persists beyond 5 or 7 days.

14. a. **True**. Many infections lead to a confusional state and/or drowsiness, including pneumonia. Remember to check the arterial gases if conscious level is poor, there is a raised respiratory rate or chest signs and/or chest radiograph infiltrate.
    b. **True**. Classical presentation with neck stiffness, often with focal neurological signs.
    c. **True**. The most important initial diagnostic consideration: presents with neck stiffness in about 90–95% (but not 100%) of patients.
    d. **False**. If conscious level is impaired, then it is *not* simply viral meningitis. If the problem is intracranial it may be bacterial meningitis, viral encephalitis, fungal meningitis, brain abscess, subdural empyema or a vascular event. Urgent admission and investigation is absolutely necessary.
    e. **False**. This would have other typical features, e.g. pinpoint pupils.

15. a. **True**. Mortality is highest in elderly people.
    b. **True**. Delays lead to increased mortality and morbidity.
    c. **True**. The CSF concentration of antibiotic needs to exceed by 20-fold the minimum inhibitory concentration of the infecting organism. This is the primary reason why intravenous therapy is necessary in meningitis.
    d. **False**. Apart from rare Gram-negative meningitis, this does not happen. However, there is an increasing problem of penicillin resistance in *Streptococcus pneumoniae* and ampicillin resistance in *Haemophilus influenzae*.
    e. **True**. *Neisseria meningitidis* has a lower mortality than *S. pneumoniae* meningitis. Furthermore about 5% of community-acquired cases are other organisms, such as *Listeria monocytogenes*. *Listeria* is intrinsically resistant to all cephalosporins,

which are now the most common primary treatment for meningitis.

Case history answers

History 1

1. The patient describes left amaurosis fugax and a left cerebral hemisphere transient ischaemic attack.
2. Major risk factors that can be targeted are hypertension, cardiac emboli in atrial fibrillation and carotid stenosis. In addition, a basic screen can be justified, which should include a full blood count (thrombocythaemia, polycythaemia rubra vera), ESR (vasculitis), lipids, urea and electrolytes (renal impairment; hypertension) and chest radiograph (cardiomegaly). A 12-lead electrocardiogram as well as careful cardiovascular examination will determine the rhythm and whether there is evidence of serious heart disease (valve, muscle) as well as hypertrophy in hypertension. The presence or absence of a **carotid bruit** is unimportant, he needs ultrasound examination of his carotid arteries. A CT or MR scan, unless there is a strong suspicion of non-vascular pathology, will not influence management.
3. The treatment will depend on the risk factors identified. Advice on lifestyle (smoking, weight, diet, etc.) is important. Remember that he is diabetic and, as such, is at greater absolute risk of an vascular event. At the very least, he should be started on low-dose aspirin (75–300 mg) and his blood pressure checked. If he is in atrial fibrillation, he should be anticoagulated unless there is a strong contraindication. If he has a 70% or greater stenosis of his left common or internal carotid artery (but not occlusion), carotid endarterectomy should be advised, whilst counselling him about the small risk of the operation resulting in a major stroke or death (3%).
4. The emergency tests for a patient with an acute stroke are outlined in Table 51.
5. He has had a major stroke: probably total anterior circulation infarction (TACI), either from occlusion of the middle cerebral or the internal carotid artery, though it is possible that he has had a major haemorrhage. The outlook is very bleak. The vast majority of patients who are unconscious at 24 hours following their stroke will die and most of the survivors will be very disabled.
6. If he survives, then the initial management will be to avoid complications. Major ones are: deep-vein thrombosis (CT scan within 7 days would exclude a cerebral haemorrhage and allow the use of prophylactic heparin therapy) and aspiration pneumonia: impairment of swallowing is very common. If present, the patient should have fluid and nutrition by another route. Other complications to consider are epilepsy, shoulder subluxation,

urinary tract infection (particularly with use of catheter). He should be assessed by a specialist for possible transfer to a stroke rehabilitation unit, but it is likely that he will remain dependent and will require long-term nursing care.

History 2

1. The history is a sub-acute progressive illness with probable paralysis of her legs. This is consistent with Guillain–Barré syndrome, which often has a prodromal minor infection and back pain. Other possibilities would be a spinal cord compression, possibly caused by an epidural abscess, but this is rare and usually there would be more systemic disturbance. Polio is now exceedingly uncommon and, in this case, the sensory symptoms are against the diagnosis. In a young woman, the symptoms may be the first manifestation of multiple sclerosis causing impairment of bladder function with transverse myelitis. Appropriate investigations should be done (including MR scan).

History 3

1. The diagnosis is motor neurone disease. The patient has dysarthria, which implies problems with articulation. This may be caused by cerebellar disease or damage to the bulbar musculature, either at the level of upper or lower motor neurones. The difficulty in swallowing and recurrent chest infections implies repeated aspiration, again pointing to impaired function of the bulbar musculature. The time course is relatively long and the disease is progressive; neither fits with cerebrovascular disease. The electrophysiological studies show denervation but relatively normal conduction velocities, implying that the damage is either to the axons of the α-motor neurones rather than demyelination. The abnormalities in the legs demonstrate a widespread disease process.
2. All of the features point to motor neurone disease. However, if sensory disturbance was present, the diagnosis becomes untenable. Another diagnostic possibility would be a non-metastatic manifestation of malignancy. Myasthenia gravis or Eaton–Lambert syndrome could be considered, but the electrophysiological studies are against these. With sensory abnormalities around the face, the very rare possibility of syringobulbia (a cavity or **syrinx** in the medulla) might be discussed.
3. The initial situation is one of breaking bad news, given that the patient has an incurable progressive disease that is going to cause paralysis (but not loss of cognition) and eventual death. The key to longer-term management is multidisciplinary (p. 203). In this case, immediate issues are communication and swallowing problems. An assessment by a speech

and language therapist is needed and the patient may need videofluoroscopic examination of swallowing. In anarthria, alternative communication aids are needed and if swallowing is severely disturbed then a percutaneous feeding gastrostomy (PEG) may be inserted endoscopically.

History 4

1. a. **False**. The travel history is important but there are other immediate priorities; however, you do want to know about recent travel.
   b. **True**. When you take blood, but blood culture and CSF are more important.
   c. **False**. Absolutely the wrong action. He represents your first priority in the whole hospital because he probably has an acute life-threatening infection and time is of the essence. If a crash call came just as you were assessing him, you should still ensure he got antibiotics immediately.
   d. **False**. Should be done, but not yet as it will not alter your immediate management.
   e. **True**. Very important to act swiftly. You should undress him so you can carefully inspect his skin for petechiae typical of meningococcal disease. Look especially around his wrists, ankles, sides of trunk and conjunctivae. Also look immediately for neck stiffness.

2. a. **True**. As quickly as possible in a large dose, e.g. 2g cefotaxime. As he is not unconscious, steroids are not indicated at present.
   b. **True**. While he is being given his first dose of antibiotics.
   c. **False**. Although coagulopathy is a contraindication to lumbar puncture, he does not have any features suggestive of disseminated intravascular coagulation or a history of haemophilia.
   d. **False**. No need as no focal neurological features. If you did the CT scan first, you would be practising defensive, not good, medicine.
   e. **False**. Anticonvulsants are not indicated routinely in patients with meningitis, unless they are already taking them or have had a fit.

3. a. **True**. You should have him put in a side room as quiet is important for these patients with severe headache, and because of the risk of transmission. With the incidence of penicillin-resistant pneumococci increasing, this is more and more important. Ideally, these patients should be admitted an infectious disease unit.
   b. **True**. For 24–48 hours, depending on your hospital's policy.
   c. **False**. Only to those sharing the same house and/or bed. The only hospital staff who require prophylaxis are those who have given mouth-to-mouth resuscitation.

d. **True**. Very important as there could be an evolving outbreak requiring public health measures immediately. **Telephone** notifications are required for meningococcal disease, typhoid and viral haemorrhagic fever.

e. **True**. On balance he will survive (90% chance) but there is still a risk of unilateral or bilateral deafness or other deficit. However, you should be cautious on your first discussion of outcome, until it is clear how he is responding to treatment.

Data interpretation answers

1. The data show impending respiratory failure. The patient has a deteriorating restrictive defect with hypoxia, hypercarbia (ventilatory failure: type 2) and a respiratory acidosis. The immediate management would be to ask a consultant in intensive care to see the patient with a view to ventilation. Action should have been taken on the first set of results.

2. **Data A**. Consistent with herpes simplex encephalitis, consider subarachnoid haemorrhage.
   Data B. Typical of viral encephalitis, possibly herpes simplex, and would still be treated with acyclovir for 10 days or until diagnosis clear.
   Data C. Most likely a subarachnoid haemorrhage or a bloody tap. Key information is missing here: namely whether xanthochromia is present or not. If it is, subarachnoid haemorrhage is most likely.
   Data D. Bacterial meningitis.
   Data E. Viral meningitis (up to 90% of white cells may be polymorphs; in bacterial meningitis over 99% are polymorphs, with the sole exception of *Listeria* meningitis).
   Data F. Tuberculous meningitis. Often the protein is higher than this. It could be fungal miningitis or, rarely, sarcoidosis.

Picture answers

1. a. The most important question is whether the weakness developed suddenly and is now improving (suggesting a vascular cause — stroke) or whether it is progressive. If it is the latter, it is very suspicious of a tumour.
   b. The patient has a irregular large lesion in the right temporoparietal region. It is predominantly low density (black) with enhancement by contrast. The surrounding brain tissue is also low density (high water content — oedema). There may be some compression of the right lateral ventricle, but there is no displacement across the midline.
   c. The appearances are caused by a tumour. The differential diagnosis is between a primary brain tumour and a solitary metastasis. When the mass is solitary, it is impossible to decide between the two diagnoses. You should consider common causes of metastatic disease, such as a bronchial carcinoma (chest radiograph).

d. The clock face shows left-sided neglect. This is caused by the tumour in his non-dominant hemisphere. Less commonly, neglect is seen in left (dominant) hemisphere lesions.

e. The drawing test simply points to a problem that is likely to have a major impact on his day-to-day function. He may deny any neurological problems (anosagnosia) and may try and walk regardless of his paralysis. He may injure his left side because of not attending to it when doing things. He may fail to register objects/people in his left visual field. Food may remain uneaten on the left-hand side of his plate. The left side of his body may not be dressed. The message is that visuospatial problems (neglect) cause a greater disability/handicap than simply weakness down one side.

2. a. The CT scan (Picture 5.4) shows areas of low attenuation (hypodensity) in both the left (most) and right occipital cortices.

b. She has had infarction in both the occipital lobes. A scan done very early (<24 hours: Picture 5.3) following infarction will be normal as the changes take time to develop. In haemorrhage, the high density (owing to the blood) is visible immediately but then becomes isodense and eventually hypodense. Therefore, a CT scan should be done immediately to diagnose haemorrhage but delayed several days to diagnose infarction. In a stroke, the compromise is to arrange a scan at around 3 days.

c. Bilateral occipital lobe damage will result in loss of vision. Patients often do not complain of profound visual loss because the 'receiving' station has been damaged and so they are unaware that they should be seeing things.

d. The occipital lobes are supplied by the posterior cerebral artery, which is the final branch of the vertebrobasilar system. The posterior cerebral artery gives off some penetrating vessels to the posterior limb of the internal capsule (anterior fibres, motor; posterior, sensory).

3. a. The patient is on anticoagulants and has become drowsy. The concern is that he has intracerebral bleeding and you may have to reverse his anticoagulation. A scan will demonstrate this.

b. The scan (Picture 5.5) shows an area of high attenuation surrounded by a rim of low attenuation deep in the left cerebral hemisphere adjacent to the basal ganglia. These appearances are caused by a cerebral haemorrhage.

c. You should measure his prothrombin time (INR) and discuss the problem with the haematologist urgently. He may need factor concentrate and the reversal of anticoagulation, with vitamin K. The problem with the latter is that it makes the patient very difficult to reanticoagulate for several days.

4. a. The CT scan (Picture 5.6) shows extensive blood in the ventricular system (lateral ventricles) and also in the subarachnoid space ('brightness' around the sulci). The appearances are caused by a large subarachnoid haemorrhage with ventricular extension. More commonly, blood will be seen in the subarachnoid space.

b. You should contact the nearest neurosurgical unit to discuss transfer. Given the severity of the bleed, her prognosis is very poor.

c. The three complications of subarachnoid haemorrhage that you should consider are: risk of rebleeding; development of vasospasm, which may produce focal neurological deficits (particularly in the territory where the aneurysm is situated); and, with extensive blood in the subarachnoid space and ventricular system, a communicating or non-communicating hydrocephalus. This is likely to present with drowsiness and vomiting owing to increasing intracranial pressure. Management is by insertion of a shunt.

5. a. The patient has a left wrist drop owing to a radial nerve lesion.

b. You should demonstrate her inability to extend her wrist. If the lesion is in the axilla (crutch palsy), then triceps will be involved and she will have weakness of elbow extension. If the damage is to the radial nerve in the spiral groove of the humerus (Saturday night palsy), then triceps is spared. When examining the rest of the hand, fixate the wrist on a flat surface, otherwise the intrinsic muscles of the hand will appear weak and you will erroneously diagnose median and ulnar nerve palsies.

c. Most likely, she has developed this problem because of pressure on the radial nerve from the wheelchair rest as the arm hangs over the side.

6. a. He has a true 'claw' hand with hyperextension of the metacarpophalangeal joints and flexion of the interphalangeal joints.

b. It is caused by weakness of the intrinsic muscles of the hand with consequent unopposed action of the long extensors of the metacarpophalangeal joints. It is probably caused by a T1 lesion rather than combined ulnar and median nerve palsies. It is not caused by an ulnar nerve lesion alone as this causes clawing confined to the fourth and fifth fingers.

c. Possible causes are a dumb-bell tumour of the T1 nerve root (schwannoma — neurofibromatosis), cervical rib, syringomyelia or Pancoast tumour.

Short note answers

1. Breaking bad news is always difficult. Here, you are being asked to provide more information to a relative, when the diagnosis has already been disclosed. Sketch out your answer using the

framework in the question. The first task would be to go over what Alzheimer's disease is. Alongside this, explain that the diagnosis is based on clinical findings, but if in doubt, you might ask for a detailed psychological assessment. The daughter may have heard of tacrine hydrochloride (anticholinesterase); make clear that the drug does not (currently) have a UK licence. Research studies have reported its usefulness in the early stages of Alzheimer's disease, but it will only ameliorate the symptoms temporarily and carries the risk of liver problems. Whilst explaining about the lack of effective drug treatment, emphasise the support that is available from the different agencies. In a general medical unit, involve the old-age psychiatrists. An important principle is to try not to remove hope. Whilst Alzheimer's disease is progressive, for many patients the course is relatively slow over a number of years.

People may feel very angry about serious illness — partly related to the apparent injustice of the condition 'picking out' either them or one of their close relatives. The anger may focus on you or of the health services in general. Acknowledge people's right to anger in the situation they find themselves in and do not react to it personally. You should remain calm, responding reasonably to questions and issues. At the end of the interview, you should offer to see the person again.

2. a. This patient is, by definition, in status epilepticus and requires senior help. The first task is to go through the 'ABC' routine: airway, breathing, circulation. The second is to control the fits; the usual treatment is with intravenous or rectal diazepam. The next step (which should start immediately) is to gather information. Is the patient a known epileptic? If yes — has there been any change in the medication or compliance? In a patient who is not a known epileptic (and even in a patient with epilepsy), the major division of causes is:

- intracranial, e.g. infection, trauma, vascular, tumour, etc.
- systemic, e.g. overdose (tricyclics), hypoglycaemia (diabetes) and metabolic disturbance (e.g. hyponatraemia).

Your history taking (witnesses, carers, etc.), examination and initial investigations should be done keeping this framework in mind.

Management is governed by your diagnostic list and your overall assessment of the patient's condition, e.g. fluid balance, ventilatory status. In a person who has not been previously diagnosed as being epileptic, you will probably need to start prophylactic anticonvulsants. A *loading dose* (much higher than maintenance dose) of phenytoin can be given i.v. (i.m. doses are very poorly absorbed). The patient may need admission to the ICU, with the fitting controlled by a chlormethiazole infusion. Some patients are managed by paralysis and ventilation.

2. b. The patient is probably in crisis: either myasthenic or cholinergic. You must consider other causes, e.g. infection (or treatment with aminoglycosides). As with (2a) above, your first task is to check ABC. In a person with myasthenia, the 'B' of the assessment is very important. You must measure and record the peak flow rate and arterial blood gases. Ask for senior help/advice; be very careful with a patient who might be tiring and will rapidly deteriorate into ventilatory failure.

3. a. In neurological disease, the first question to ask is 'where is the anatomical site of the problem?' In this case the symptoms point to the retina/optic nerve. The second question relates to the time course. If the problem was vascular, then the history would be of a sudden onset; here it is more gradual and would suggest something evolving. The description best fits with optic neuritis, probably caused by multiple sclerosis.

b. The description is of a left homonymous hemianopia. In the optic tracts and radiation this is usually complete, but in the occipital cortex, the macula may be spared.

c. The bitemporal hemianopia is characteristic of damage around the chiasma. When the problem starts with the *lower* fields, it relates to compression from *above* (think of opposites), possibly because of a craniopharyngioma.

d. The history is consistent with cytomegalovirus retinitis in AIDS. The retinal appearances are characteristic, with white exudates and haemorrhage: 'cottage cheese and ketchup' or 'pizza' (p. 339).

4. In the initial description, there are a number of facts which put the case into context. In a man of this age, think of the common pathologies, for example ischaemic heart disease. The dizziness followed by a seizure implies cerebral anoxia, especially when coupled with the bradycardia post event. Going down this path, the description is in keeping with a **Stokes–Adams attack** (see p. 26). Another possibility would be a dysrhythmia/reduction in cardiac output in association with an acute myocardial infarction. The initial management would be to obtain a 12 lead electrocardiogram (not simply a rhythm strip), take blood for cardiac enzymes (NB in a seizure, the skeletal muscle isoenzyme of creatinine phosphokinase — MM — may be elevated) and consider monitoring on the coronary care unit.

The second path is to think about intracranial causes and examine for focal neurological signs. In a patient with raised intracranial pressure, a bradycardia may occur in conjunction with rising blood pressure. Acutely, this could be caused by bleeding; longer term, the patient may have an intracranial tumour, either primary or secondary.

You should obtain more information Is the patient a diabetic? In any case, a blood glucose must be done. Is the patient a known epileptic? Has the patient taken an overdose? Tricyclic antidepressants usually cause a tachycardia, but digoxin could cause heart block.

Viva answers

Remember that viva questions are very similar in thought processes to short notes. One is writing the material down, the other is giving your thoughts orally. In both, it is important to be logical.

1. The question is asking you to focus your examination on the particular signs that you might expect. The answer is not a 'full neurological examination'.

   You need to check for evidence of raised intracranial pressure: drowsiness, loss of retinal vein pulsation, papilloedema, bradycardia, hypertension. Damage to the right hemisphere is going to cause symptoms on the left side of the body: hemiparesis, hemisensory loss, hemianopia. Particular problems with the right (non-dominant) hemisphere would be inattention and neglect of the left side (visual/sensory). In association with this, the patient may deny any problems (anosagnosia) and may have problems with dressing. Is the patient right or left handed? If left handed then, in 20% of patients, there might be impairment of language.

   If the lesion is in the parietal lobe, there may be particular problems (does not depend on the side of the lesion). Check for arm drift, **astereoagnosis** (inability to integrate the sensory and motor systems to identify an object in the hand), **graphaesthesia** (inability to identify numbers drawn on the hand) and impaired **two-point discrimination.**

   You should also consider the rest of the patient. Is this a brain abscess or a tumour? Are there any clues to the aetiology on general physical examination?

2. Details for this question are given on page 202 and in Table 49. Remember that anticholinergic drugs are used to ameliorate the tremor (limited effect). Side-effects include blurred vision, dry mouth, urinary retention and constipation (blockage of cholinergic receptors). The main aim of therapy is to preserve/boost transmission at the dopamine receptor either by using L-dopa or a dopamine agonist (in the later stages these may be combined). The side-effects are listed in Table 52. Discuss the pharmacokinetics of the drugs in relation to the dosage regimens, for example the phenomena of **on–off** and **peak dose effects**.

3. The question is emphasising the importance of being able to assess conscious level using the Glasgow coma scale (Table 47). Terms such as semiconscious, stuporose, etc. mean different things to different people and you should not use them. The number of possible causes are huge. Consider two steps. First, division into 'brain' causes and 'non-brain' causes. Second, filter these by incidence, i.e. causes in a middle-aged woman; see Box 9.

Haematology

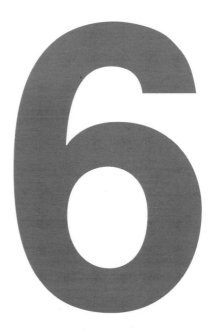

6.1 Background

Introduction

This chapter is structured around disorders of:

- red cells
- white cells
- platelets
- coagulation.

Remember, however, that individual diseases may affect more than one of them.

Learning objectives

You need:

- to know what to ask about in the haematological history and what to look for on examination
- to feel confident in looking at a full blood count result and know what each of the major parameters implies
- to understand the other main haematological investigations and when to carry them out
- to know which situations commonly confront a house officer and understand how to manage them
- to know enough about the other major haematological diseases to recognise them, to make appropriate and timely referrals and to explain them to your patients.

Physiology

The marrow is a large organ, approaching the size of the liver. In adults, most of it is in the flat bones, including the sternum, pelvis and vertebrae. White blood cell precursors form 75% of the marrow and most of the rest consists of erythroid precursors. Megakaryocytes (from which platelets are formed) are scattered throughout. It may seem surprising that so much of the marrow is devoted to the white cell series, given that there are 500 times as many red cells as white cells in the circulation. However, erythrocytes have a mean life of 120 days whereas white cells have a circulating lifespan measured in hours. Even in health, marrow is an extremely active tissue which is able to respond to sudden stresses like haemorrhage and infection. All blood cells are derived from multipotent, uncommitted stem cells. These differentiate into the lines of committed stem cells from which red cells, platelets, monocytes, granulocytes and lymphocytes are formed. The processes of differentiation and proliferation are controlled by growth factors, including interleukins, colony-stimulating factors and erythropoietin.

Clinical assessment

This begins as the patient walks into the room or you go to the bedside:

- look for pallor and signs of bruising/bleeding
- is the patient unkempt or thin and is there a smell of alcohol?
- take note of racial origin and gender

History

Specific symptoms

Anaemia. The symptoms include:

- tiredness
- breathlessness
- chest pain
- ankle swelling.

Tiredness is thought of as the classical symptom of anaemia but most tired people are not anaemic and some patients (particularly elderly ones) have few symptoms despite profound anaemia. This is usually because the anaemia has developed slowly and their lifestyle does not make heavy demands for oxygen. Apart from tiredness, impaired oxygen delivery causes breathlessness, light-headedness and faints. It worsens angina and can precipitate heart failure, especially if it is superimposed on coronary artery disease.

Red cell excess (polycythaemia). The symptomatology is covered on page 238.

Leucopenia. The symptoms of leucopenia include:

- mouth ulceration
- infective symptoms.

Mouth ulceration must always be taken seriously in an at-risk patient. Infective symptoms occur with both neutropenia and lymphopenia.

White cell excess (Leukaemia and lymphoma). The symptomatology is relatively specific to individual diseases which are covered on pages 240–244.

Platelet/coagulation disease. Symptoms include:

- easy bruising
- bleeding
- thromboses.

Thrombocytopenia causes petechial haemorrhages and bruising. When it is severe, it also causes bleeding from the gums or into the gut. Impaired coagulation more commonly causes bleeding into soft tissues than overt external bleeding. Haemophilia and other hereditary clotting disorders may cause prolonged bleeding from minor injuries, but they usually present with bleeding into joints. Remember to ask about menorrhagia and bleeding problems after dental extractions and surgery. Thrombophilia (increased tendency to clot) causes recurrent venous and arterial thromboses.

General history

You should take a detailed drug history from every patient. Remember not just the prescription drugs but also medicines bought over the counter. Take a family history if the patient has haemolytic anaemia, a bleeding tendency or thrombophilia and construct a family tree if it is positive. Take a dietary and alcohol history. Note the length of history and take particular note if the symptoms suggest that more than one aspect of haematological function is affected (e.g. symptoms of infection, bruising *and* anaemia). Be alert to symptoms of systemic disease, such as weight loss, dyspepsia, change in bowel habit, night sweats and pruritus.

Examination

Your examination (Fig. 43) should include

- a thorough and systematic examination of the skin
- careful palpation of all groups of lymph nodes (including deep palpation of the abdomen)
- inspection of the conjunctivae and mouth
- palpation of the spleen and liver
- a thorough search for signs of infection.

Red cell disorders

The physical signs of anaemia are extremely subjective. Examine the conjunctivae which are less affected by variations in capillary blood flow than the skin or nail beds. Examine the sclerae carefully for jaundice

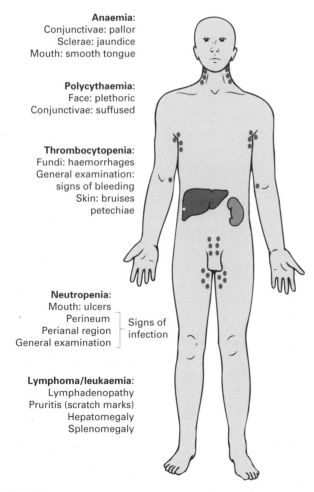

Anaemia:
Conjunctivae: pallor
Sclerae: jaundice
Mouth: smooth tongue

Polycythaemia:
Face: plethoric
Conjunctivae: suffused

Thrombocytopenia:
Fundi: haemorrhages
General examination:
signs of bleeding
Skin: bruises
petechiae

Neutropenia:
Mouth: ulcers
Perineum
Perianal region } Signs of infection
General examination

Lymphoma/leukaemia:
Lymphadenopathy
Pruritis (scratch marks)
Hepatomegaly
Splenomegaly

Fig. 43
Physical signs of haematological disease. Uncommon signs are omitted.

(not detectable until serum bilirubin is raised to three times normal); this is present in haemolytic but not other types of anaemia. Look at the patient's face: a plethoric complexion with suffusion of the conjunctivae is a sign of polycythaemia. Examine the abdomen for splenomegaly, which is a prominent feature of chronic extravascular haemolysis.

White cell disorders

Neutropenia should be considered in any patient with severe oral ulceration/candidiasis. Examination for lymphadenopathy requires skill, not just in knowing where and how to palpate but in interpreting the findings. If there are palpable lymph nodes, record:

- whether they are hard, firm or soft
- whether they are tender or non-tender
- their approximate size
- whether they are mobile and discrete or matted together.

Axillary and inguinal lymphadenopathy is commonly found in normal people, particularly if they have a history of injury or infection. Pathological lymph nodes are larger, present in the neck and epitrochlear region of the elbow and sometimes coalescent or matted. Lymph nodes which are enlarged because of infection are smaller than those of lymphoma (usually less than 2 cm) and more likely to be discrete. The distribution of lymphadenopathy in Hodgkin's and non-Hodgkin's lymphoma is considered on page 242. Assess the size of the spleen and liver and search for para-aortic and pelvic nodes. Mild splenomegaly may be caused by an infection but moderate or massive splenomegaly suggests lymphoma, myelofibrosis or chronic leukaemia. Hepatomegaly may be found in myeloproliferative diseases. Tissue infiltration (particularly of the gums) occurs in some leukaemias.

Platelet and coagulation disorders

Petechial haemorrhages are a sign of thrombocytopenia. They are characteristically seen first over the lower legs, where capillary pressure is highest. Later they become generalised, and may coalesce as bruises (ecchymoses), particularly over the arms. Inspect the gums for bleeding and the fundi for retinal haemorrhages, which should be taken very seriously as a sign of impending cerebral haemorrhage.

Thrombocytosis and other hypercoagulable states have no specific physical signs other than those of arterial or venous thrombosis.

Investigation

Learning objectives

You should know when to measure and how to interpret:
- a full blood count, film, differential white count, platelet count and erythrocyte sedimentation rate (ESR)

- haematinics: iron and total iron-binding capacity, ferritin, vitamin B$_{12}$, folate and red cell folate
- coagulation tests: international normalised ratio (INR), prothrombin time (PT), activated partial thromboplastin time (APTT), fibrin degradation products.

You should know the indications for, and the information which can be gained from:

- bone marrow examination
- lymph node biopsy.

Blood count and film

When you take blood, you can affect the result by:

- excessive cuffing: a prolonged increase in venous pressure artificially increases the haematocrit
- being slow to put blood in the tube or not mixing it thoroughly: coagulation in the tube gives a falsely low platelet count.

Automated counters measure concentrations (per unit volume) of red cells, haemoglobin, platelets and leucocytes (lymphocytes, monocytes, neutrophils, eosinophils and basophils). They also measure the percentage of red cells present as reticulocytes (newly released cells) and calculate indices which describe the size of red cells and platelets and the degree of haemoglobinisation. Normal values for adults are shown in Table 1 (p. 4). In addition, a dried and stained blood film can be inspected to assess the morphology of the cells and detect abnormal cells. Some of the terms you will come across on blood film reports are given in Table 53.

Interpreting the haemoglobin and red cell indices

Anaemia is diagnosed when there is a reduction in the concentration of haemoglobin caused by a reduced number of red cells or a reduced amount of haemoglobin within the cells. An *increase* in haemoglobin concentration resulting from an increased number of red cells per unit volume is termed erythrocytosis.

Whenever you are told that a patient is anaemic, you should ask for the mean cell volume (MCV), by which anaemias are classified (explained further on page 231). The cell counter also tells you how similar the red cells are to one another in size. This is expressed as the red cell distribution width (RDW). A low RDW signifies a normal, homogeneous population of cells. An increasing RDW signifies heterogeneity in cell size as a result of:

- active haemopoiesis, because immature red cells (reticulocytes) are large
- treatment of iron deficiency, due to a mixture of microcytic and normocytic cells
- mixed deficiency, giving both small and large 'diseased' cells.

Reticulocytes can be counted automatically and are expressed as a percentage of the total red cell count.

White cells and platelets

Changes in cell counts are diagnosed by the automated counter. Examination of the film gives an accurate dif-

Table 53 Terms used to describe abnormalities of red blood cells

Term	Description
Hypochromia	Defective haemoglobinisation, as in some anaemias
Anisochromia	Variable haemoglobinisation, as in haemolysis
Polychromasia	Bluish tinge to the red cells, reflects increased haemopoiesis
Microcytosis	Small size (p. 231)
Macrocytosis	Large size (p. 231)
Anisocytosis	Variable size, as in iron deficiency
Poikilocytosis	Abnormal shape; as in myelofibrosis (p. 000)
Erythrocytosis	Increased number of red cells
Spherocytosis, elliptocytosis	Abnormal shape resulting from congenital or acquired cell membrane defect
Sickle cells	Abnormal shape resulting from abnormal haemoglobin
Target cells	Increased surface: volume ratio; as in liver disease
Fragmented or damaged cells	Trauma to red cells (p. 248)
Inclusions	
Basophilic stippling	Immature cells resulting from accelerated haemopoiesis
Iron granules (siderocytes)	Seen with special stain in sideroblastic anaemia
Howell–Jolly bodies	Nuclear remnants seen after splenectomy

ferential count and detects cells such as leukaemic blast cells. It also detects morphological changes such as the degree of lobulation of the neutrophil nuclei, which depends on their age. In infection, neutrophils are relatively immature and may appear as bands rather than with the normal multilobulated appearance; a 'left shift'. Conversely, the neutrophils are hypermature ('right shifted') in megaloblastic anaemia because vitamin B$_{12}$ deficiency impairs haemopoiesis (p. 233). There may also be cytoplasmic abnormalities, e.g. vacuolation or heavy granulation of neutrophils during bacterial infection.

Platelets

A simple platelet count is the clue to most platelet diseases.

Erythrocyte sedimentation rate

The erythrocyte sedimentation rate (ESR) is a very crude test which measures the rate (in mm/h) at which red cells sediment. Abnormal proteins in inflammatory conditions and myeloma cause rapid sedimentation. The ESR is, therefore, a non-specific marker of infection, inflammation and neoplasia. In some hospitals, blood viscosity or **acute-phase proteins** are measured as more reliable markers of inflammation.

Haematinics

The blood count must always be checked before measuring haematinics because it is unlikely that a patient has significant iron, vitamin B_{12} or folate deficiency if the count is normal. An extremely high index of suspicion (e.g. suspected subacute combined degeneration of the cord, p. 210) would be needed to justify these extra measurements in the face of a normal blood count. Similarly, it is wasteful to measure serum iron or ferritin if the diagnosis of iron deficiency is obvious from the clinical context and blood count. With those provisos, measure:

- vitamin B_{12} and folate in patients with macrocytic anaemia
- iron in patients with microcytosis
- all three in a patient with anaemia and a normal MCV (to rule out a mixed deficiency although a high RDW would normally make that obvious).

The diagnosis of iron, vitamin B_{12} and folate deficiency are considered on pages 231 and 233.

Tests of coagulation and fibrinolysis

These are discussed on page 246.

Bone marrow examination

Bone marrow can be examined either as an aspirate from the sternum or iliac crest or as a trephine biopsy from the iliac crest. Marrow aspirate is useful for detailed cytology, cell counts and assessment of iron stores. Trephine biopsies are useful for judging cellularity, detecting tumour and diagnosing myelofibrosis (p. 242).

Remember that marrow examination is not infallible in detecting tumour deposits because they may be absent from the area sampled. Marrow aspiration is a painful procedure which should not be done without good indications. These include:

- to confirm iron deficiency or megaloblastic anaemia, if the diagnosis is in doubt or the patient does not respond to treatment
- to investigate unexplained anaemia
- to investigate suspected leukaemia, myeloma or other haematological malignancy
- to monitor response to the treatment of leukaemia
- to diagnose cancer, where there is circumstantial evidence of marrow involvement
- to investigate agranulocytosis or thrombocytopenia
- to stain and obtain cultures for suspected tuberculosis, histoplasmosis and leishmaniasis.

In some conditions — notably myelofibrosis and aplastic anaemia — bone marrow aspiration may be unsuccessful. A 'dry tap' is pathological and of diagnostic value.

Lymph node biopsy

Lymph node biopsy is the definitive investigation to diagnose lymphoma and identify its histological type. It is also used to diagnose disseminated cancer and other causes of lymphadenopathy. The features of lymph nodes which make them 'suspicious' are described on page 229, and other clinical features suggesting lymphoma are described on page 242. Which node should

be biopsied is partly a surgical decision and partly determined by their 'feel'. Lymph node biopsies are usually taken under general anaesthesia. The specimen will be ruined for some analyses if it is put straight into formalin. It should be promptly handled by a skilled histology technician. Remember to request culture if tuberculosis is suspected.

6.2 Red cell disorders

Erythropoiesis:

- is controlled by erythropoietin, which is secreted by the kidneys
- is stimulated by hypoxia
- requires an adequate supply of folic acid, vitamin B_{12} and iron
- is inhibited by poor nutrition, systemic disease and local disease within the marrow.

Learning objectives

You should understand:
- the range of diseases which cause anaemia
- how they do so
- how to diagnose and treat them
- what polycythaemia is, what can cause it and how it causes symptoms and signs.

Anaemias

Think of anaemias in terms of:

- decreased red cell production
- increased loss.

This classification is expanded in Table 54. Note that the commonest form, iron-deficiency anaemia, often results from a combination of both. The MCV is central to the diagnosis of anaemia. Remember that:

- iron deficiency causes microcytosis
- B_{12} and folate deficiency cause macrocytosis (other causes are covered on p. 233)
- the anaemia of marrow suppression is often normocytic.

Exceptions to these rules are discussed under individual diseases. Given the haemoglobin and MCV, white cell count, platelet and reticulocyte counts and a description of the blood film, you can make a working diagnosis in most cases.

Iron-deficiency anaemia

This is the most common and, to the generalist, most important anaemia because it:

- is a significant public health problem
- may be the presentation of an occult GI carcinoma at a curable stage
- is eminently treatable whatever its cause.

Iron deficiency is caused by an imbalance between dietary availability and blood loss, so much of the population is iron deficient in areas of the developing world where GI parasites are endemic. Active growth, pregnancy and lactation increase the demand for iron and may unmask deficiency. The prevalance of depleted iron stores in women of menstrual age may be as high as 20% and that iron deficiency can persist into the postmenopausal years if they have a poor diet and do not replete their iron stores. Iron deficiency is much less prevalent in adult men and, therefore, more likely to be caused by an occult carcinoma or other underlying disease.

There are sizeable iron stores in the liver, reticuloendothelial system and marrow, as well as in the erythrocytes themselves, so negative iron balance must exist for some time before anaemia develops. For the same reason, replenishment of iron stores takes longer than the restoration of haemopoiesis, and iron treatment should be continued after the haemoglobin has returned to normal.

Causes
These are:

- blood loss
- dietary deficiency
- malabsorption.

Iron may be malabsorbed as a result of small intestinal disease or after gastrectomy.

Sources of blood loss, in order of frequency, are:

- menstruation
- the GI tract (Chapter 3)
- the urinary tract.

Table 54 A classification of the anaemias

	Decreased production	Increased destruction/ loss
Acute haemorrhage		+
Haematinic deficiency		
Iron deficiency	+	±
B$_{12}$ deficiency	+	
Folate deficiency	+	
Hypoplastic anaemias		
Idiopathic	+	
Secondary	+	
Anaemia of chronic disease	+	
Marrow replacement		
Leukaemias	+	
Myeloma	+	
Other tumours	+	
Congenital haemolysis		
Spherocytosis and elliptocytosis	±	+
Sickle cell disease		+
Thalassaemia		+
Glucose 6-phosphate dehydrogenase deficiency		+
Acquired haemolysis		
Autoimmune		+
Microangiopathic		+
Hypersplenism		+

In practice, it may be difficult to decide whether menorrhagia is the sole cause of blood loss. If in doubt, suspect another disease.

Common causes of GI blood loss are:

- gastritis, peptic ulcer or oesophagitis, particularly in patients on aspirin, NSAIDs or steroids
- diverticular disease
- carcinoma of the stomach, caecum or colon
- angiodysplasia of the colon, an increasingly recognised cause in elderly people
- oesophageal varices.

A less common cause is Meckel's diverticulum.

Although a small minority of iron-deficient patients have GI tumours, it is worthwhile identifying them because diagnosis at the stage of a predominantly mucosal lesion may allow curative surgery.

Clinical and haematological signs
Symptoms and signs were covered earlier and in Figure 45. Early signs on the blood film are variability in size and shape of the red cells. In established iron deficiency, they are hypochromic and microcytic and 'pencil cells' may be seen.

Diagnosis and further investigation
Iron deficiency is overwhelmingly the most common UK cause of microcytosis but it also occurs in thalassaemia trait and, sometimes, in the anaemia of chronic disease. If there is doubt, iron deficiency is diagnosed by measuring serum iron and total iron-binding capacity. These are measured together because binding protein deficiency may lower the serum iron concentration without signifying true iron deficiency; <10% saturation of iron-binding capacity is diagnostic of iron deficiency. Measurement of serum ferritin is a better reflection of iron stores (particularly to detect iron overload, as in haemachromatosis). Absence of stainable marrow iron stores and a reticulocyte response to iron replacement are definitive evidence of iron deficiency.

Stool samples are often tested for occult blood to confirm or exclude the GI tract as the site of blood loss, but they may be falsely positive or negative. Dietary assessment and tests for malabsorption (p. 112) may be indicated. The investigations are not complete until a patient with undiagnosed iron deficiency has had gastroscopy, colonoscopy and/or barium studies to look for a site of blood loss.

Management
There is little to choose between the many formulations of oral iron. Ferrous sulphate is usually prescribed. It may cause nausea, abdominal pain, diarrhoea or constipation, in which case the dose should be reduced or a different iron salt given. A response should be seen within 1 week of starting treatment and a rise in haemoglobin of 10 g/l each week is to be expected. Treatment is continued for 3 months after the haemoglobin has returned to normal to replenish iron stores.

Megaloblastic anaemias

Vitamin B_{12} (cobalamin) and folic acid are coenzymes for cellular metabolism, particularly haemopoiesis. Deficiency affects DNA synthesis in all marrow cell lines and the red cell precursors develop 'megaloblastic' morphological changes. Ineffective erythropoiesis reduces the production of mature red cells and they are enlarged (macrocytic). Formation of platelets and granulocytes is also impaired.

Vitamin B_{12} and folate deficiency are not the only causes of macrocytosis; others, in approximate order of frequency, are:

- common causes
  - alcohol abuse
  - liver disease
  - active haemopoiesis (immature red cells are large): haemolytic anaemias, blood loss
- less common causes
  - myelodysplasia
  - aplastic anaemia
  - antifolate drugs: methotrexate, phenytoin.

However, vitamin B_{12} and folate deficiency are the only common conditions to produce the typical megaloblastic bone marrow appearances. They have identical haematological features but differ in their causes and non-haematological manifestations. This section will first present the common features and then the differences between them.

Clinical and haematological features

Patients typically present with symptoms of anaemia and malaise.

These develop insidiously and the anaemia may be very severe by the time the diagnosis is made. Elderly people, in particular, may tolerate it surprisingly well until they present with heart failure or angina resulting from tissue hypoxia. There may be

- mild jaundice caused by haemolysis of the defective red cells
- fever
- glossitis
- splenomegaly (very unusually).

Although moderate neutropenia and thrombocytopenia are common, they are not usually symptomatic. Vitamin B_{12} deficiency may, uncommonly, present with its neurological complications (see Chapter 5). There may be features of an underlying GI disease in either vitamin B_{12}, folate or a mixed deficiency anaemia.

Whatever the cause, the blood film shows:

- pancytopenia
- macrocytosis: large oval red cells
- hypersegmentation of the neutrophil nuclei (termed a 'right shift')
- megaloblasts in peripheral blood in severe cases.

This haematological picture is so characteristic that the diagnosis can generally be made without bone marrow examination, but that is the definitive way of demonstrating megaloblastic change.

Vitamin B_{12} deficiency

Vitamin B_{12} is present in meat and dairy produce. It is absorbed as a complex with intrinsic factor (IF) produced by the gastric parietal cells. Pure dietary deficiency is exceptionally rare because there are large hepatic stores. It can occur in alcoholics. More commonly, deficiency is caused by

- autoimmune damage to the gastric parietal cells: pernicious anaemia
- destruction of vitamin B_{12} by bacterial overgrowth in diverticulae, blind loops or fistulae
- disease of the terminal ileum where the B_{12}–IF complex is absorbed: usually Crohn's disease
- pancreatic exocrine deficiency
- gastrectomy.

Pernicious anaemia

Pernicious anaemia is an organ-specific autoimmune disease caused by antibodies to gastric parietal cells and intrinsic factor. It

- is commoner in women than men
- may develop from adolescence onwards but is most common in middle to old age.

It is associated with:

- blood group A
- failure of gastric acid secretion
- an increased risk of gastric carcinoma
- an increased incidence of the other organ-specific autoimmune diseases, including vitiligo, diabetes mellitus, hypothyroidism and Addison's disease.

The diagnosis is made by demonstrating a reduced serum vitamin B_{12} concentration, and intrinsic factor antibodies. It is confirmed by the Schilling test, in which radiolabelled B_{12} is given on two occasions, first on its own and then with oral intrinsic factor. Urinary excretion of the label is measured. In pernicious anaemia, there is malabsorption which is correctable by intrinsic factor. Other causes of malabsorption are not correctable.

Neurological effects of B_{12} deficiency

Full blood counts are now so widely available that B_{12} deficiency is usually recognised and treated before it has any significant neurological effects; however, some individuals may develop neurological effects with little or no anaemia. These include:

- optic atrophy
- dementia
- subacute combined degeneration of the cord (Chapter 5).

Treatment

One simple rule is that folate and vitamin B_{12} should always be given together in megaloblastic anaemia, at least until the haematinic results are known, because folate treatment alone can increase haemopoiesis in patients with pure vitamin B_{12} deficiency and actually precipitate neurological complications. Patients with vitamin B_{12} deficiency should be given injections of vitamin B_{12} weekly for 6 weeks and then 3-monthly indefinitely thereafter. The reticulocyte response should be checked after 7 days. Potassium supplements are needed in some cases, as well as iron and folate, because cellular anabolism requires potassium. Whether or not patients with severe megaloblastic anaemia should be transfused is controversial because even careful transfusion can precipitate heart failure. If it is done, it should be slow and with diuretic cover and should not aim to restore haemoglobin immediately to normal.

Folate deficiency

Folate is absorbed in the upper small intestine. The body stores are relatively small so folate deficiency develops earlier in malabsorption syndromes than does iron or vitamin B_{12} deficiency. For the same reason, folate deficiency is more likely to have a purely dietary cause, to develop during pregnancy or to be precipitated by active haemopoiesis in haemolytic states. Folate metabolism is vulnerable to a wide range of drugs and is actually the target of some chemotherapeutic agents, e.g. methotrexate. These are the main causes of folate deficiency:

- dietary, for example in:
  — alcoholism
  — elderly or neglected people
- increased demand
  — pregnancy
  — active haemopoiesis, e.g. haemolytic anaemia
- malabsorption
  — coeliac disease
  — pancreatic insufficiency
  — postgastrectomy
  — Crohn's disease
- drugs which interfere with folate absorption: phenytoin
- drugs which interfere with folate metabolism: methotrexate, phenytoin, trimethoprim.

Investigation of the cause of folate deficiency will depend on the context in which it is diagnosed. If there is a clear dietary or drug cause, no further investigation is needed. Otherwise, investigation for malabsorption is indicated.

Diagnosis
A low serum or red cell folate concentration confirms the diagnosis. Of the two, red cell folate more accurately reflects total body folate stores.

Prevention and treatment
Pregnant women are routinely given prophylactic oral folate. Alcoholic or poorly nourished patients should be given folate as part of their rehabilitation. Proven folate deficiency is treated with oral folic acid. As explained above, this must never be given alone in macrocytic anaemia unless vitamin B_{12} deficiency has been excluded. If there is evidence of iron deficiency, oral iron should also be given.

Aplastic/hypoplastic anaemia

Aplastic anaemia is a rare condition which may be congenital or acquired. It may be primary (no cause identified) or secondary to:

- drugs, e.g. chloramphenicol, chemotherapy, zidovudine, ganciclovir, phenylbutazone
- irradiation
- chemicals
- infection, e.g. viral hepatitis
- autoimmune disease.

There is usually leucopenia and thrombocytopenia as well as anaemia, although pure red cell aplasia may occur. The aplasia may be *transient* or *chronic*, and *partial* (hypoplastic) or *complete* (aplastic). The symptoms and signs depend on the relative degrees of anaemia, thrombocytopenia and neutropenia. The red cells are normocytic or slightly macrocytic. The marrow trephine biopsy is hypoplastic. The differential diagnosis is with other causes of pancytopenia, particularly marrow replacement/fibrosis. Severe aplastic anaemia has a high mortality. A significant number of patients respond to antilymphocyte globulin, but the best chance of cure lies in bone marrow transplantation from an HLA-identical sibling donor. Androgens and corticosteroids have occasionally been effective. Supportive care of the neutropenic patient (p. 239) and transfusions of platelet and red cells are needed. With time, platelet and red cell antibodies develop and may complicate management.

Leucoerythroblastic anaemia

This term is used to describe a blood film showing immature leucocytes and erythroblasts. It has many causes, notably marrow infiltration with a solid tumour, myeloma, lymphoma, leukaemia or myelofibrosis. It is investigated by marrow aspiration/biopsy.

Anaemia of chronic disease

This is, second to iron deficiency, the most common anaemia you are likely to encounter. Common causes are:

- chronic infection
- renal failure
- liver disease
- malignancy
- autoimmune disease.

The typical pattern is a normocytic or microcytic anaemia with reduced serum iron and total iron-binding capacity, intact marrow iron stores and reduced erythroblast haemosiderin. It is usually caused by suppressed erythropoiesis, although other mechanisms such as haemolysis may contribute. The anaemia is often relatively mild. There is no specific treatment other than management of the causative disease.

Haemolytic anaemias

Destruction of red cells by a disease process either intrinsic or extrinsic to the cell causes:

- shortened red cell survival
- increased erythropoiesis
- anaemia if erythropoiesis cannot keep pace with red cell destruction.

There may be morphological changes in the red cells, giving a clue to the cause of haemolysis.

In most haemolytic anaemias, red cells are removed by macrophages of the reticuloendothelial system, chiefly in the spleen. This process is termed **extravascular haemolysis**. Breakdown of haemoglobin increases the plasma level of unconjugated bilirubin, causing clinically overt jaundice in severe haemolysis. Splenomegaly and pigment gall stones may occur.

When there is rapid breakdown of red cells within the circulation (**intravascular haemolysis**), haemoglobin is liberated. Initially, it is bound to plasma proteins called haptoglobins. When the binding capacity of haptoglobins is exceeded, free haemoglobin is filtered in the kidneys and converted to haemosiderin in renal tubular cells. Haemosiderin can be detected in urine.

The haemolytic anaemias are a heterogeneous group of disorders which can be classified into congenital and acquired forms. Congenital haemolytic anaemias include:

- haemoglobinopathies
  — sickle cell disease
  — thalassaemia
- membrane defects
  — spherocytosis
  — elliptocytosis
- red cell enzyme defects
  — glucose 6-phosphatase deficiency.

Acquired haemolytic anaemias include:

- autoimmune (p. 236)
- non-immune
  — microangiopathic haemolytic anaemia
  — prosthetic heart valve
  — drug or toxin induced.

Diagnosis

The clinical features of haemolytic anaemias are those of the anaemia, the sequelae of haemolysis and any underlying cause. Patients with chronic haemolytic anaemia are prone to leg ulceration and may develop pigment gall stones.

Laboratory features of haemolysis are:

- evidence of increased erythropoiesis: reticulocytosis, polychromasia, erythroid hyperplasia of bone marrow
- evidence of increased red cell breakdown: increased plasma unconjugated bilirubin and urinary urobilinogen, reduced plasma haptoglobin.

Congenital haemolytic anaemias

The only situations covered here are those that you might expect to encounter as a house officer.

Sickle syndromes

Sickle syndromes are caused by a recessively inherited amino acid substitution in the haemoglobin A molecule, which causes it to become insoluble and cross-link under hypoxic conditions. This causes haemolysis, 'stickiness' and microvascular occlusion.

Africans are most often affected, so heterozygotes are common in areas with a high African population. They may develop symptoms during any illness which causes hypoxia or after surgery.

'Sickle trait' can be diagnosed by the in vitro 'sickle test' and by haemoglobin electrophoresis.

Homozygotes are more severely affected. They have a chronic haemolytic anaemia and may have sickling crises precipitated by:

- hypoxia
- dehydration
- infection
- other systemic stresses.

During crises, microvascular occlusion causes infarcts of bone and soft tissues. Patients experience severe pain, fever and malaise. Splenic infarcts lead to hyposplenism and an increased risk of pneumococcal septicaemia. Salmonella osteomyelitis is common in areas of infarcted bone. There may be soft tissue complications, including retinopathy, acute renal papillary necrosis and leg ulcers. Pigment gall stones are common. Pregnancy is hazardous. Prophylactic penicillin is required to prevent pneumococcal septicaemia.

Sickling crises are treated by

- keeping the patient warm
- oxygen
- intravenous fluids
- opiate analgesia
- antibiotics.

The thalassaemias

The thalassaemias are a group of congenital haemolytic anaemias caused by mutations or gene deletions affecting the α- and β-globin chains (α- and β-thalassaemia, respectively). They vary in severity from a chance finding in an asymptomatic individual to a disease which is incompatible with life. Synthesis of abnormal haemoglobin causes 'ineffective erythropoiesis'. There is microcytosis and the cells are irregular in size, shape and degree of haemoglobinisation.

Heterozygotes (thalassaemia trait) usually remain asymptomatic but may become mildly anaemic during intercurrent infection or pregnancy. Remember thalassaemia trait in the differential diagnosis of microcytic anaemia. Thalassaemia major is not considered further here.

Acquired haemolytic anaemia

Autoimmune haemolytic anaemia

Autoimmune haemolytic anaemia (AIHA) is most commonly idiopathic but may be caused by:

- autoimmune disease, e.g. SLE
- neoplasia, e.g. chronic lymphocytic leukaemia
- infection, e.g. infectious mononucleosis, mycoplasma
- drugs, e.g. methyldopa.

The anti-red cell antibody involved may cause haemolysis at body temperature ('warm AIHA': usually IgG) or only at temperatures well below 37°C ('cold AIHA': usually IgM) and the clinical picture varies accordingly.

Cold AIHA (cold haemagglutinin disease). Haemolysis is mediated by complement and usually intravascular, classically causing episodes of dark urine (haemoglobinuria) after cold exposure. At the same time, agglutination of red cells in peripheral capillaries may cause peripheral cyanosis, Raynaud's-like symptoms and even gangrene. Cold haemagglutinin disease may occur as a transient problem after infectious diseases such as infectious mononucleosis or mycoplasma pneumonia. Red cell agglutinates can be seen on a blood film at room temperature.

Warm AIHA. Haemolysis is usually extravascular, particularly in the spleen, and leads to jaundice and splenomegaly. The blood film shows spherocytosis.

Direct antiglobulin test. In either case, the definitive test for AIHA is the direct antiglobulin test, in which antibodies are demonstrated on the red cell surface by the addition of anti-human globulin, which will cause agglutination.

Management of warm AIHA. Warm AIHA can be treated with:

- steroids
- splenectomy
- immunosuppressive therapy.

Management of cold AIHA. Patients with cold agglutinins should be kept warm; they respond less well to steroids and splenectomy. Blood transfusion may be needed for haemolytic crises, but cross-matching can be difficult.

Non-immune acquired haemolytic anaemias

The non-immune acquired haemolytic anaemias are caused by:

- fibrin deposited in the microcirculation, as in DIC (p. 248)
- heart valves or other mechanical prostheses
- toxic causes, including uraemia, lead poisoning and some drugs.

In the case of DIC and mechanical red cell damage, schistocytes (fragmented red cells) are seen on the blood film.

Blood transfusion

There are two quite distinct indications for blood transfusion:

- to restore volume after acute blood loss
- to restore the red cell mass in a patient with anaemia and a normal blood volume (compensated anaemia).

Acute blood loss

Acute blood loss is caused by trauma, haemorrhage, usually from the GI tract, and surgery. If haemorrhage is severe, there is circulatory collapse. The physical signs are from the blood loss itself and from volume depletion (p. 167).

You should ideally transfuse whole blood and give it as quickly as necessary to restore the circulation, monitoring the pulse, blood pressure and urine output. Remember that the haemoglobin concentration is no guide to the severity of acute blood loss because it takes time for haemodilution to occur.

Transfusion for anaemia

In this situation, plasma volume is normal despite lack of red cells. This process of compensation takes hours or days after acute blood loss. The indications for transfusion are less strong than after acute blood loss because:

- the patient is not shocked
- treating the underlying cause of anaemia is a more permanent (albeit slower) solution than transfusing red cells, which have a short lifespan
- transfusion increases blood volume and may cause heart failure.

Transfusion may nevertheless be indicated to:

- relieve symptoms
- prepare anaemic patients for surgery
- increase the red cell mass in case of further bleeding.

As a rule of thumb, blood transfusion:

- is rarely indicated if the haemoglobin concentration is above 100 g/l
- may be indicated between 80 and 100 g/l
- is most likely to be needed below 80 g/l.

Iron deficiency — which is usually the result of blood loss — is a much clearer indication than vitamin B_{12} or folate deficiency, which should be treated with haematinics. Transfusion for anaemia is particularly hazardous if the patient is in heart failure, when packed red cells should be given with an i.v. loop diuretic and close observation of the patient's haemodynamic state. Blood transfusion is expensive and potentially hazardous. It should not be 'dished out' carelessly.

Blood groups

The main ABO system consists of two markers inherited as Mendelian dominant traits from the parents. The red cells of an individual may carry the A antigen (group A), the B antigen (group B), both (group AB) or neither (group O). The antigens are carried on many tissues other than red cells and individuals are exposed early in life to those antigens which they do not carry. Thus group A individuals have agglutinins to the B antigen and vice versa; group O individuals have agglutinins to both antigens and group AB individuals have agglutinins to neither. The importance of this system to blood transfusion is that donated cells may be lysed by host agglutinins; lysis of host cells by donor agglutinins is not usually a significant problem. Table 55 summarises the system and reminds you that group O subjects are 'universal donors' because their cells have neither antigen and will not be lysed if they are transfused into group A, B or AB recipients. Group AB subjects are 'universal recipients' because they have agglutinins against neither antigen.

The rhesus (D) blood group system is also conceptually very simple. About 85% of the Caucasian population (and a higher proportion of Asians) carry the D (or rhesus) antigen on their red cells. Those who are rhesus negative may develop antibodies against the D antigen but only if exposed to it by blood transfusion or, in pregnancy, by placental leakage.

Cross-matching

The first step in cross-matching is to determine the patient's ABO and rhesus blood groups. Donor blood of an appropriate group is then cross-matched both at room temperature and 37°C, to detect cold and warm antibodies. There is an increasing move towards storing the patient's own blood in preparation for elective surgery, eliminating the risks of cross-infection and incompatible transfusion (autologous transfusion).

Complications of transfusion

The major risks of HIV and hepatitis B and C infection can be effectively eliminated by careful screening of donor blood. Other potential complications are:

- minor febrile reactions
- haemolytic reactions
- hypocalcaemia
- chronic iron overload.

Minor febrile reactions

Minor febrile reactions are not uncommon, particularly in patients who have developed platelet and/or white cell antibodies from repeated transfusions. They may be prevented by washing the red cells before transfusion, or using a filter to trap white cells and platelets.

Acute, severe haemolytic reactions

These are fortunately rare, invariably caused by ABO incompatibility (e.g. a group O recipient receiving group A blood) and almost always caused by elementary errors like the incorrect labelling of blood samples or incomplete pretransfusion checks. They are likely to lead to undefendable litigation. The patient may develop pyrexia, chest or abdominal pain and pass black urine, rapidly progressing to shock, acute renal failure and disseminated intravascular coagulation. If a haemolytic reaction is suspected, you should:

- stop the transfusion immediately
- give intravenous hydrocortisone and chlorpheniramine
- check the patient's identity and details of the donor blood
- return the blood to the transfusion laboratory with a fresh sample of the patient's blood
- call for senior help and resuscitate as needed.

Hypocalcaemia

This may occur in patients who receive massive blood transfusions as a result of the chelating action of citrate, particularly if there is liver disease which impairs citrate metabolism.

Iron overload

Repeated blood transfusions can eventually lead to cardiac, liver and endocrine damage.

Table 55 The ABO and rhesus blood group systems

Blood Group	Relative frequency (%)	Alleles	Agglutinins present	Plasma will agglutinate cell types	Comment
O	45	Null, null	Anti-A, Anti-B	A, B, AB	Universal donor
A	40	A, A or A, null	Anti-B	B, AB	
B	10	B, B or B, null	Anti-A	A, AB	
AB	5	A, B	None	None	Universal recipient
Rh+	85	D+	None	None	
Rh-	15	D-	None or anti-D	None or Rh+	

Polycythaemia

Polycythaemia is defined as an increased red cell mass. You will recognise it on the blood count as an increased haemoglobin concentration, red cell count and haematocrit. It may be *absolute,* or *relative* to a reduced plasma volume.

Absolute polycythaemia may be:

- primary: termed polycythaemia vera
- secondary to increased erythropoietin.

Causes of secondary polycythaemia include:

- compensatory increased erythropoietin secretion as a result of:
  — tissue hypoxia
  — lung disease
  — cyanotic heart disease
  — altitude
  — hypoventilation (Pickwickian syndrome)
- non-compensatory increased erythropoietin secretion from:
  — renal tumour or cysts
  — other tumours.

Only lung disease is a common cause of clinical polycythaemia.

Polycythaemia increases the oxygen-carrying capacity of blood but it also increases viscosity and impairs blood flow. Many of its clinical effects are the result of stasis and impaired tissue oxygenation.

Polycythaemia vera

Polycythaemia vera is a neoplastic stem cell proliferation which increases the formation primarily of red cells but also of leucocytes and platelets. Clinical manifestations result from:

- hyperviscosity
- tissue hypoxia
- vascular occlusive events resulting from stasis and thrombocytosis.

Paradoxically, patients may also bleed easily because their platelets are dysfunctional.

Clinical presentation
Patients may present with:

- systemic symptoms such as pruritus (particularly after a warm bath) or malaise
- an arterial or deep venous thrombosis
- neurological symptoms, including headache, tinnitus and visual disturbance
- cardiovascular symptoms, including angina and intermittent claudication
- dyspepsia or non-specific abdominal pain signifying GI mucosal ulceration
- episodes of epistaxis or GI haemorrhage
- gout.

On examination, there is plethora, cyanosis, injection of the conjunctivae and, in most cases, splenomegaly. There may also be hepatomegaly. The blood count shows a haematocrit in the range 50–70%, with leucocytosis and an increased platelet count. The red cell mass, measured isotopically, is increased. The marrow is active but normoblastic. Serum uric acid and vitamin B_{12} are usually raised.

Management
Treatment is with:

- venesection to reduce hyperviscosity
- phosphorus-32 or an alkylating agent to reduce stem cell proliferation.

The aim is to reduce both the haematocrit and the platelet count. Life expectancy is reduced despite treatment, and the disease may transform into acute leukaemia or myelofibrosis.

Relative polycythaemia

Relative polycythaemia is far more common than polycythaemia vera. It is a disorder often seen in middle-aged hypertensive men who drink and smoke too much. The primary abnormality is a reduced plasma volume. The aetiology is unknown.

Faced with an apparently polycythaemic patient:

- measure the haematocrit more than once to be sure the apparent erythrocytosis is not an artefact
- consider the possibility of secondary polycythaemia, of which the common cause is chronic lung disease; measure the blood gases
- check that the patient is truly polycythaemic (i.e. exclude *relative* polycythaemia) by measuring the red cell mass and plasma volume.

If the patient has a leucocytosis, thrombocytosis or splenomegaly, the diagnosis is likely to be polycythaemia vera.

6.3 **White cell disorders**

Physiology

Granulocytes
Granulocytes are the most abundant white cells in peripheral blood.

Neutrophils. Most granulocytes are neutrophils, a key element of defence against most bacteria and some fungi. Most neutrophils in the normal person are present in the blood loosely adherent to the walls of vessels (marginating pool). When the appropriate stimulus comes along (such as a bacterial infection) they are released from the marginating pool and attracted to sites of inflammation by chemotactic factors including complement. Once a neutrophil comes into contact with a microbe or a foreign body it attaches itself, ingests it into a vacuole called a phagosome and kills it.

Eosinophils. These are the next most abundant form. They attack parasites which are too large to be phagocytosed and also have a role in mucosal immunity.

Basophils. These are the least abundant form. They release histamine and other inflammatory mediators during immediate hypersensitivity reactions.

Monocytes

Monocytes are large non-granulated white cells which are released from the bone marrow, circulate for several days and then enter tissues to become the tissue macrophages, including pulmonary alveolar macrophages, osteoclasts and the Kupffer cells of the liver. They engulf and kill bacteria in tissues and, as antigen-presenting cells, play a key role in immunity.

Lymphocytes

Lymphocytes are derived from the same stem cells of the bone marrow as the other cell lines. During fetal development, they migrate out to populate the thymus, liver, spleen, lymph nodes and other lymphoid tissues. In adult life, some lymphocytes are formed in the marrow but most are formed in lymphoid tissues elsewhere. There are two distinct cell lines, morphologically identical but distinguishable by cell-surface markers. The B cells — plasma cells and memory cells — are responsible for humoral immunity. T cells are responsible for cell-mediated immunity and for activating B cells. The sub-types of T cells are not discussed further here but an understanding of them is crucial to an understanding of AIDS (p. 335).

Learning objectives

You should understand:
- the causes of neutropenia
- what infections to be concerned about in the neutropenic patient and what to do if such a patient gets a fever
- the diseases of white cell proliferation and how they are diagnosed and treated.

A simple way of approaching white cell disorders is to think in terms of white cell numbers. They may be:
- reduced, in which case the problem is increased susceptibility to infection
- increased, signifying systemic disease or marrow proliferation.

Leucopenia

Leucopenia is a reduction in the number of white blood cells.

Lymphopenia is caused by:

- HIV infection
- autoimmune disease
- irradiation.

Neutropenia is caused by:

- Decreased production
  — drugs, e.g. cytotoxic therapy, carbimazole, phenylbutazone
  — vitamin B_{12} or folate deficiency
  — irradiation
  — marrow aplasia, fibrosis, malignant invasion
  — marrow dysplasia (p. 241)
  — infection.

- Increased consumption
  — hypersplenism
  — antineutrophil antibodies.

Neutropenia is relatively rare except in haematological malignancies and as a result of their treatment, the subject of the next section.

Management of neutropenia

The normal neutrophil count is around $2000 \times 10^6/l$. There is an increasing risk of infection when the count falls below 1000 and the risk of invasive infections rises substantially when the count falls below $500 \times 10^6/l$. A longer duration of neutropenia (e.g. more than 7 days) also puts the patient at substantially greater risk of life-threatening infection. Infections include:

- streptococci
- Gram-negatives, including *Pseudomonas aeruginosa*
- *Staphylococcus epidermidis* (usually related to indwelling central venous lines, and not immediately life-threatening)
- mucosal and invasive candidiasis
- invasive pulmonary aspergillosis
- herpes simplex virus (especially mouth ulcers).

A typical clinical scenario is that you are on call for haematology patients and summoned to the ward because a patient with no circulating neutrophils has developed a new fever 7–14 days after chemotherapy for leukaemia. You need to:

- assess whether there are any localising symptoms such as cough, skin rash, nasal symptoms, abdominal pain, etc.
- examine the mouth, chest, skin and rectal area and any other sites that are symptomatic
- assess whether the patient is in shock or going into respiratory failure
- order a portable chest X-ray if there are any respiratory features to the illness
- check the notes and recent results for any positive microbiology
- take at least one blood culture and collect any other microbiological specimens that are indicated by the patient's symptoms
- start broad-spectrum intravenous antibiotics according to the policy of the unit; typically these will include coverage for *Pseudomonas aeruginosa*

and streptococcal infections as a minimum (e.g. ceftazidime)

- if there are any unusual features, or the patient is very ill, you should contact the consultant or other senior member of staff primarily responsible for the patient.

Expert microbiological advice is needed if the patient remains profoundly neutropenic and has persistent fever.

Ceasing therapy. Antibiotics can usually be stopped when the neutrophil count has risen above $500 \times 10^6/\text{l}$.

Leucocytosis

Causes of leucocytosis include:

- neutrophilia
  - infection, usually bacterial
  - inflammation
  - connective tissue disease
  - myeloproliferative disease
  - non-haematological malignancy
  - corticosteroid therapy
  - diabetic ketoacidosis
- eosinophilia
  - parasitic infection
  - allergy
  - connective tissue disease, e.g. polyarteritis nodosa
- lymphocytosis
  - viral infection
  - connective tissue disease
  - lymphoproliferative disease
- basophilia: rare and usually caused by myeloproliferation
- monocytosis
  - infection, particularly during convalescence
  - connective tissue disease
  - myeloproliferative disease.

In many cases, the cause is obvious. In others, detailed haematological investigation is needed. Remember the common causes and remember that diabetic ketoacidosis and steroid therapy cause leucocytosis in the absence of infection.

The leukaemias, myeloproliferative disorders and lymphomas

These neoplastic diseases may seem hard to understand and remember but a few simple principles provide a skeleton on which the diseases hang:

- all of them are neoplastic clonal proliferations but they differ in their degree of malignancy
- the more chronic diseases tend to become increasingly malignant with time
- a distinction can be drawn between *lymphoproliferative* and *myeloproliferative* diseases
- the myeloproliferative group, particularly the more

chronic types (polycythaemia vera, essential thrombocythaemia and chronic granulocytic leukaemia) usually involve proliferation of more than one cell line

- other marrow tissues that are not derived from stem cells proliferate reactively to myeloproliferation and lymphoproliferation, as in myelofibrosis and lymphoma.

Figure 44 shows the relationship between the diseases. In general, the more malignant the disease, the more intense the treatment required and the higher the chance of cure. Low-grade diseases tend to be chronic and incurable.

The acute leukaemias

Classification and risk factors

There are two broad categories of acute leukaemia, **acute lymphoblastic leukaemia (ALL)** and **acute myeloblastic leukaemia (AML)**, the latter including several subtypes, shown in Figure 44. The incidence of ALL peaks in childhood. It is more common in males. AML is a disease of both children and adults, with a rapidly rising incidence in old age and no gender difference. Radiation exposure, genetic factors, viral infections and toxins, including chemotherapeutic drugs, have been implicated as risk factors for leukaemia, although the cause in an individual case is usually unknown.

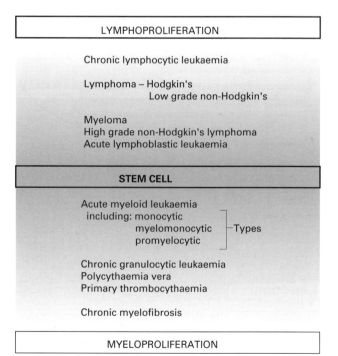

Fig. 44
Schematic representation of the lymphoproliferative and myeloproliferative diseases. The darkest shading indicates the highest degree of malignancy.

Clinical and haematological features

Acute leukaemia may arise de novo or in patients with chronic myeloproliferative disease. The clinical manifestations result from marrow dysfunction and tissue infiltration. They include:

- symptoms and signs of anaemia
- bruising, bleeding and purpura
- increased susceptibility to infection.

Tissue infiltration may cause:

- bone and joint pain
- gum infiltration.

There is occasionally hepatosplenomegaly and, in ALL, lymphadenopathy. The diagnosis is made on blood film and bone marrow examination. There is usually anaemia and thrombocytopenia. There may be leucopenia or a leucocytosis with blasts (primitive cells) in peripheral blood. The marrow is hypercellular and infiltrated with blasts. AML and ALL are distinguished on morphological, cytochemical, immunological and cytogenetic characteristics. Rod-shaped cytoplasmic bodies, named Auer rods, are a virtually pathognomonic feature of AML.

Management

The treatment of ALL has been one of the success stories of oncology because two-thirds of children (fewer adults) are cured. Most forms of acute leukaemia are amenable to chemotherapy, but equally important is the intensive supportive treatment with antibiotics and blood products, and sympathetic management of the patient and his/her family. The aim is to eliminate the abnormal clone from blood, bone marrow and other sites and allow repopulation with normal haemopoietic cells. This is termed **remission**. A discussion of the specific drugs and regimens is beyond the scope of this chapter but treatment may include the following phases:

1. Remission induction: elimination of neoplastic tissue, allowing recovery of normal marrow
2. Consolidation of remission
3. Prevention of recurrence in extramedullary sites (as in ALL) and maintenance of remission
4. Treatment of relapses.

It may also include bone marrow transplantation to repopulate the marrow with healthy tissue after obliteration of malignant cells, if a suitable donor is available.

There are some important differences between the treatment of ALL and AML. More myelosuppression is needed in AML so the risks of infection and bleeding are higher. Induction therapy in ALL usually fails to eliminate malignant tissue from extramedullary sites including the brain, spine and testes, so cranial irradiation and intrathecal chemotherapy are given. Maintenance therapy is continued for 2–3 years in ALL. In AML, induction is followed by several further courses of very intensive chemotherapy in which different drugs are introduced in an attempt to maintain remission. If an HLA-identical sibling is available, bone marrow transplantation improves the prognosis of AML and ALL in younger patients who have achieved remission, although it may often be unnecessary in children with ALL. An **autograft**, using the patient's own bone marrow after intensive treatment, is also possible but carries the risk of reintroducing malignant tissue. Over 90% of children and 80% of adults with ALL achieve remission; the 5-year survival for children is over 60%. AML has a worse prognosis, with a remission rate of 70% in younger patients and a 25% 5-year survival rate. Increasing age has an adverse effect in all types of acute leukaemia and a high white count at presentation predicts a bad outcome.

Myelodysplastic syndrome

Myelodysplastic syndrome describes a group of disorders characterised by cytopenias of one or more cell lines with a cellular marrow and morphological abnormalities in both marrow and peripheral blood. The cytopenias are presumed the result of ineffective haemopoiesis. Myelodysplastic syndrome progresses at a variable rate to leukaemia. Management is supportive until leukaemia develops, when cytotoxic therapy may be indicated although the outlook is poor at this stage. Many patients are elderly and unsuitable for intrusive treatment.

Myeloproliferative diseases

Chronic granulocytic leukaemia

Chronic granulocytic leukaemia (CGL) is an uncommon disease with a peak incidence in young to middle-aged adults. It is characterised by uncontrolled proliferation of myeloid progenitor cells, generally most noticeable in granulopoietic cells but also affecting red cells and platelets. The characteristic feature, present in all affected cells, is the **Philadelphia chromosome**, an abnormality of chromosome 22 caused by translocation to the long arm of chromosome 9.

These are the clinical features and some modes of presentation of CGL:

- patients typically present with symptoms of anaemia, weight loss or abdominal discomfort
- there is splenomegaly, which may be massive, and there may be symptomatic splenic infarction
- there may be symptoms and signs of haemorrhage
- the diagnosis may be made by chance on a blood count.

There is marked leucocytosis including, especially, neutrophils and myelocytes and, in many cases, basophils and eosinophils. The platelet count is usually normal or raised at presentation. The bone marrow shows granulopoietic hyperplasia.

CGL can be distinguished from other causes of leucocytosis by:

- symptoms and signs
- blood film
- Philadelphia chromosome
- reduced leucocyte alkaline phosphatase score on a blood film.

CGL progresses after about 3 years from the chronic to an accelerated phase. This may be sudden, causing death within weeks, or more gradual. The accelerated phase is marked by:

- systemic symptoms
- weight loss
- increased susceptibility to infection
- anaemia
- bruising
- blasts on the blood film
- unresponsiveness to treatment
- a very poor prognosis.

During the chronic phase, treatment is with hydroxyurea or busulphan, an alkylating agent. Because the prognosis of the accelerated phase is so poor, bone marrow transplantation in the chronic phase is indicated in younger patients with a suitable donor.

Polycythaemia vera and thrombocythaemia

Although these are myeloproliferative disorders, they are described in the red cell (p. 238) and platelet (p. 245) sections of this chapter because their clinical features are determined by the predominant cell type in peripheral blood rather than their progenitor cell.

Myelofibrosis

Myelofibrosis describes a disease in which proliferation of fibrous tissue in the marrow is the main feature. It may be the final result of other myeloproliferative diseases or may present as a primary disorder in middle-aged or elderly people. There is anaemia — which may be leucoerythroblastic (p. 234) — and massive splenomegaly. It can be impossible to aspirate marrow. Trephine biopsy shows extensive fibrosis. The treatment is supportive, sometimes with splenectomy to improve red cell, white cell and platelet survival. It may progress to acute leukaemia.

Lymphoproliferative diseases

Hodgkin's disease

There are incidence peaks of Hodgkin's disease in early adulthood and old age. The two main clinical characteristics of lymphomas are lymphadenopathy and systemic symptoms.

A cardinal feature of Hodgkin's disease (which distinguishes it from non-Hodgkin's lymphoma) is that, when more than one group of nodes is involved, they are always contiguous, suggesting lymphatic spread of malignant cells. The cervical nodes are most often involved. With disseminated disease, there may be hepatosplenomegaly and extralymphatic involvement.

Systemic symptoms include pruritus, fever, night sweats and weight loss. Anaemia is common. There may be neutrophilia and eosinophilia. Impaired cell-mediated immunity predisposes to infection, most typically herpes zoster.

The diagnostic feature on lymph node biopsy is the presence of multinucleated **Reed–Sternberg cells.** Hodgkin's disease is subclassified by the relative proportions of lymphocytes and reactive elements into two histological grades:

- lymphocyte predominant: good prognosis
- lymphocyte depleted: poor prognosis.

Three other factors are associated with a worse prognosis:

- increasing age
- presence of systemic symptoms: fever, weight loss and night sweats
- more extensive disease (higher 'stage').

Staging is the most important determinant of treatment and prognosis but cannot be discussed in detail here. It is done by:

- a careful history and physical examination
- chest X-ray
- liver function tests
- bone marrow trephine biopsy
- ultrasound and CT or MR scanning to assess involvement of the spleen and the extent of lymphadenopathy.

Treatment is with radiotherapy for local disease and chemotherapy for disseminated disease. Depending on stage and histological type, Hodgkin's disease has a 50–90% 5-year survival.

Non-Hodgkin's lymphoma

Non-Hodgkin's lymphoma (NHL) is a more heterogeneous group of disorders with varying malignancy and prognoses. It differs from Hodgkin's disease in three ways:

- higher prevalence
- older mean age at diagnosis
- non-contiguous, multicentric spread
- extranodal involvement is more common.

Several types of NHL are known to be caused by viruses, including Epstein–Barr virus (Burkitt's lymphoma), human T cell leukaemia-1 virus and HIV. Like Hodgkin's disease, NHL presents with lymphadenopathy and systemic symptoms.

Remember that lymphadenopathy must always be taken seriously. In younger people, it is more likely to be caused by infection than malignancy. In older people, there is a high likelihood of cancer (usually localised lymphadenopathy), lymphoma or chronic lymphocytic leukaemia (generalised lymphadenopathy). The diagnosis of NHL is made by biopsy and it is staged as for Hodgkin's disease.

There are two broad histological categories.

Low-grade NHL. This is indolent, usually untreatable and may become more aggressive with time.

High-grade NHL. This form carries a much higher early mortality but is more responsive to treatment, with an approximately 30% 5-year disease-free survival.

Treatment. Because NHL is usually more widespread than Hodgkin's disease at presentation, treatment is more often with chemotherapy, although localised disease is treated with radiotherapy. Stem cell or bone marrow transplantation is used in some patients.

Chronic lymphocytic leukaemia

Chronic lymphocytic leukaemia (CLL) is the least malignant of the leukaemias and is characteristically a disease of elderly people. It is more common in men than women. It may be a chance finding on a blood film or may present with lymphadenopathy or anaemia. Typically, there is hepatosplenomegaly. The blood film shows (sometimes massively) increased numbers of mature lymphocytes. Because the lymphocytes are B cells in over 95% of patients, there may be:

- a 'paraprotein' (see Myeloma, below)
- depression of normal immunoglobulins and increased susceptibility to infection
- autoimmune haemolytic anaemia.

Cytotoxic therapy or corticosteroids may be given for symptoms or complications, although the disease is so benign that many patients need no treatment. Progressive disease causes:

- worsening lymphocytosis
- increasing hepatosplenomegaly and lymphadenopathy
- eventually, bone marrow failure.

There is a 50% five-year survival.

Multiple myeloma

Multiple myeloma is a monoclonal malignant proliferation of plasma cells (B cells) which are relatively highly differentiated and secrete immunoglobulin. Like most lymphoproliferative diseases, myeloma is predominantly a disease of old people, although it may arise at any time in adult life. The plasma cells may secrete:

- IgG, with or without free light chains (50% of patients)
- IgA (20%)
- free light chains only (20%)
- Other patterns of paraprotein (10%).

The clinical features result from:

- plasma cell proliferation
- systemic effects of the paraprotein
- impairment of normal haematological function.

There is bone destruction caused by humorally mediated activation of osteoclasts without the normal osteoblastic response. This may cause diffuse osteopenia or, radiologically, punched-out lesions at the site of plasma cell deposits. Such deposits may present as mass lesions: plasmacytomas. Bone destruction mobilises calcium, so hypercalcaemia (p. 317) is a common complication of myeloma.

Apart from its skeletal features, two other characteristics of myeloma are hyperviscosity and renal failure. Hyperviscosity occurs because the paraprotein alters the surface charge of the red cells and thus leads to aggregation. It may impair cerebral and peripheral blood flow, typically causing lethargy, confusion and impaired consciousness. It is particularly seen in **Waldenström's macroglobulinaemia**, a rare plasma cell proliferative disease with an IgM paraprotein. Renal failure in myeloma results from:

- a direct nephrotoxic effect of the paraprotein
- hypercalcaemia
- hyperuricaemia and urate nephropathy
- infection
- amyloid deposition in the kidneys.

The effects upon normal haematological function include:

- increased susceptibility to bacterial infection (typically septicaemia or pneumonia) as a result of the reduced leucocyte numbers or function together with reduced secretion of normal immunoglobulins
- anaemia or pancytopenia because of marrow replacement or suppression of haemopoiesis.

Clinical presentation

Patients may present with bone pain or fractures (particularly involving the spine and ribs), weight loss, anaemia, infective episodes and renal failure. Other typical symptoms include thirst, polyuria, nocturia (owing to hypercalcaemia and/or renal failure), constipation (from hypercalcaemia), lethargy and confusion.

The diagnosis is based upon finding:

- a high ESR (except in those cases with only light chain secretion)
- the paraprotein, by immunoelectrophoresis of blood and/or urine
- reduced concentrations of normal immunoglobulins (immune paresis)
- radiological evidence of generalised osteopenia or local bone destruction
- increased plasma cell numbers in a bone marrow aspirate.

Other laboratory features include:

- anaemia, thrombocytopenia and leucopenia
- renal failure
- hypercalcaemia.

It should be noted that the term **Bence–Jones proteinuria** is of historical interest only. It describes the behaviour of light chains in boiled urine, now superseded by immunoelectrophoresis of concentrated urine.

Management

Patients may become caught in a vicious spiral of hypercalcaemia, volume depletion and renal failure. The first step for such patients is i.v. fluid therapy (described under acute renal failure, p. 157). Infection should be sought and treated, pain controlled, and hypercalcaemia treated with corticosteroids and/or bisphosphonates if fluid alone does not control it. Plasma exchange may occasionally be needed to control hyperviscosity. Long-term treatment is with chemotherapy such as oral melphalan, an alkylating agent, or more aggressive regimens in younger patients. Bone pain may be controlled with radiotherapy. Despite treatment, the 50% survival is about 2 years.

6.4 **Platelet disorders**

Physiology

The role of platelets is to 'plug' defects in damaged vessels, initiate coagulation and promote healing. They:

- adhere to the vessel wall
- become activated
- degranulate
- aggregate.

This can best be thought of as a cascade process, which becomes self-perpetuating as they activate one another.
The trigger of the cascade may be:

- damage to the vessel wall, which exposes platelets to collagen and von Willebrand factor (vWF)
- blood coagulation, which leads to thrombin formation
- the activation of other platelets, which causes discharge of ADP, thromboxane A_2 and platelet-derived growth factor
- inflammation, which leads to release of platelet-activating factor from neutrophils and monocytes.

The process of adherence and aggregation is promoted by the prostaglandin thromboxane A_2. This is derived from arachidonic acid within platelets and is held in check by prostacyclin which is synthesised from arachidonic acid in the endothelium.
Adherence leads to platelet degranulation. The contents of the granules attract other platelets, cause platelet aggregation and trigger blood coagulation. Uncontrolled platelet adhesion and thrombosis are prevented by secretion of prostacyclin and activation of protein C (p. 246) from adjacent healthy endothelium.
Whilst platelet numbers can easily be measured with an automated counter, their function can only be assessed crudely by measuring how long a patient bleeds after 'nicking' the skin (bleeding time).
Conceptually, platelet disorders are straightforward. Patients may have too many platelets, too few platelets or platelets which do not work properly. Changes in platelet number are caused by increased or reduced thrombopoiesis or platelet consumption. Moderate thrombocytopenia (e.g. count $<50 \times 10^9/l$) or decreased platelet function may result in easy bruising. Severe thrombocytopenia (e.g. count $<10 \times 10^9/l$) can cause mucosal or intracerebral haemorrhage, in which case urgent platelet transfusion is indicated. Transfused platelets have such a short life that transfusions may need to be repeated daily. Thrombocytosis or increased platelet activity raise the coagulability of blood, causing arterial and venous thromboses. Thrombocytosis is treated with antiplatelet drugs or chemotherapy.

Learning objectives

You should:
- be able to understand the clinical presentations of platelet disorders
- understand the indications for platelet transfusions
- understand how increased platelet numbers can cause thrombophilia.

Thrombocytopenia

Decreased platelet production is usually caused by one of the major haematological diseases or its treatment. Other causes include:

- bone marrow infiltration
- myelosuppressive drugs
- radiation exposure
- megaloblastic anaemia.

Increased platelet loss may be caused by:

- increased activity of the spleen causing 'sequestration' of platelets
- entrapment of platelets in fibrin deposited in small vessels (see DIC, p. 248)
- immunity or autoimmunity.

The two immune mechanisms of platelet destruction are:
- antibodies formed against platelet antigens
- antigen–antibody complexes (e.g. precipitated by a drug) which bind to platelets and accelerate their destruction.

Idiopathic (immune) thrombocytopenic purpura, marrow suppression and DIC are the most important conditions to know about.

Idiopathic thrombocytopenic purpura

Idiopathic thrombocytopenic purpura may occur acutely, often in infants or young adults, sometimes soon after a viral infection and with a self-limited course. It may also have a less acute presentation, typically in a young adult or middle-aged woman, and a chronic course.
The presentation is with purpura and bleeding, which may be severe. In its subacute form, it may be a

chance laboratory finding. The disease is benign unless there is a cerebral haemorrhage, which is very rare. Platelet antibodies can be demonstrated in some patients and the marrow is active, signifying compensatory thrombopoiesis. Steroids or high-dose immunoglobulin infusions may be used. In the chronic form, steroid therapy may induce a lasting remission. If it does not and thrombocytopenia is severe, splenectomy may be effective by removing the site of platelet destruction.

Thrombocytosis

Decreased platelet consumption occurs after splenectomy, although there is usually only a transient thrombocytosis. Increased production may be secondary to any marrow stimulus such as bleeding, haemolysis or surgery. The one primary disease is **essential thrombocythaemia**, an uncommon myeloproliferative disease characterised by increased numbers of variably active platelets. As has been explained above, patients may either develop arterial/venous thromboses or bleed. It is characteristically a disease of middle or old age. As well as thrombocytosis, there may be normocytic anaemia and leucocytosis (caused by myeloproliferation) and either splenomegaly or hyposplenism owing to splenic infarction. The marrow shows megakaryocyte proliferation with other myeloproliferative features. Treatment is with antiplatelet drugs or chemotherapy. Leukaemic transformation or myelofibrosis may be late complications.

Antiplatelet therapy

Particularly in ischaemic heart disease and transient ischaemic attacks, antiplatelet therapy is of proven value in preventing arterial thromboses. Recent evidence suggests that it may also protect against venous thromboembolism. Aspirin is the most effective drug. It works by irreversible inhibition of cyclo-oxygenase, the key enzyme in prostaglandin synthesis. Since cyclo-oxygenase inhibition prevents synthesis of endothelial prostacyclin as well as platelet thromboxane, aspirin has prothrombotic as well as antithrombotic effects. These effects are dose related and the balance can be shifted towards antithrombosis by giving lower doses. The main side-effects are dyspepsia, peptic ulceration and GI haemorrhage. Other platelet inhibitors such as sulphinpyrazone and dipyridamole may also be used but there is less evidence that they are clinically effective.

Whether **antiplatelet** or **anticoagulant** therapy is more appropriate depends on the pathophysiology of the disease in question: platelet activation is central to the arterial thrombo-embolism of cerebrovascular (p. 196) and ischaemic heart disease (p. 14), so aspirin is the treatment of choice to prevent them. Intra-cardiac thrombosis and venous thrombo-embolism are more dependent on the coagulation pathways and are, therefore, treated with anticoagulants.

6.5 Coagulation disorders

Learning objectives

You should understand:

- how coagulation defects are acquired
- how warfarin and heparin work, when to use them, and their potential dangers
- the concept of hypercoagulability (thrombophilia) and its causes.

Physiology

The functions of the coagulation and fibrinolytic system are to:

- maintain the fluidity of blood
- plug damaged vessels
- prevent the uncontrolled propagation of blood clot
- remove clot as healing proceeds.

Coagulation is a complex process, trigggered by damage to the vessel wall. This exposes collagen and tissue thromboplastin, which activate the coagulation cascade, summarised in Figure 45. Platelet activation also triggers coagulation. The final result is conversion of fibrinogen to an insoluble fibrin plug. This is catalysed by thrombin formed from its precursor prothrombin. Within the cascade, there are the intrinsic and extrinsic systems. These converge on a common pathway which activates the final two steps of thrombin and fibrin formation. Calcium is essential to coagulation.

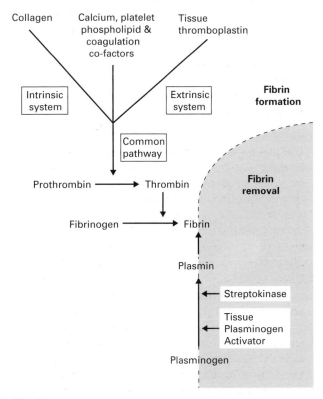

Fig. 45
The coagulation and fibrinolytic systems.

The coagulation factors are synthesised in the liver; many of them are dependent on vitamin K.

There are also mechanisms which restrain coagulation, notably the thrombin inhibitor, antithrombin III. Protein C is another. This protein is activated by thrombin formation and feeds back to suppress the coagulation cascade. Protein S is a cofactor for that inhibitory pathway.

Once formed, clots are lysed by plasmin with the release of fibrin degradation products. The conversion of plasminogen to plasmin is promoted by tissue plasminogen activator (tPA). The dynamic equilibrium between the formation of fibrin and its removal maintains haemostasis.

Warfarin inhibits coagulation by preventing the hepatic synthesis of vitamin K-dependent clotting factors. Heparin potentiates antithrombin III. Fibrinolytic drugs include **streptokinase** and **recombinant tPA**, both of which potentiate plasmin formation and the breakdown of fibrin.

Tests of coagulation and fibrinolysis

Two tests are in general use (Fig. 46): the prothrombin time (PT) and activated partial thromboplastin time (APTT). The PT tests the extrinsic system, common pathway and fibrin formation. It is sensitive to deficiency of the vitamin K-dependent clotting factors and is prolonged by:

- warfarin
- hepatocellular dysfunction
- fat malabsorption
- consumption of clotting factors in DIC.

When the prothrombin time is used to measure the effect of warfarin, it is performed with standardised reagents (so that it is reproducible from one laboratory to another) and expressed as the international normalised ratio (INR).

The APTT tests the intrinsic system, common pathway and fibrin formation. It is affected by:

- liver disease
- circulating anticoagulants, including heparin
- DIC.

The APTT is prolonged by deficiency of the vitamin K-dependent clotting factors but less so than the PT and can be 'corrected' by mixing normal plasma (replete with those factors) with the patient's plasma. It is more sensitive than the PT to circulating anticoagulants and is used to monitor heparin therapy.

The only fibrinolytic test which is widely used is measurement of fibrin degradation products (FDPs). This detects excess fibrinolysis but is so insensitive that it can only detect DIC. There is also a sensitive test for a specific breakdown product of fibrin, D-dimer.

Coagulation defects

Inherited disorders are uncommon and are cared for in specialist units so they are not discussed here.

Acquired coagulation defects

The causes of acquired coagulation disorders are listed under the coagulation tests above. You should remember that any GI disease which affects fat absorption may cause vitamin K deficiency. Hepatocellular dysfunction impairs coagulation factor synthesis to such an extent that the PT is a very sensitive test of hepatocellular failure. Clinical implications of this are considered under liver disease (p. 122).

The effects of warfarin and heparin are discussed in the next section and 'consumption coagulopathy' under DIC (p. 248). Vitamin K is given parenterally to treat malabsorption and to reverse the action of warfarin. It may also improve clotting factor synthesis in mild liver disease. Otherwise, the treatment for coagulation defects is infusion of fresh frozen plasma (FFP).

Anticoagulation and fibrinolytic therapy

These therapies are primarily used in cardiovascular disease. Anticoagulation is considered here and fibrinolysis under acute myocardial infarction (p. 18).

Heparin

Heparin consists of natural polysaccharides of various molecular weights which have an almost immediate anticoagulant effect. It has to be given parenterally, and either by continuous infusion or as several injections per day because it has a short half-life. It prevents the formation of new clot and shifts the balance of fibrin formation/lysis in the direction of lysis but is not primarily a fibrinolytic drug. It is indicated whenever an immediate anticoagulant effect is required. It may also be used to prevent (usually venous) thrombosis. There are two common schedules:

- prophylaxis: heparin 5000 units subcutaneously 8 or 12 hourly
- treatment: heparin 5000 units as an i.v. loading dose followed by 1000–2000 units hourly by continuous i.v. infusion.

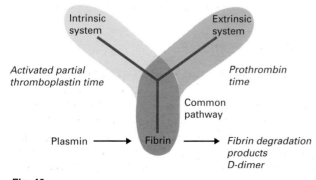

Fig. 46
Tests of coagulation and fibrinolysis.

Sensitivity to heparin varies from patient to patient. You should check the APTT every 6–12 hours until it is prolonged approximately two-fold (depending upon the indication) and stable. Warfarin can be introduced while the patient is on heparin. Heparin should be continued at least until the patient is stabilised on warfarin, and for a minimum of 5 days in venous thromboembolism. Prolonged heparin treatment (> 5 days) can cause thrombocytopenia. More prolonged treatment (as in pregnancy) can cause osteoporosis. Although more expensive, the new low molecular weight heparin preparations are likely to be used widely because they can be given by once or twice daily injection, do not need laboratory monitoring, do not require hospitalisation and are proven effective, for e.g. deep venous thrombosis.

Warfarin

Warfarin and other coumarins are used for long-term anticoagulation. They take about 48 hours to become effective, governed by the half-lives of the vitamin K-dependent factors. Warfarin is strongly protein bound. Anything which affects this binding will affect sensitivity to it. Liver function and levels of the vitamin K-dependent factors also affect sensitivity to warfarin to such an extent that patients may be 'autoanticoagulated'. Because of this, you must always check the PT before starting therapy. Warfarin is given as loading doses over 2 days and a maintenance dose adjusted to prolong the PT (reported as the INR, see p. 246) by a factor of 1.5–4 (depending upon the indication). The effect of warfarin is unpredictable in alcoholism and liver disease. Important drug interactions are:

- potentiation of warfarin by displacement from protein binding, e.g. salicylates, sulphonamides
- potentiation of warfarin by inhibiting warfarin metabolism, e.g. metronidazole, amiodarone, cimetidine, isoniazid
- potentiation of the effect of warfarin on the liver, e.g. tetracycline
- reduced effect of warfarin by inducing warfarin metabolism, e.g. phenobarbitone, carbamazepine, rifampicin.

Indications for anticoagulation

- Short-term prophylaxis (usually low-dose heparin)
  — prolonged recumbency
  — immobilisation, e.g. traction
  — severe heart failure
  — malignant pelvic disease or impediment to venous flow
- Acute (usually heparin)
  — venous disease: deep venous thrombosis, pulmonary embolism
  — arterial disease: peripheral arterial thrombosis or embolism, cardiac mural thrombo-embolism, unstable angina
- Chronic (usually warfarin)
  — continued treatment of acute indications
  — prophylactically in cardiac dysrhythmia (e.g. AF, especially if intermittent or associated with mitral stenosis), poor cardiac function (cardiomyopathy), prosthetic heart valve or vascular prosthesis, after full-thickness anterior myocardial infarct.

Contraindications to anticoagulation

- Absolute
  — cerebral haemorrhage
  — GI, urinary tract or other haemorrhage
  — active peptic ulceration
- Relative
  — liver disease
  — alcoholism
  — likely poor compliance
  — concomitant drug therapy likely to cause instability.

Side-effects of anticoagulation

Even if the contraindications listed above are observed, over-anticoagulation may occur and directly cause haemorrhage from the mucosae, into the skin or into the tissues (e.g. cerebral haemorrhage). That should be rare provided the dosage schedule and degree of anticoagulation are appropriately chosen and monitored. Warfarin can be reversed in an emergency by intravenous vitamin K. Heparin action will wear off after about 4 hours. If more immediate reversal of anticoagulation is needed, FFP should be given.

Sometimes, a decision has to be taken to anticoagulate a patient at risk of haemorrhage because the risk of not providing anticoagulation is even more unacceptable. Your responsibilities as a prescriber are to:

- vet *all* patients' suitability for anticoagulation in terms of compliance and understanding
- screen for underlying diseases which may complicate treatment
- advise patients about the risks and benefits of treatment and the need to abstain from alcohol and drugs (including over-the-counter drugs) which may complicate anticoagulation
- ensure adequate monitoring of the INR.

Thrombophilic states

Thrombophilic states may be inherited or acquired.

Inherited thrombophilia

The most common cause of inherited thrombophilia is a defect in the factor V gene (factor V Leiden), which causes resistance to activated protein C. Antithrombin III deficiency is an autosomal dominant condition which is incompatible with life in its homozygous form. The prevalence of heterozygosity is about 1 per 2000. Protein C and protein S deficiency are similarly inherited but are less common. The mechanism by which these disorders predispose to thrombosis is discussed on page 246.

Acquired thrombophilia

Antiphospholipid syndrome is an uncommon autoimmune disorder in which an autoantibody triggers coagulation. It may be associated with lupus (lupus anticoagulant) and can cause recurrent fetal loss in young women. Anticardiolipin antibodies are often present. Lesser degrees of thrombophilia occur in women taking the oral contraceptive, during pregnancy and in any illness which increases fibrinogen levels.

Clinical presentation

Inherited thrombophilia presents with thrombosis at an early age, recurrent thrombosis and/or a positive family history. The thromboses are usually venous but may be arterial.

Screening for thrombophilia

The following are indications to screen a patient for thrombophilia:

- venous or arterial thrombo-embolism in a young person (aged < 40 years)
- recurrent venous thrombosis
- family history of venous thrombo-embolism
- recurrent fetal loss.

Investigation

You should check a full blood count to exclude erythrocytosis (p. 238) and thrombocytosis (p. 245): measure plasma fibrinogen and the PT and APTT. Other investigations include anticardiolipin antibodies and direct measurements of protein C, protein S and antithrombin III. These should be done before starting anticoagulants.

Management

Significant thrombophilia requires lifelong anticoagulation.

6.6 Disseminated intravascular coagulation

Pathophysiology

DIC describes widespread activation of the coagulation pathways secondary to a severe illness. There is intravascular fibrin deposition, which may cause microvascular occlusion. Clotting factors and platelets are consumed and may become so depleted that the patient bleeds. Fibrin in the microvasculature may cause mechanical damage to the red cells (microangiopathic haemolysis) leading to haemolytic anaemia, with schistocytes (fragmented cells, p. 230) on the blood film.

Causes of DIC
- Septicaemia
- incompatible blood transfusion (p. 237)
- crush injury or other trauma
- disseminated malignancy
- acute pancreatitis
- amniotic fluid embolism.

These factors all have in common the systemic release of toxins which trigger coagulation.

Clinical effects

The dominant clinical features are usually those of the underlying illness. Often a fall in the platelet count is the first sign that the patient is developing DIC. The features of DIC can be worked out if you think system by system of the effects of small vessel occlusion:

CNS. Impaired consciousness, fits, focal neurological signs.

Lungs. Acute respiratory distress syndrome.

Kidneys. Acute renal failure.

Gut. Bowel infarction.

Skin. Ischaemic ulceration, digital gangrene.

In addition, there may be haemorrhage into any or all of these tissues. Petechial skin haemorrhages, purpura and bleeding from the mucosae may develop.

Investigations

The investigations follow directly from the pathophysiology. The diagnostic features of DIC are:

- thrombocytopenia ($<100 \times 10^9/l$)
- prolonged PT and APTT
- raised FDPs and D-dimer
- reduced plasma fibrinogen
- signs of microangiopathic haemolytic anaemia (p. 235).

Treatment and natural history

The development of DIC is a bad prognostic sign in a disease which already has a bad prognosis. The main aim of treatment is to control the underlying disease; without this, treating the DIC is unlikely to be of value. The treatment of DIC consists of replacing the coagulation factors (as FFP) and platelets. This narrative has described severe, fulminating DIC. Low-grade DIC may develop in association with malignant disease, vasculitis and other illnesses. Again, treatment is aimed at the underlying disease, and prognosis is determined by the disease itself more than the DIC.

Other related diseases

Detailed knowledge of the haemolytic uraemic syndrome, thrombotic thrombocytopenic purpura and other such rare diseases is not 'core'. You should simply be aware that the pathophysiological processes of consumption coagulopathy and microangiopathic haemolysis can occur in settings other than classical DIC.

Self-assessment: questions

Multiple choice questions

1. The following statements are true:
   a. Hypocalcaemia causes prolongation of the prothrombin time
   b. The prothrombin time is a sensitive test of hepatocellular dysfunction
   c. The activated partial thromboplastin time (APTT) is prolonged by heparin therapy
   d. The effect of heparin is reversed by vitamin K
   e. Deep venous thrombosis can be reliably diagnosed by measuring fibrin degradation products (FDPs)

2. In a patient with severe thrombocytopenia:
   a. Rectal bleeding is usually the first symptom
   b. Examination of the optic fundi should be performed regularly
   c. There is a risk of cerebral haemorrhage
   d. Corticosteroids are given to prevent haemorrhage, whatever the cause
   e. Platelet transfusions can be expected to cause prompt normalisation of the platelet count

3. The following may cause a microcytic anaemia:
   a. Sickle cell disease
   b. The thalassaemias
   c. Anaemia of chronic disease
   d. Anticonvulsant therapy
   e. Haemolysis, whatever the cause

4. In lymphoma:
   a. If a newly presenting patient has generalised lymphadenopathy, the diagnosis is more likely to be non-Hodgkin's lymphoma than Hodgkin's disease
   b. Early stages of Hodgkin's disease can be cured by radiotherapy alone
   c. Lymphocyte predominance is a favourable histological sign in Hodgkin's disease
   d. Pain in lymph nodes after alcohol is very typical of non-Hodgkin's lymphoma
   e. Bone marrow transplantation has greatly improved the prognosis of low-grade non-Hodgkin's lymphoma

5. The following statements are true:
   a. A neutrophil count of only $800 \times 10^6/l$ is a major risk for infection
   b. A neutrophil count in a febrile patient of $25\,000 \times 10^6/l$ reflects mostly the production of new neutrophils from the bone marrow
   c. In a patient with less than $100 \times 10^6/l$ neutrophils and a fever, treatment with antibiotics should await the results of blood culture
   d. Neutropenia is common in AIDS
   e. Neutropenia can be caused by carbimazole therapy

Data interpretation

1. Suggest a cause for the findings described in Table 56 for each of six patients.
2. A 22-year-old patient is admitted to hospital 48 hours after a paracetamol overdose, complaining of haematuria. The prothrombin time is 60 s (control 18 s). What is the likely diagnosis?
3. A 70-year-old man is referred to hospital because he is anaemic (Hb 82 g/dl, MCV 90, Platelets $150 \times 10^9/l$ ESR 130 mm/hr. Name a possible haematological diagnosis. What biochemical tests should be performed?

Table 56 Data obtained for six patients

	1	2	3	4	5	6
Hb (g/dl)	42	78	185	91	87	84
MCV (Fl)	123	69	96	85	80	86
WBC ($\times 10^9/l$)	2.3	13.6	15.3	8.7	63.0	1.7
Platelets ($\times 10^9/l$)	60	200	600	180	140	48

Case history questions

History 1

Your consultant is concerned that a 73-year-old man in atrial fibrillation is at risk of stroke and asks you to anticoagulate him. You are aware that the patient is vaguely confused and the nursing staff on the ward have received a telephone call from a neighbour stating that he has become increasingly reclusive. He has often been noted to be unsteady on his feet and has once been found lying in the road. At visiting time you have a chance to meet his wife to discuss the plan to use anti-coagulation therapy and to give further information.

1. Suggest two important questions which you should ask
2. Name two haematological investigations which it would be appropriate to perform
3. Name two possible contraindications to anticoagulation in this case
4. If a decision were made to proceed with anti-coagulation, describe two pieces of advice which you would give to the patient and his wife

History 2

You are called on a Sunday to see a 63-year-old man with non-Hodgkin's lymphoma and a fever of 38.6°C. He is in reverse barrier nursing because his total white cell count is $0.2 \times 10^9/l$ and his platelets are $15 \times 10^9/l$ despite daily platelet transfusions. He received intensive chemotherapy (fludarabine) 15 days previously and has been leukopenic for 7 days. You put on your gown, mask and gloves to examine the patient and finds that he has no symptoms except those of the fever, mild headache, sweating and an uncomfortable feeling around his bottom.

1. Which of the following actions would be appropriate:
   a. Order a chest X-ray
   b. Take a blood culture
   c. Do a blood count
   d. Do a digital rectal examination
   e. Start him on oral amoxycillin

The senior sister on the ward encourages you to start him on the 'usual' antibiotics (ceftazidime and gentamicin). His fever is still elevated 6 hours later despite antibiotics and he looks more toxic. The consultant suggests that you add metronidazole to his regimen. Four days later you are also on call and are asked to see him again. He has had fever up to 38.3°C for four days despite ceftazidime, gentamicin, metronidazole and 2 days of vancomycin. He now has a dry cough, in addition to a painful bottom.

2. What actions should you now take?
   a. Look at his white cell and platelet counts from that morning
   b. Arrange for transfer to intensive care
   c. Examine him again carefully
   d. Treat him for a possible fungal infection
   e. Do blood cultures, including a special fungal blood culture

On examination, you find crackles at the left base which do not clear on coughing and a black and red perianal area about 2 cm across with surrounding erythema.

3. Should you:
   a. Speak to his consultant at home
   b. Arrange a chest X-ray
   c. Arrange an induced sputum
   d. Call the physiotherapist in
   e. Arrange for a special mattress to help his developing pressure sore

4. Give a differential diagnosis and your thoughts on management

Picture questions

1. This skull X-ray (Picture 6.1) was taken from a 73-year-old patient who presented in acute renal failure.
   a. What abnormality do you see?
   b. How could the skull X-ray be relevant to the renal failure? Be as precise as you can.
   c. Name one rapid biochemical test which might establish a link.
   d. What would be your immediate management?

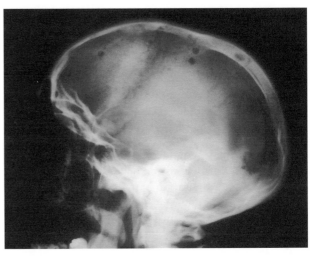

Picture 6.1.

2. A previously fit 28-year-old woman has lost weight. She has night sweats, pruritus and weight loss. She has noticed pain in the cervical region after drinking alcohol. Her GP arranged a chest radiograph which was thought to show hilar enlargement. Pictures 6.2A and B show thoracic computed scans before (A) and after (B) an intravenous contrast agent. T, trachea; A, aortic arch, B, left brachiocephalic vein.
   a. What abnormality is shown?
   b. Suggest, in order of likelihood, a differential diagnosis

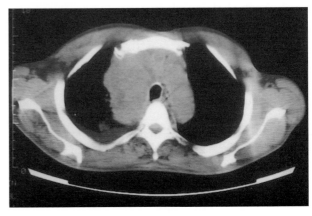

Picture 6.2A.

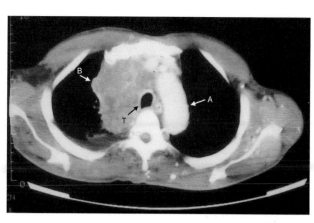

Picture 6.2B.

Viva questions

1. What complications might you expect in a patient with aplastic anaemia and how would you prevent them?
2. How would you decide whether to use antiplatelet or anticoagulant therapy?

Self-assessment: answers

Multiple choice answers

1. a. **False**. This is true in vitro but hypocalcaemia severe enough to have the same effect in vivo would be incompatible with life.
   b. **True**. Because hepatocellular dysfunction impairs the synthesis of vitamin K-dependent clotting factors.
   c. **True**. This is used as a measure of heparinisation.
   d. **False**. Vitamin K reverses the action of warfarin; protamine reverses heparin action.
   e. **False**. FDPs are raised by massive intravascular fibrin formation, as in DIC, and may be increased in thrombotic conditions but are not sensitive or specific enough to be a useful diagnostic test. Measurement of D-dimer is sensitive enough to detect venous thrombosis.

2. a. **False**. A purpuric rash or easy bruising on the limbs or trunk are more likely first symptoms.
   b. **True**. The appearance of retinal haemorrhages indicates that the patient is at risk of haemorrhage.
   c. **True**.
   d. **False**. Corticosteroids are given to some patients with idiopathic thrombocytopenic purpura but thrombocytopenia is often not steroid responsive.
   e. **False**. The goal is to prevent bleeding, not to normalise the blood count.

3. a. **False**.
   b. **True**. Thalassaemia is one of the causes of microcytosis.
   c. **True**.
   d. **False**. Anticonvulsants may cause macrocytosis.
   e. **False**. Haemolysis increases the reticulocyte count which, since reticulocytes are large, causes macrocytosis.

4. a. **True**. In Hodgkin's disease, the lymphadenopathy is often confined to a single site, most commonly the neck, at presentation.
   b. **True**.
   c. **True**.
   d. **False**. Alcohol-related pain is typical of Hodgkin's disease.
   e. **False**. Low-grade NHL responds poorly to treatment of any type.

5. a. **False**. A minor risk. It is when the count falls below $500 \times 10^6/l$ and particularly $100 \times 10^6/l$ that the risk becomes major.
   b. **False**. Mostly neutrophil release from the marginating pool. The left shift (or band forms) is the proportion of new neutrophils from the marrow.
   c. **False**. Immediate intravenous broad-spectrum antibiotics are indicated.
   d. **True**. Especially caused by the drugs zidovudine and ganciclovir.
   e. **True**. Neutropenia occurs in 1:10 000 patients treated with carbimazole for thyrotoxicosis.

Data interpretation answers

1. **Patient 1.** This is a fairly typical picture of megaloblastic anaemia caused by vitamin B_{12} or folate deficiency with severe macrocytosis, leucopenia and thrombocytopenia; hypersegmented neutrophils on the blood film would confirm the diagnosis, as would bone marrow aspiration although this is not done as a routine. Haematinics should be measured.

   Patient 2. This is a moderately severe microcytic anaemia (the differential diagnosis is given on p. 232). Iron deficiency is the most likely cause. The leucocytosis may be caused by infection or inflammation but could signify acute or subacute blood loss, a possible cause for the iron deficiency.

   Patient 3. There is erythrocytosis, thrombocytosis and leucocytosis, suggestive of polycythaemia vera. The red cell mass is likely to be increased and bone marrow examination should be diagnostic.

   Patient 4. There is a normocytic anaemia with normal white cell and platelet counts. This would be typical of the anaemia of chronic disease (e.g. renal failure) but could also be caused by a mixed deficiency. This would be suggested by an increased RDW and a 'dimorphic' blood film. You should examine and investigate the patient for an underlying disease.

   Patient 5. Here, there is a normochromic anaemia with mild thrombocytopenia, but the striking abnormality is the marked leucocytosis; this is typical of a chronic leukaemia. A differential white cell count and blood film would be crucial.

   Patient 6. This shows moderate pancytopenia. This could be seen in a patient with acute leukaemia, hypoplastic anaemia or after chemotherapy (see p. 234 for a fuller list of causes).

2. Prolongation of the prothrombin time may be caused by warfarin, consumption of clotting factors as in DIC, vitamin K deficiency or deficiency of the vitamin K-dependent clotting factors owing to liver disease. At 48 hours after a massive paracetamol overdose is about the time when hepatocellular damage becomes apparent, and the prothrombin time is quite a sensitive test for this. The likely

diagnosis is acute hepatocellular necrosis caused by paracetamol.

3. An extremely high ESR is usually caused by multiple myeloma, giant cell arteritis or chronic/severe infection/inflammation. This patient also has a moderate normochromic anaemia. Multiple myeloma is a likely diagnosis. Renal failure and hypercalcaemia are common in myeloma. You should measure plasma urea, creatinine and calcium. The definitive diagnosis is made by plasma and urine immunoelectrophoresis.

Case history answers

History 1

1. Whilst anticoagulation is indicated to prevent cerebral embolism in patients with atrial fibrillation, you must not initiate it unless you are sure it will be safe. Age, in itself, is not a contraindication, but there are aspects of the history which suggest there are other contraindications. There are strong hints that he may be abusing alcohol. The confusion is worrying because someone who is having falls and becomes confused could have a subdural haematoma, which is an absolute contraindication to anticoagulation. You should ask about:
   • his alcohol intake
   • dyspepsia or history of blood loss
   • his likelihood of taking tablets and attending for anticoagulant monitoring reliably.
2. You should measure his prothrombin time *before starting anticoagulants*; autoanticoagulation is common and would affect your choice of loading dose. It would also increase your anxiety about the possibility of alcohol abuse (prolonging the PT by causing hepatocellular damage). You should also check the haemoglobin concentration; anaemia would be a relative contraindication to anticoagulation or should, at least, be investigated before anticoagulation.
3. These might include
   • alcohol abuse
   • dementia (if it would interfere with compliance)
   • difficulty attending for anticoagulant monitoring
   • inability of wife or carer to supervise treatment
   • history of GI bleeding or anaemia
   • history of cerebral haemorrhage
   • concomitant drug therapy affecting the stability of warfarin levels
   • falls.
4. Advice would include:
   • avoid alcohol
   • avoid nonsteroidal analgesics and aspirin
   • report any excessive or unusual bleeding immediately
   • attend regularly for anticoagulant monitoring.

You should give the patient and his wife an information sheet about anticoagulants, listing drugs to be avoided.

History 2

1. a. **True**. This is always appropriate in neutropenia, even in the absence of chest signs or symptoms.
   b. **True**. Very important.
   c. **False**. Unnecessary if done that morning, which it will have been to see whether platelet transfusions were required.
   d. **False**. You must inspect his anal area as he has a symptom there, but a formal rectal examination is not appropriate as it may cause bacteraemia.
   e. **False**. Not appropriate; i.v. therapy required with broader coverage.
2. a. **True**.
   b. **False**. He is not that ill and you would take him out of protective isolation. In fact, even if he were so ill and requiring ventilation, neutropenic leukaemic patients do so badly in ITU that it is used rarely.
   c. **True**. Always true in this group of patients. Especially mouth, chest, skin and rectal area (p.239).
   d. **True**. Candidaemia or invasive aspergillosis are now more likely. This group of patients with persistent fever have a 30% mortality, mostly as a result of fungal infection.
   e. **True**. It is always worth repeating blood cultures, even though he is on antibiotics, as these patients get breakthrough bacteraemia.
3. a. **True**. Now you have a complex problem with two possible sites of infection.
   b. **True**. Even though one was done only 4 days ago. He also needs a CT scan of his chest.
   c. **False**. Not useful in lymphoma patients (unlike AIDS), although pneumocystis pneumonia is a diagnostic possibility.
   d. **False**. As the cough is not productive, of no benefit.
   e. **False**. His lesion is almost certainly not a pressure sore but a developing infection called icthyma gangrenosum (*Pseudomonas aeruginosa*).
4. He probably has two focal infections: one in his lungs and the other perirectally. The perirectal infection is likely to be caused by *Pseudomonas aeruginosa*, other bacteria including anaerobes, *Aspergillus* or mucormycosis. His lung disease may be caused by any of these or other bacteria or possibly *Pneumocystis*. He needs large doses of antifungals (amphotericin B), a CT scan of the lung, which is helpful diagnostically, and a biopsy of his rectal lesion as soon as possible.

Picture answers

1. a. Picture 6.1 shows multiple 'punched-out' lesions, in keeping with multiple myeloma or another cause of osteolytic metastases.

b. Hypercalcaemia is a common cause of acute renal failure in multiple myeloma. Volume depletion is an important and reversible effect of hypercalcaemia. 'Myeloma kidney' may cause renal failure without hypercalcaemia. This is because of tubular damage by the paraprotein, secondary hyperuricaemia, amyloidosis and infection.

c. With the history given, you should immediately measure serum calcium. You should also arrange serum and urine immunoelectrophoresis to identify a paraprotein but that is not an emergency investigation.

d. You should assess the patient's volume status, using a central venous pressure line if necessary, and give saline to increase urinary calcium excretion. Corticosteroid and/or bisphosphonate therapy may be needed as second-line treatment for hypercalcaemia.

2. a. There is a large soft tissue attenuation mass within the mediastinum abutting the trachea and aortic arch and compressing the superior vena cava (which cannot be seen). This is almost certainly a large lymph node mass.

b. Although you are not told that she has cervical lymphadenopathy, the scenario makes it very likely that she is describing alcohol-related lymph node pain, which is very specific to Hodgkin's disease. The combination with mediastinal lymphadenopathy makes the diagnosis of Hodgkin's by far the most likely diagnosis. Other causes of a mediastinal soft tissue mass include non-Hodgkin's lymphoma (unlikely in a young person and not associated with alcohol-related pain) or sarcoidosis (the second most likely possibility in this case). Unlikely causes are tuberculosis, retrosternal thyroid (unlikely), thymic tumour, dermoid or lung cancer nodes (especially small cell).

Viva answers

1. Aplastic anaemia usually affects the red cells, white cells and platelets. Patients are anaemic, thrombocytopenic and neutropenic. The anaemia may be symptomatic; it may precipitate symptoms of coronary, cerebrovascular or peripheral vascular ischaemia and may cause heart failure. Thrombocytopenia may cause purpura, bruising and — in severe cases — mucosal or GI bleeding or cerebral haemorrhage. Neutropenia causes mouth ulceration, perineal infection and susceptibility to opportunistic infection. Anaemia is treated with periodic blood transfusions. Platelet transfusions are given if the patient is severely thrombocytopenic and at risk of haemorrhage. Granulocyte transfusions are relatively ineffective and so the treatment of neutropenia is prophylaxis against infection and aggressive treatment of the earliest signs of it.

2. The choice of antiplatelet or anticoagulation therapy depends upon the pathophysiology of the disease (see p. 245).

Endocrinology and metabolism

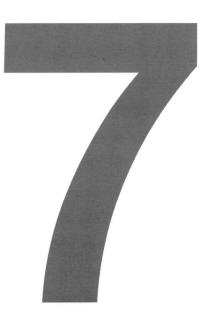

7.1 General introduction

Endocrinology may seem a large and disjointed subject because there are many glands each with its own diseases and symptomatology. There are, however, some unifying principles of pathology, investigation and management which make learning easier. Remember that glands malfunction in three ways:

- by enlarging
- by becoming overactive
- by becoming underactive.

Sometimes, enlargement is combined with underactivity or overactivity. The pituitary gland has a central, controlling function. Remember that there are six anterior pituitary and one posterior pituitary hormone which control the endocrine 'axes' described in Figure 47. The main endocrine diseases are shown in Table 57.

Learning objectives

You need to:
- know the range of common endocrine diseases
- understand the relationship between the pathological processes of autoimmunity and neoplasia and those diseases
- understand how biochemical testing and imaging are used to diagnose endocrine disease
- understand how to approach a patient with 'a lump in the thyroid'
- know the main clinical features, investigation and treatment of thyroid, adrenal and pituitary overactivity and underactivity

- know the main causes and clinical features of hypogonadism
- understand the common hyperlipidaemias and their relationship to cardiovascular disease.

Pathology

Endocrine underactivity is usually autoimmune (e.g. hypoparathyroidism, hypothyroidism, Addison's disease, insulin-dependent diabetes mellitus (IDDM)). The exception is hypopituitarism, which is usually caused by a tumour. Endocrine overactivity usually results from a tumour (e.g. acromegaly, hyperprolactinaemia, Cushing's and Conn's syndromes, phaeochromocytoma, hyperparathyroidism and insulinoma). The exception is hyperthyroidism which is often (but not always) autoimmune. Most endocrinologically active tumours are benign, because malignant tumours behave in a primitive way and grow at the expense of hormone synthesis. That does not apply to ectopic hormone production; some extremely malignant tumours which are not derived from an endocrine gland synthesise hormones, e.g. adrenocorticotrophic hormone (ACTH), antidiuretic hormone (ADH), parathyroid hormone (PTH)-related peptide (p. 316) from small cell carcinoma of the bronchus.

Investigations

There are three main types of investigation:

- measurement of hormone concentrations or responses
- imaging
- autoantibody measurement.

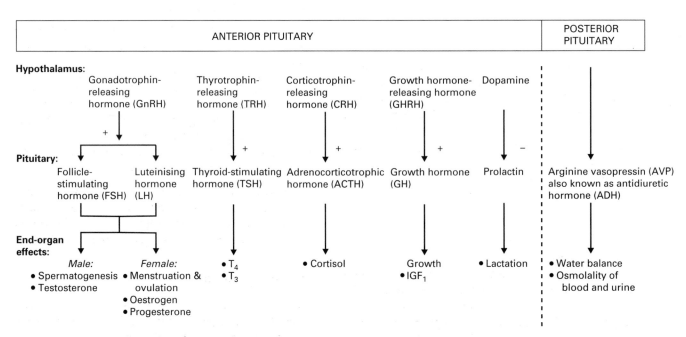

Fig. 47
Hypothalamic and pituitary hormones and their effects.

Table 57 A scheme for revising endocrine diseases

	Overactivity	Underactivity	Enlargement
Thyroid	Hyperthyroidism	Hypothyroidism	Thyroid nodule
Pituitary	Acromegaly, hyperprolactinaemia	Hypopituitarism, diabetes insipidus	Pituitary tumour
Adrenal			
HPA axis	Cushing's syndrome	Hypoadrenalism (including Addison's disease)	
RAA axis	Conn's syndrome		
Medulla	Phaeochromocytoma		
Parathyroid	Hyperparathyroidism[a]	Hypoparathyroidism[a]	
Pancreas	Insulinoma	Diabetes mellitus	

HPA, hypothalamo–pituitary–adrenal; RAA, renin–angiotensin–aldosterone.
[a]See Chapter 8 (p. 319).

Biochemistry

There are two types of biochemical test: static and dynamic. Static tests are single tests measuring blood hormone levels at one point in time. Dynamic tests measure how that hormone level responds to a stimulus. Static tests are used first and may be sufficient. For example, demonstrating that the serum cortisol is unmeasurably low in a patient with a large pituitary tumour and clinically obvious hypopituitarism is diagnostic of hypoadrenalism. Some static tests (e.g. thyroid-stimulating hormone (TSH) measurement) are now so sensitive that they have made dynamic tests redundant. Dynamic tests are more sensitive but more complex and expensive. If there was doubt that the patient described above was hypoadrenal, he would be challenged by adrenocorticotrophic hormone (ACTH) stimulation or insulin hypoglycaemia to see if he could produce cortisol under stress. Dynamic tests have a simple underlying principle:

- if you suspect that a gland is overactive, try to suppress its function
- if you suspect that it is underactive, stimulate it.

Imaging

Ultrasound, CT and MR imaging are the most sensitive methods of finding and delineating mass lesions and showing their consistency. Radionuclide scanning is generally less sensitive but can show that tissue is endocrinologically active and can find lesions which cannot be found in any other way (e.g. metastases of thyroid cancer located by labelled iodine scanning or use of labelled somatostatin analogue to locate an endocrinologically active tumour).

Immunology

Immunology plays a limited part, usually secondary to clinical diagnosis and biochemistry. Thus, high titres of adrenal or thyroid microsomal antibodies support clinical and biochemical diagnoses of autoimmune Addison's disease and Hashimoto's thyroiditis, respectively. They can also predict that a patient is at risk of developing them.

Management

Overactive glands can be treated surgically, with a drug which reduces hormone synthesis or by radiotherapy. If a gland is underactive, the treatment is to replace the missing hormone or give a synthetic analogue.

The efficacy of treatment can be monitored in three ways:

- the end-organ effects (health and wellbeing)
- plasma level of the replaced hormone
- levels of a trophic hormone; for example, measurement of TSH to check the adequacy of thyroid replacement therapy (p. 261).

This chapter will go through diseases, gland by gland, and consider their pathology, clinical features, investigation, management and prognosis.

7.2 Thyroid disease

Normal thyroid function

The synthesis of thyroid hormone (thyroxine (T_4) and triiodothyronine (T_3)) is controlled by a sequence of hormonal signals:

- Thyrotrophin-releasing hormone (TRH) secreted by the hypothalamus into the hypophysial portal system
- Thyroid-stimulating hormone (TSH) secreted by the pituitary into the systemic circulation
- Feedback inhibition exerted by thyroid hormones on the pituitary and hypothalamus.

Thyroxine and triiodothyronine are largely protein bound. Thyroxine is converted to triiodothyronine by deiodination in the thyroid and peripheral tissues. The level of thyroid hormone determines tissue metabolic activity.

Hyperthyroidism

This is a better term than thyrotoxicosis because overproduction of thyroid hormone is the fundamental abnormality and the clinical expression (toxicosis) of the disease is secondary to it and remarkably variable.

Pathology

The common causes of hyperthyroidism are Graves' disease and toxic nodular goitres.

Graves' disease. This is also known as diffuse toxic goitre and is the classical cause of hyperthyroidism. It is caused by antibodies formed within the thyroid which bind to TSH receptors on follicular cells and stimulate thyroid hormone synthesis and secretion; other autoantibodies promote thyroid growth and eye disease (see below). It is possible to have ophthalmic signs of Graves' disease without hyperthyroidism and vice versa, presumably because there are different antibodies in different individuals.

Toxic nodular goitres. These are autonomous solitary or multinodular goitres which are probably not autoimmune in origin; they are not associated with autoimmune skin and eye signs and tend to present in older patients. They are investigated and managed in much the same way as Graves' disease and will be described with it.

Uncommon causes of hyperthyroidism include:

* subacute thyroiditis (p. 262)
* Hashimoto's thyroiditis (p. 260)
* amiodarone therapy.

Extremely rarely, hyperthyroidism can be caused by a TSH-secreting pituitary tumour, but this is the exception to a general rule that hyperthyroidism is a primary disease of the thyroid.

Graves' disease is at least five times as common in women as men and may present at any age but is most common between 40 and 60. Toxic nodular goitres are also more common in women but usually present in later life.

Clinical features

Hyperthyroidism causes symptoms by increasing cell metabolism and by sensitising the tissues to catecholamines, hence the similarity between hyperthyroidism and the adrenergically mediated symptoms and signs of anxiety. The classical staring eyes and lid lag of hyperthyroidism are caused by adrenergic stimulation of levator palpebrae superioris. Hyperthyroid patients usually present with the symptoms listed in Figure 48 or with abnormal thyroid function tests found coincidentally. Elderly patients may present with atrial fibrillation or heart failure. The symptoms and signs are of:

* hyperthyroidism and its complications

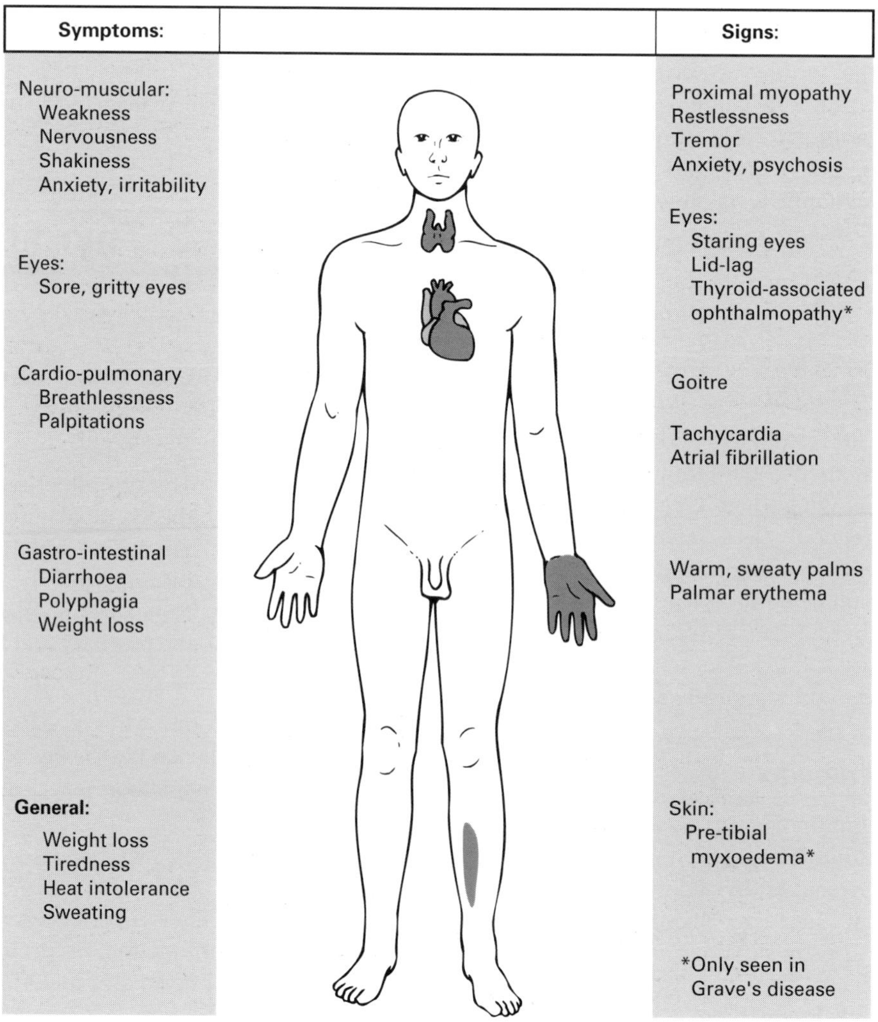

Symptoms:		Signs:

Neuro-muscular:
  Weakness
  Nervousness
  Shakiness
  Anxiety, irritability
		Proximal myopathy
		Restlessness
		Tremor
		Anxiety, psychosis

Eyes:
  Sore, gritty eyes
		Eyes:
		  Staring eyes
		  Lid-lag
		  Thyroid-associated
		  ophthalmopathy*

Cardio-pulmonary
  Breathlessness
  Palpitations
		Goitre
		
		Tachycardia
		Atrial fibrillation

Gastro-intestinal
  Diarrhoea
  Polyphagia
  Weight loss
		Warm, sweaty palms
		Palmar erythema

General:
  Weight loss
  Tiredness
  Heat intolerance
  Sweating
		Skin:
		  Pre-tibial
		  myxoedema*

		*Only seen in Grave's disease

Fig. 48
Symptoms and signs of hyperthyroidism.

- the goitre, if present (p. 262)
- other autoimmune features, notably eye disease.

Thyroid-associated ophthalmopathy

Any hyperthyroid patient may have sore, gritty eyes, lid retraction, lid lag and a staring appearance. Only those with Graves' disease develop the more severe inflammatory changes of thyroid-associated ophthalmology which include enlargement and (later) fibrosis of ocular muscles.

The symptoms are watering eyes, photophobia, retro-orbital pain, double vision and (in a few cases) visual loss. Patients are very self-conscious of their abnormal appearance. They have proptosis, which may be asymmetrical, and conjunctival and periorbital oedema. They may develop corneal ulceration and/or diplopia with decreased visual acuity. Physical examination should include measurement of visual acuity, fields and fundoscopy. CT scan is indicated, particularly if the disease is asymmetrical, to demonstrate the swollen eye muscles and exclude a retro-orbital tumour.

Treatment is with artificial tears, sunglasses and diuretics for severe oedema. Raising the head of the bed at night helps reduce periorbital oedema. In severe cases, the treatment is high-dose steroids, orbital radiotherapy and/or surgical decompression.

Investigations

Investigation of hyperthyroidism has been greatly simplified by the sensitive and reliable assays now available. In most cases, both total thyroxine and triiodothyronine are raised. Occasionally only triiodothyronine is raised (termed T_3 toxicosis). Measurement of total thyroxine can be misleading because increased thyroid-binding globulin (as in patients who are pregnant or on the pill) gives a raised total thyroxine suggesting hyperthyroidism, when the 'free' (unbound) fraction of thyroxine is normal. Many laboratories measure free thyroxine routinely to avoid this catch.

Measurement of TSH gives extra information because:

- thyroid autonomy causes feedback suppression of TSH; serum TSH may be low before the thyroid

hormones are measurably increased, making it a very sensitive test for hyperthyroidism
- serum TSH will be normal if total thyroxine is artificially raised by an increased level of thyroid-binding globulin (see previous paragraph)
- it will detect the very rare cases in which thyrotoxicosis is caused by increased pituitary TSH secretion.

Table 58 summarises some common abnormalities of thyroid function tests.

Neither immunology nor imaging have any part in the routine investigation of hyperthyroidism because:

- measurement of the thyroid-stimulating immunoglobulins of Graves' disease is not routinely available
- a goitre (if present) is extremely unlikely to be malignant in a thyrotoxic patient and the exact nature of the goitre rarely influences management.

The only exception is the solitary toxic nodule, which can be diagnosed by an isotope scan in a patient with hyperthyroidism and a clinically obvious solitary nodule; this might be treated surgically out of choice.

Management

Antithyroid drugs

Most patients are treated with antithyroid drugs first and later with **ablative treatment**, usually radioiodine but sometimes surgery. Antithyroid drugs (carbimazole and propylthiouracil) work by preventing iodine-trapping and suppressing antithyroid autoimmunity. Their main side-effect is neutropenia, which is not dose related and usually occurs in the first 8 weeks of treatment. Skin rashes, nausea and cholestatic jaundice are other side-effects. Graves' disease may remit and is more likely to do so after treatment with antithyroid drugs, so it is common practice to give drug treatment for a period and then withdraw it. It is usual to start a moderately large dose and taper it once hyperthyroidism is controlled. The drug is continued for up to 2 years, although the optimum duration of treatment is

Table 58 Typical thyroid function test results in a range of diseases

	Thyroxine		Triiodothyronine	TSH
	Total	Free		
Primary hypothyroidism	↓	↓	↓	↑
Secondary hypothyroidism	↓	↓	↓	↔ or ↓
'Euthyroid sick' syndrome	↔ or ↓	↔ or ↓	↓	↔ or ↓
Hyperthyroidism	↑	↑	↑	↓
T_3 toxicosis	↔ or ↓	↔ or ↓	↑	↓
Raised TBG (e.g. pregnancy, the pill)	↑	↔	↔ or ↑	↔

TBG, thyroid-binding globulin.
↓ fall; ↑, increase; ↔ no change from normal

controversial. Sometimes antithyroid drugs and thyroxine are given together (block-replace regimen). The long-term results are disappointing, since only one half of cases remit and, of those who do, one half relapse. Causes of hyperthyroidism other than Graves' disease do not usually remit. Long-term antithyroid drug therapy is a treatment option which may occasionally be used, for example, in elderly patients who refuse radioiodine or do not respond to it. Since many thyrotoxic symptoms (particularly tremor and palpitations) are adrenergic, beta-blockers give very rapid and effective symptom relief at the start of treatment.

Radioiodine

Radioiodine treatment is non-invasive and relatively free of immediate side-effects, although it can precipitate a hyperthyroid crisis in an inadequately prepared patient. It is slow to act, taking months or sometimes years to have its full effects. For that reason, a dose of radioiodine which produces an acceptable rate of early euthyroidism (e.g. 95% cured within 12 months of treatment) carries a 50% likelihood of hypothyroidism within 12 months and a 90% or higher lifetime risk. If a first dose of radioiodine fails to control hyperthyroidism, for example in patients with multinodular goitres, it can be given more than once. Radioiodine is absolutely contraindicated in children, nursing mothers and women likely to become pregnant within 3 months because of the risks of thyroid cancer, transmission in breast milk and congenital malformations, respectively.

Surgery

Surgery is indicated for a small number of patients including those who have large goitres, or respond poorly to other modalities of treatment. Surgery may be complicated by recurrent laryngeal nerve palsy, permanent hypoparathyroidism and hypothyroidism. Patients whose thyrotoxicosis is inadequately controlled may have a thyroid crisis during surgery. A small number of patients are uncontrolled by surgery and late relapse of hyperthyroidism may also occur. There is a trend for fewer patients to be treated with surgery.

Whichever form of ablative therapy is chosen, it is usual to pretreat all but the mildest cases with antithyroid drugs and/or beta-blockers for rapid symptom relief and to prevent hyperthyroid crisis. All successfully treated patients, whichever treatment they have received, need annual thyroid function tests for the rest of their lives to detect late hypothyroidism or relapse.

Prognosis

Hyperthyroidism can usually be cured without serious sequelae. Many patients, particularly those who have received radioiodine, eventually become hypothyroid. The most severe acute effects are hyperthyroid crises, psychoses and cardiac dysrhythmias. Paroxysmal atrial fibrillation is a particularly important complication because it may cause embolic stroke. Patients with hyperthyroidism and atrial fibrillation should be given anticoagulation therapy unless there are strong contraindications. Every patient with atrial fibrillation should have thyroid function tests to exclude hyperthyroidism.

Hypothyroidism

Pathology

Hypothyroidism is *commonly* primary or secondary to radiotherapy or surgery, and *uncommonly* secondary to pituitary tumours.

Primary hypothyroidism is now almost always autoimmune, although iodine deficiency used to be the most common cause. The most common diagnosis is **primary atrophic hypothyroidism** and so the majority of hypothyroid patients have no palpable goitre; **Hashimoto's thyroiditis**, a more florid autoimmune disease with a firm rubbery goitre, lymphocytic infiltration and high-titre thyroid autoantibodies, is less common. Rarely, patients with Hashimoto's thyroiditis may go through a short phase of hyperthyroidism (Hashitoxicosis). Hashimoto's disease is 10 times more common in women than men and usually presents in middle age. **Previous ablative therapy** for hyperthyroidism is another common cause of hypothyroidism. Less common causes include viral thyroiditis and amiodarone or lithium treatment. Hypothyroidism is not a presenting feature of thyroid cancer.

Clinical features

Figure 49 summarises the specific clinical features of hypothyroidism. It may also cause non-specific symptoms; thyroid function tests are cheap, reliable and often performed, so many cases of hypothyroidism are found almost by chance. A particularly high yield is in women with gynaecological complaints, because menorrhagia and infertility can be caused by hypothyroidism. Hypothyroidism rarely *presents* with obesity (p. 274), although patients often admit to weight gain.

Investigations

Like hyperthyroidism, hypothyroidism is easily diagnosed from the serum thyroxine and TSH concentrations (Table 58). Patients with *primary* hypothyroidism have a low serum thyroxine with a compensatory increase in TSH. Deficiency of thyroid-binding globulin causes a low serum thyroxine, but this is not accompanied by a raised TSH. *Secondary* (pituitary) hypothyroidism should be suspected if the patient is truly hypothyroid (low free thyroxine concentration, p. 259) with no compensatory increase in serum TSH. Serum triidothyronine adds nothing to the information given by serum thyroxine and TSH and is actually unhelpful

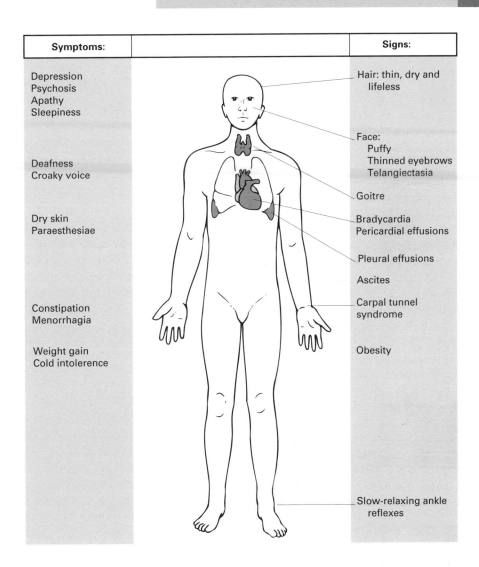

Symptoms:		Signs:
Depression Psychosis Apathy Sleepiness		Hair: thin, dry and lifeless
		Face: Puffy Thinned eyebrows Telangiectasia
Deafness Croaky voice		Goitre
Dry skin Paraesthesiae		Bradycardia Pericardial effusions
		Pleural effusions
		Ascites
Constipation Menorrhagia		Carpal tunnel syndrome
Weight gain Cold intolerence		Obesity
		Slow-relaxing ankle reflexes

Fig. 49
Clinical features of hypothyroidism.

because it can be reduced by non-specific intercurrent illness (low T_3 syndrome or 'euthyroid sick syndrome'). The serum thyroxine and TSH will invariably be abnormal in true primary hypothyroidism.

Imaging the thyroid is not indicated in uncomplicated primary hypothyroidism, even if accompanied by a diffuse goitre. Rarely, pressure symptoms or a suspicious-feeling nodule justify aspiration cytology and/or ultrasound scanning (p. 262).

Management

Thyroxine deficiency is treated by thyroxine replacement. Unless hypothyroidism has come on suddenly (as after surgery), a small dose is started and increased at 2–4 weekly intervals. It has a long half-life and is given once daily. The serum thyroxine and TSH concentrations often normalise before patients feel back to normal, so biochemical monitoring is essential.

The longer the history and more severe the symptoms, the more cautiously thyroxine replacement should be given because hypothyroidism causes hypercholesterolaemia and coronary artery disease. Speeding up metabolism with injudicious doses of thyroxine can cause myocardial infarction and death. Even if thyroxine is started in a small dose, angina may be precipitated or worsened; however, that is not a reason for stopping treatment, because untreated hypothyroidism leaves patients feeling unwell and the persistently high serum cholesterol causes progression of the coronary artery disease. By analogy with other lipid-lowering treatments, it is to be hoped that thyroxine replacement will cause regression of coronary atherosclerosis.

Prognosis

Hypothyroidism, left untreated, is a risk factor for ischaemic heart disease. If diagnosed and treated early, life expectancy is good.

Myxoedema coma
This is a rare medical emergency caused by longstanding and severe hypothyroidism. It presents with coma and, usually, hypothermia. It is fatal in over 50% of patients despite treatment. This consists of:

- intensive nursing care
- nasogastric suction
- cautious fluid therapy

- passive rewarming
- corticosteroid therapy
- intravenous triiodothyronine
- treatment of underlying infection.

Goitre

Thyroid swelling matters because it may be:

- unsightly
- a cause of pressure symptoms
- accompanied by hypothyroidism or hyperthyroidism
- caused by a tumour (in up to 10% of patients).

The clinical approach is determined by:

- the context: thyroid enlargement in patients with hypothyroidism, hyperthyroidism, pregnancy or puberty rarely needs investigation
- feel: diffuse goitres are rarely malignant
- history: onset in childhood, a rapid onset at any age, or a history of previous thyroid radiation are suggestive of malignancy.

Even benign thyroid enlargement may need surgery for cosmetic reasons, for comfort or to control hyperthyroidism. If the goitre extends retrosternally, surgery may be needed for pressure symptoms. In most cases, the aim is to exclude or treat malignancy. Table 59 shows causes of thyroid enlargement.

Pathology of thyroid tumours

Thyroid tumours are typically unifocal and solid; apart from toxic adenomas, they are non-functioning ('cold') on isotope scanning.

Papillary carcinoma. This constitutes about 60% of thyroid cancers and is the most differentiated and least aggressive of the malignant tumours. It may present in children.

Follicular carcinoma. Follicular carcinoma (20%) is less differentiated and more likely to metastasise (typically to lung or bone).

Medullary carcinoma. This form (5%) may arise as a lone abnormality or part of the syndrome of **multiple endocrine neoplasia**; it is relatively slow-growing but prone to recur and spread locally. Its biochemical hallmark is calcitonin secretion.

Anaplastic carcinoma. Anaplastic carcinoma (10%) affects elderly people and is extremely invasive locally.

Lymphomas (<5%). These may arise in longstanding autoimmune thyroid disease.

Investigation and treatment

The investigation and treatment of thyroid swelling is summarised in Figure 50. Having decided that a thyroid swelling is a suspicious nodule rather than an innocent diffuse goitre, relevant investigations are:

- fine needle aspiration cytology
- thyroid ultrasound
- surgical biopsy.

Isotope scintigraphy is only useful to demonstrate that a solitary solid nodule is functional and, therefore, not malignant. Aspiration cytology can give an index of suspicion of malignancy. Ultrasound can demonstrate that a lesion is cystic, multinodular, solid and/or invasive. It can also be used to guide a biopsy needle. The definitive investigation/treatment is surgical removal of a nodule, partial or total thyroidectomy.

Papillary and follicular carcinomas are treated by total thyroidectomy with high-dose radioactive iodine for metastases. Anaplastic carcinoma is so invasive that it is untreatable. Lymphoma is treated with chemotherapy.

Thyroiditis

A number of conditions can present as subacute thyroiditis, which is characterised by:

- pain in some patients
- swelling
- thyroid dysfunction in some patients.

Table 59 Causes of thyroid enlargement

	Hypothyroid	Euthyroid	Hyperthyroid
Diffuse	Iodine deficiency Hashimoto's thyroiditis	Simple goitre Pregnancy Puberty	Graves' disease
	Subacute thyroiditis (tender)	Subacute thyroiditis (tender)	Subacute thyroiditis (tender)
Nodular/asymmetrical		Thyroid cyst Adenoma Nodular goitre Carcinoma: papillary, follicular, medullary, anaplastic Lymphoma Metastasis	Adenoma Nodular goitre

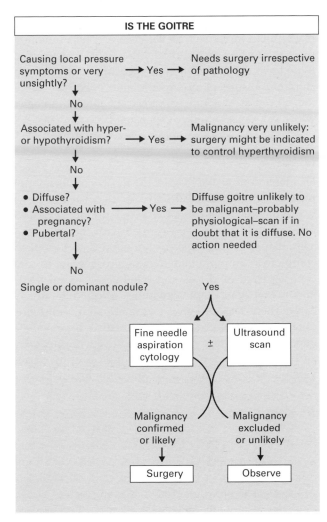

IS THE GOITRE

Causing local pressure symptoms or very unsightly? → Yes → Needs surgery irrespective of pathology

No ↓

Associated with hyper- or hypothyroidism? → Yes → Malignancy very unlikely: surgery might be indicated to control hyperthyroidism

No ↓

- Diffuse?
- Associated with pregnancy? → Yes → Diffuse goitre unlikely to be malignant–probably physiological–scan if in doubt that it is diffuse. No action needed
- Pubertal?

No ↓

Single or dominant nodule? ——— Yes

Fine needle aspiration cytology ± Ultrasound scan

Malignancy confirmed or likely | Malignancy excluded or unlikely

Surgery | Observe

Fig. 50
An approach to the investigation and treatment of thyroid enlargement.

Commoner syndromes include:

- postpartum thyroiditis
- Hashimoto's thyroiditis
- subacute (de Quervain's or viral) thyroiditis.

Very uncommon forms of thyroiditis are acute suppurative thyroiditis and Riedel's (invasive fibrous) thyroiditis.

Hashimoto's disease
Hashimoto's disease may present with classical thyroiditis but far more often presents with painless goitre and thyroid dysfunction.

Subacute thyroiditis
This is a distinctive syndrome which, though less common than Hashimoto's disease, is prevalent enough to be important, because it can be treated if recognised. It causes rapid, painful thyroid enlargement, sore throat with dysphagia, systemic malaise and myalgia. The gland is enlarged and tender. There is fever and a high ESR. Thyroid function progresses over days or weeks

from euthyroidism to hyperthyroidism, then hypothyroidism before spontaneously returning to normal. The aetiology is thought to be a viral infection with release of stored thyroid hormone causing hyperthyroidism, and impaired synthesis causing hypothyroidism. The gland shows greatly reduced uptake on an isotope scan. The condition resolves spontaneously with time but a short course of high-dose prednisolone rapidly relieves systemic symptoms and speeds recovery.

7.3 Pituitary disease

Normal anatomy and physiology

The pituitary is located in the pituitary fossa, bounded by the anterior and posterior clinoid processes, diaphragma sellae and (laterally) cavernous sinuses. A narrow plate of bone separates the pituitary fossa from the sphenoid sinus, which is readily accessible to the surgeon.

The pituitary gland is connected to the hypothalamus by the pituitary stalk. It is composed of the anterior pituitary, which synthesises and secretes the anterior pituitary hormones (see Fig. 49) and the posterior pituitary, an extension of neurones of the hypothalamus, which secretes arginine vasopressin (AVP, antidiuretic hormone (ADH)). ADH diffuses down these neurones but is not synthesised in the posterior pituitary; therefore, pituitary damage does not necessarily cause ADH deficiency.

Secretion of all the anterior pituitary hormones except prolactin is stimulated by hypothalamic trophic hormones. Prolactin secretion is under the *inhibitory* control of hypothalamic dopamine. These controlling hormones reach the anterior pituitary through the blood vessels of the hypophysial portal system. Signalling by hormones is a complex process and some of its intricacies have a bearing on clinical practice. For example, gonadotrophin-releasing hormone (GnRH) is secreted by the hypothalamus in a pulsatile fashion. Pulsatile GnRH infusion stimulates gonadotrophin secretion and can be used as a treatment for infertility, whereas non-pulsatile GnRH therapy downregulates the GnRH receptors and actually inhibits gonadotrophin secretion. Long-acting GnRH analogues can be used, for example, to suppress 'precocious puberty' or treat carcinoma of the prostate.

Pituitary tumours

Pathology

The significance of the anatomical location of the pituitary in the development of symptoms from pituitary tumours is shown in Figure 51. At postmortem, up to

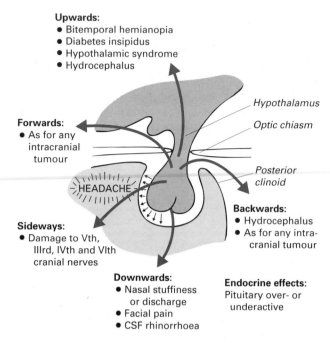

Upwards:
- Bitemporal hemianopia
- Diabetes insipidus
- Hypothalamic syndrome
- Hydrocephalus

Forwards:
- As for any intracranial tumour

Hypothalamus

Optic chiasm

HEADACHE

Posterior clinoid

Backwards:
- Hydrocephalus
- As for any intra-cranial tumour

Sideways:
- Damage to Vth, IIIrd, IVth and VIth cranial nerves

Downwards:
- Nasal stuffiness or discharge
- Facial pain
- CSF rhinorrhoea

Endocrine effects:
Pituitary over- or underactive

Fig. 51
How expanding pituitary tumours cause symptoms.

one-third of pituitary glands contain microscopic or macroscopic adenomas. They are known about in life only if they grow large enough to compress adjacent structures (e.g. the optic chiasm) or overproduce a hormone which causes symptoms. Most do neither. Even tiny tumours can cause serious disease if they are secretory (e.g. Cushing's disease). Hyperprolactinaemia is the most common pituitary overactivity, usually presenting in women during their menstrual years. Most such women have **microadenomas** (< 1 cm diameter). Pituitary tumours can secrete any anterior pituitary hormone and sometimes several, but prolactin, growth hormone (GH) and ACTH are the most clinically important. Tumours need to be over 1 cm in diameter to present with 'mass effects'. Most pituitary tumours are benign, but the pituitary fossa is so small and so close to important structures that relatively modest expansion can cause serious damage. They can expand (Fig. 51):

- **upwards:** towards the optic chiasm, hypothalamus and third ventricle
- **sideways:** into the cavernous sinus, compressing the cranial nerves in its walls
- **downwards:** into the base of skull, sphenoid sinus and nasopharynx
- **forwards:** exceptionally, into the anterior cranial fossa
- **backwards:** exceptionally, into the middle and posterior fossae.

Secondary tumours can deposit in or near the pituitary fossa and several types of primary intracranial tumour can affect the pituitary and its hypothalamic connections. Of these, craniopharyngiomas are the most

important; their embryonic origin from Rathke's pouch places them in the suprasellar cistern. The commonest presentations of such tumours are visual impairment, hypothalamic dysfunction, hypopituitarism and (in children) disorders of growth and puberty. Granulomata, cysts and tuberculomas are rare pathologies which can cause pituitary expansion.

Clinical features

Headache and visual loss are the most common symptoms of an expanding pituitary tumour. The headache is frontal or retro-orbital. As the tumour expands upwards and comes into contact with the optic chiasm, it first causes superior temporal field loss, then complete bitemporal hemianopia, progressing to concentric visual field loss and blindness. Central fields and visual acuity are sometimes affected relatively early. There may be some asymmetry, but both fields are usually affected. Later, the optic discs become pale and atrophic. Optic nerve function can be saved by early decompression; established optic atrophy is irreversible. Other symptoms are shown in Figure 51.

Investigations

Investigation includes assessment of:

- optic nerve damage
  — perimetry
  — visual acuity
  — visual evoked potentials
- endocrine status, testing for
  — hypopituitarism
  — overactivity (prolactin and GH in particular)
- the tumour mass
  — high-resolution CT and/or MR scan
  — angiography, sometimes needed to exclude an aneurysm mimicking a tumour.

Management and prognosis

There are three types of treatment:

- medical treatment
- surgery
- radiotherapy.

If the optic nerves are compromised by a large pituitary tumour, urgent action is needed. Two classes of drug — dopaminergic agonists (bromocriptine, cabergoline and quinagolide) and a somatostatin analogue (octreotide) — can shrink some types of pituitary tumours. Dopaminergic agonists are highly effective for prolactinomas and may also shrink GH-secreting tumours. Octreotide is mainly used for GH-secreting tumours. In practice:

- your first step when presented with a large pituitary tumour is to measure serum prolactin
- if it is high (> 5000 mU/l), the first-line treatment is to give an oral dopaminergic agonist, which act so

rapidly that they can be used for a 'medical' optic nerve decompression without the need for surgery

- in all other patients, urgent decompressive neurosurgery is needed.

If visual acuity and fields are normal, there is less urgency and medical therapy, surgery and radiotherapy are tailored to the individual patient. Dopaminergic agonists are so effective for prolactin-secreting tumours that surgery is usually only indicated in patients who cannot tolerate them. Surgery is the best choice for other secretory *micro*adenomas, because the surgeon can directly inspect the gland, remove the tumour and cure the endocrine disease without necessarily causing hypopituitarism. It may also be indicated to debulk *macro*adenomas (see previous paragraph). Radiotherapy is slow to act and likely to damage residual normal pituitary function, so it is reserved for tumours of any size where drugs and/or surgery have failed to control overactivity or there is a residual large tumour mass. The advent of high-quality non-invasive imaging, less invasive neurosurgical techniques and effective medical therapies means that most patients, even with large pituitary tumours, have a good prognosis. This is highly specialised medicine, not for the generalist.

Hypopituitarism and diabetes insipidus

Hypopituitarism may present out of the blue or develop in a patient with known pituitary disease as a result of surgery or radiotherapy. Transient diabetes insipidus and hypopituitarism are common immediately after pituitary surgery and may resolve within days or weeks. If they last longer than 1 month, they are likely to be permanent. In contrast, radiotherapy causes hypopituitarism months, years or decades later. In patients with hypopituitarism as their first presentation of pituitary disease, CT and MR scanning have revolutionised management. Together with a careful clinical history, they can usually narrow the diagnosis down to just one of the following:

Common causes:

- pituitary and hypothalamic tumours
  — primary: intra- and extrasellar
  — secondary
- iatrogenic
  — surgery
  — radiotherapy
- idiopathic: empty sella syndrome.
  Rare causes:
- cysts, granulomata
- autoimmune: lymphocytic hypophysitis
- vascular: Sheehan's syndrome.

Since AVP is secreted by hypothalamic neurones, diabetes insipidus (DI) is a symptom of hypothalamic damage. It may occur without anterior pituitary underactivity and vice versa. Extensive damage is needed to cause simultaneous anterior and posterior pituitary underactivity.

Clinical features

Anterior pituitary underactivity

The symptoms and signs of anterior pituitary underactivity are determined by which hormones are deficient. Prolactin differs from the others in that it is under the *inhibitory* control of hypothalamic dopamine. Hypoprolactinaemia rarely occurs and is clinically unimportant when it does. The other anterior pituitary hormones are under *stimulatory* hypothalamic control. With progressive anterior pituitary dysfunction, they are usually lost in the order:

1. GH
2. gonadotrophins
3. ACTH
4. TSH.

GH deficiency causes growth failure in children and non-specific lethargy in adults. Gonadotrophin deficiency (like hyperprolactinaemia, p. 266) causes amenorrhoea in women and impotence/infertility in men. ACTH deficiency causes hypoadrenalism (p. 268) and TSH deficiency causes hypothyroidism.

The hypoadrenalism of hypopituitarism differs from primary adrenal failure in that the patient does not become pigmented and is not aldosterone deficient.

The hypothyroidism of pituitary disease differs from primary hypothyroidism in that it rarely causes weight gain because there is accompanying hypoadrenalism.

The patient with panhypopituitarism is pale, hypotensive, impotent, weak and lethargic. Advanced disease may present with collapse, hyponatraemic fits (as a result of cortisol and thyroxine deficiency) or symptoms of an underlying tumour. A tumour which oversecretes one hormone (typically prolactin or GH) may cause deficiency of the others, although tumours presenting with hypopituitarism are more often than not non-functioning.

Diabetes insipidus

The symptoms are overwhelming thirst, polyuria (often over 4 litres/day), frequency and nocturia. Patients have to get up and drink during the night. One patient of mine used to fantasise about drinking whole swimming pools before he received treatment. The diagnosis is obvious if these symptoms develop suddenly after neurosurgery or a head injury but are harder to recognise if they develop slowly and spontaneously.

Investigation

Anterior pituitary underactivity

Hypopituitarism is confirmed by 'static' and 'dynamic' tests (p. 257). Examples of helpful static tests are:

- hypothyroidism without a compensatory rise in TSH, strong presumptive evidence of pituitary or hypothalamic underactivity
- hypogonadotrophic hypogonadism
- lack of appropriately high gonadotrophins in postmenopausal women.

Cortisol, GH and ACTH have short half-lives and their plasma levels are very variable in health, so random measurements are of limited value. GH and ACTH deficiency can be shown by measuring the cortisol and GH response to insulin-induced hypoglycaemia. This is unpleasant, potentially dangerous and contraindicated in

- elderly people (age > 70 years)
- patients with histories of ischaemic heart disease or epilepsy
- patients who appear profoundly hypopituitary.

Alternative tests are increasingly used. Glucagon can be used to stimulate ACTH and GH secretion and a short synacthen test can detect longstanding (> 3 months) secondary hypoadrenalism. If a patient with suspected hypopituitarism undergoes insulin stress testing, the dose of insulin should be kept small (0.1 unit/kg) to avoid dangerous hypoglycaemia.

Diabetes insipidus

The diagnosis is obvious if a patient develops polyuria after pituitary surgery or a head injury (provided he or she is not clearing an iatrogenic fluid load). Treatment is with desmopressin, a synthetic ADH analogue.

If diabetes insipidus develops insidiously and/or the diagnosis is uncertain, a 'water deprivation test' is performed. The patient is given nothing to drink for 8 hours and then has an injection of desmopressin. Urine volume, urine osmolality and plasma osmolality are measured. The test distinguishes between:

- normal: urine volume falls, urine osmolality rises and plasma osmolality remains normal
- diabetes insipidus: there is no fall in urine volume, no rise in urine osmolality and plasma osmolality rises.

Patients with **nephrogenic diabetes insipidus** have no response to injected desmopressin because their kidneys are insensitive to it. Patients with **cranial diabetes insipidus** respond as normal (see above) to desmopressin.

Management and prognosis

Cortisol and thyroxine are replaced as described under hypoadrenalism (p. 269) and hypothyroidism (p. 261). GH is of proven value in children with short stature but its role in adults has yet to be fully evaluated. Gonadotrophin deficiency is treated by sex-steroid replacement and diabetes insipidus by intranasal or oral desmopressin. Patients newly presenting with panhypopituitarism should receive corticosteroids for at least a week before thyroxine is started because increasing the metabolic rate can precipitate a hypoadrenal crisis. Sex steroid therapy can safely be deferred (but must not be forgotten). If diabetes insipidus is proven, it should be treated without delay because starting corticosteroids will exacerbate diabetes insipidus in a patient with panhypopituitarism.

The most serious risk to the hypopituitary patient is a hypoadrenal crisis because of either non-compliance or inadequate therapy, particularly during intercurrent illness (p. 268). Even with adequate replacement treatment, there is an increased risk of cardiovascular disease in hypopituitary patients.

Pituitary overactivity

Hyperprolactinaemia

Hyperprolactinaemia most commonly presents as galactorrhoea, menstrual disturbance and/or infertility in a young woman and is usually caused by a **microadenoma** or **lactotroph hyperplasia** (no tumour seen on scan). In men, hyperprolactinaemia causes impotence/infertility. Male reproductive function is less sensitive to hyperprolactinaemia so men usually present later in life and have larger tumours. **Macroprolactinomas** can present at any age and are the second most common pituitary macroadenoma (after non-functioning tumours). Particularly in elderly people, there may be no symptoms directly related to the hyperprolactinaemia. There are many causes of hyperprolactinaemia.

Primary hyperprolactinaemia is caused by a pituitary tumour or lactotroph hyperplasia.

Secondary causes include:

- mass lesions preventing inhibitory control of prolactin secretion: intra- or suprasellar tumours or granulomata
- Drugs: metaclopramide, phenothiazines, antidepressants, H_2-antagonists
- endocrine: primary hypothyroidism, polycystic ovarian syndrome
- systemic illness: renal failure
- chest wall/breast stimulation or disease
- fear, anxiety or fitting.

Secondary hyperprolactinaemia is most commonly a chance biochemical finding but it can cause the same symptoms and signs as idiopathic hyperprolactinaemia. Once it has been excluded, investigation consists of CT or MR scanning and pituitary function testing. Treatment is with dopaminergic agonists, which are very successful at relieving galactorrhoea, menstrual disturbance and infertility and reducing tumour size. The place of surgery and radiotherapy have been discussed earlier (pp. 264–265).

Acromegaly and gigantism

Pathology

GH oversecretion is the second most common pituitary overactivity and almost invariably results from a pituitary adenoma, usually large enough to expand the pituitary fossa and often to extend outside it. A minority of GH-secreting tumours also secrete prolactin.

Extremely rarely, acromegaly may be caused by an ectopic tumour secreting GHRH. There are two distinct presentations:

- most often, GH excess presents in middle or later life as acromegaly
- rarely, GH excess before epiphyseal fusion presents with the syndrome of gigantism.

The mass effects, investigation and treatment of macro-adenomas have been covered earlier (p. 264).

Clinical features and investigation

Figure 52 shows the symptoms and signs of acromegaly other than those caused by tumour expansion and accompanying hypopituitarism or hyperprolactinaemia. Enlargement of the hands and feet is the classical symptom. Most patients admit to the symptom and there are few other causes in adults. However, that is rarely how

the diagnosis is made. It is usually a chance observation by a doctor.

GH excess is confirmed by glucose tolerance testing. In normal people, serum GH suppresses to unmeasurable levels after oral glucose whereas it is not suppressed and may actually rise in acromegaly/gigantism. Serum prolactin must always be measured and pituitary function tests performed to exclude hypopituitarism. In almost every patient, CT or MR scanning will demonstrate a pituitary adenoma, usually a macroadenoma.

Management and prognosis

Surgery is the first-line treatment for most cases of acromegaly. Trans-sphenoidal surgery can cure 80% of microadenomas with little morbidity; however, it is less effective for macroadenomas. Bromocriptine can suppress GH secretion and alleviate symptoms but is rarely

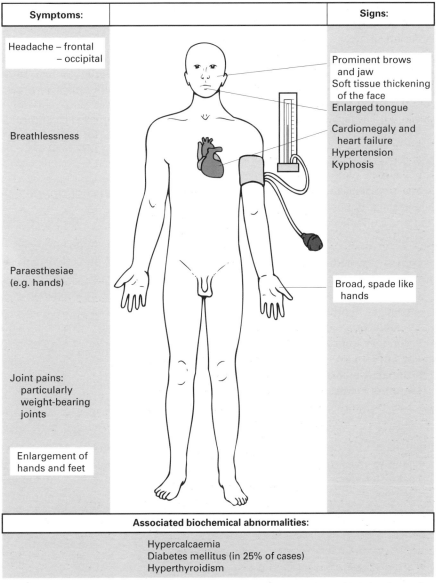

Fig. 52
The symptoms and signs of acromegaly.

* The signs and symptoms shown unshaded are the most reliable for making the diagnosis curative. A newer drug, the somatostatin analogue octreotide, is much more effective but

- is extremely expensive
- has to be given by injections or continuous infusion
- has many side-effects, including gall stone formation owing to stasis of bile.

Radiotherapy is also effective but is slow to act; it is indicated for patients not cured by surgery. Acromegaly causes unpleasant symptoms and major morbidity from joint, heart and respiratory disease and increased mortality from cardiorespiratory and malignant disease, so there are strong arguments for treating it aggressively.

7.4 Adrenal disease

Normal anatomy and physiology

The two adrenal glands are situated at the upper poles of the kidneys. There are three main adrenal hormones:

- cortisol (cortex), controlled by the hypothalamo–pituitary–adrenal axis
- aldosterone (cortex), controlled by the renin–angiotensin–aldosterone system
- adrenaline (from the medulla).

Hypoadrenalism

Adrenaline deficiency does not cause disease. The clinical effects of hypoadrenalism are caused by glucocorticoid and mineralocorticoid deficiency. Adrenal cortical underactivity may be:

- primary, i.e. because of disease in the adrenal itself, in which case both glucocorticoid and mineralocorticoid secretion are likely to be impaired
- secondary to pituitary disease, in which case mineralocorticoid secretion is unimpaired
- secondary to prolonged corticosteroid therapy and suppression of the hypothalamo–pituitary–adrenal axis, in which case mineralocorticoid secretion is unimpaired

The main clinical syndrome described here is primary hypoadrenalism or **Addison's disease**. Iatrogenic hypoadrenalism is the cause you are most likely to encounter (or have to prevent) and is considered later. Isolated hypoaldosteronism is a rare condition not discussed in this chapter.

Pathology

Over 80% of cases of primary hypoadrenalism are autoimmune, caused by a lymphocytic adrenalitis and associated (in about half the patients) with measurable adrenal antibodies in plasma. Other causes are:

- infectious
  - tuberculosis is an important cause in developing countries, now rare in developed countries
  - AIDS, cytomegalovirus and histoplasmosis
  - the Waterhouse–Friedrichson syndrome, adrenal haemorrhage complicating meningococcal septicaemia
- tumour: tumours often metastasise to the adrenals but hypoadrenalism is uncommon because both glands have to be destroyed before this occurs.

Clinical features

The symptoms of hypoadrenalism are non-specific and include weight loss, lethargy, weakness, nausea and abdominal pain. Both glucocorticoid and mineralocorticoid deficiency cause hypotension, particularly on standing. Pigmentation (caused by a compensatory increase in ACTH secretion and, therefore, absent in *secondary* hypoadrenalism) affects the nipples, recent scars, face and neck, palmar skin creases and buccal mucosa. Patients with incipient hypoadrenalism are often precipitated into 'hypoadrenal crisis' by intercurrent illness because the failing adrenals cannot mount an appropriate response. Treatment with rifampicin, which induces hepatic enzymes and increases cortisol metabolism, can have the same effect. The clinical picture of hypoadrenal crisis is collapse and vomiting with characteristic changes in electrolytes (see below).

Investigation

The biochemical signs of hypoadrenalism are:

- hyponatraemia
- hyperkalaemia
- a raised urea concentration
- mild acidosis.

Random cortisol measurements are unreliable because what appears 'normal' may be inappropriately low for someone who is 'ill'; however, a markedly low cortisol concentration with raised ACTH in an ill patient is diagnostic. All patients should have the following investigations.

A synacthen test. This tests the ability of the adrenals to increase cortisol secretion in response to (synthetic) ACTH stimulation. The short synacthen test measures the response over 1 hour. If there is no response, ACTH can be given for 48 hours to exclude temporary adrenal suppression (long synacthen test).

Abdominal CT scan. This will exclude tuberculous calcification and adrenal tumours.

Adrenal antibody measurement. This is a pointer to autoimmune Addison's disease if positive but is unhelpful if negative.

Renin and aldosterone levels. These can be measured to test the integrity of the renin–angiotensin–aldosterone axis.

Treatment

The treatment of adrenal crisis is saline repletion and intravenous hydrocortisone. You should look for evidence of underlying infection and treat it. Maintenance treatment is with oral hydrocortisone. Most, but not all, patients are also mineralocorticoid deficient and need oral fludrocortisone. Patients with tuberculous hypoadrenalism should receive antituberculous chemotherapy. *All patients should be taught to increase their steroid doses during intercurrent illness and advised to carry a security disc or steroid card at all times. They must receive parenteral steroid if they are vomiting or seriously ill.*

Iatrogenic adrenal suppression

Corticosteroid therapy suppresses the hypothalamo–pituitary–adrenal axis. When it is stopped, there may be a delay before the axis recovers. After prolonged suppression, it may never do so. If corticosteroids are withdrawn from people whose axis is permanently suppressed, or withdrawn too quickly from those who have the potential to recover, hypoadrenalism results. It may also result if patients do not increase their steroid dose during intercurrent illness. You should follow the rules below:

- remember the risk of adrenal suppression in any patient who has had prolonged corticosteroid therapy, e.g. >1 month
- reduce steroid doses slowly in patients who have had prolonged therapy and warn them of the risk and symptoms of hypoadrenalism
- teach all patients to increase 'maintenance' steroid doses during intercurrent illness and report symptoms of hypoadrenalism immediately.

Withdrawal of steroids in patients who have received them long-term can be difficult and requires expert supervision.

Congenital adrenal hyperplasia

A number of inherited adrenal enzyme defects affect cortisol and/or aldosterone biosynthesis. The commonest of these is 21-Hydroxylase deficiency, which is inherited as an autosomal recessive trait. The homeostatic response to cortisol deficiency is increased ACTH secretion. This cannot overcome the enzyme deficiency but does increase androgen synthesis. There may also be mineralocorticoid deficiency. 21-Hydroxylase deficiency often presents in the first week of life with salt-losing crises caused by hypoadrenalism. It causes virilisation of female infants and can cause precocious puberty in males. Treatment is with glucocorticoid and mineralocorticoid replacement, as for Addison's disease. Congenital adrenal hyperplasia can also present with hirsutism in adult women. Serum 17-hydroxyprogesterone concentration (the steroid 'upstream' of the enzyme block) is the definitive investigation.

Cushing's syndrome

Pathology

Cushing's syndrome has the following characteristics:

- two-thirds of cases are caused by pituitary disease, usually microadenomas
- the remainder of cases split roughly equally between adrenal tumours and ectopic ACTH secretion, usually from carcinoid tumours
- prolonged corticosteroid therapy can cause a similar clinical picture, but the aetiology is obvious
- alcohol abuse can give a similar clinical picture: 'alcohol-induced pseudo-Cushing's'
- obesity and depression can produce changes in cortisol metabolism which are almost indistinguishable from Cushing's.

Clinical features

The clinical features of Cushing's syndrome are given in Figure 53. It is impossible to distinguish between Cushing's caused by a pituitary adenoma, an adrenal tumour or carcinoid ectopic ACTH secretion on clinical grounds. Ectopic ACTH secretion from *malignant* tumours (see respiratory disease, p. 75) presents quite differently because the patients are very ill, wasted and heavily pigmented.

Investigations

The diagnosis is made by demonstrating increased plasma or urinary cortisol levels. There is loss of the normal circadian rhythm of plasma cortisol (lowest at midnight) and it remains inappropriately high after dexamethasone; this corticosteroid is used because it does not cross-react with cortisol in the laboratory assay.

Having demonstrated unsuppressible hypercortisolism, the next step is to measure plasma ACTH. If this is suppressed, the presumptive diagnosis is an adrenal adenoma, which can be confirmed by abdominal CT or MR scanning.

If ACTH is unsuppressed, the patient may have either an ectopic or pituitary source of ACTH. MR scanning of the pituitary may show an adenoma and MR or CT scan of the thorax may show an occult carcinoid tumour.

Most patients with 'high-ACTH Cushing's' will also need bilateral simultaneous inferior petrosal sinus sampling with corticotrophin-releasing hormone (CRH) stimulation. This involves placing catheters in the veins draining both sides of the pituitary and stimulating ACTH secretion with CRH. Although complex to perform, it is the best way to distinguish between pituitary and ectopic Cushing's syndrome. In pituitary Cushing's,

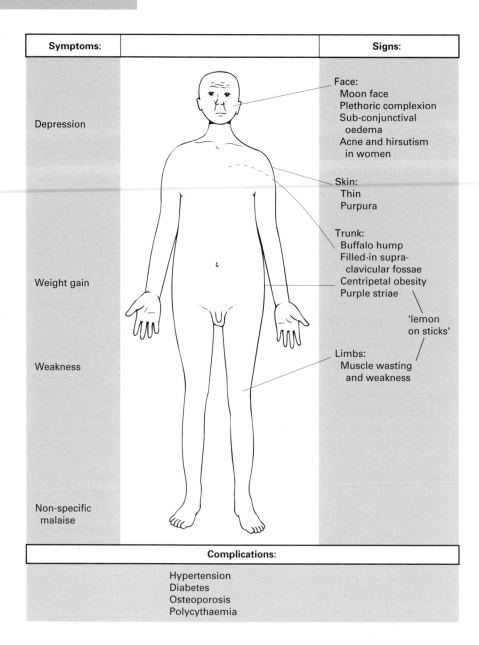

Symptoms:		Signs:

Face:
Moon face
Plethoric complexion
Sub-conjunctival
 oedema
Acne and hirsutism
 in women

Depression

Skin:
Thin
Purpura

Trunk:
Buffalo hump
Filled-in supra-
 clavicular fossae
Centripetal obesity
Purple striae

Weight gain

'lemon
on sticks'

Limbs:
Muscle wasting
 and weakness

Weakness

Non-specific
malaise

Complications:

Hypertension
Diabetes
Osteoporosis
Polycythaemia

Fig. 53
The clinical features of Cushing's
syndrome.

ACTH levels are higher in pituitary venous effluent than peripheral blood and rise further after CRH injection. In Cushing's syndrome secondary to an ectopic tumour, pituitary ACTH secretion is suppressed and unresponsive to CRH stimulation.

Management

Adrenal adenomectomy is the definitive treatment for adrenal Cushing's. Likewise, tumours secreting ectopic ACTH should be excised. Selective adenomectomy is the first-line treatment for pituitary Cushing's. Whatever the cause, patients need to be prepared for surgery with a drug such as metyrapone, mitotane, aminoglutethimide or ketoconazole, which blocks cortisol biosynthesis. If pituitary surgery for ACTH-dependent Cushing's fails to cure the patient, bilateral adrenalectomy is an option but it carries a risk of late pituitary tumour expansion and optic nerve compression (Nelson's syndrome). Radio-

therapy is indicated for pituitary tumours which have not been cured by neurosurgery.

Prognosis

Cushing's is a disabling disease which often causes irreversible physical and psychological morbidity before it is diagnosed and may respond poorly to treatment. Pituitary microsurgery has improved the prognosis but is not always successful and tumours may recur.

Hyperaldosteronism

Secondary hyperaldosteronism, caused by reduced effective arterial volume/reduced renal perfusion, is a homeostatic response which causes saline retention in heart failure and hypoalbuminaemic states (p. 167).

Primary hyperaldosteronism (**Conn's syndrome**) is a rare disorder which:

- presents with hypokalaemia and mild-to-moderate hypertension
- may be caused by a discrete adrenal adenoma or bilateral hyperplasia of the zona glomerulosa
- accounts for less than 1% of cases of hypertension.

Patients with Conn's syndrome may have symptoms of hypokalaemia (muscle weakness, cramps, polyuria) but are usually asymptomatic. The disease can be screened for by measuring plasma electrolytes in all hypertensive patients before they start treatments which affect potassium (diuretics, ACE inhibitors etc.). The diagnosis is confirmed by measuring renin and aldosterone after overnight recumbency and again after 4 hours in the upright posture:

- patients with adrenal adenomata have suppressed renin and a raised serum aldosterone concentration which does not change with posture
- those with bilateral hyperplasia also have hyporeninaemic hyperaldosteronism but plasma aldosterone rises with posture.

Adrenal adenomata can be demonstrated by CT, MR or ultrasound. Bilateral hyperplasia can be confirmed by catheterising the renal veins and demonstrating that aldosterone levels are similar on both sides.

All forms of hyperaldosteronism can be treated with spironolactone. Adrenal adenomata are treated surgically, with a 50% chance of complete remission of hypertension.

Phaeochromocytoma

Phaeochromocytoma is the one disease of the adrenal medulla. Like Conn's syndrome, it is a cause of secondary hypertension but it is even rarer than Conn's. It is an important disease to recognise because it causes florid and potentially fatal hypertensive crises. The diagnosis is often made postmortem, patients dying of haemorrhagic stroke or cardiovascular complications. It is usually caused by a solitary adrenal adenoma but there are exceptions which lead to the nickname 'the 10% tumour':

- 10% are bilateral
- 10% malignant
- 10% extra-adrenal.

The tumours usually secrete noradrenaline. Symptoms are classically paroxysmal, the commonest being the triad of:

- headache
- sweating
- palpitations.

Nervousness, panic attacks and flushing may also occur. Hypertension can be paroxysmal or sustained. Patients may be hypotensive between paroxysms and on standing. This hypotension results from two homeostatic responses: downregulation of catecholamine receptors and plasma volume contraction. The diagnosis is made:

- first and foremost by thinking of it
- by measuring urinary or plasma catecholamines in patients with suggestive symptoms, severe or labile hypertension or a positive family history.

Once a biochemical diagnosis is made, the adrenals are imaged, as for Conn's syndrome. In addition, radionuclide scanning with a labelled precursor of catecholamine synthesis can demonstrate hormone synthesis in the tumour.

Treatment is first with i.v. then with oral alpha-blockers (phentolamine and phenoxybenzamine, respectively). Intravenous fluids should be given to stabilise blood pressure once alpha-blockade has been instituted. Beta-blockers are often added later. A period of stabilisation on antihypertensives precedes surgery.

7.5 Hypogonadism

Hypothalamic and pituitary diseases commonly disrupt gonadotrophin secretion and cause sex-steroid deficiency either by:

- a direct effect on the hypothalamo–pituitary–gonadal axis
- causing hyperprolactinaemia which suppresses the axis secondarily.

Hypogonadism may also be caused by ovarian/testicular failure. The presentation, investigation and management of female hypogonadism is covered in gynaecology textbooks. This section describes male hypogonadism although the same general principles can be applied to female hypogonadism.

Male impotence and infertility are rarely due to hypogonadism but that should be suspected if the patient has:

- loss of drive and libido
- reduced beard growth
- erectile failure
- anorgasmia
- a reduced volume of ejaculate
- reduced testicular volumes.

Hypogonadism may be caused by hypothalamic or pituitary failure; in both instances serum testosterone and gonadotrophins will be low (*hypo*gonadotrophic hypogonadism). It may also result from testicular failure (*hyper*gonadotrophic hypogonadism). Prolactin should also be measured, as hyperprolactinaemia causes hypogonadism by interfering with gonadotrophin secretion. A full list of causes is given in Box 10.

Hyperprolactinaemia is treated with a dopaminergic agonist (p. 266). Otherwise, treatment is by testosterone replacement therapy, which can be given:

Box 10
Causes of hypogonadism

Hypogonadotrophic causes

Hypopituitarism (see p. 265)
Hyperprolactinaemia
Hypothalamic tumours
Kallman's syndrome
Haemochromatosis

Hypergonadotrophic causes

Testicular injury
Klinefelter's syndrome

- orally
- by monthly injection
- transdermally
- as a 6-monthly subcutaneous implant.

Induction of spermatogenesis requires gonadotrophin injection or infusion therapy. Untreated hypogonadism predisposes to osteoporosis and may cause non-specific lethargy and weakness, so testosterone treatment should be offered even to patients who do not wish to be sexually active.

7.6 Hyperlipidaemia

Hyperlipidaemia can seem a very confusing subject. This discussion follows a simple, pragmatic approach, emphasising key points. These are:

- hyperlipidaemia is an important public health problem because it increases the risk of cardiovascular disease

- severe hyperlipidaemia may, in addition, cause skin lesions and pancreatitis
- hyperlipidaemia may be secondary to systemic disease or may be primary (genetic)
- treatment is first with diet and second with one of a limited range of drugs.

You should be familiar with the consensus guidelines which are used to decide when to start treatment.

Investigation

To diagnose hyperlipidaemia and assess cardiovascular risk, you need to measure:

- serum total cholesterol
- high-density lipoprotein cholesterol (HDL)
- low-density lipoprotein cholesterol (LDL)
- triglyceride.

Ideally, lipids should be measured after a 12-hour fast (necessary for triglycerides but not cholesterol). LDL cholesterol increases cardiovascular risk. HDL (involved in cholesterol disposal) reduces it. The result should be interpreted in the light of the patient's age and gender and the presence or absence of cardiovascular disease. Lipids should not be measured between 24 hours and 3 months after a severe illness (e.g. myocardial infarct), which will make them artificially high. Table 60 summarises the main primary and secondary types of hyperlipidaemia.

Lipids and coronary risk

Hypercholesterolaemia is one of the three main factors, together with smoking and hypertension (the 'unholy trinity'), which predispose to cardiovascular disease. Serum cholesterol accounts for as much as two-thirds of the variance in cardiovascular risk between different

Table 60 Types of hyperlipidaemia

Primary	Cholesterol	Triglycerides	Prevalence
Primary (genetic)			
Polygenic hypercholesterolaemia	↑		++++
Familial hypercholesterolaemia			
Heterozygous	↑		++
Homozygous	↑↑		Rare
Familial combined hyperlipidaemia	↑	↑	+++
Familial hypertriglyceridaemia		↑	+
Remnant hyperlipoproteinaemia	↑↑	↑↑	+
Hyperchylomicronaemia		↑↑	Rare
Secondary to systemic disease			
Obesity	↑	↑	
Hypothyroidism	↑		
Nephrotic syndrome	↑	(↑)	
Liver disease	↑		
Diabetes		↑	
Alcohol abuse		↑	

↑, increased.

populations. There is no such thing as a *normal* cholesterol because cardiovascular risk rises progressively with increasing serum cholesterol, particularly above 6.5 mmol/l. Presence of more than one major risk factor increases cardiovascular risk multiplicatively. Triglycerides are a weaker risk factor for coronary artery disease but can cause acute pancreatitis in high concentration (> 20 mmol/l). There is an inverse relationship between triglyceride and HDL-cholesterol concentrations and it is controversial how far this accounts for the apparent protective effect of HDL.

Clinical presentation

Symptoms and signs
Hyperlipidaemia is usually detected by screening. Hypercholesterolaemia may cause:

- corneal arcus: a white ring at the junction of cornea and sclera
- xanthelasmata: subcutaneous cholesterol deposits at the inner margins of the eyelid
- xanthomata: thickening of tendons.

Hypertriglyceridaemia can cause:

- eruptive xanthomata: subcutaneous deposits of triglyceride
- lipaemia retinalis: milky appearance of the retinal vessels on ophthalmoscopy.

Specific syndromes
Primary hypercholesterolaemia is usually inherited in a simple polygenic pattern. Heterozygous autosomal dominant familial hypercholesterolaemia is less common and causes moderate hypercholesterolaemia. Homozygous familial hypercholesterolaemia causes extremely severe hypercholesterolaemia which is usually fatal in early adult life. Hypercholesterolaemia may be secondary to hypothyroidism, obstructive jaundice or nephrotic syndrome.

Hypertriglyceridaemia may be caused by obesity, alcoholism, uncontrolled diabetes or the uncommon condition of familial hypertriglyceridaemia. Familial combined hyperlipidaemia is dominantly inherited and may produce different patterns of hyperlipidaemia in different family members.

Management

Clinical trials have shown that, whatever the starting cholesterol level, lowering it by 1 mmol/l lowers the incidence of coronary heart disease by 50%; however, the improvement in overall mortality has been less impressive. Those with the highest cardiovascular risk benefit most from treatment. Table 61 shows practical guidelines for when to lower serum cholesterol as proposed by the British Hyperlipidaemia Association.

Other cardiovascular risk factors such as smoking and hypertension should be corrected. Diet is always the first and, for many patients with mild hyperlipidaemia, only line of treatment. If diet fails, there are two classes of drug which are well tolerated and widely used:

- fibric acid derivatives: bezafibrate, fenofibrate, gemfibrozil; these are generally well tolerated, effective at lowering triglycerides and cholesterol and widely used when diet fails
- statins: simvastatin, pravastatin, lovastatin; these are the most potent cholesterol-lowering agents, increasingly widely used as second-line treatment after diet.

Two other classes of drug are available but less well tolerated and with more limited indications:

- bile acid sequestrants: cholestyramine and colestipol; these are effective at lowering cholesterol but are expensive, and usually reserved for familial hypercholesterolaemia
- nicotinic acid and derivatives (e.g. acipimox): primarily lower triglycerides; facial flushing is the main side-effect.

Table 61 British Hyperlipidaemia Association: priorities and cut-off values for lipid-lowering drug therapy for hypercholesterolaemia persisting after institution of dietary treatment

Priority	Patient category	Total cholesterol (mmol/l)	LDL cholesterol (mmol/l)
First	Patients with established CHD, including post-CABG, angioplasty or cardiac transplant, or with other significant atherosclerosis	>5.2	>3.5
Second	Patients with genetically determined hyperlipidaemia (e.g. familial hypercholesterolaemia) or with multiple risk factors (family history, diabetes mellitus, hypertension, long smoking history)	>6.5	>5.0
Third	Men without evidence of atherosclerosis or other risk factors	>7.8	>6.0
Fourth	Postmenopausal women[a] without evidence of other risk factors	>7.8	>6.0

CHD, chronic heart disease; post-CABG, after coronary artery bypass graft
[a]Take account of premature menopause or low HDL cholesterol. Hormone replacement therapy may be appropriate before consideration of lipid-lowering medication.

7.7 Obesity

It is a common lay belief that obesity is caused by 'something wrong with the glands'. Do not fall into the trap of thinking that obesity is an 'endocrine disease'. Obese patients may deposit their food more readily into their fat stores than non-obese people but they also eat more and exercise less. There are few organic causes of obesity, and patients with those diseases do not usually present with obesity. Those organic causes include:

- hypothyroidism
- Cushing's syndrome
- hypothalamic tumours causing polyphagia
- insulin or sulphonylurea treatment of diabetes
- insulinoma.

Some of these causes are common and obvious, others are exquisitely rare. Investigation of obese patients for endocrine disease is generally unrewarding. It is important to convince patients that there is not 'something wrong with their glands' rather than entrench their belief by investigating them fruitlessly.

The management of obesity is sympathetic dietary advice, emotional support and exercise. The one licensed drug for the management of obesity is **dexfenfluramine**. This causes modest weight loss during the 3 months that it can be taken but long-term results are disappointing. Drug treatment of obesity may do more harm than good by distracting from the real challenge of modifying eating behaviour.

7.8 Diabetes mellitus and spontaneous hypoglycaemia

Diabetes

Diabetes mellitus is the most common endocrine disease. It is caused by insulin deficiency and/or insulin resistance, the relative contributions of which vary between different types of diabetes. The net effect is hyperglycaemia. The metabolic disturbance ranges from an asymptomatic biochemical abnormality to a fatal metabolic emergency. Over months or years, diabetes causes tissue damage, seen clinically as diabetic complications. Diabetes:

- shortens life expectancy by up to one-third
- increases the risk of ischaemic heart disease three-fold
- increases the risk of amputations 15-fold; it is responsible for nearly half of lower limb amputations
- is the most common cause of blindness in middle age
- is responsible for one in ten cases of renal failure requiring dialysis or transplantation.

Much of this morbidity is preventable by well-structured medical care, with an emphasis on good gly-caemic control and detection of complications at an early stage. Diabetic patients have to take responsibility for much of their own care and need good education and support. You will inevitably care for diabetic patients early in your career because over 5% of UK hospital bed-days are associated with diabetes.

Learning objectives

You need to:

- know the main types of diabetes and understand their causes and the rationale for their treatment
- be able to describe the management of the common metabolic emergencies of diabetes (hypo- and hyperglycaemia)
- understand what is meant by 'diabetic tissue complications' and know their features and management.

Normal carbohydrate metabolism

Think of insulin as a 'storage hormone' which is secreted by the pancreatic β cell when blood glucose rises after a carbohydrate meal. Insulin causes:

- increased glucose uptake in many tissues by activation of glucose transporter molecules
- increased glycolysis
- decreased gluconeogenesis
- storage of glucose in liver and muscle as glycogen.

Insulin also affects protein and fat metabolism:

- protein synthesis is stimulated and protein breakdown inhibited
- lipid synthesis is increased
- ketogenesis is reduced.

Insulin is formed by cleavage of a connecting peptide (C-peptide) from the precursor proinsulin. C-peptide can be measured as a marker of endogenous insulin secretion. Glucagon, adrenaline, cortisol and growth hormone have opposite metabolic effects and are sometimes termed the 'anti-insulin hormones'.

During starvation, insulin levels fall and increased levels of the anti-insulin hormones maintain blood glucose by glycogenolysis, and gluconeogenesis from the substrates alanine, lactate and glycerol.

Reduced insulin action also causes release of amino acids from protein, and glycerol and fatty acids from adipose tissue. Free fatty acids are metabolised to the ketones acetoacetate, β-hydroxybutyrate and acetone, which can be used as a fuel.

In health, continuous variation in the rate of insulin secretion maintains plasma glucose within narrow limits. The brain, in particular, has a high demand for glucose and is absolutely reliant on an adequate blood glucose level. Even a modest fall impairs cognitive function. A plasma glucose <2.8 mmol/l is defined as hypoglycaemia. Profound hypoglycaemia (<2 mmol/l) causes coma and, ultimately, permanent neurological damage or death.

Abnormal carbohydrate metabolism

Diabetes is caused by insulin deficiency from one or more of:

- insufficient insulin secretion as a result of β cell failure
- tissue resistance to insulin caused by a receptor or postreceptor defect
- excess of one or more anti-insulin hormones.

The earliest abnormality is an increased blood glucose after ingesting carbohydrate. The **glucose tolerance test** — in which blood glucose is measured before and 2 hours after 75 g oral glucose — is a sensitive test for impaired insulin secretion/action. At this early stage, the feedback loop between glucose and insulin is able to maintain a normal fasting blood glucose but, with worsened insulin action, fasting hyperglycaemia (>7 mmol/l) develops. This is the biochemical hallmark of diabetes. Symptoms do not develop until there is quite marked fasting hyperglycaemia. With severe insulin deficiency, excessive ketone body formation and acidosis develop, as well as severe hyperglycaemia (diabetic ketoacidosis). Impaired glucose tolerance, insulin-dependent (IDDM) and non-insulin-dependent diabetes (NIDDM) represent three points on a spectrum of insulin deficiency. Impaired glucose tolerance, non-insulin-dependent diabetes (NIDDM) and insulin-dependent diabetes represent three points on the spectrum of insulin deficiency.

Hypoglycaemia is caused by:

- excessive insulin given to treat diabetes
- excessive insulin secretion from an insulin-secreting pancreatic tumour or from sulphonylurea therapy (see below)
- underproduction of the anti-insulin hormones, for example in hypoadrenalism or hypopituitarism
- starvation or liver disease, in which the glycogen stores are depleted and/or gluconeogenesis fails.

Glycation and other metabolic effects of hyperglycaemia

Glucose attaches to proteins throughout the body by the process of glycation. This is not dependent on enzymes and occurs in proportion to blood glucose levels averaged over the life of the protein. This process is important because:

- glycation damages tissues and is one of the processes causing diabetic complications
- measuring the degree of glycation gives a time-averaged measure of hyperglycaemia.

Haemoglobin is a readily accessible protein with a long half-life. Glycation alters the electrophoretic mobility of haemoglobin A. This glycated form of haemoglobin A is termed haemoglobin A_{1c} (HbA_{1c}). The percentage of haemoglobin A in this glycated form (usually <5%) is a measure of blood glucose control and a predictor of diabetic complications. Fructosamine is a measure of the degree of glycation of plasma proteins. It is a less precise and less stable measure of glycaemic control than HbA_{1c}.

Diabetic patients have many other metabolic abnormalities which predispose to vascular disease including hyperlipidaemia, increased fibrinogen levels, increased blood viscosity and high insulin levels.

Epidemiology

Diabetes affects 2% of Caucasians, up to a quarter of whom are insulin dependent. Its prevalence rises to 10% in elderly people and is three to four times higher in Asians than Caucasians in the UK. Some non-UK populations have prevalences as high as 50%.

Types of diabetes

In temperate countries there are two main types of diabetes (Table 62): **IDDM** and **NIDDM**. Internationally, 'tropical diabetes' is another important type which may be insulin-treated or non-insulin-treated. It is not discussed here.

The stereotypes in Table 62 are far from absolute. Patients with NIDDM may present in young adult life and IDDM may present in old age. That is why the terms maturity-onset and juvenile-onset diabetes have been abandoned. There is another terminological problem in that about 10% of patients with NIDDM per year after diagnosis become uncontrollable with tablets and progress to insulin treatment without becoming ketosis prone. Such patients are best described as insulin-treated rather than insulin-dependent, giving a third abbreviation: **ITDM**.

Causes

IDDM is caused by autoimmunity against the β cells of the pancreas, which eventually destroys them completely and causes absolute insulin deficiency. It is thought that this process may be triggered by a viral

Table 62 Characteristics of the two main types of diabetic mellitus[a]

	IDDM	NIDDM
Age of onset	Younger: peak incidence in late teenage	Older: incidence increases progressively with age
Weight	Lean	Obese
Treatment	Absolute dependence on insulin therapy	Treatable initially with diet alone or tablets
Ketosis	Develops if insulin not given	Not ketosis prone

[a] These stereotypes are not absolute.

infection or some other environmental insult. It can be halted by immunotherapy (for example, with cyclosporine A) but over 90% of β cells are destroyed by the time a patient presents with IDDM, so immunotherapy gives no lasting benefit. NIDDM is less well understood: insulin is still produced but the response to an increase in plasma glucose is 'too little and too late', probably because the capacity of the β cells to recognise and respond to hyperglycaemia is impaired. Likewise, the responsiveness of insulin's target tissues is impaired. NIDDM is, therefore, an effect of both insulin deficiency and insulin resistance: **relative insulin deficiency**. Since neither the feedback loop between plasma glucose and the β cell nor the capacity to secrete insulin are lost completely, hyperglycaemia is not usually as severe as in IDDM and ketosis does not occur. Why patients with NIDDM progress to insulin treatment is unexplained by this mechanism; a leading theory is that deposits of amyloid in the islets of Langerhans progressively (but incompletely) destroy the β cells, a process quite distinct from the lymphocytic inflammation which destroys the islets in IDDM.

Primary and secondary diabetes

Diabetes can be caused by any process which interferes with the production or action of insulin. IDDM and NIDDM, as described above, could be termed *primary* or idiopathic diabetes. There are many causes of *secondary* diabetes, which can be insulin-dependent or non-insulin-dependent, depending on the degree of insulin deficiency. Secondary diabetes may be accompanied or unaccompanied by pancreatic exocrine deficiency. Causes can be categorised by the underlying mechanism:

Failure of insulin secretion

- Common
  — pancreatitis, pancreatectomy
  — pancreatic carcinoma
  — alcohol abuse
  — drugs: beta-blockers, thiazides (including diazoxide)
- rare
  — haemachromatosis.

Insulin resistance

- Common
  — steroid therapy
  — gross obesity
- rare
  — endocrine diseases: Cushing's disease, acromegaly, thyrotoxicosis, phaeochromocytoma.

Associated with congenital syndromes. These are all rare and the causes unknown. They are not discussed here.

Gestational diabetes. This is a special case, which will be considered below (p. 283).

Clinical presentation

Symptoms

Mild to moderate hyperglycaemia can be asymptomatic or can cause any or all of these symptoms:

- thirst, polyuria and polydipsia
- blurred vision
- balanitis in men and pruritis vulvae in women
- lethargy and somnolence
- weight loss and weakness
- anorexia and nausea
- recurrent skin infections.

Severe hyperglycaemia causes:

- severe thirst
- drowsiness or coma
- vomiting.

Ketosis causes:

- nausea, vomiting
- breathlessness.

It is important to think of the ways in which diabetes may present. There are four main ways.

1. Classically, IDDM presents with a short history (days or weeks) of severe symptoms, sometimes culminating in ketoacidosis.
2. NIDDM can also cause severe hyperglycaemic symptoms but more typically presents with less severe symptoms over a longer time (months or even years)
3. Even quite severe hyperglycaemia may cause no symptoms at all and NIDDM is commonly diagnosed by screening (e.g. well-person checks, insurance or employment medicals). Even if found by chance, diabetes must be taken seriously because asymptomatic hyperglycaemia can cause complications (see below).
4. Finally, diabetes may present with its complications:
- infections, e.g. staphylococcal skin infections, foot ulcers, thrush
- visual impairment caused by cataract or retinopathy
- arterial disease, e.g. myocardial infarction, peripheral vascular disease
- neuropathy, e.g. mononeuritis multiplex or polyneuropathy
- renal failure.

Investigations

You can infer that patients have diabetes if they have glycosuria, but different people 'spill' glucose into the urine at different levels of blood glucose (renal threshold) so you can neither make a diagnosis of diabetes nor exclude it on the result of a urine test.

- Typical symptoms and a grossly raised non-fasting blood glucose (venous whole blood concentration >10 mmol/l) confirm the diagnosis

- If asymptomatic, two abnormal blood glucose concentrations are needed to exclude laboratory error or other spurious causes; the appropriate investigation is the *fasting* blood glucose, because random measurements are influenced by the timing and size of the most recent meal
- A *glucose tolerance test* (GTT) is needed occasionally, usually in an asymptomatic patient with borderline fasting or random blood glucose values.

The GTT can define a second category of abnormality in which fasting blood glucose is normal but there is an abnormally high level after oral glucose: **impaired glucose tolerance**. Such patients do not have diabetes and are not at risk of its microvascular complications but are at increased risk of coronary heart disease.

Diagnostic criteria for diabetes:

diabetes: fasting whole venous blood glucose concentration ≥ 7 mmol/l and/or ≥ 10 mmol/l 2 hours after a 75 g oral glucose load

impaired glucose tolerance: fasting glucose <7 mmol/l; 2-hour value 7–9.9 mmol/l.

These figures are 1 mmol/l higher if measured on venous plasma rather than whole blood; consult your laboratory if in doubt.

Management

The principles of treatment follow directly from the pathophysiology. IDDM and ITDM can only be treated by insulin replacement. NIDDM is treated by lessening insulin resistance and/or boosting insulin secretion.

Diet

This is central to the management of all types of diabetes. Patients with NIDDM are usually obese and their insulin resistance can be improved by weight loss. Many can be treated by diet alone. For those on tablets or insulin, diet is an essential adjunct. The aim of the diet is to:

- optimise glycaemic control
- combat hyperlipidaemia and minimise the risk of vascular disease
- minimise the risk of hypoglycaemia if on tablets or insulin.

For all types of diabetes, the approach is similar:

- restrict calories if overweight
- take starchy and high-fibre foods in preference to simple sugars to prevent violent swings in blood glucose
- take frequent and small meals and snacks to match the sluggish insulin response from the diseased pancreas and/or the slow absorption of injected insulin
- limit total fat intake and encourage mono- and polyunsaturates in preference to animal fat to aid weight loss and reduce plasma lipids.

Patients with diabetic nephropathy are recommended to take a low-protein diet.

Tablets

Oral treatment is indicated in NIDDM if diet fails to achieve satisfactory glycaemic control. There are three types:

> *biguanides:* metformin, which works by reducing hepatic gluconeogenesis
> *sulphonylureas:* tolbutamide, chlorpropamide, glibenclamide, glipizide, gliclazide, which work by increasing insulin secretion
> *α-glucosidase inhibitors:* acarbose, which works by inhibiting intestinal brush border saccharidases and delaying glucose absorption.

Metformin does not increase insulin secretion and, therefore, does not cause weight gain. Since many patients with NIDDM are obese, this makes it the treatment of choice for those who cannot be controlled with diet alone. It is as effective as sulphonylureas but causes intolerable side-effects (nausea, anorexia and diarrhoea) in up to 20% of patients. It can cause lactic acidosis, a fatal metabolic complication, in patients with severe heart failure, liver disease and renal failure and is, therefore, contraindicated in them.

Although sulphonylureas cause weight gain by increasing insulin secretion, they are effective, well tolerated and widely used. Hypoglycaemia is their main complication. Patients over 70, particularly if they live alone, should not be given long-acting sulphonylureas like glibenclamide and chlorpropamide, which can cause profound, prolonged and potentially fatal hypoglycaemia.

Acarbose is used as first-line or adjunctive treatment for NIDDM. The actions of all three classes of drug are different so they can be used in combination.

Insulin

Insulin is indicated in patients who present with classical IDDM or who, having originally presented with NIDDM, become ketosis prone or hyperglycaemic despite sulphonylureas. The mystique which surrounds insulins is largely unjustified and can be dispelled if they are thought of generically rather than by trade name; insulin preparations differ in their:

- species of origin: beef, pork or human
- length of action: short (soluble), medium/long (isophane, lente), long (ultralente).

Almost all patients can be controlled with human soluble and isophane in various combinations, usually:

- once or twice daily isophane
- twice daily premixed soluble and isophane
- the same combination drawn up separately and mixed together in the syringe
- three-times daily soluble, with isophane before bed.

Most of these regimens can be given with pen-injectors, which are more convenient than a conventional syringe.

The choice of regimen depends on the preferences of patient and physician and, sometimes, trial and error.

Monitoring

This can be divided broadly into self-monitoring and clinic monitoring:

- home urine and blood testing are the common forms of self-monitoring
- clinic monitoring is by enquiry about hyperglycaemic and hypoglycaemic symptoms, measurement of weight and fasting blood glucose and measurement of a glycated protein such as HbA_{lc} or fructosamine.

All patients who are able should at least do home urine tests. A typical recommendation is to do one test per day on three days per week and in addition whenever they feel unwell. Home blood glucose testing is usually reserved for those who are younger, on insulin or more inquisitive about their control. How often patients test is a matter of individual choice. One test per day minimum, varying the time, is a safe rule.

Education

Responsibility for controlling diabetes rests primarily with the patient. It may involve complex day-to-day decisions about insulin doses. Education of the patient and ready availability of advice are key aspects of diabetes management. Some common issues are:

- Hypoglycaemia. All patients on sulphonylureas or insulin and their partners must be acquainted with the symptoms and know how to prevent and treat them. The partners of patients with IDDM should be provided with glucagon (p. 283) and taught how to use it.
- Exercise. Advice is needed on how to tailor the regimen to regular or unexpected exercise by taking extra carbohydrate and/or reducing insulin doses.
- Illness. Every patient should be taught never to reduce insulin doses during illness, given instructions how to manage their diabetes if their tests are high and/or they cannot eat and advised who to contact if they lose control.
- Shift work and travel across time zones.
- Pregnancy. Every diabetic woman of child-bearing potential must be educated about the need for good control at the time of conception, and other aspects of pregnancy (p. 282).
- Employment, careers, etc.
- Insurance.
- Complications. In particular, the reasons not to smoke and the need for retinal screening and preventive foot care.

The multidisciplinary diabetes team

Diabetes care is most effectively delivered by a team of doctors, nurses, dietitians, chiropodists and other professionals working closely together. In particular, diabetes specialist nurses are key members of this multidisciplinary team, available to educate and advise students and doctors in training as well as diabetic patients.

Complications of diabetes

The effects of diabetes include:

- tissue complications
- pregnancy-related complications
- metabolic complications (hypoglycaemia and hyperglycaemia)
- psychosocial complications (a major cause of morbidity which will not be further considered here)
- increased susceptibility to infections.

Tissue complications. These are largely caused by vascular disease:

- *macrovascular* (large vessel) complications include cardiovascular disease, peripheral vascular disease and stroke: these are more prevalent in diabetes but not specific to it
- *microvascular* complications include retinopathy, nephropathy and neuropathy; these are specific to diabetes.

Macrovascular complications and hypertension

Figure 54 lists the manifestations and causes of macrovascular disease. The important point to remember is that diabetes is a potent risk factor for all types of large vessel disease, which may present at younger ages and is diffuse, affecting smaller as well as larger arteries. Apart from the surgical difficulties posed by diffuse disease, there is nothing special about the management of arterial disease in diabetes.

Hypertension

Hypertension and diabetes are linked in a number of ways:

- hypertension is so common in NIDDM that it is thought the two diseases have a pathophysiological link, either genetic or acquired in utero or in early life. Many hypertensive patients with NIDDM are also hyperlipidaemic and hyperinsulinaemic. This cluster of factors is potently atherogenic and sometimes termed **syndrome X**
- the treatment of hypertension with beta-blockers or thiazide diuretics may precipitate NIDDM by impairing insulin secretion and causing insulin resistance
- hypertension increases the risk of both microvascular and macrovascular disease
- patients with nephropathy may be caught in a vicious circle of rising blood pressure and worsening renal function; this can be broken by antihypertensive therapy

EFFECTS	CAUSES

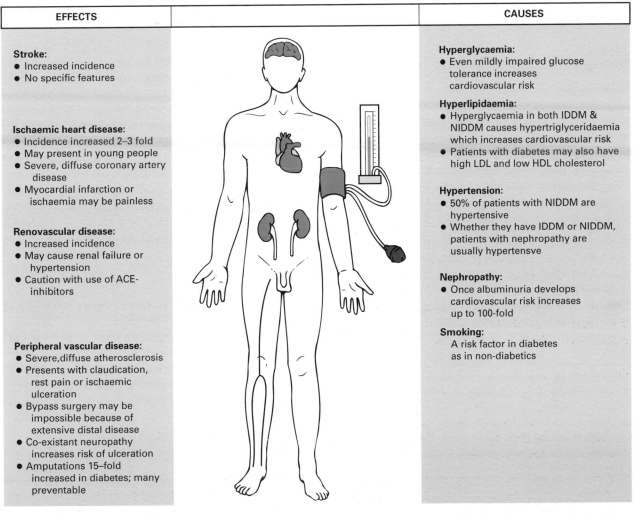

Stroke:
- Increased incidence
- No specific features

Ischaemic heart disease:
- Incidence increased 2–3 fold
- May present in young people
- Severe, diffuse coronary artery disease
- Myocardial infarction or ischaemia may be painless

Renovascular disease:
- Increased incidence
- May cause renal failure or hypertension
- Caution with use of ACE-inhibitors

Peripheral vascular disease:
- Severe,diffuse atherosclerosis
- Presents with claudication, rest pain or ischaemic ulceration
- Bypass surgery may be impossible because of extensive distal disease
- Co-existant neuropathy increases risk of ulceration
- Amputations 15–fold increased in diabetes; many preventable

Hyperglycaemia:
- Even mildly impaired glucose tolerance increases cardiovascular risk

Hyperlipidaemia:
- Hyperglycaemia in both IDDM & NIDDM causes hypertriglyceridaemia which increases cardiovascular risk
- Patients with diabetes may also have high LDL and low HDL cholesterol

Hypertension:
- 50% of patients with NIDDM are hypertensive
- Whether they have IDDM or NIDDM, patients with nephropathy are usually hypertensve

Nephropathy:
- Once albuminuria develops cardiovascular risk increases up to 100-fold

Smoking:
A risk factor in diabetes as in non-diabetics

Fig. 54
Macrovascular disease in diabetics.

The prevalence of hypertension is not increased in uncomplicated IDDM, unless nephropathy has developed. The clinical presentation and investigation of hypertension are as described on page 40. There are some specific points about its treatment in diabetes:

- diabetic patients should be regarded as high-risk hypertensives; apply the principles shown on page 43 but err on the side of treating rather than not treating, irrespective of age
- hypertension should be treated aggressively in patients with nephropathy; unless there is evidence of renal artery stenosis (p. 161) or a possibility of pregnancy, use ACE inhibitors
- the presence of macrovascular complications may influence the choice of antihypertensive drug. Heart failure is common in diabetes and ACE inhibitors are proven to improve life expectancy. Likewise, beta-blockers and calcium antagonists are indicated in patients with myocardial infarction or angina
- thiazides (particularly in inappropriately high doses) and beta-blockers worsen glucose tolerance

and hyperlipidaemia. Their role as first-line antihypertensives in NIDDM is debated.

Prevention of macrovascular disease. This consists of primary prevention, the early identification and correction of risk factors, and secondary prevention, the management of established disease. All patients should have as good glycaemic control as possible, although this has not yet been *proven* to prevent macrovascular disease. All risk factors, including hypertension, should be treated because their effects are additive:

- hyperlipidaemia is common in diabetes and should be treated aggressively (p. 273)
- smoking is even more dangerous than in the general population
- blood pressure should be monitored regularly and treated early (see above).

Patients who already have macrovascular disease have a very high risk of disease progression and mortality, so secondary prevention should be even more strenuous than primary prevention. These topics are also covered under Hyperlipidaemia (p. 272), Hypertension (p. 40) and Ischaemic heart disease (p. 12).

Microvascular complications

Retinopathy

Diabetes is the most common single cause of blindness in middle age and a cause of visual loss at all ages. Retinopathy may be present when diabetes is diagnosed, particularly in old people, and becomes increasingly prevalent with longer durations of diabetes. Clinical features are summarised in Figure 55. Diabetic retinopathy results from occlusion and leakage of retinal capillaries. There are two causes of visual loss:

- **maculopathy** is loss of visual acuity caused by background retinopathy involving the fovea
- **proliferative retinopathy** is the formation of new blood vessels or fibrous tissue on the surface of the retina in response to retinal ischaemia; ultimately, those vessels bleed and/or the fibrous tissue related to them contracts.

Blindness is caused by progressive macular damage, bleeding from new vessels, contraction of fibrous tissue leading to retinal detachment and 'rubeotic glaucoma'

(obstruction of the filtration angle in the anterior chamber by new vessels).

Retinopathy can be prevented in IDDM (and probably in NIDDM, although the evidence does not yet exist) by excellent glycaemic control. Once maculopathy or proliferative retinopathy have developed, visual loss can usually be prevented by laser photocoagulation. Vision may be salvaged by vitrectomy surgery for advanced proliferative retinopathy. Patients with proliferative retinopathy may have normal visual acuities until their new vessels bleed and patients with maculopathy may not complain of visual loss. If you wait until the patient has symptoms, you will detect diabetic retinopathy too late. It should be detected by regular (at least annual) eye examination consisting of:

- measurement of visual acuity
- retinal examination by an experienced observer through dilated pupils, or retinal photography.

Presence of anything more than mild background retinopathy and/or *any* degree of visual impairment are indications for immediate ophthalmic referral.

Cataracts and glaucoma. These are not microvascular complications but are mentioned here because they are part of 'diabetic eye disease'.

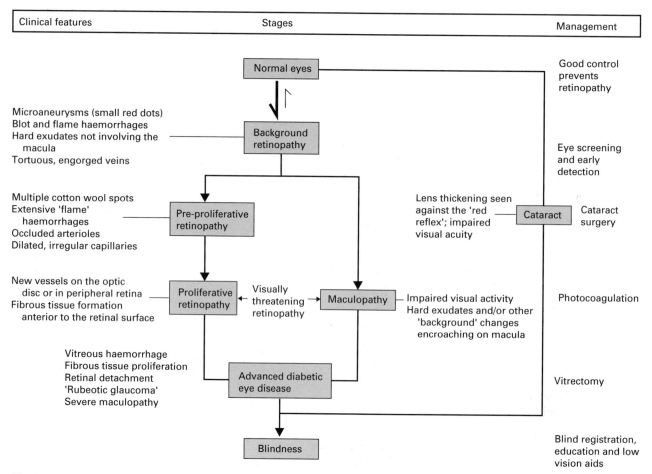

Fig. 55
Diabetic eye disease: progression and management.

Cataracts. These are more prevalent in diabetes and present at younger ages, but their clinical features are little different from cataracts in non-diabetics. The association is so strong that all patients with cataracts should be screened for diabetes. Treatment is by lens extraction. Many old people go blind needlessly because their diabetic cataracts are not treated.

Glaucoma. Various types of glaucoma are more common in diabetes and can cause visual loss.

Nephropathy

Diabetes is one of the most common causes of chronic renal failure. Up to one-third of patients with IDDM and 10% with NIDDM develop it. Once nephropathy is established, it is likely to progress to renal failure. Also, it increases the risk of ischaemic heart disease up to 100-fold. The stages are illustrated in Figure 56.

Nephropathy can be prevented by good control. Proteinuria is the first sign and is virtually diagnostic of nephropathy if the patient has retinopathy (signifying microvascular disease elsewhere in the body) and no other cause for proteinuria (such as a urinary tract infection). Occasionally, a renal biopsy is needed to distinguish diabetic nephropathy from other causes of proteinuria. Once nephropathy is established, ACE inhibitors reduce proteinuria and delay progression. Dietary protein restriction has a similar effect. Other antihypertensives are less effective than ACE inhibitors. Many patients with nephropathy die of ischaemic heart disease, so all cardiovascular risk factors (smoking and hyperlipidaemia as well as hypertension) should be treated. Diabetic patients with end-stage renal failure are treated by dialysis or transplantation.

Neuropathy

Neuropathy is caused by small vessel disease within the nerves and a direct metabolic effect of diabetes on them. Clinical presentations are summarised in Figure 57 and include:

- motor and sensory polyneuropathy in a 'glove and stocking' distribution, affecting the legs more than the arms
- mononeuritis multiplex, causing sudden dysfunction of peripheral nerves or nerve roots, typically painful and resolving spontaneously over time. Typical examples include cranial mononeuropathy causing isolated oculomotor palsies, radiculopathy (diabetic amyotrophy) or peripheral nerve lesions (peroneal mononeuropathy causing foot drop).

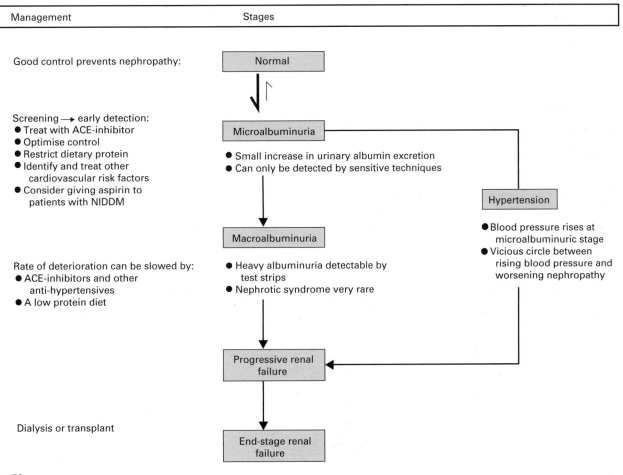

Fig. 56
Stages of nephropathy

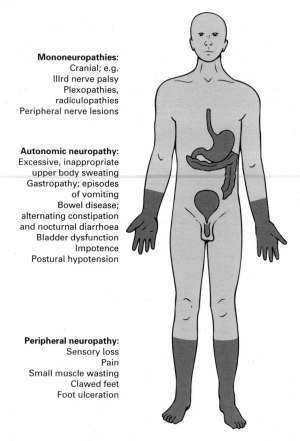

Mononeuropathies:
Cranial; e.g.
IIIrd nerve palsy
Plexopathies,
radiculopathies
Peripheral nerve lesions

Autonomic neuropathy:
Excessive, inappropriate
upper body sweating
Gastropathy; episodes
of vomiting
Bowel disease;
alternating constipation
and nocturnal diarrhoea
Bladder dysfunction
Impotence
Postural hypotension

Peripheral neuropathy:
Sensory loss
Pain
Small muscle wasting
Clawed feet
Foot ulceration

Fig. 57
Clinical presentations of diabetic neuropathy.

- autonomic neuropathy, including excessive upper body sweating, postural hypotension, atonia of the bladder, gastropathy (episodic vomiting), bowel involvement (episodic nocturnal diarrhoea) and erectile impotence.

Diabetic foot disease. This may be caused by neuropathy, peripheral vascular disease (see above) or both. Neuropathy is usually painless but can sometimes cause deep 'toothache' or burning superficial leg pain, often worse at night. There is loss of pinprick and vibration sense. Motor involvement causes 'clawing' of the toes and callus formation or ulceration under the metatarsal heads. Every patient should have:

- an annual foot examination
- education about the risks of foot disease and how to prevent it
- access to preventive chiropody
- appropriate footwear.

Ulceration. This results from:

- accidental damage owing to insensitivity
- foot deformity caused by motor neuropathy
- autonomic neuropathy, which causes loss of sweating, dry skin and fissuring
- impaired resistance to infection
- disordered neurogenic control of the distal circulation.

Ulceration requires immediate expert attention and, often, hospital admission. It is treated with chiropody, rest, debridement and antibiotics. Amputation is needed for severe infection, osteomyelitis or chronic, disabling ulceration. These problems often result from late presentation or inadequate care. Painful neuropathy is treated with a tricyclic antidepressant (imipramine) and/or carbamazepine.

Diabetes and pregnancy

Established diabetes is the most common medical disorder complicating pregnancy in the UK, occurring in about 4/1 000 pregnancies. This is because many patients with IDDM are of childbearing age. In addition, pregnancy can precipitate transient or permanent diabetes (see below).

Complications

Several decades ago, diabetes was usually lethal to the fetus and sometimes also to the mother. With good control *throughout pregnancy*, the outlook is now almost as good in diabetic as in non-diabetic women.

Glucose crosses the placenta. Hyperglycaemia is teratogenic in early pregnancy and stimulates excessive fetal insulin secretion as pregnancy progresses. Complications are associated with poor glycaemic control.

In early pregnancy. Major congenital malformations are two to three times more common than in non-diabetic women and include neural tube and cardiovascular defects; the main risk factor for them is poor glycaemic control *at the time of conception.*

In later pregnancy. Complications include:

- intrauterine death, hydramnios and pre-eclampsia
- fetal macrosomia (large-for-dates)
- neonatal complications, including hyaline membrane disease and hypoglycaemia.

Other complications. Nephropathy and retinopathy may deteriorate during pregnancy and must be monitored carefully. Women with these complications have a worse fetal outcome.

Management

There are three stages, all requiring good glycaemic control: at conception, during pregnancy and during labour.

At conception. All diabetic women who are 'at risk' of pregnancy should be informed of the increased risk of congenital malformations if they become pregnant when poorly controlled. Some hospitals run prepregnancy clinics to counsel women, give contraceptive advice, optimise control and advise on the timing of pregnancy.

During pregnancy. Blood glucose levels and HbA_{1c} should be kept as close to normal as possible. Insulin doses have to be increased as pregnancy progresses because the hormones of pregnancy cause insulin resistance. Women who are treated with twice-daily insulin outside pregnancy are often treated with four injections per day. Dietary advice is reinforced. Blood glucose needs to be measured several times each day. Tight control increases the risk of hypoglycaemia, so the patient's partner should be instructed in the use of glucagon (p. 274). Hypoglycaemia, though unpleasant to the mother, is not known to be harmful to the fetus. Patients are seen every 2–4 weeks, ideally in a joint diabetic/antenatal clinic. If good control is achieved and pregnancy progresses well, the aim is a spontaneous vaginal delivery at term.

During labour. As during surgery (p. 284), blood glucose is kept within normal limits by constant infusion of glucose and insulin.

Gestational diabetes

Just as pregnancy hormones increase insulin requirements in women with established diabetes by causing insulin resistance, they can actually precipitate diabetes, usually in the third trimester. This is termed gestational diabetes if it remits after delivery. Remember also that IDDM may first present during pregnancy. Women at risk of gestational diabetes are those with a history of

- large-for-dates babies
- previous gestational diabetes
- diabetes in the family.

Gestational diabetes increases the risk of macrosomia and perinatal complications. It is usually asymptomatic and diagnosed by measuring random blood glucose levels backed up by glucose tolerance testing. It is treated with a sugar-free diet and, in many cases, insulin. Good glycaemic control has been shown to improve the fetal outcome. Within 10 years of delivery, 50% of women with gestational diabetes have developed permanent diabetes, usually NIDDM.

Metabolic complications

Hypoglycaemia

Hypoglycaemia in diabetes only occurs in patients on insulin or sulphonylureas. Sulphonylurea-induced hypoglycaemia is usually the result of over-aggressive treatment and should, therefore, be an infrequent occurrence. Hypoglycaemia on insulin, however, can occur despite the best care because

- insulin is absorbed erratically from injection sites
- sensitivity to it varies with the patient's emotional state, menstruation, drugs and many other factors
- variations in exercise and eating habits also cause hypoglycaemia.

Hypoglycaemia is disruptive to the patient, family and friends but rarely has lasting sequelae unless it causes injury. The incidence of severe hypoglycaemia can be reduced by good education, regular home blood glucose monitoring and regular eating habits. Patients are particularly vulnerable to it if, as may occur with long-standing diabetes, the early warning symptoms are lost

(hypoglycaemia unawareness). This is particularly likely to occur in those with the best glycaemic control because frequent, low blood glucose levels desensitise the hypothalamus to hypoglycaemia. Sulphonylurea-induced hypoglycaemia can be prevented by starting on small doses of drugs and not increasing them too quickly. Long-acting sulphonylureas (glibenclamide, chlorpropamide) should not be used in patients over the age of 70 because they can cause fatal hypoglycaemia.

Whatever the cause, the symptoms of hypoglycaemia include

- **the adrenergic, anti-insulin response:** sweating, shaking, pallor, anxiety, headache
- **neuroglycopenia:** loss of concentration, personality change, drowsiness and coma.

It is loss of the adrenergic response which causes patients to go into coma without warning.

Except in patients with hypoglycaemia unawareness, the adrenergic symptoms come first. Mild hypoglycaemia is treated by taking extra carbohydrate. All patients on insulin should be encouraged to carry glucose tablets at all times, particularly when driving. Severe hypoglycaemia is best treated with intramuscular glucagon, which can be given by relatives, friends or ambulance personnel and acts within 5 minutes. Intravenous glucose is harder to give and damaging to veins. Emergency treatment of hypoglycaemia is described in the box below.

Spontaneous hypoglycaemia — not treatment-induced — is discussed below.

Severe hyperglycaemia/ketoacidosis

Although often described as two distinct conditions, there are more similarities than differences between diabetic ketoacidosis (DKA) and the diabetic hyperosmolar non-ketotic state (HONKS). Ketoacidosis occurs in patients with IDDM or those with NIDDM who have unusually high levels of anti-insulin hormones caused by intercurrent illness, such as myocardial infarction or severe infection. The hyperosmolar non-ketotic state develops slowly in patients with some residual insulin

---

Emergency treatment: management of hypoglycaemia

- Diagnosed by typical symptoms in a known diabetic
- May be confirmed by finger-prick testing
- If able to cooperate, treat with oral glucose
- More severe hypoglycaemia can be treated with proprietary glucose solution or syrup squirted or smeared in the mouth
- If comatose or uncooperative, give glucagon 1 mg i.m.
- If still unresponsive, 25 g glucose (50 ml, 50%) i.v.
- Feed as soon as conscious
- Consider how to prevent recurrence

secretion (NIDDM) and is characterised by profound depletion of sodium and water. Ketoacidotic patients are also dehydrated because of an uncontrolled osmotic diuresis. The diagnosis and management of DKA and HONKS are similar and described together here.

Causes are divided roughly equally between:

- newly presenting diabetes
- intercurrent illness (particularly bacterial infection)
- mistakes with insulin doses
- no cause identified, sometimes a result of deliberate manipulation.

Presenting features. These include vomiting, hyperglycaemic symptoms, unexplained unconsciousness or the symptoms of a precipitating illness. Hyperglycaemic symptoms come on over hours or days, compared with the symptoms of hypoglycaemia which come on over minutes. There are signs of volume depletion unless the illness is complicated by cardiac or renal failure. If ketoacidotic, there is deep, sighing respiration and a smell of acetone on the breath.

Management. Your priorities are to:

- confirm the diagnosis
- search for and treat any precipitating cause
- assess hydration and give fluid
- give insulin
- monitor the biochemistry and clinical signs.

Immediate clinical assessment. Take a quick history, examine carefully for signs of a precipitating illness and assess hydration (p. 167). The emergency treatment of ketoacidosis/hyperosmolar non-ketotic states is given in the box below.

Immediate investigations. Measure glucose, urea, electrolytes and bicarbonate; record an ECG, culture blood and urine and arrange a chest X-ray.

Emergency treatment: management of ketoacidosis/hyperosmolar coma

- Put up a drip
- If comatose, protect the airway; consider nasogastric tube and urinary catheter
- Establish the diagnosis: measure glucose, venous bicarbonate and urine or plasma ketones
- Quick history and examination. What has caused it?
- Assess hydration: give saline (see text)
- Start insulin infusion (e.g. soluble insulin 6 units/hour)
- Urgent ECG, chest X-ray, blood and urine cultures
- Give potassium (see text) from the second bottle of fluid onwards
- Observe state of hydration, urine output and conscious level repeatedly
- Monitor plasma glucose and potassium repeatedly
- Infuse dextrose when plasma glucose reaches 15 mmol/l

Immediate management. Set up a drip, give saline and start an insulin infusion or hourly i.m. insulin injections. If central venous pressure is uncertain, a central venous pressure (CVP) line may be inserted and fluid replacement adjusted to maintain a CVP of approximately 10 cm H_2O.

Fluid therapy. Initial resuscitation is with isotonic saline. If the patient is hypernatraemic, some of the fluid should be hypotonic saline. Potassium is given, even if the plasma level is high initially, because insulin lowers it by driving it into cells. Patients with profound acidosis complicated by shock or cardiac dysrhythmias may be given sodium bicarbonate, but this will cause an even greater potassium shift into cells and can precipitate severe hypokalaemia. Once plasma glucose is at or below 15 mmol/l, the infusion is changed to 5% dextrose.

General care. Patients who are comatose and cannot protect their airways should have a naso-gastric tube to prevent vomiting and aspiration and, if necessary, an airway. Severely ill and/or oliguric patients should have a urinary catheter. Antibiotics are given if there is evidence of infection or the patient is severely ill; such patients should be treated on an intensive care unit.

Monitoring. Careful and repeated observation of the conscious level and state of hydration is essential. Plasma glucose and electrolytes should be measured 1–2 hourly initially and less frequently thereafter. Once the intravenous fluid is changed to dextrose, bedside glucose monitoring can be used to adjust the insulin infusion rate.

Prevention of recurrence. Severe hyperglycaemia carries a mortality of 50% in old people and can be lethal at any age so it is important to search for causes. A common preventable cause of ketoacidosis is to reduce the insulin dose misguidedly during intercurrent illness. All diabetic patients should be advised against this when they are first started on insulin.

Surgery and special situations

In hospital, managing diabetes perioperatively or during intercurrent illness is the skill most commonly required of non-specialists. The subject is too complex to be discussed in detail; however, the general principles are:

- insulin rather than tablets should be used to control hyperglycaemia in all acute situations
- if a patient is fasting or too ill to eat, a constant infusion of insulin (given through a syringe pump or added to isotonic dextrose and potassium) is the best approach
- unless the volume of intravenous fluid has to be minimised because of heart failure, it is always best to infuse dextrose simultaneously with insulin to achieve stable glycaemic control; potassium should be added to the infusion
- patients who are well enough to eat can usually be managed with four-times daily subcutaneous insulin given before meals and before bed; doses

need to be reviewed regularly and adjusted according to four-times daily glucose measurements
- in less acute situations, twice-daily insulin or sulphonylureas can be used.

Spontaneous hypoglycaemia

Hypoglycaemia is defined as:

- a plasma glucose <2.8 mmol/l *and*
- typical symptoms *and*
- relief of the symptoms by carbohydrate.

Patients who are not diabetic and not on insulin or sulphonylureas may become spontaneously hypoglycaemic through:

- excessive secretion of insulin from the B-cells
- other insulin-like hormones (sometimes secreted by mesenchymal tumours)
- antibodies with insulin-like activity.

Hypoglycaemia may also result from:

- excessive sensitivity to insulin, as in hypoadrenalism
- surreptitious abuse of insulin or sulphonylureas.

The classical cause of spontaneous hypoglycaemia is an insulinoma: a rare, usually benign, pancreatic tumour. Table 63 gives a more complete list of causes of spontaneous hypoglycaemia, all of which are rare.

Suspected hypoglycaemia must be confirmed biochemically; blood taken at the time of hypoglycaemia is crucial in determining the cause. Your tasks are to:

- recognise hypoglycaemia when it presents with confusion, coma or a fit; a bedside glucose test gives you a working diagnosis

Table 63 Causes of spontaneous hypoglycaemia

Cause	Biochemical profile
Excessive insulin	
Insulinoma	High insulin, high C-peptide
benign	
malignant	
Sulphonylurea abuse	High insulin, high C-peptide
Insulin abuse	High insulin, low C-peptide
Excessive sensitivity to insulin	Low insulin, low C-peptide
Hormone deficiency	
hypoadrenalism	
hypothyroidism	
hypopituitarism	
Impaired gluconeogenesis	
liver disease	
alcoholism	
Other insulin-like factors	Low insulin, low C-peptide
Hormones	
Antibodies with agonist activity	

- recognise that it is spontaneous, i.e. the patient is not known to be on treatment for diabetes
- measure blood glucose on a fluoride sample (yellow tube) to confirm the diagnosis of hypoglycaemia
- obtain blood at the time of hypoglycaemia for insulin, C-peptide and other measurements
- treat the hypoglycaemia.

Insulinomas are located by CT scanning, angiography and transoesophageal ultrasound. Removal of the tumour can be curative. Diazoxide can be used as a medical treatment in patients who are not fit for surgery.

Self-assessment: questions

Multiple choice questions

1. Prognosis of diabetes:
   a. Cardiovascular mortality is higher in diabetic than in non-diabetic people up to the age of 80
   b. Diabetic patients with proteinuria have a higher cardiovascular risk than those without it
   c. When sulphonylureas became available, there was a noticeable improvement in cardiovascular mortality
   d. Good glycaemic control, on the balance of available evidence, can reduce cardiovascular mortality in both IDDM and NIDDM
   e. Even mildly 'impaired glucose tolerance' increases cardiovascular risk

2. Epidemiology of diabetes:
   a. Asian people in the UK have a more than two-fold increased prevalence of diabetes
   b. The incidence of diabetes peaks at the age of 60
   c. If you are going to develop IDDM, you will do so by the age of 30
   d. The prevalence of IDDM and NIDDM is increasing in the UK
   e. There are more insulin-treated people in the UK over the age of 30 than below it

3. In secondary diabetes:
   a. A patient can be assumed not to be ketosis-prone
   b. A patient is more than 85% likely to have clinical pancreatic exocrine deficiency
   c. Classical diabetic complications do not occur
   d. Thiazide diuretics and beta-blockers can both impair insulin secretion
   e. Most patients with acromegaly are diabetic

4. In hypoglycaemia:
   a. Insulin-dependent patients may recover from hypoglycaemic coma without treatment
   b. Sweating and shaking are always late symptoms of insulin-induced hypoglycaemia
   c. Insulin-dependent patients may lose their warning symptoms of hypoglycaemia after many years of diabetes
   d. Metformin is responsible for as many cases of hypoglycaemia as sulphonylureas
   e. The symptoms characteristically come on over hours rather than minutes

5. Diabetic retinopathy:
   a. Characteristically causes arterio-venous nipping
   b. Should be referred to an ophthalmologist only if the patient has visual symptoms
   c. Inevitably causes blindness
   d. May cause cotton wool spots (soft exudates)
   e. Is more likely to cause blindness in IDDM than in NIDDM

6. In the treatment of NIDDM:
   a. Most patients gain weight when they are started on metformin
   b. Glibenclamide is the sulphonylurea of choice in people aged over 70 years
   c. Acarbose improves blood glucose levels after meals by delaying the breakdown of complex carbohydrates in the gut
   d. All but the most symptomatic patients should first be treated by diet alone
   e. Fewer than 2% of patients treated with tablets are switched to insulin in their diabetic lives

7. In insulin treatment:
   a. Pen injectors are reserved for the small minority who take four or more injections per day
   b. Only patients who cannot be controlled with once-daily insulin should have two or more injections
   c. Insulin should be started without delay in a thin hyperglycaemic patient with ketonuria
   d. Insulin may sometimes be needed during short periods of illness in patients with NIDDM
   e. All patients on insulin should be discouraged from changing their doses without first checking with the doctor or nurse

8. Instituting intensive insulin treatment aiming to normalise HbA_{1c} in IDDM:
   a. Increases the risk of severe hypoglycaemia
   b. Reduces the incidence of diabetic retinopathy
   c. Reduces the incidence of diabetic nephropathy
   d. Increases the mortality of IDDM
   e. May be hazardous if the patient does not do regular home blood glucose monitoring

9. Hypertension in diabetes:
   a. Is more prevalent in IDDM than NIDDM
   b. Its treatment slows the deterioration of nephropathy in IDDM
   c. Thiazide diuretics should not be used in diabetes
   d. Beta-blockers may increase the risk of severe hypoglycaemia in insulin-treated patients
   e. Increases the risk of stroke in diabetes

10. In diabetic pregnancy:
    a. Insulin-dependent women should be advised not to contemplate pregnancy
    b. Diabetes increases the risk of neural tube defects
    c. Poor glycaemic control at conception increases the risk of congenital malformations

d. There is a less than 10% chance that an episode of ketoacidosis will cause intrauterine death

e. Sulphonylureas are the treatment of choice for gestational diabetes

11. Diabetic foot ulceration:
    a. Is best treated by keeping the patient weight-bearing
    b. Is more likely to lead to amputation if caused by peripheral vascular disease than if caused by neuropathy
    c. Is usually caused by patients reporting pain in their feet too late
    d. May require prolonged (> 2 weeks) antibiotic treatment
    e. Can be prevented in many cases by chiropody

12. Which of the following are true?
    a. Most tumours causing overactivity or underactivity of endocrine glands are malignant
    b. Surgery can cure many diseases of endocrine overactivity
    c. Autoimmunity is a common cause of endocrine underactivity
    d. The best way to tell if an endocrine gland is overactive is to stimulate it and test how it responds
    e. Most endocrine diseases can be managed without radionuclide imaging.

13. The following are true of hyperthyroidism:
    a. Goitres in hyperthyroid patients are rarely (< 5%) malignant
    b. More patients are treated surgically than by any other form of treatment
    c. Proptosis is caused by hyperthyroidism
    d. Patients on carbimazole should be warned that it may cause neutropenia
    e. An isotope scan should be done in every case of hyperthyroidism

14. The following are true of hypothyroidism:
    a. Thyroid cancer sometimes (> 20% of patients) causes hypothyroidism
    b. It may be caused by pituitary tumours
    c. Most cases are autoimmune
    d. Ultrasound scanning is usually indicated
    e. It predisposes to ischaemic heart disease

15. Thyroid function tests:
    a. Serum TSH is a sensitive test of hyperthyroidism
    b. Serum TSH can distinguish primary from secondary hypothyroidism
    c. Serum triiodothyronine can be an unreliable test for hypothyroidism
    d. Hyperthyroid patients may have a raised serum triiodothyronine with a normal thyroxine

e. Treatment with the contraceptive pill artificially increases the serum free thyroxine concentration

16. Thyroid nodules:
    a. Are best investigated by isotope scanning followed by surgery
    b. Are usually (> 50%) malignant
    c. May be associated with hyperthyroidism
    d. Can be ignored if they present in children
    e. Can be investigated by aspiration cytology

17. In pituitary tumours:
    a. Surgery is the treatment of choice for patients with hyperprolactinaemia
    b. The early visual field defect of chiasmal compression is superior temporal hemianopia
    c. Diabetes insipidus suggests hypothalamic damage
    d. Optic atrophy may be an effect of pituitary tumours
    e. Radiotherapy may cause hypopituitarism up to 10 years later

18. Acromegaly:
    a. Has no effect on life expectancy
    b. Often causes headaches
    c. Can be cured by surgery
    d. Can be treated medically if surgery is impossible or unsuccessful
    e. Is associated with an increased risk of malignant disease

19. Cushing's syndrome:
    a. Causes osteoporosis
    b. The diagnosis is made by a high-dose dexamethasone test
    c. Serum ACTH is important in diagnosing the underlying cause
    d. The classical 'lemon-on-sticks' appearance may be caused by small cell carcinoma of the bronchus
    e. Can only be cured by bilateral adrenalectomy

20. In hyperlipidaemia:
    a. Hypertriglyceridaemia is not a risk factor for cardiovascular disease
    b. Bezafibrate is the first-line treatment for hypercholesterolaemia
    c. Lipid-lowering has not been shown to reduce the incidence of cardiovascular disease
    d. Hypercholesterolaemia is always a congenital abnormality
    e. There is no indication to treat hyperlipidaemia in smokers

Case history questions

History 1

> A 23-year-old woman with IDDM since the age of 10 has attended clinics infrequently. She has recently married and attends clinic at her husband's insistence. Her blood pressure, averaged over three measurements at weekly intervals, is 162/94. She has a 24-hour urine protein excretion of 2 g and her haemoglobin A$_{1c}$ high.

1. List three key components of the physical examination.
2. What diagnosis and action should be considered as a result of her urine protein excretion?
3. Apart from discussing her current treatment regimen, what else should she be counselled about?

History 2

> A 68-year-old diabetic man who has been on glibenclamide and frusemide for 5 years presents breathless, vomiting and collapsed 12 hours after an episode of precordial chest pain. His blood glucose stick test is unrecordably high.

1. Which of the following are true?
   a. Intravenous fluid should be given before the patient is examined or any investigations are done
   b. The fact that he has diabetes and has had chest pain makes a diagnosis of myocardial infarction unlikely
   c. An ECG should be done soon after presentation
   d. If he is able to take tablets, his hyperglycaemia should be controlled with glibenclamide

> His ECG confirms acute myocardial infarction and his biochemistry shows him to be in ketoacidosis with a serum potassium of 3 mmol/l.

2. Which of the following are true?
   a. His relatives should be told that he is critically ill and may not survive
   b. Acidosis should be corrected with bicarbonate as a first priority
   c. He may eventually return to tablet therapy
   d. Insulin should not be given without a dextrose infusion

History 3

> A 78-year-old patient has had NIDDM for 1 year treated with glipizide. She is very thin and continuing to lose weight. She has become incontinent.

1. Suggest how these problems may be linked and what investigations you would do.

History 4

> You are an on-call medical house officer and receive a telephone call from the husband of a 48-year-old insulin-dependent patient who has caught a heavy cold. His wife is normally well controlled on two injections per day. It is teatime and she is due for her injection. She is not sure that she can face a cooked meal. Her finger-prick glucose is 9 mmol/l.

1. What advice would you give?

History 5

> You are a casualty officer. At 10 p.m., a young man with IDDM is brought in by the police having been found wandering and confused. He is pale and sweating and has a finger-prick glucose < 2 mmol/l. He is aggressive and agitated.

1. How would you manage him?

> Once he has recovered, you want to know the cause.

2. Name four points you would enquire about.

> You cannot identify a cause for his attack. His diabetes is normally well controlled. He is fully recovered and ready to go home.

3. Suggest one action that you should take.

History 6

> A 48-year-old woman presents with irritability, restlessness and poor energy. She has a palpable goitre. Plasma thyroxine is 200 nmol/l (normal up to 150) and triiodothyronine 3.4 nmol/l (normal up to 2.9).

1. What other biochemical abnormality would confirm your suspected diagnosis of hyperthyroidism?

> The diagnosis of hyperthyroidism is confirmed biochemically.

2. What investigations would be useful in elucidating the pathology of the condition?

> A diagnosis of solitary toxic nodule is made.

3. How might the patient be treated?

History 7

> A 35-year-old diabetic man complains of impotence.

1. What organic causes should be considered and what points are important in the clinical assessment?
Serum testosterone is reduced.
2. What possible causes are there for the reduced testosterone and what further biochemical information would be helpful?
Serum prolactin is grossly reduced.
3. What further investigations and treatment are indicated?

Data interpretation

1. In an oral glucose tolerance test with 75 g glucose, the venous whole blood glucose values (in mmol/l) for three patients were as follows:

	Fasting	2 hours after glucose
A	5	8
B	8	12
C	3	4

How would you interpret the results?

2. A 45-year-old who has had IDDM for 20 years presents with swollen hands and feet. Biochemical results are as follows:
plasma urea   24 mmol/l
creatinine   250 mmol/l

albumin   24 g/l
24 hour urine protein excretion 15 g

What is your diagnostic formulation?

3. A 60-year-old man with NIDDM of 5 years duration is taking no regular treatment and has the following results:
HbA$_{1c}$ 9.5% (normal up to 5%)
total cholesterol   6 mmol/1 (see Table 2, p. 000)
triglycerides   6 mmol/l

   a. Comment on the results
   b. What other information would help to interpret these results?
   c. How would you treat him?

4. A young woman with no history of diabetes was brought to Casualty having had a fit. Her previous health had been good but she had gained weight over the last year. Her fingerprick glucose was < 2 mmol/l. Laboratory glucose was 1.1 mmol/l. Her serum insulin and C-peptide were both found to be high. What is the differential diagnosis?

5. Interpret the three sets of thyroid function test results given in Table 64.

6. In a water deprivation test, a patient is not allowed to drink for 8 hours and the hourly urine volume, plasma and urine osmolalities are measured hourly. Intramuscular desmopressin (ADH analogue) is then given and the measurements are continued for 2 hours more during which time the patient is allowed to drink. Interpret the three sets of results given in Table 65.

Table 64 Thyroid function test for three patients

	Total thyroxine (nmol/l)	Total triiodothyronine (nmol/l)	TSH (mU/l)
A	48	–	2.4
B	210	5.3	< 0.1
C	30	–	> 50
Normal range	50–150	1.9–2.9	0.5–5.0

Table 65 The results of a water deprivation test

		After 8 hours of water deprivation	Two hours after desmopression
Expected results	Serum osmolality[a]	≤ 295	≤ 295
	Urine osmolality[a]	> 750	> 750
Patient A	Serum osmolality[a]	302	298
	Urine osmolality[a]	180	800
	1-hour urine volume (ml)	100	0
Patient B	Serum osmolality[a]	294	293
	Urine osmolality[a]	820	900
	1-hour urine volume (ml)	15	10
Patient C	Serum osmolality[a]	298	300
	Urine osmolality[a]	200	200
	1-hour urine volume (ml)	80	85

[a]Osmolality in mosmol/kg.

Picture questions

1. Picture 7.1 is the coronal magnetic resonance image taken in a young woman complaining of amenorrhoea, infertility and galactorrhoea. The pituitary gland is in the midline immediately above the sphenoid sinus, which shows black. To the left of the midline is an oval lesion.
   a. What is this lesion likely to be?
   b. How would you confirm the diagnosis ?
   c. How would you treat her?

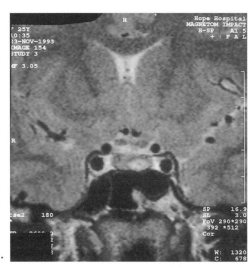

Picture 7.1.

2. Picture 7.2 is a sagittal MR image showing a huge 'cottage loaf' pituitary tumour, part within the pituitary fossa and part extending up into the suprasellar cistern. The 'waist' around the tumour corresponds to the position of the diaphragma sellae. The base of the tumour is outlined by the sphenoid sinus, which shows black on this image. How could this tumour have presented?

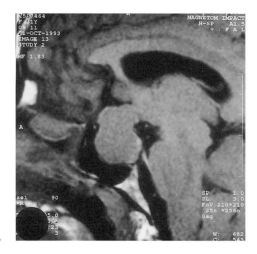

Picture 7.2.

3. A 65-year-old cigarette smoker is admitted to hospital so weak that he cannot stand. He complains of cough and a painful right upper arm. He has lost 2 stone in weight over the last 3 months. He is pigmented. His serum potassium is 1.8 mmol/l.

   a. Picture 7.3a shows his thoracic CT scan. What abnormality does it show?
   b. Picture 7.3b shows his right humerus. Describe the abnormality shown.
   c. Suggest a diagnosis and give your reasons
   d. Assuming the diagnosis was confirmed, how would you treat him?

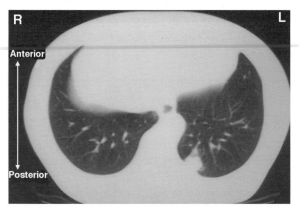

Picture 7.3a.

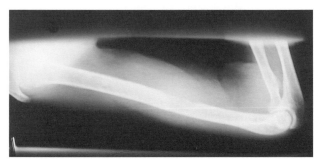

Picture 7.3b.

4. Picture 7.4 is a radiograph of the foot of a 58-year-old man with NIDDM. He has a painless discharging ulcer under the forefoot.
   a. What abnormality is shown?
   b. What is the likely diagnosis?
   c. How should it be treated?

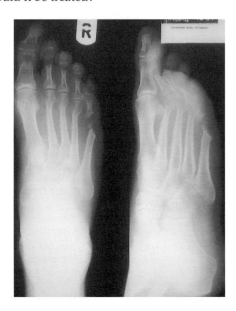

Picture 7.4.

Short notes

Write short notes on the following:

1. The treatment options and factors affecting the choice of therapy for a 24-year-old woman presenting with classical hyperthyroidism and a diffuse goitre
2. An obese patient is referred by her general practitioner to exclude organic causes of her continuing weight gain.
3. Hypoadrenal crisis.

Viva question

1. Why do some diabetic patients need insulin and others do not?

Self-assessment: answers

Multiple choice answers

1. a. **True.** A three-fold increase.
   b. **True.** It is indicative of nephropathy, which increases the risk of cardiovascular disease up to 100-fold.
   c. **False.** No treatment for diabetes has been proven to prevent cardiovascular disease. One clinical trial even suggested that sulphonylureas increased the risk.
   d. **False.** See above.
   e. **True.**

2. a. **True.**
   b. **False.** It increases progressively with age and there is no peak.
   c. **False.** IDDM can present at any age.
   d. **True.** Both are becoming more prevalent.
   e. **True.** Many patients with NIDDM (which is much commoner than IDDM) need insulin and IDDM itself may present after the age of 30. Almost all of those who present before age 30 survive well into middle age.

3. a. **False.** If secondary diabetes causes complete pancreatic failure, the patient will be prone to ketosis.
   b. **False.** Many causes of secondary diabetes only affect endocrine function. Even those which can cause both do not always do so.
   c. **False.** Secondary diabetes causes all the same complications as idiopathic diabetes.
   d. **True.**
   e. **False.** Fewer than 30% are diabetic.

4. a. **True.** The anti-insulin hormones can bring the patient round and the insulin which caused the coma can 'wear off'.
   b. **False.** They are early warning symptoms for many patients.
   c. **True.** About 50% of patients who have had IDDM for 20 years or more develop 'hypoglycaemia unawareness'.
   d. **False.** Metformin does not cause hypoglycaemia.
   e. **False.** Hypoglycaemic symptoms typically come on over minutes rather than hours.

5. a. **False.** This is a sign of hypertensive retinopathy.
   b. **False.** Ophthalmic referral for laser photocoagulation is often made in asymptomatic patients with visually threatening retinopathy seen on ophthalmoscopy but without symptoms.
   c. **False.** Provided it is detected early, even visually threatening retinopathy should not cause blindness.

   d. **True.** These may also occur in hypertension and other ischaemic retinopathies.
   e. **False.** It may cause visual loss in patients with all types of diabetes. It is wrong to think of NIDDM as 'mild diabetes'; its complications can be anything but 'mild'.

6. a. **False.** It is sulphonylureas and insulin, not metformin, which cause weight gain.
   b. **False.** It is contraindicated in patients over the age of 70. On account of side-effects, it is arguable whether glibenclamide is the drug of choice in any diabetic patient.
   c. **True.** It inhibits brush border saccharidases and so delays glucose absorption.
   d. **True.** Provided you are sure (e.g. by testing the urine for ketones) that the patient does not have IDDM.
   e. **False.**

7. a. **False.** Pen injectors can be used by most patients on insulin.
   b. **False.** Twice-daily insulin is the first-line regimen for most patients.
   c. **True.** These are signs of IDDM.
   d. **True.**
   e. **False.** Almost every insulin-treated patient should be taught how to alter their doses independently.

8. a. **True.**
   b. **True.**
   c. **True.**
   d. **False.**
   e. **True.**

9. a. **False.** Hypertension is associated with NIDDM more strongly than with IDDM.
   b. **True.**
   c. **False.** There is no absolute contraindication to their use, particularly in IDDM and if used in low dose.
   d. **True.** This is true primarily of non-cardioselective beta-blockers.
   e. **True.**

10. a. **False.** IDDM is rarely a contraindication to pregnancy.
    b. **True.** Neural tube defects are two to three times more common.
    c. **True.** Hyperglycaemia is teratogenic in early pregnancy; major congenital malformations are two to three times more common.
    d. **False.** Ketoacidosis carries a high risk of intra-uterine death.

e. **False.** If the patient is significantly hyperglycaemic on a sugar-free diet, insulin is given.

11. a. **False.** Ulcers will only heal if the weight is taken off them. This requires rest. Special footwear is needed to keep pressure off the ulcer.
    b. **True.**
    c. **False.** This is nonsensical because foot ulceration is more often than not painless when caused by neuropathy.
    d. **True.**
    e. **True.**

12. a. **False.** Most are benign.
    b. **True.** Apart from hyperthyroidism, which is usually treated with drugs or radioiodine, and hyperprolactinaemia, which is treated with dopaminergic agonists, surgery is the most likely treatment to cure endocrine overactivity.
    c. **True.**
    d. **False.** Suppression tests are used to confirm overactivity.
    e. **True.** Radionuclide scans are used occasionally to locate elusive tumours or to demonstrate overactivity but are less often useful than ultrasound, MR or CT.

13. a. **True.** If a patient is hyperthyroid, it is relatively unlikely that a thyroid swelling is malignant.
    b. **False.** Most patients are first treated with antithyroid drugs. Many have radioiodine as second-line therapy. Only a minority have surgery.
    c. **False.** Proptosis only occurs with Graves' disease and is caused by the immunological process. The patient need not be hyperthyroid.
    d. **True.** This serious side-effect has an incidence of 1:10 000 in patients taking carbimazole.
    e. **False.** Isotope scans are only useful in the hyperthyroid patient to confirm that a solitary nodule is functional.

14. a. **False.** Thyroid cancer would have to destroy the entire gland to cause hypothyroidism and this rarely occurs.
    b. **True.** Pituitary tumours cause secondary hypothyroidism.
    c. **True.**
    d. **False.** Imaging is rarely required in hypothyroidism.
    e. **True.** Hypothyroidism causes hypercholesterolaemia, which predisposes to ischaemic heart disease.

15. a. **True.** Suppression of TSH is the first biochemical sign of hyperthyroidism.
    b. **True.** In primary hypothyroidism, TSH is high; in secondary hypothyroidism, it is low.

    c. **True.** Low triiodothyronine may result from intercurrent illness, particularly in elderly people, and can be misleading.
    d. **True.** The condition of 'T$_3$ toxicosis'.
    e. **False.** Oestrogen increases plasma thyroid-binding globulin which increases plasma total thyroxine and can lead to a mistaken diagnosis of hyperthyroidism; *free* thyroxine is not affected by changes in thyroid-binding globulin.

16. a. **False.** Isotope scans are often unhelpful. Fine needle aspiration cytology and isotope scanning usually make surgery unnecessary.
    b. **False.** 10% or less are malignant.
    c. **True.** 'Toxic nodular goitre'.
    d. **False.** Nodules in children should be taken seriously as they may be malignant.
    e. **True.**

17. a. **False.** Hyperprolactinaemia, even if the patient has a large pituitary tumour, is best treated medically.
    b. **True.**
    c. **True.** Pituitary tumours usually do not cause diabetes insipidus unless there is hypothalamic involvement or the patient has had surgery.
    d. **True.** Optic atrophy is a late effect of optic nerve compression.
    e. **True.** Radiotherapy is slow acting and can have an effect decades later.

18. a. **False.** Acromegaly reduces life expectancy significantly.
    b. **True.** Headache is common and hard to treat effectively.
    c. **True.** The cure rate for smaller tumours (≤ 1 cm) is approximately 80%.
    d. **True.** Dopaminergic agonists and octreotide are effective.
    e. **True.** Also cardiorespiratory disease.

19. a. **True.**
    b. **False.** A high-dose dexamethasone test distinguishes between pituitary Cushing's and ectopic ACTH syndrome. The low-dose test is used to diagnose Cushing's in the first place.
    c. **True.** Patients with primary adrenal Cushing's have unmeasurably low serum ACTH.
    d. **False.** Patients with ectopic ACTH from small cell carcinoma of the bronchus do not have the typical body habitus of Cushing's. They usually lose weight rather than gain it. The ectopic ACTH in Cushing's syndrome is from less malignant tumours.
    e. **False.** Pituitary microsurgery cures many cases of pituitary Cushing's. Resection of a thoracic carcinoid tumour, for example, can cure the ectopic ACTH syndrome.

20. a. **False.** Hypertriglyceridaemia is not as predictive of cardiovascular disease as cholesterol but is associated with it.
    b. **False.** Diet is the first-line treatment for all types of hyperlipidaemia. Bezafibrate lowers cholesterol but not as effectively as simvastatin. Bezafibrate is more effective at lowering triglycerides than cholesterol.
    c. **False.** It has been shown to reduce coronary events although the effect on overall mortality is much weaker.
    d. **False.** There are numerous acquired causes of hypercholesterolaemia (p. 273).
    e. **False.** Smoking and hyperlipidaemia greatly increase the risk of cardiovascular disease; there are stronger arguments for treating smokers than non-smokers.

Case history answers

History 1

1. The following should form part of the examination:
   - examine fundi through dilated pupils
   - test for peripheral neuropathy (light touch, pinprick, cold metal and vibration sense)
   - test for peripheral vascular disease
   - examine for foot ulceration
   - examination for left ventricular hypertrophy/failure.
2. She probably has diabetic nephropathy as the cause of her proteinuria; the diagnosis is even more likely if she also has severe retinopathy. She needs antihypertensive therapy. An ACE inhibitor is most beneficial to the kidneys but contraindicated if she is contemplating pregnancy.
3. She should be counselled about pregnancy including:
   - the risks to the fetus if she becomes pregnant while poorly controlled
   - the risk that her diabetic nephropathy may worsen during pregnancy
   - the increased fetal loss in diabetic women with nephropathy
   - the dangers of fetal malformations associated with ACE inhibitors.

History 2

1. a. **False.** Since it sounds as though he has had a myocardial infarct, he may be in heart failure, in which case intravenous fluid would be contraindicated. Assessment of his fluid status must be done first.
   b. **False.** Diabetes may cause painless myocardial infarction but painful infarction is more common.
   c. **True.** An ECG is needed urgently.
   d. **False.** Tablet treatment of diabetes has no place in the management of acutely ill patients.
2. a. **True.** Diabetic ketoacidosis at his age has a mortality of 50% and myocardial infarction has a mortality of 30% in diabetic patients. The two together are a serious combination.
   b. **False.** There is a high risk of heart failure and sodium-containing fluids must be given cautiously. In addition, correcting his acidosis with bicarbonate will further lower serum potassium (by shifting potassium into cells) and could cause cardiac arrest.
   c. **True.** Just as diabetic ketoacidosis can be caused by intercurrent illness, so patients can sometimes return to tablets when they have recovered.
   d. **False.** Insulin is given without a glucose infusion during the initial management of diabetic ketoacidosis. If there is a risk of fluid overload (as in a patient with acute myocardial infarction), it may be safer to give insulin without infusing glucose even when hyperglycaemia has been controlled, although more stable control is achieved if both are infused together.

History 3

1. She may have:
   - IDDM or ITDM which has not been recognised and is causing weight loss and osmotic diuresis
   - carcinoma of the pancreas causing diabetes and weight loss
   - urinary tract infection, possibly causing hyperglycaemia
   - thyrotoxicosis, which exacerbates diabetes and causes weight loss.

Other possibilities include dementia, depression or other psychiatric or social problems. Other organic diseases include tuberculosis, occult neoplasia, renal failure, hypercalcaemia.

Investigations that could be done include:
- fasting or random glucose
- HbA_{1c}
- test urine for ketones
- TFTs
- renal, hepatic function and calcium
- chest X-ray
- urine culture
- abdominal ultrasound scan.

History 4

1. She should:
- test her urine for ketones
- take her normal evening insulin dose; she *should not reduce it*
- take whatever carbohydrate calories she can up to her normal amount as milk, biscuits or glucose tablets/drink
- test her urine for ketones and blood glucose before bed.

She will need to be admitted to hospital if she starts vomiting or develops uncontrolled hyperglycaemia or ketosis.

History 5

1. Try to persuade him to take carbohydrate, e.g. glucose tablets or drink. If this is unsuccessful, he should be given i.m. glucagon. Avoid i.v. 50% dextrose if possible because it is difficult to give to an agitated patient and may permanently thrombose veins.
2. Enquire about:
   - whether he had eaten normally
   - had he drunk alcohol? (note the time of his admission)
   - had he taken different insulin doses from normal?
   - his physical activity before the hypoglycaemic attack
   - previous history of hypoglycaemia
   - whether he does or does not experience hypoglycaemic warning symptoms
3. Notify his normal carers, e.g. general practitioner or diabetes centre. On the evidence given here, there is no reason to adjust his insulin doses and you should feel no obligation to do so. A hypoglycaemic attack may be a 'one-off'.

History 6

1. Serum TSH. This is likely to be suppressed.
2. If the goitre is diffuse, no other investigation is indicated. If it seems clinically to be nodular, isotope scanning may be of value to identify a solitary toxic nodule.
3. First, her thyrotoxicosis should be controlled with antithyroid drugs. Surgical removal of the toxic nodule will be curative. Alternatively the patient may be treated with radioiodine.

History 7

1. Disease of the iliac arteries can cause impotence, as can autonomic neuropathy. Symptoms and signs of peripheral vascular disease and neuropathy should be sought. Impotence is rarely caused by endocrine disease but evidence of testosterone deficiency (reduced beard growth and testicular atrophy) would suggest hypogonadism. This might be caused by a pituitary tumour so evidence of optic nerve compression and hypopituitarism should also be sought.
2. Low serum testosterone may result from gonadal or pituitary failure (p. 271 for causes). Serum gonadotrophins distinguish between these causes. If raised and there is no evidence of testicular injury, his karyotype should be checked as Klinefelter's syndrome may present in adulthood. If gonado-trophins are reduced, pituitary function tests should be performed and serum prolactin measured.
3. Pituitary CT or MR scan should be arranged and visual fields/acuities checked. First-line treatment is with a dopaminergic agonist (bromocriptine).

Data interpretation

1. **Patient A.** Impaired glucose tolerance.
   Patient B. Diabetes.
   Patient C. Normal.
2. The patient has nephrotic syndrome (oedema, albuminuria and hypoalbuminaemia) and renal failure (raised urea and creatinine). Diabetic nephropathy is the likely cause but there is insufficient information here to make that diagnosis.
3. a. Glycaemic control is poor and he is hypertriglyceridaemic, probably because of his poor control but possibly also because of obesity and/or alcohol excess.
   b. His body mass index.
   c. The best treatment would be to control his hyperglycaemia and hypertriglyceridaemia by diet. Only if that fails should he use drugs.
4. She is not known to be diabetic; she has 'hyperinsulinaemic hypoglycaemia'. The insulin could be endogenous (from her own pancreas) or injected. C-peptide is released when endogenous proinsulin is processed to insulin so the fact that it is high tells you that her insulin excess is endogenous. She probably has an insulinoma. People with insulinomas often gain weight as she has done. Sulphonylurea abuse causes oversecretion of insulin so that should also be considered.
5. **Patient A.** Secondary hypothyroidism. Serum TSH should rise as thyroxine falls. If it does not, the patient should be investigated for hypothalamic or pituitary disease.
   Patient B. Thyrotoxicosis.
   Patient C. Primary hypothyroidism, with an appropriate rise in TSH.
6. **Patient A.** The patient has a high plasma osmolality and continues to pass dilute urine; this is diagnostic of diabetes insipidus. There is a good response to desmopressin so the diagnosis is cranial diabetes insipidus.
   Patient B. Normal.
   Patient C. This patient differs from patient A because there is no response to desmopressin; the diagnosis is nephrogenic diabetes insipidus.

Picture answers

1. a. A prolactin-secreting pituitary tumour.
   b. Measure serum prolactin; there is no need to do a stimulation or suppression test. A raised serum prolactin with this history and radiological appearance would confirm the diagnosis of prolactinoma.
   c. She should be treated medically; with bromocriptine, cabergoline or quinagolide. The tumour does not extend outside the pituitary fossa and is not causing mass effects. Even if it were, the treatment would be medical rather than surgical in the first instance because

dopaminergic agonists can relieve symptoms, restore fertility and shrink even large tumours.

2. The tumour may have presented with endocrine and mass effects.

Endocrine effects. Large pituitary tumours may be non-functioning, prolactin-secreting or growth hormone-secreting. Hyperprolactinaemia causes impotence and hypogonadism in men and galactorrhoea/amenorrhoea in women. The symptoms of acromegaly are given on page 266.

Mass effects. The scan shows encroachment of the tumour into the suprasellar cistern. The patient is likely to have visual impairment and visual field defects, typically a bitemporal hemianopia. Lateral extension into the cavernous sinus may cause ophthalmoplegias.

3. a. Picture 7.3a is of a small mass lesion lying in the posterior left lower lobe. Magnified images of the mediastinum after contrast.

  b. There is a lucency on the medial side of the humerus. This lytic lesion extends through the cortex into the medulla.

  c. He has a nodular lesion on the thoracic CT scan, a subcarinal node and a lytic bone lesion elsewhere. He is a smoker with a cough. He probably has a malignant lung tumour with distant metastases. The muscle weakness is probably caused by his severe hyperkalaemia. The picture is strongly suggestive of ectopic ACTH secretion from a malignant tumour.

  d. First, he should receive potassium supplements and analgesics. If the diagnosis of small cell carcinoma is confirmed, you should consider chemotherapy. Local radiotherapy may help to relieve the pain in his arm. If he has ectopic ACTH secretion (confirmed by measuring his serum cortisol and ACTH), you may improve his symptoms by giving a treatment to suppress cortisol secretion. Metyrapone is rapidly effective and usually the first choice.

4. a. There is loss of the right fifth metatarsal head.

  b. Osteomyelitis secondary to a penetrating, neuropathic foot ulcer.

  c. Surgical exploration, removal of necrotic bone, prolonged bed rest and antibiotic treatment.

Short note answers

1. Surgery is rarely used as first- or second-line treatment of Graves' disease, the diagnosis in this patient. Radioiodine may be used as first-line or,

more commonly, second-line treatment after antithyroid drug therapy. Since she is aged 24, radioiodine should not be considered if there is any possibility of pregnancy within 3 months of giving it. Antithyroid drug therapy is usually given to control hyperthyroidism before 'ablative therapy' and this is what she should be offered. Beta-blockers may also be used initially to control symptoms.

2. Obesity is rarely caused by organic disease. Hypothalamic tumours are a very rare cause of hyperphagia but should be obvious from the clinical history and examination. Cushing's disease and hypothyroidism cause weight gain but rarely present with obesity and are likely to be clinically obvious. Obesity is almost always caused simply by over-eating and inactivity.

3. Causes of hypoadrenal crisis in a patient on long-term corticosteroids include non-compliance, failure to take an adequate dose during intercurrent illness or over-rapid reduction of high-dose, long-term steroids. Other causes include vomiting or non-absorption of oral steroid or the introduction of rifampicin (or other enzyme-inducing) therapy. Alternatively it could be a new presentation of adrenal (p. 268) or pituitary failure (p. 265).

The **symptoms** are collapse and vomiting with characteristic changes in electrolytes: low sodium, high potassium a raised urea concentration and mild acidosis.

Treatment of hypoadrenal crisis is with parenteral corticosteroid, i.v. fluid, intensive care and treatment of the precipitating cause.

All patients on corticosteroids should be warned of the risk of a hypoadrenal crisis, advised to take adequate steroid doses during intercurrent illness, carry a card or identity bracelet stating that they are on steroid therapy and advised to seek immediate medical help if 'ill'.

Viva answer

1. The need for insulin is governed by the degree of insulin deficiency. A patient with NIDDM has some residual β-cell function and can be treated by lessening insulin resistance (by diet and weight loss) and/or enhancing secretion (with a sulphonylurea). IDDM is caused by complete failure of the β-cells so it can only be treated by insulin replacement. Remember that some patients with NIDDM eventually develop β-cell exhaustion and need insulin.

Musculoskeletal disease

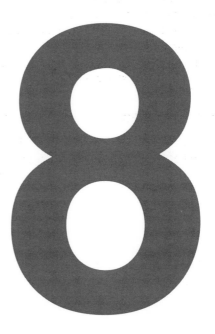

8.1 Clinical aspects

Learning objectives

You must:
- be able to formulate a differential diagnosis based on the history and examination findings and the results of investigations; this must take into account the pattern of joint and other organ involvement
- know the key investigations for particular diseases and why these are important
- understand the principles of management.

Normal structure and function

You need to know the basic structure and working of a joint in order to follow what happens when a joint becomes inflamed and/or damaged. A synovial joint consists of two articular surfaces, enclosed by a fibrous capsule lined with synovium. The space between the articular cartilages is filled with synovial fluid acting as a lubricant. Surrounding the joints are tendon insertions on bone (**enthesis**), muscles, ligaments and bursae. Any of these may be affected by an inflammatory process.

The **articular** surface is covered by avascular hyaline cartilage. The **synovium** is a specialised vascular membrane whose main function is to produce synovial fluid. The cells can be divided into two types: A cells, which are phagocytic and B cells, which are secretory. The fluid is derived from plasma and has a high concentration of hyaluronic acid giving a high viscosity. Joint sensation and pain come from the capsule, periosteum and ligaments.

Common symptoms

You should think of symptoms in terms of:
- joints
- bone
- muscles and their connections
- systemic features
- whether the problem is acute or chronic.

The age of the patient is important. Giant cell arteritis (p. 311) is extremely rare before the age of 60 years; osteoarthritis is much more common in elderly people. Rheumatoid arthritis, systemic lupus erythematosus (SLE) and Reiter's syndrome are more common in younger people.

Joints

Arthritis is characterised by:
- pain
- swelling
- increased local heat
- deformity.

In the absence of any joint changes, the pain is described as **arthralgia.**

Swelling is common in arthritis and may be identified from either the history or the examination. It may be caused by:
- synovial thickening
- joint effusion
- bony overgrowth.

Furthermore the pattern of joint involvement must be noted when talking to the patient and during your examination; is it monoarticular (e.g. gout), oligoarticular (less than five joints, e.g. reactive arthritis) or polyarticular (five or more, e.g. rheumatoid disease)? Is the arthropathy symmetrical (e.g. rheumatoid disease) or asymmetrical (e.g. psoriatic)? Does it involve small joints — hands (Fig. 58) wrists, toes — large joints and/or the spine (Fig. 59). Is there evidence of an active arthritis, with local heat, effusion and synovial thickening? How is the range of movement affected?

A combination of this information will frequently point to the diagnosis. For example, if the patient is a middle-aged woman with a symmetrical polyarthritis affecting the proximal interphalangeal (PIP) joints and metacarpophalangeal (MCP) joints with marked synovial involvement and systemic disturbance, then she has an inflammatory arthropathy, probably rheumatoid disease. In contrast, an elderly woman with a slowly progressive problem involving the right hip with pain on exercise, short-lived stiffness after resting and marked limitation of movement, particularly rotation, probably has osteoarthritis.

Back pain

Back pain is a very common symptom. As with many diagnostic problems, a rewarding approach is to consider a number of options and target the questions accordingly, gradually homing in on a probable cause. Above all, does the pain represent a serious underlying problem such as infection or malignancy? Clues may be recent onset, unremitting severe pain with marked localised tenderness and associated symptoms such as weight loss and fever.

Examples of diseases causing back pain are:
- an inflammatory arthropathy such as ankylosing spondylitis, which may be differentiated by the age of the patient, pattern of joints affected, effect of exercise and rest and systemic features
- osteoporosis, which is seen in older people and may present with increasing kyphosis, loss of height and episodes of severe pain resulting from vertebral collapse
- intervertebral disc prolapse, in which the onset of pain is sudden with marked muscle spasm and radiation of pain if there is radicular involvement; neurological symptoms and signs may be present.

By means of exclusion, the residual diagnosis may be non-specific back pain. It is necessary to decide at which point to stop: after taking a history and performing an examination, or following a few basic tests or, in a small

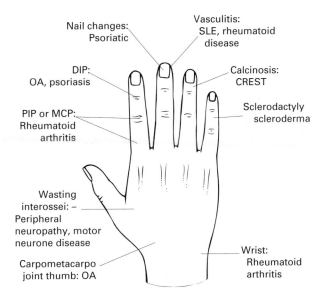

Nail changes:
Psoriatic

Vasculitis:
SLE, rheumatoid
disease

DIP:
OA, psoriasis

Calcinosis:
CREST

PIP or MCP:
Rheumatoid
arthritis

Sclerodactyly
scleroderma

Wasting
interossei: –
Peripheral
neuropathy, motor
neurone disease

Carpometacarpo
joint thumb: OA

Wrist:
Rheumatoid
arthritis

Fig. 58
Involvement of the joints and soft tissues in the hand in various
musculoskeletal diseases.

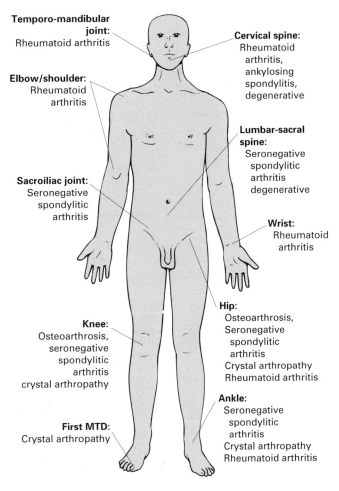

**Temporo-mandibular
joint:**
Rheumatoid arthritis

Cervical spine:
Rheumatoid
arthritis,
ankylosing
spondylitis,
degenerative

Elbow/shoulder:
Rheumatoid
arthritis

**Lumbar-sacral
spine:**
Seronegative
spondylitic
arthritis
degenerative

Sacroiliac joint:
Seronegative
spondylitic
arthritis

Wrist:
Rheumatoid
arthritis

Hip:
Osteoarthrosis,
Seronegative
spondylitic
arthritis
Crystal arthropathy
Rheumatoid arthritis

Knee:
Osteoarthrosis,
seronegative
spondylitic
arthritis
crystal arthropathy

Ankle:
Seronegative
spondylitic
arthritis
Crystal arthropathy
Rheumatoid arthritis

First MTD:
Crystal arthropathy

Fig. 59
Common involvement of the major joints in the body in
musculoskeletal disease.

number of cases, more complex investigations. In reaching a diagnosis of non-specific back pain, the important points are that you have considered other possible causes and reassured the patient.

Bone

In bone, the common symptoms are pain/tenderness and deformity.

Bone pain is often deep and poorly localised. It may be very severe and unremitting, particularly if caused by malignancy. The history of the pain will be a clear pointer to its cause. If the patient is an elderly female and the pain was sudden in onset, localised in the middle of the lower back and then has gradually improved over several days/weeks, this points to osteoporotic collapse. However, if the pain radiates down a leg and is associated with neurological signs and symptoms, it is more likely to be a disc prolapse.

The other symptom (and sign) is deformity. If localised, it may imply a fracture or a malignant process. If the whole bone is involved in an older patient, Paget's disease may be suspected. Rarely, it may be caused by osteomalacia.

Muscle

Patients often complain of fatigue, but unless this is accompanied by a onset and other symptoms, it is often very difficult to make a specific diagnosis. If the patient has a pattern of increasing weakness during repetitive exercise, myasthenia gravis can be considered (see p. 212). Proximal weakness might suggest a myositis (occasionally with pain/tenderness) in association with a connective tissue disease. The major effects of proximal weakness are related to activities such as climbing stairs or getting up out of a chair.

Stiffness of muscles or joints is a very important symptom and patients need to be asked directly about this. Common causes are:

- osteoarthrosis
- rheumatoid arthritis
- polymyalgia rheumatica.

In osteoarthrosis, the stiffness is usually shortlived and improves within about 15–30 minutes even after prolonged resting. In contrast, stiffness is a dominant and disabling feature of an inflammatory process such as rheumatoid arthritis or polymyalgia rheumatica. **Morning stiffness** may take a few hours to disappear and improvement in the duration of stiffness is a clear sign of remission.

Systemic features

In your assessment, it is very important to inquire about systemic disturbance. Connective tissue disease cannot be regarded as confined to joints. The concept is, for example, rheumatoid *disease* rather than rheumatoid

arthritis. Patients feel generally unwell, may lose weight as well as having specific problems such as breathlessness (lung involvement) or a peripheral nerve lesion.

Other symptoms

Within the history, there are a number of other features that should be sought as they may provide a key to the diagnosis. Gout and Reiter's syndrome are *uncommon* in women, but rheumatoid arthritis and SLE are more common. Repeated stress and minor trauma on joints, such as in professional sport, may cause osteoarthritis in later life. A recent viral illness or episode of diarrhoea may have been triggers for arthritis.

In the family, there may be a history of rheumatoid arthritis (and other autoimmune disease), psoriasis or ankylosing spondylitis (with HLA-B27).

In addition to the symptoms, it is very important that particular attention is paid to the effect the disease/problem is having on the patient's lifestyle. You have to be able to describe the patient's disability as well as document the examination findings. You should also carefully go through the drug history, documenting which drugs have been taken for how long, the patient's response and any side-effects.

Investigations

Learning objectives

You should:
- know which investigations to request according to the suspected rheumatological problem
- be able to interpret the results of these investigations.

Haematology

A full blood count is mandatory in musculoskeletal disease. **Anaemia of chronic disease** is seen in many of these (p. 234). In the inflammatory arthritides, anaemia is common and broadly reflects disease activity. The level of haemoglobin may fall to around 9 g/dl and the anaemia has characteristically a normochromic normocytic pattern. The serum iron is normal and total iron-binding capacity reduced, reflecting impaired iron utilisation. Serum ferritin cannot be used to reflect iron stores as it is an acute-phase reactant and will be elevated in any inflammatory process. In some patients, there may be iron deficiency secondary to blood loss from the GI tract (peptic ulcer: NSAIDs). If the MCV is low, you should investigate for a cause. Red cell aplasia rarely occurs in SLE.

A **leucocytosis** may be seen in a number of different diseases, including gout and bacterial infection. Remember that corticosteroid therapy commonly causes a granulocytosis. A high white cell count, with eosinophils, is sometimes seen in polyarteritis nodosa.

A low white cell count can occur. In active SLE, **lymphopenia** is characteristic. **Felty's syndrome** is seen in rheumatoid disease where hypersplenism (spleno-megaly with associated lymphadenopathy) causes pan-cytopenia. **Thrombocytosis** is seen in patients with active rheumatoid disease, whereas thrombocytopenia is observed in SLE.

In addition, you should consider the effects of drugs. Not only may cytotoxic agents such as azathioprine cause bone marrow depression, but others, including NSAIDs, can cause haematological disturbance.

Measures of inflammation

Erythrocyte sedimentation rate (ESR). The ESR is a non-specific marker for an inflammatory process and, like **plasma viscosity** (PV), reflects changes in fibrino-gen and other globulins. Unlike PV, the ESR is influ-enced by age, gender (normal values, p. 4, Table 1) and haematocrit, with reduced values in erythrocytosis and higher values in anaemia. It can be used to monitor dis-ease activity.

C-reactive protein (CRP). This is one of a family of acute-phase proteins, others being fibrinogen, hap-toglobin, caeruloplasmin, ferritin and α₁-antitrypsin. They increase in concentration in active inflammatory

joint disease. Like ESR, the C-reactive protein is used to monitor response to treatment.

Biochemistry

The key biochemical abnormalities are disturbances in renal function, particularly in SLE and the vasculitides. Rheumatoid disease may cause renal amyloidosis (renal impairment and nephrotic syndrome) and many of the drugs used can affect renal function. In addition to serum urea, creatinine and urinalysis, measurement of 24-hour protein excretion and creatinine clearance may be indicated.

In any patient with suspected crystal arthropathy, you must measure serum urate. A low value makes the diagnosis unlikely, but a raised value does not necessar-ily confirm the diagnosis (need joint aspiration).

Immunology

The diagnosis of most autoimmune diseases can be sup-ported with an antibody test (Table 66). This does not mean that the antibody causes the damage. There are

Table 66 Useful autoantibody tests

Antibody	Interpretation
Nuclear and nucleic acid antigens	
ANA	High titre: SLE
Double-stranded DNA	Diagnostic of SLE, some correlation with disease activity
Single-stranded DNA	Drug-induced SLE
Ro and La	SLE, Sjögren's syndrome
Ro	SLE with sclerodactyly and lung fibrosis
Jo-1	Fibrosing alveolitis, Raynaud's syndrome
Extractable nuclear antigen (RNA) (ENA)	Mixed connective tissue disease
Centromere	CREST syndrome
Phospholipids	
Cardiolipin, lupus anticoagulant	Antiphospholipid syndrome
Mitochondria	
Antimitochondrial antibodies	Primary biliary cirrhosis
Neutrophils	
Cytoplasmic-ANCA	Generalised or limited Wegener's granulomatosis
Perinuclear-ANCA	Microscopic polyarteritis, idiopathic glomerulonephritis, Churg–Strauss syndrome
Circulating proteins	
Rheumatoid factor (Fc portion of IgG)	Low titre: normal, connective tissue disease, rheumatoid arthritis High titre: erosive rheumatoid arthritis
Thyroglobulin	Hashimoto's thyroiditis
Structure-specific antibodies	
Basement membrane	Goodpasture's syndrome
Acetylcholine receptors	Myasthenia gravis, Eaton–Lambert syndrome
Cell (organ)-specific antibodies	
Adrenal cortex	Addison's disease
Intrinsic factor cells	Pernicious anaemia
Epidermal cells	Pemphigus vulgaris
Red cells, specific blood group antigens	Haemolytic anaemia
Platelets	Idiopathic thrombocytopenic purpura
Islet cell antibodies	Diabetes mellitus
Spermatozoa	Male infertility

two major immunopathological processes involved in autoimmunity:

- direct antibody attack with complement activation, e.g. Goodpasture's syndrome, myasthenia gravis, Hashimoto's thyroiditis and organ-specific autoimmune diseases
- formation of immune complexes (type III hypersensitivity) (Table 67).

There is a relatively strong genetic component to the development of autoimmune disease. In all of them, T cell involvement appears to be critical. In addition, there is small subset of B1 lymphocytes responsible for autoantibody production. Continuous exposure to the inciting antigen (exogenous or endogenous) is probably important for perpetuating the disease.

Autoimmune diseases vary from highly specific single organ diseases (as in male infertility, Hashimoto's thyroiditis or pemphigus vulgaris) to multisystem disease. As a general rule, the greater the specificity of the antibody for an organ or tissue, the more the autoimmune disease is confined to a single site. Antibodies to cellular targets present in all cells, such as cardiolipin or antinuclear antibody, lead to multisystem disease.

For more detailed explanation of abnormalities of the immune system see Chapter 9.

Rheumatoid factors (RF). These are autoantibodies which are directed against the Fc fragment of IgG. They are predominantly IgM. Seropositivity is defined as agglutination in the latex test at a serum dilution of 1:20 (1:32 in the sheep cell agglutination test: SCAT). Rheumatoid factors can be found in the normal population (increasing with age), a whole range of other connective tissue diseases (e.g. Sjögren's syndrome, SLE, PAN, systemic sclerosis), chronic infections and other immunological disorders (e.g. sarcoidosis). You must *not*, therefore, interpret the presence of rheumatoid factor as diagnostic of rheumatoid disease. In the early stages of rheumatoid disease, the test may be negative; however, strong seropositivity (high dilutions) is associated with severe disease.

Antinuclear antibodies (ANA). As with rheumatoid factors, there are a wide range of conditions in which these antibodies are found. Antibodies against *double*-stranded DNA have a high specificity for SLE, whereas antibodies against *single*-stranded DNA are a feature of drug-induced lupus erythematosus. Antibodies against *extractable nuclear antigen* are characteristic of mixed connective tissue disease (p. 312).

Complement. A detailed explanation of complement function is given on page 332. Low serum levels of C3 or C4 (or total haemolytic complement) are found in SLE. Particularly low concentrations are found in **lupus nephritis**, with consumption of complement. Serial measurements can help in monitoring disease activity and response to treatment.

Imaging

Other than requesting plain radiographs of affected joints, you should order radiographs of the hands and feet, since diagnostic features may be present despite the *absence* of symptoms and signs. The common features seen with specific conditions are given in the separate sections. In certain instances, other imaging may be useful, including CT or MR scan and arthrography.

Bone scanning

Bone scans are useful for diagnosing acute and chronic osteomyelitis and metastatic disease of bone. Patients receive a small dose of labelled technetium linked to phosphate and the whole skeleton is imaged after 2–4 hours. False positives are sometimes caused by healing fractures or arthritis.

Joint aspiration

The two key diagnoses that *require* joint aspiration are:

- crystal arthropathy
- septic arthritis.

The aspirate is divided into three portions for:

- white cell count and differential
- Gram stain and culture
- polarised light microscopy for crystals.

Table 68 gives details of the findings in different diseases.

Management

With any disease, you should have a broader view of management than simply drug therapy. All patients need to have three things discussed with them:

Table 67 Examples of diseases linked to immune complex deposition

	Sites of deposition of immune complex and inflammatory processes						
	Brain	Kidney	Vessels	Joints	Skin	Lungs	Muscle
SLE	+	+	+	+	+	+	
Rheumatoid arthritis			+	+			
Vasculitis			+		+		
Polyarteritis nodosa		+	+				+
Polymyositis and dermatomyositis			+		+		+
Cryoglobulinaemia		+	+	+	+		

- What is it? Explanation and discussion of the disease process
- What will happen? Explanation of natural history, prognosis for morbidity (including disability) and any threat to life
- What can be done? Discussion of treatment options and recommendations.

Management is aimed at the person, not just the disease. Consequently, the major end-points are survival, disability (p. 182) and handicap (p. 182). You need to know when and how to involve the professions allied to medicine (including physiotherapists and occupational therapists). Other medical disciplines may need to be consulted and surgery may be required. A doctor in training may only see the person for a short time, but their relationship with the multidisciplinary team is likely to extend over a number of years.

Common drugs

Learning objectives

You should:
- have a working knowledge of the main classes of drug used in rheumatological disorders
- know the broad indications for their use
- know the potential harm.

Non-steroidal anti-inflammatory drugs

The NSAIDs are important in the management of inflammation. There are a whole range of drugs available; you need to know their common properties. The prime action is to block the **cyclo-oxygenase** pathway, producing various inflammatory mediators (prostaglandins). One potential consequence of blockade is an overactivity of the **lypo-oxygenase** pathway, with increase in leucotrienes. As the leucotrienes include powerful bronchoconstrictors, the disturbance in balance between the two systems can produce bronchoconstriction. In aspirin-induced asthma, there is a hypersensitivity reaction over and above this mechanism.

Another consequence of cyclo-oxygenase blockade is a reduction of **intrarenal** generation of prostaglandins. This can have deleterious affects on intrarenal vascular control, causing a deterioration in renal function and hyperkalaemia.

The third, and most important, problem associated with the use of NSAIDs is an increased risk of the complications of peptic ulcers. Numerous epidemiological studies have shown a clear relationship between NSAIDs and perforation, bleeding and risk of death, particularly in older people. The use of rectal preparations, prodrugs, or enteric coated drugs do *not* protect against gastric damage.

Of the currently available drugs, **ibuprofen** appears safest, with diclofenac and naproxen being relatively safe despite stronger anti-inflammatory action. The mechanism of gastric mucosal damage is linked, like the renal changes, to alteration in prostaglandin production. **Misoprostol**, which is a prostaglandin analogue, helps prevent damage to the mucosa (p. 108).

There are other problems with NSAIDs, for example fluid retention and resistance to treatment for heart failure or hypertension (particularly indomethacin). Individual drugs have their own spectrum of side-effects.

The main use of NSAIDs is in inflammation. They can bring marked relief in inflammatory arthropathies, including osteoarthritis, if there is an inflammatory component. They do *not* influence the underlying disease process. The principle should always be to initiate treatment with ibuprofen in moderate doses. Only if there is no relief at high doses of ibuprofen, should you change to one of the more potent drugs (such as diclofenac or naproxen). It is better to be familiar with two or three drugs, getting to know these well.

There are other situations in which NSAIDs are of benefit:

- bone pain from metastatic disease
- renal and biliary colic (**diclofenac sodium** is as efficacious as narcotic analgesics).

Table 68 Synovial fluid abnormalities with different joint disorders

	Appearance	White cells (10^6/1)	Culture	Crystals (polarising light)
Normal	Clear viscous	< 200	Sterile	None
Rheumatoid arthritis	Green/yellow, very low viscosity, may be turbid	Very high (20 000–40 000)	Sterile	None
Osteoarthritis	Viscosity preserved	Raised (2000–4000)	Sterile	Small (< 5%), pyrophosphate
Crystal arthritis	Clear, reduced viscosity	High (8000–12 000)	Sterile	Negatively birefringent: urate — gout Weakly positive birefringent: pyrophosphate — pseudogout
Septic arthritis	Turbid, reduced viscosity	Extremely high (100 000)	Positive (may be on Gram stain)	None

Simple analgesics

The use of simple analgesics in musculoskeletal disease is often not fully exploited. They are the drugs of choice in osteoarthritis. The order of potency is paracetamol, codeine, dihydrocodeine and morphine. Patients should always be on the full dose of the least potent drug before moving onto the next one. Compound preparations are frequently used and you need to be aware of their constituents and dose. All narcotic analgesics cause constipation and a laxative should be prescribed as a preventative measure.

Corticosteroids

Corticosteroids are effective in suppressing inflammatory disease activity. Recent evidence has also shown that, in regular low dose, they improve the outcome in rheumatoid disease. Corticosteroids have many long-term adverse effects, including osteoporosis, cataracts, skin atrophy, susceptibility to infection and adrenal suppression. When used as intra-articular therapy, repeated injection of the same joint may result in joint destruction.

Potential disease-modifying drugs

Early treatment with chloroquine, gold, penicillamine, or sulphasalazine over time may modify the underlying disease. Initiation of therapy and monitoring of response and side-effects are best done within a specialised unit.

Chloroquine. Chloroquine and hydroxychloroquine are antimalarial drugs which coincidently suppress disease activity in rheumatoid disease. The main toxicity occurs in the retina, with deteriorating visual acuity.

Gold. Gold therapy (either by injection or orally) takes 2–3 months to have any impact on disease activity. At least one-third of patients develop side-effects, many of which are serious. These include rashes, thrombocytopenia, leucopenia, aplastic anaemia and glomerulonephritis (nephrotic syndrome). Consequently, it is necessary to monitor the patient's full blood count and renal function (particularly for proteinuria).

Penicillamine. The indications for use of D-penicillamine and the side-effects are similar to gold therapy. Particular problems are a loss of, or a metallic, taste and, rarely, a myasthenia gravis-like syndrome. The bone marrow and renal problems necessitate surveillance.

Sulphasalazine, 5-aminosalicylic acid. Sulphasalazine is a compound of sulphapyridine and 5-aminosalicylic acid. These are better tolerated than either gold or D-penicillamine, with a lower incidence of serious adverse effects. Main problems are with GI upset and depression. A reversible oligospermia also occurs.

Immunosuppressives. Azathioprine and cyclophosphamide are commonly used though methotrexate is sometimes prescribed. The last drug may cause intrahepatic fibrosis and a pneumonitis. Because of bone marrow suppression, monitoring of the blood count is necessary.

Surgery

The two aims of surgery are prophylactic, to prevent further damage and reconstructive, to restore function and stability. Procedures include synovectomy, tendon reconstruction, arthroplasty and arthrodesis. Surgery has an important role in the management of musculoskeletal disease.

8.2 Infection

Learning objectives

You should:
- be able to recognise the clinical features of an acutely inflamed joint
- be able to initiate appropriate investigations for an acutely inflamed joint
- be familiar with the common organisms causing septic arthritis and appropriate initial investigation and management
- know how both acute and chronic osteomyelitis present clinically, which investigations are useful and the management strategies.

Septic arthritis

Septic arthritis is an infection (usually bacterial) of one or more joints. Bacteria invade the synovial membrane and fluid and the inflammatory response (especially neutrophils) leads to cartilage and joint destruction. It is a medical emergency and the immediate, appropriate management of septic arthritis is critically important to the preservation of function of the joint over the long term, as the infecting organisms and the neutrophil response will lead to substantial damage to cartilage in 1 to 2 days. As part of your management, you should always exclude other causes of an acutely inflamed joint (such as gout or an inflammatory arthritis).

Clinical presentation

The primary symptoms of septic arthritis are
- fever
- acute joint pain
- acute joint swelling.

In your initial evaluation of the patient, you should establish whether the problem is a monoarthritis, oligoarthritis or polyarthritis Monoarthritis is caused particularly by *Staphylococcus aureus*, β-haemolytic streptococci and *Mycobacterium tuberculosis*. The first two commonly present more acutely than the last. Previously damaged joints are at greater risk of infections.

Oligoarthritis or polyarthritis has a wider aetiology, including *Neisseria gonorrhoeae*, postinfectious or reactive arthritis, rheumatic fever (p. 365), parvovirus or rubella infection (p. 364) or Henoch–Schönlein purpura.

Investigations

The key investigation is joint aspiration (arthrocentesis). You may be able to aspirate fluid from the knee relatively easily, but most other joints require specialist help, particularly small joints such as the elbow or sternoclavicular joint. If the area of inflammation is large and fluid has collected above or directly over a smaller joint, then direct aspiration is appropriate. If on aspirating the joint, the fluid is obviously turbid, then the joint should be aspirated to dryness as this is an important part of the management regardless of the organism. The fluid should be examined for total cell count, differential white cell count and by Gram stain and culture (see Table 68).

It is important to try to do the aspiration before antibiotics are started, although these should not be delayed for very long waiting for appropriate expertise.

The white cell count is usually raised. Serology for parvovirus and rubella and ASO titre for rheumatic fever are appropriate for an oligo- or polyarthritis, as may be rheumatoid factor and other autoimmune antibody tests. In toxic patients or those with systemic manifestations, a blood culture should be done.

Management

The principles of management are:

- appropriate intravenous antibiotics (e.g. flucloxacillin 2 g every 6 hours for *S. aureus*)
- repeated aspiration of joints (at least once a day) or arthroscopy and joint washout to prevent cartilage destruction
- complete rest of the affected joint, particularly if weight-bearing, until there is substantial improvement
- pain relief.

In some patients, septic arthritis is a manifestation of disseminated or systemic infection. This is particularly true of staphylococcal septic arthritis if there has been no injury. You should seek other sites of infection (e.g. endocarditis) and treat appropriately. Septic arthritis may also be the presentation of SLE, sarcoidosis and a number of other rare diseases. Expert advice should be sought if there are other clinical features suggesting a generalised disease.

Osteomyelitis (osteitis)

Osteomyelitis is infection of bone. It may be acute or chronic. The presentation and management of acute and chronic osteomyelitis are substantially different.

Acute osteomyelitis

Acute osteomyelitis occurs following a bacteraemic episode usually with *S. aureus*, but occasionally with Gram-positive, Gram-negative (e.g. *Salmonella*) or anaerobic bacteria. The most common site is the vertebral column, but no bone in the body is exempt.

Clinical presentation

The patient almost always has fever and localised pain. Sometimes patients are very ill when bacteraemia develops and do not complain of pain. Often the osteomyelitis presents days or weeks after the episode of bacteraemia that precipitated it. In other slightly less acute cases, complaints such as back pain caused by acute osteomyelitis are shrugged off by patients and doctors. There are two features that are will help you:

- the pain is persistent
- usually palpation over the affected area is painful.

Investigations

There may be a raised white cell count and the ESR or C-reactive protein is almost always extremely high. Blood cultures are often positive for *S. aureus*. Plain radiographs are normal for at least the first 10 days of infection and may then show lucency and bone destruction. Bone scan and white cell scans show abnormalities earlier than radiographs.

Management

The principles of management are:

- establish the extent of infection by radiology and isotope scanning of the affected site
- ascertain the bacterial cause using direct needle puncture under radiographic control
- i.v. antibiotic therapy with large antibiotic doses as bony penetration is poor
- immobilisation of the area, particularly if a critical part of the vertebral column is involved or there is evidence of epidural compression
- a review by an orthopaedic surgeon of the need for surgery; if there is extensive involvement or localised abscess formation impinging on important structures such as the spinal cord, then surgery is often mandatory.

Chronic osteomyelitis

Chronic osteomyelitis presents with symptoms over months or years. Typical forms of infection include:

- tuberculous osteomyelitis
- osteomyelitis of the metatarsals or other bones in the feet in diabetic patients with chronic foot ulcers
- chronic discharging sinus overlying a prior fracture or injury involving foreign bodies (e.g. shrapnel)
- fracture site with infected metalwork within it
- chronic vertebral osteomyelitis caused by fungi (such as *Aspergillus* or *Coccidioides*), which is often initially mistaken for bony metastases
- osteomyelitis of the head or neck related to chronic sinus or ear infections.

Clinical presentation

The clinical presentation falls into two groups: those with chronic pain or deformity (such as patients with tuberculous osteomyelitis who develop Pott's disease of the spine) and patients with a chronically discharging sinus overlying an area of osteomyelitis. Unlike in acute osteomyelitis, where plain radiographs are often normal, in chronic osteomyelitis the plain radiographs are almost always abnormal. The primary exception is diabetic foot osteomyelitis, in which the area of involvement is often small. White cell scans or bone scans also show areas of infection. Most patients do not have a raised white cell count although they usually have a raised sedimentation rate and C-reactive protein.

Management

The principles are:

- determine the cause by needle biopsy or surgery; submit cultures for aerobic, anaerobic, mycobacterial and fungal culture
- if bacterial in origin, complete debridement and removal of all dead bone (sequestrum), metalwork, foreign bodies, etc.
- high-dose i.v. antibiotic therapy for at least 3 weeks, followed by long-term oral antibiotic therapy
- if caused by *M. tuberculosis* or fungi, medical therapy is used initially unless the deformity is so extensive or dangerous that surgery is required.

The prognosis of chronic osteomyelitis is poor, partly because of the underlying disease and partly because of the chronicity and difficulty in removing all dead infected bone. Exceptions include tuberculous osteomyelitis, which has a good outlook, although it takes weeks or even months for pain and symptoms to improve. You will find chronic osteomyelitis to be a major therapeutic challenge and accurate determination of the cause together with susceptibility testing are critical to a good outcome.

8.3 Arthropathies

Rheumatoid disease

Rheumatoid disease is the most common disorder of the connective tissues and is characterised by:

- a symmetrical chronic polyarthritis that often results in joint damage
- disease affecting many body systems (see Fig. 60)
- usually the presence of rheumatoid factor.

Epidemiology

Rheumatoid disease has prevalence of around 2–3% and a male to female ratio of 1:3. The onset is most commonly between the ages of 30 and 60 years. Within families, approximately 10% have a first-degree relative affected and there may be up to 50% concordance in identical twins. A strong association exists between the disease and HLA-DR4 and HLA-D4. The relative risk for development of the disease is increased 6–12-fold for an individual with one of the antigens.

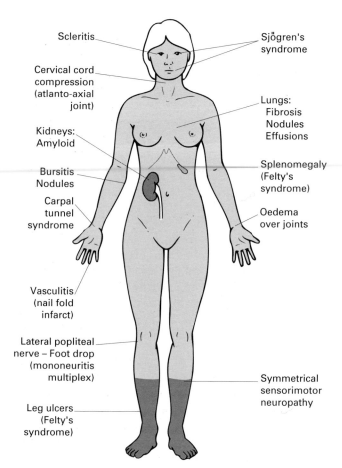

Fig. 60
Systemic manifestations of rheumatoid disease.

Pathology and pathogenesis

The cause of rheumatoid disease is unknown, but there is strong evidence of disordered immunity. Rheumatoid factors (particularly IgG) play a part in forming immune complexes which are found in the circulation and within the synovium. These can activate the complement cascade, generating inflammatory and chemotactic factors (p. 332).

The vascularity of the synovium increases, and the membrane thickens and becomes oedematous with infiltration by T lymphocytes, plasma cells and macrophages. Within the synovial fluid there are large numbers of granulocytes. A chronic inflammatory **pannus** is formed in the synovium, which encroaches from the joint margins leading to cartilage and joint destruction.

Changes are also found in other tissues. Rheumatoid nodules, which are pathognomonic, show *palisading* macrophages (histiocytes) around a central zone of hyaline necrosis.

Clinical features

Rheumatoid disease usually comes on insidiously over a few months, though in a minority there is an acute onset with marked systemic disturbance. In some patients, an episodic arthralgia may have been present for months/years (**palindromic rheumatism**).

Joints

Characteristically, the joint involvement is symmetrical and affects the small joints of the hands (PIPs, MCPs, wrists) and feet. In a smaller proportion, the large weight-bearing joints are affected and this causes more disability. The natural history is usually involvement of increasing numbers of joints. The main symptoms are joint pain and swelling together with marked morning stiffness. In the early inflammatory phase, there may be tenderness and swelling over a greater area than simply the joints. As the disease progresses, permanent joint damage occurs, with bone and cartilage damage and rupture of tendons resulting in joint subluxation and dislocation. In the hands this produces typical changes (Fig. 61).

Small joints: hands and feet. Rheumatoid disease characteristically affects the small peripheral joints. The wrists, MCPs, PIPs and, occasionally, the dorsal interphalangeal (DIP) joints show swelling, increased warmth, tenderness and, sometimes, skin discoloration. Disease activity over years leads to limitation of movement, wrist subluxation, ulnar styloid resorption, ulnar deviation of the fingers and swan neck and boutonnière deformity of the fingers (Fig. 61); most of these are caused by tendon displacement or damage. Wasting of the interossei muscles may be apparent. In the feet, there is tenderness over the metatarsal heads and eventually subluxation. The patients often complain that it feels as though they are walking on pebbles.

Large joints. The knees may be warm and swollen, because of effusions, synovial thickening or, in the later stages, bony overgrowth. A varus or a valgus deformity may result. Quadriceps wasting is often prominent and the joint may be unstable owing to damage to the cruci-ate and lateral ligaments. The ankles, elbows, shoulders and hips may be involved.

Other joints. Rheumatoid disease may affect the temporomandibular joint, giving pain on mastication. Damage to the atlanto-axial joint may cause odontoid peg destruction and instability. Symptoms include:

- pain radiating to the occiput (C1, C2 dermatome): most common
- paraesthesia, sensory loss
- sudden deterioration in hand function
- abnormal gait
- urinary retention or incontinence.

If the patient requires intubation for a general anaesthetic, care has to be taken not to hyperextend the neck. The lower cervical vertebra can be involved, again with cord problems. Management initially involves stabilisation using a *firm* collar and a neurosurgical opinion.

Periarticular involvement. Rheumatoid nodules are associated with high titres of rheumatoid factor and are found over the extensor surfaces of the elbows, pressure points and, sometimes, along tendons. They are usually not fixed and are not painful, though they can sometimes ulcerate. They are pathognomonic for the disease.

Tenosynovitis and bursitis. These are common. The latter involves the olecranon, prepatella, subacromial and trochanteric bursa.

Systemic involvement

You must think rheumatoid *disease* rather than *arthritis* (see Fig. 60). Patients feel unwell when the disease is active; they lose weight and are anaemic. They are also more susceptible to infection, especially if treated with corticosteroids.

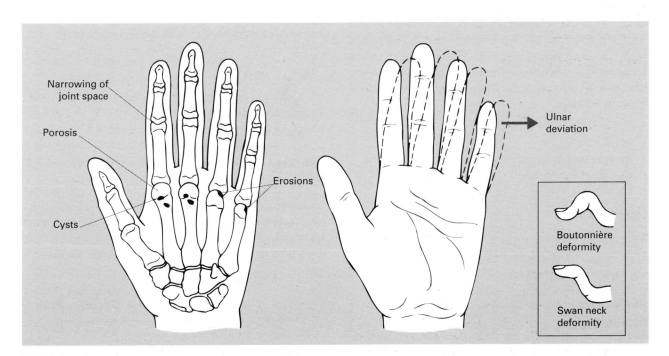

Fig. 61
Schematic representation of (a) radiographic changes in rheumatoid arthritis and (b) hand deformities.

Pulmonary involvement. Rheumatoid disease frequently affects the lung and pleura. Effusions occur and can mimic empyema. Pulmonary nodules may be difficult to differentiate from other causes (p. 77). They may predate the arthropathy and are associated with aggressive disease and high titres of rheumatoid factor. Pulmonary fibrosis occurs, particularly affecting the lower zones and causing a restrictive defect.

Nervous system. A sensorimotor neuropathy may develop, with predominantly sensory disturbance. A vasculitis can affect individual nerves causing a mononeuritis (multiplex). Common nerves affected are the median, ulnar, lateral popliteal, tibial and the oculomotor nerves. There may be *entrapment* neuropathies in which nerves are compressed by the swelling and tissue thickening around joints. The ulnar, median, lateral popliteal and tibial nerve are the usual ones affected. Disease involvement of the **cervical spine** with cord and root signs has been discussed.

Vascular involvement. Vasculitis is one of the hallmarks of aggressive disease with high rheumatoid factor titres. It can affect all sizes of vessels:

- small end-arteries: nailfold and small areas of skin infarction
- large arteries (rarely affected): stroke, mesenteric ischaemia or limb ischaemia
- medium (and small calibre) arteries: mononeuritis multiplex (through involvement of the vasa nervorum) and patchy muscle ischaemia.

The renal vasculature is *spared*.

Eye. Main ocular complications are:

- Sjögren's syndrome
- uveitis and scleritis.

Primary Sjögren's syndrome is a combination of keratojunctivitis sicca (dry eyes) and xerostomia (dry mouth). The salivary and lacrimal glands are infiltrated with lymphocytes. The syndrome is seen in association with other connective tissue diseases (e.g. SLE). Diagnosis is by **Schirmer's test** for impaired tear secretion, or a lip salivary gland biopsy. Dry eyes are helped by artificial tears.

Other complications. Rheumatoid disease can affect most body systems. The **kidney** may be affected by

- amyloidosis (severe disease): nephrotic syndrome and renal impairment
- the drugs used (see above).

Lymphadenopathy is occasionally seen but is more common in juvenile arthritis. Splenomegaly can lead to hypersplenism and pancytopenia (**Felty's syndrome**). There is also an association with leg ulceration (vasculitis). Often a pericarditis occurs with a small effusion.

Investigations

The investigation of a symmetrical inflammatory polyarthritis has been described (p. 300). Additional considerations are monitoring of disease activity and drug therapy. Disease activity is measured using a composite of different indices: clinical assessment, ESR, C-reactive protein, full blood count and rheumatoid factor.

Radiological assessment must always be carried out, including radiographs of the hands and feet. The typical features are shown in Figure 61. **Erosions** occur and are associated with high rheumatoid factor titres. An important consideration is the change in radiographic appearances over time.

Management and prognosis

The management of musculoskeletal disease has been outlined. Patients should be started on low-dose prednisolone to improve the long-term outlook (not to ameliorate the symptoms). The prognosis is variable, with only around 1 in 10 patients becoming severely disabled. A worse prognosis is predicted by:

- male gender
- HLA-DR4
- insidious onset
- systemic disease
- high antibody titre
- early appearance of erosions.

Seronegative spondyloarthropathies

Learning objectives

You should:
- know the differences between the seronegative spondyloarthritides and seropositive rheumatoid disease
- be aware of the range of conditions within the seronegative spondyloarthritides and the similarities and differences between them.

The seronegative spondyloarthropathies are a group of conditions that share several common features:

- *absence* of rheumatoid factor in the serum
- a peripheral arthritis which is usually *asymmetrical*
- sacroiliitis
- extra-articular manifestations
- linkage with HLA-B27.

The term *spondyl* refers to involvement of a spinal joint. Radiological examination may show asymmetric bony ankylosis (fusion) and marginal periostitis. The main histopathological abnormalities are at insertion of tendons and ligaments (**enesthopathy**) rather than in the synovium.

There is a strong familial tendency. The proportion of those with the **HLA-B27** histocompatibility antigen ranges from almost all with ankylosing spondylitis to approximately half with psoriatic arthropathy.

The cause of the seronegative spondyloarthritides is unclear apart from the association with HLA-B27.

Psoriatic arthropathy

Many of your patients will have psoriasis (usually it is incidental to the reason for which they are consulting) and about 1 in 10 will have an arthropathy. The skin disease often predates the arthropathy by many years. There is no close correlation between the severity of the skin problem and the joint disease; the exception is the association between nail psoriasis and arthritis of the DIP.

The arthritis may take different forms:

- arthritis mutilans with severe deformity of the fingers and hands
- an asymmetrical oligoarthritis affecting the hands and feet and sometimes larger joints
- spondylitis with evidence of sacroiliitis (one-third)
- nail and DIP disease together.

The treatment is similar to that of rheumatoid arthritis and the prognosis is *better*.

Ankylosing spondylitis

Ankylosing spondylitis is approximately three to four times more common in men; in women it tends to be mild. In most patients, the disease will have started in young adulthood. Around 95% of patients are HLA-B27 positive and a child of an affected parent has about a 1 in 3 chance of developing the disease.

The most important pathological changes are seen in *cartilage* rather than synovium. The joints of the spine are affected with damage to the discs and ligament attachments. Eventually ankylosis occurs with calcification of intervertebral ligaments and annulus fibrosus.

Clinical presentation

Most patients present with back pain and may be systemically unwell. The pain is worse after rest, may wake the patient during the night and is usually associated with marked morning stiffness. Unlike other arthropathies, symptoms *improve* with exercise.

On examination, you will commonly find that the lumbar lordosis is lost and that there is sacroiliac tenderness. In late, severe cases, there is a typical posture with marked kyphosis, stiff pelvis and limited back movement, making the diagnosis easy.

Other large joints are involved, particularly lower limb, in approximately 20–30% of patients. Tenderness at the insertions of tendons is common.

There are extra-articular manifestations:

- constitutional upset
- upper lobe fibrosis: restrictive pulmonary function
- aortic incompetence and conduction problems
- iritis, which may lead to blindness
- amyloidosis (renal impairment, peripheral neuropathy)
- cauda equina syndrome.

Investigations

Investigations fall into several groups:

- haematology: raised ESR in active disease, anaemia (normochromic, normocytic)
- biochemistry: renal impairment, features of nephrotic syndrome (amyloidosis)
- radiology: sacroiliitis, characteristic syndesmophytes (calcification around the intervertebral disc) giving a **bamboo spine** and **squaring** of the vertebra
- tissue typing: HLA-B27.

Management

The treatment plan is continued activity (patients may need the help of a physiotherapist for an exercise programme) together with NSAIDs (p. 303). Long periods of bed rest are *avoided* as much as possible.

Prognosis. For most patients, the outlook is good, with severe progressive disease in only a small minority.

Reiter's syndrome and reactive arthritis

Reiter's syndrome and reactive arthritis refer to different aspects of the same condition.

Reiter's syndrome is defined as an episode of peripheral arthritis of more than 1 month's duration in association with urethritis, cervicitis or both.

Reactive arthritis is defined as a non-specific arthritis strongly linked to a recognised episode of infection with no viable microorganisms in the affected joint.

Reactive arthritis may follow a lower genital tract or bowel infection. The dysenteric form is associated with *Shigella flexneri*, *Yersinia enterocolitica* and *Salmonella typhimurium*. *Chlamydia trachomatis* is often the responsible organism in genital tract infection.

Clinical presentation

Most urogenital cases occur in young men; the postdysenteric syndrome has an equal sex incidence. Often the first element to appear is urethritis. There are superficial ulcers that coalesce as a **circinate balanitis** of the glans penis. The skin manifestation on the palms of the hands and soles of the feet looks identical to pustular psoriasis and is called **keratoderma blenorrhagica.** Commonly a **sterile conjunctivitis** occurs, and occasionally a severe anterior uveitis. Cardiac complications include heart block, aortic valve disease and pericarditis.

The arthritis ranges from mild synovitis to a chronic progressive arthropathy. It is usually asymmetrical in the fingers and toes, with some large joint involvement. The problem usually lasts for a few months.

Investigations

The ESR is elevated when the disease is active and there may be juxta-articular osteoporosis and, characteristically, **periostitis. Plantar spurs** occur in about one-third of patients and may be painful. Spondylitis may develop together with sacroiliitis.

Management

Most patients are treated with NSAIDs. Eye disease should be managed by an ophthalmologist; treatment includes corticosteroid drops.

Enteropathic arthropathy

Enteropathic arthropathy is defined as an arthritis associated with inflammatory bowel disease. Both sacroiliitis and synovitis (affecting weight-bearing joints) occur. About half of patients are HLA-B27 positive.

With ulcerative colitis, the arthritis tends to occur at times of flares of the bowel disease and in patients with severe involvement. A pan-colectomy cures the arthropathy. Similarly, in Crohn's disease, the synovitis correlates with disease activity.

The back can be involved with typical changes of ankylosing spondylitis. This may predate the bowel disease and does not follow the disease activity.

8.4 Systemic lupus erythematosus

Learning objectives

You should:
- know that SLE is a multisystem disorder with an autoimmune basis and, from this, be able to predict its manifestations
- know how to investigate a person with possible SLE and be able to intepret the results
- understand the principles of management.

Epidemiology and immunopathogenesis

SLE can affect virtually any organ, but skin, joints, kidneys and brain are most often involved. It affects women 10 times more often than men and there is likely to be a hormonal (probably oestrogenic) component to the pathogenesis. It is more common in the Afro-Caribbean population. Within families, there is a higher than expected incidence and a significant concordance between identical twins.

Patients with the disease undoubtedly have a disordered immune response. There is activation of B lymphocytes, leading to hyperglobulinaemia, impaired T cell regulation of the immune response and production of autoantibodies. Immune complexes are formed and deposited widely, particularly in the blood vessels (vasculitis) and kidney (glomerulonephritis). The formation of immune complexes leads to consumption of complement. Pathologically, SLE is characterised by widespread vasculitis and deposition of fibrinoid.

Clinical presentation

The onset of SLE is usually between 20 and 40 years. The criteria used for the diagnosis and classification of SLE are the presence of any four of the following together or separately in time:

- malar rash
- discoid rash
- photosensitivity

- oral ulcers
- arthritis
- pleurisy or pericarditis
- renal disease
  - cellular casts
  - proteinuria > 0.5 g in 24 hours
- seizures or organic psychosis without other cause
- blood dyscrasia
  - haemolytic anaemia
  - leucopenia
  - lymphopenia
  - thrombocytopenia
- raised antinuclear antibody titre
- immunological features, e.g. raised double-stranded DNA antibody titre.

Classical initial presentations of SLE include the following:

- joint pain without arthritis but with positive ANA
- butterfly rash over the bridge of the nose with or without other features of photosensitivity
- pleurisy with other features to suggest a multisystem disease
- haematological abnormalities.

Your assessment of the patient with possible SLE depends to some extent upon the presentation. All patients require a thorough physical examination, including individual joint assessment. Consideration of other associated diseases such as Sjögren's syndrome and antiphospholipid syndrome is important.

Investigation

Investigations should include antinuclear antibody and double-stranded DNA antibodies, complement levels with assessment of renal function and haematology. Measurement of C-reactive protein can help to distinguish between active disease (normal) and infection (high).

Management

Once the diagnosis is established, the patient should be referred to physicians who specialise in SLE. The patient will need lifelong supervision. As the disease waxes and wanes over time, the intensity of support varies. There should be regular assessments of renal function. General treatment measures include:

- rest when the disease is active
- low-fat diet
- protection from photosensitivity with sun-block creams
- NSAIDs for symptoms.

Management of the more serious complications includes corticosteroids, azathioprine and cyclophosphamide for accelerating renal disease. Chloroquine (or hydroxychloroquine) is the mainstay of treatment for skin or joint disease; the main complication is ocular toxicity. Renal and cerebral disease are the major determinants of outcome. Without these, the disease is usually relatively mild and has a good long-term outcome, e.g. > 90% survival over 5 years.

8.5 Vasculitides

In many connective tissue diseases, vasculitis occurs and can have serious consequences in terms of morbidity and mortality. There is also a range of conditions in which vasculitis is the major feature. The simplest classification is to think of the calibre of the vessel affected:

- large, e.g. temporal arteritis
- medium, e.g. polyarteritis nodosa
- small, e.g. SLE.

Temporal arteritis and polymyalgia rheumatica

It is very important for you to recognise these overlapping clinical problems because:

- temporal arteritis poses a major threat to vision and is easily treated with corticosteroids
- polymyalgia rheumatica is debilitating and easily treated with corticosteroids.

They are diseases of later life, so be very wary of making the diagnosis in a person aged under 60 years; look for other causes of their symptoms. Histopathological examination shows a vasculitis with giant cells ('giant cell arteritis'); characteristically the inflammatory process 'skips' certain sections of an affected artery whilst damaging others.

In temporal arteritis, it is the arteries of the scalp and the ophthalmic artery that are predominantly affected, though occasionally it can cause a stroke through intracranial involvement, particularly of the vertebro-basilar system.

In polymyalgia rheumatica, it is the arteries within the muscle bed that bear the brunt of the inflammation.

Temporal arteritis

Headache and scalp tenderness are the dominant features. The headache is usually severe and the patient will say that it is unlike any previous ones (p. 183). Sometimes the first manifestation is monocular blindness (p. 184), which is often permanent. In a few, vision may be impaired temporarily. The patient will often complain of general malaise. On examination, you may find tender temporal arteries which may be thickened and non-pulsatile. You should make full visual assessment (e.g. visual fields, acuity, ophthalmoscopy, eye movement).

Polymyalgia rheumatica

It is easy to miss this diagnosis because the features are non-specific. Patients complain of general ill-health, with anorexia, weight loss and fatigue. The cardinal feature is *morning stiffness*. It is important to ask specifically about the symptoms of temporal arteritis.

Diagnosis

The diagnosis is based on the clinical features supported by a high ESR, plasma viscosity or C-reactive protein, indicating a general inflammatory process. You should consider a temporal artery biopsy using the following criteria:

- it is most useful in temporal arteritis (but one-third are negative), much less in polymyalgia rheumatica
- when diagnosis is in doubt
- do not delay treatment in patients with a high probability of having the condition
- the yield is greatest when performed within 24 hours of starting treatment (after a week only 10% of biopsies are positive)
- a negative result does not exclude the diagnosis
- a positive result may help if the diagnosis is questioned later (lack of response to treatment or complications of treatment).

Management

Treatment is the immediate administration of corticosteroids. In temporal arteritis, this should be 60 mg prednisolone and the patient should obtain symptomatic relief within 24–48 hours. In polymyalgia rheumatica, a lower dose (20 mg) is used and improvement may take 1–2 weeks. The disease activity is monitored by the patient's wellbeing and changes in the ESR (or plasma viscosity). The dose of steroids is gradually reduced over weeks or months to the lowest maintenance dose that keeps the disease in remission; ideally this should be less than 10 mg prednisolone to prevent long-term side-effects. Corticosteroids *suppress* but do not cure the condition; the natural history is for the arteritis to burn itself out over 2 or more years.

Polyarteritis nodosa

Polyarteritis nodosa is characterised by a patchy vasculitis of medium and large vessels, with fibrinoid necrosis and small aneurysm formation. It is more common in males and usually starts in middle age; 50% of the patients are hepatitis surface antigen positive.

Clinical presentation

The symptoms and signs depend on the vessels affected, but most patients present with non-specific malaise and weight loss. Abdominal pain caused by bowel ischaemia is common. Involvement of the renal vasculature leads to renal failure and malignant hypertension. Elsewhere, brain and limb ischaemia develops. As with all the vasculitides affecting the vasa nervorum, mononeuritis multiplex occurs.

Investigation

The ESR may be raised and there may be a polymorphonuclear leucocytosis. Arteriography of the renal or GI vasculature will demonstrate the microaneurysms. A firm diagnosis may be established by biopsy.

Management

Treatment is with corticosteroids and immunosuppressives. Untreated, the outlook is bleak with death commonly from renal failure.

Small vessel vasculitis

Many connective tissue diseases have a small vessel vasculitis. **Henoch–Schönlein purpura** and mixed cryoglobulinaemia (globulins which may cause agglutination below a certain temperature) have, as a major feature, a small vessel vasculitis. In the skin, this causes a purpura which is *palpable* (cf. thrombocytopenia). Features of mixed cryoglobulinaemia are abdominal pain, haematuria, polyarthritis and a mononeuritis. Cases are often self limiting.

Vasculitis with granulomata

In **Wegener's granulomatosis,** there is a vasculitis with granulomata affecting the respiratory tract (p. 86), nasopharynx and the kidneys. It often presents with a bloody nasal discharge and haemoptysis. Renal failure supervenes. A chest radiograph shows multiple ill-defined nodules that may cavitate. Untreated, most patients will die within 12 months; the use of cyclophosphamide has dramatically altered this.

A variant of the above is Churg–Strauss syndrome, with asthma, pulmonary infiltrates and a very high eosinophil count.

8.6 Systemic sclerosis

Systemic sclerosis is a rare condition that is more common in females and has an onset between the third and fifth decade. It is characterised by connective tissue fibrosis. It is often called **scleroderma** because of the skin involvement, but it is a multisystem disease.

Pathology

The cause of the condition is unknown. The histopathological sequence is inflammation, followed by fibrosis and atrophy. As well as the connective tissue changes, there is concentric proliferation and thickening of the intima within the vascular bed. The pattern of organ involvement varies, but occasionally the changes are localised to a patch of skin (**morphoea**).

Clinical presentation

In the skin, the disease starts with painless oedema, which is followed by thickening of the fingers, hands and face; sometimes more widely. As atrophy develops, the face becomes 'pinched', with a beaked nose, small mouth (microstomia) and widespread telangiectasiae. There is also alopecia, pigmentation and vitiligo. Subcutaneous calcification occurs in nodules, particularly around the fingertips, and these may ulcerate. In almost all patients, **Raynaud's phenomenon** (see below) is present, which may predate the other changes.

The second most common system affected is the GI tract. In the oesophagus, there is decreased/absent peristalsis with dilatation. Patients may be asymptomatic or may have marked dysphagia and heartburn. In the small bowel, stasis and dilatation occur with bacterial overgrowth and malabsorption.

In the musculoskeletal system, there are flexion and spindling deformities of the fingers. Other problems are myositis and myocardial fibrosis (conduction defects and arrhythmias). The lungs may show fibrosis and honeycombing leading to a restrictive defect. Sjögren's syndrome may be present.

The most serious problems are progressive renal failure and malignant hypertension owing to an obliterative endarteritis.

Investigation

A positive speckled or nucleolar antinuclear antibody is present in the majority of patients and rheumatoid factor is found in up to one-third. Many have a normochromic normocytic anaemia with a raised ESR. Careful monitoring of the blood pressure and renal function is required. Radiographs show deposits of calcium and erosion of the tufts of the distal phalanges. A barium swallow will show oesophageal involvement and a barium meal and follow-through may demonstrate dilatation and flocculation.

Management

There is no treatment. Control of blood pressure is important and oesophageal problems are managed symptomatically. Around half of patients will survive 5 years.

CREST Syndrome

A benign variant of systemic sclerosis is known by the acronym Calcinosis, Raynaud's, Esophagitis, Sclerodactyly and Telangectasia. Anticentromere antibodies are specific to this condition (now termed **limited cutaneous scleroderma**).

Mixed connective tissue disease

In a tiny number of patients, there is an overlap between the features of systemic sclerosis, SLE and myositis. They do not have anti-DNA antibodies but are strongly positive for antibodies against extractable nuclear antigen (RNA protein) and have a speckled pattern on antinuclear antibody tests.

Dermatomyositis and polymyositis

These are covered on page 213.

Raynaud's phenomenon

Raynaud's phenomenon is characterised by:

- episodic colour change of fingers (toes less common) in response to cold
- the colour changes are: white (ischaemia) then blue (stasis) then red (reactive hyperaemia).

Raynaud's phenomenon is common, affecting about 5% of the population. Over 90% of sufferers are female. It can be associated with connective tissue disease, but this is very uncommon (< 5%). The associations are with:

- scleroderma (most common)
- SLE, Sjögren's syndrome, myositis
- rheumatoid disease (least common).

The presence of antinuclear antibodies is helpful in predicting the probability of an underlying connective tissue disease.

8.7 Crystal arthropathies

Learning objectives

You should:
- know how gout and pseudogout commonly present
- understand the metabolism of uric acid and how abnormalities lead to gout
- know the principles of acute treatment and long-term management.

Gout

Uric acid is produced by the breakdown of purine bases. The enzyme responsible is xanthine oxidase which metabolises xanthine. The main pathway for uric acid excretion is in the kidney with filtration at the glomerulus. The uric acid is then reabsorbed in the proximal tubule and subsequently excreted in the distal tubule. *Low-dose* aspirin blocks this distal secretion and causes hyperuricaemia; *high-dose* aspirin blocks proximal reabsorption and, as this is of greater magnitude, the net effect is urate excretion.

Classical gout with monoarthritis affecting the big toe is seen predominantly in men. The first attack is severe, but subsequent attacks are less severe and involve joints other than the big toe. There may be systemic disturbance, including pyrexia. Gout is very uncommon in premenopausal females; in older women it may cause a chronic polyarthritis.

The underlying problem is excess urate production, which cannot be excreted by the kidney. The urate is deposited as crystals in the joints and also in the tissues as **tophi**. Gout can occur secondary to some other process. Factors affecting the balance between production and excretion are illustrated in Figure 62.

GOUT	
Increased production:	Reduced excretion:

- myeloproliferative disorders
- lymphoproliferative disorders (chemotherapy can exacerbate these)
- starvation

- chronic renal disease
- drugs:
  – diuretics
  – low-dose salicylates

Fig. 62
Factors affecting the balance between production and excretion of uric acid.

Management

Management involves:

- identifying any cause, such as drugs; most cases will be idiopathic
- treating the acute attack with an NSAID such as diclofenac; occasionally colchicine is used
- unless there is a definite precipitating factor which can be removed, starting *prophylactic* treatment.

Prophylaxis is usually with **allopurinol**, which acts by blocking the enzyme xanthine oxidase. Xanthine is much more water soluble and can be excreted by the kidneys. You must remember to continue NSAID treatment for a few months because allopurinol treatment allows mobilisation of the urate that was deposited in the tissues and this may precipitate a further attack of gout.

Extremely rapid rises of urate (e.g. in the treatment of leukaemia) can precipitate renal failure, not gout. Consequently, leukaemic patients only require allopurinol prophylaxis rather than NSAID treatment.

Pseudogout

Pseudogout is predominantly a disease of older people. Like gout it is a crystal arthropathy, but it tends to occur in the knees and ankles. The patients often present with a monoarthritis. A radiograph may show a line of calcification within the joint space and examination of the joint aspirate under a polarising microscope will show the crystals of pyrophosphate (Table 68). The principles of management are:

- rest the joint
- analgesics, particularly NSAIDS, for the inflammatory component.

8.8 Degenerative arthropathies

Osteoarthritis

Many texts use the terms osteo*arthrosis* to mean signs and symptoms of joint damage without a marked inflammatory component and osteo*arthritis* to indicate the presence of inflammation. This can be a difficult distinction (cf. diverticulosis and diverticulitis). You should be aware of why the terms are used and stick to one of them.

Osteoarthritis is the most common arthropathy in the UK. The prevalence rises with age, affecting the great majority of patients over the age of 75 years. Most cases are *primary*, that is no cause can be found, though you should always ask yourself whether one can be identified, in which case the problem is *secondary* osteoarthritis.

Primary osteoarthritis has a strong familial tendency and is associated with increasing age and obesity.

Learning objectives

You must:
*   know how to diagnose osteoarthritis, distinguish it from rheumatoid arthritis and establish whether it is primary or secondary
*   be able to outline the principles of management.

Pathogenesis and pathology

The cause of osteoarthritis is not known. It is a metabolically active condition that shows a variable balance between anabolic and catabolic processes. At different times, there is increased activity in all the joint tissues. The primary problem seems to be either mechanical damage to cartilage or a biochemical abnormality of the cartilage itself. The chondrocyte releases enzymes which can degrade collagen and proteoglycans. Crystals released into the synovial fluid initiate and perpetuate inflammation. With repair comes remodelling, producing the characteristic osteophyte.

The list of conditions associated with secondary osteoarthritis is long but can be categorised into:

*   mechanical joint damage: occupational, inflammatory arthritis, neuropathic joints, congenital dysplasia, fracture through the joints
*   abnormal cartilage: pyrophosphate arthropathy, haemochromatosis.

The joint shows **fibrillation** of the superficial cartilage layer with deeper **fissures**. With advanced disease there is complete cartilage loss and **eburnation** ('polishing') of bone. The synovium is infiltrated with mononuclear cells and the subchondral bone is thickened and may contain cysts.

Clinical features

The joints most often affected are the knees and hips. Particularly in **primary generalised osteoarthritis,** the small joints of the hands are involved. **Heberden's nodes** occur in the DIPs (which can be hot and painful when they first arise) and **Bouchard's nodes** in the PIPs. The first carpo-metacarpal joint is commonly damaged with *squaring* of the hand at the base of thumb. The

apophyseal joints in the cervical and lumbar spine may be involved. Rarely affected, unless there is pre-existing joint abnormality, are the elbows, shoulders and ankles.

The characteristic features of osteoarthrosis are:

*   pain that is worse in the evenings and is aggravated by use
*   stiffness following rest, lasting for only 15–30 minutes, unlike that caused by inflammatory arthritis
*   reduced mobility
*   disability as the disease progresses.

On examination, the joint is swollen either through bony overgrowth or an effusion. During an exacerbation, the joint may be hot. There is limitation of movement, crepitus, deformity and instability.

One important complication, associated with any chronic arthropathy, is the formation of a **Baker's cyst** in the knee. This consists of a degenerative outpouching of the synovium, which can be palpated in the popliteal fossa. It can rupture, allowing tracking of synovial fluid into soleus and gastrocnemius muscles. The fluid sets up an inflammatory response, the signs of which closely mimic those of a deep vein thrombosis. The use of anticoagulants makes the situation worse. It can be diagnosed by an arthrogram or ultrasound.

Investigation and management

There are no haematological or biochemical abnormalities in primary osteoarthritis. The radiological features are shown in Figure 63.

The mainstay of drug therapy is simple analgesia (p. 303). The use of NSAIDS should be limited, particularly in elderly people, because of potential gastrotoxicity. NSAIDs do have a place in those patients with either an acute or a chronic inflammatory component.

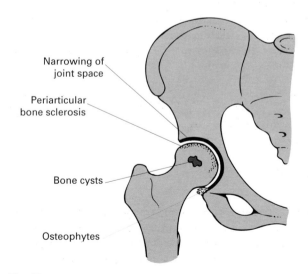

Narrowing of joint space

Periarticular bone sclerosis

Bone cysts

Osteophytes

Fig. 63
Schematic representation of radiographic changes in osteoarthrosis.

Physiotherapists can help by giving guidance on muscle-strengthening exercises (e.g. quadriceps), local therapy (e.g. heat), provision of walking aids and rehabilitation after surgery.

For many patients with severe disability and pain, surgery has been a major advance. Joint replacement of the hip is extremely successful and replacement of other joints, for example the knee, gives good results. Other options are arthrodesis and osteotomy.

8.9 Calcium metabolism and metabolic bone disease

Calcium and phosphate are measured routinely on multiple channel analysers so you will encounter abnormalities from the start of your career. Hypercalcaemia and hypocalcaemia are important — if uncommon — medical emergencies. Amongst bone diseases, osteoporosis is a a major and potentially preventable cause of debility in old age. Metabolic bone disease is *par excellence* an area of learning where command of simple anatomical and physiological principles makes learning easy.

Learning objectives

You must:
- understand calcium metabolism in terms of control mechanisms (principally parathyroid hormone (PTH) and vitamin D) and intestinal and renal calcium and phosphate handling
- understand the processes of bone formation and resorption in relation to the bone matrix, the 'remodelling unit' of osteoblast and osteoclast and the process of mineralisation
- be able to interpret serum calcium, phosphate and alkaline phosphatase and related parameters (urea, creatinine and albumin)
- understand the causes and management of hypercalcaemia and hypocalcaemia
- understand the causes, clinical presentations and prevention of osteoporosis
- know about some other disorders of bone including Paget's disease.

This section will combine a problem-orientated (hypo- and hypercalcaemia) and disease-orientated approach to metabolic bone disease. Table 69 shows the relationships between them.

Functional anatomy of bone

Bone is composed of a collagen matrix (osteoid) impregnated with calcium phosphate (hydroxyapatite crystals). It has a dense cortex and a less dense medulla composed of trabecular bone. Long bones have a central marrow cavity. Bone is vascular and contains:

- osteoblasts that form the osteoid and initiate the process of crystallisation

Table 69 Bone diseases related to serum calcium

	Serum calcium		
	Low	High	Normal
Parathyroid			
Hyperparathyroidism		*	
Hypoparathyroidism	*		
Vitamin D			
Vitamin D excess		*	
Osteomalacia/rickets	*		
Malignant hypercalcaemia		*	
Renal bone disease	*	*	*
Osteoporosis			*
Paget's disease			*

- osteoclasts: multinucleate cells that erode and resorb mineralised bone.

It is important to conceive of bone as a dynamic structure in a constant state of turnover, adapting to injury and mechanical stress. About 10% of its mass is remodelled each year. The remodelling unit, consisting of osteoclasts and osteoblasts, moves slowly through bone completing remodelling in about 100 days. Alkaline phosphatase is an enzyme secreted by the osteoblasts which indicates the activity of remodelling units.

Calcium and phosphate metabolism

Calcium comprises 1.5% of body weight and 99% of it is within the skeleton. A small fraction of skeletal calcium is in a rapidly exchangeable pool, but the majority can only be released by increased osteoclast activity. In blood, calcium is about 50% albumin-bound (and biologically inactive). Most unbound calcium is ionised and this is the biologically active fraction, essential to blood coagulation and nerve and muscle function. An important practical point is that a low plasma albumin reduces the total calcium concentration reported by the biochemistry laboratory without any change in the ionised fraction, and vice versa. Moreover, the ionised fraction (which cannot easily be measured) increases with acidosis and falls with alkalosis. That is why hyperventilation causes hypocalcaemic tetany without any change in total plasma calcium.

Calcium is actively absorbed from the gut under the control of vitamin D. There is obligatory reabsorption of calcium in the proximal renal tubule and variable reabsorption in the distal tubule controlled by PTH.

Like calcium, most phosphate is in a skeletal pool. It is absorbed from the gut in direct proportion to dietary intake and reabsorbed from the glomerular filtrate in the proximal tubule, a process inhibited by PTH. Apart from the hormonal control mechanism described below, there is a direct relationship between plasma calcium and phosphate concentrations because calcium phosphate comes out of solution once the product of their concentrations exceeds a critical value.

Vitamin D and PTH

These two interrelated hormone systems control calcium absorption and excretion and influence the balance between bone deposition and resorption. There are two sources of 'parent' vitamin D:

- the skin, where it is formed in response to sunlight
- intestinal absorption.

It undergoes two hydroxylation steps (25-hydroxylation in the liver and 1-hydroxylation in the kidneys) to become the biologically active 1,25-dihydroxycholecalciferol (calcitriol). Active vitamin D increases intestinal calcium absorption.

PTH is secreted by the parathyroid glands in direct response to changes in plasma calcium and phosphate and is under negative feedback control from 1,25-dihydroxycholecalciferol. Its effects are to increase plasma calcium and lower phosphate by:

- increasing osteoclast activity
- increasing 1-hydroxylation of vitamin D
- increasing renal calcium reabsorption
- reducing renal phosphate reabsorption.

The actions of vitamin D and PTH are intimately interrelated and conjointly regulate serum calcium and phosphate within tight limits.

Other hormones and the skeleton

Calcitonin. It is secreted by the parafollicular cells of the thyroid in response to hypercalcaemia and reduces bone resorption. It does not have a major physiological role, as illustrated by the fact that diseases of calcitonin deficiency and excess do not disrupt calcium metabolism; however, pharmacological doses can be used to reduce bone remodelling in Paget's disease and net bone resorption in malignant hypercalcaemia.

Glucocorticoids. They reduce calcium and phosphate absorption (an important therapeutic effect in vitamin D excess) and inhibit net bone formation; the basis for steroid-induced osteoporosis.

Thyroid hormones. They reduce bone mineral density and can cause osteoporosis in hyperthyroidism.

Sex steroids. They increase bone formation over resorption by a direct effect on osteoblasts.

PTH-related peptide (PTH-rp). This hormone is produced by some malignant tumours. It is chemically related to native PTH and causes malignant hypercalcaemia (see p. 318) but is not detected by PTH assays.

Clinical presentation

Symptoms and signs can be caused by:

- hypocalcaemia
- hypercalcaemia
- bone pain, deformity and/or fractures.

Hypocalcaemia

Clinical manifestations result from irritability and dysfunction of nerves and muscles and include:

- paraesthesiae in the hands and around the mouth
- weakness
- spasms of skeletal muscles (tetany); laryngeal stridor and asphyxia in severe cases
- mental confusion and fits.

Signs can be precipitated by:

- tapping the facial nerve over the parotid gland; a positive response is twitching of the ipsilateral facial muscles (Chvostek's sign)
- occluding the brachial artery by inflating a sphygmomanometer above systolic pressure for 3 minutes; a positive response is carpal spasm (Trousseau's sign).

These signs are, at best, a stop-gap and cannot substitute for measuring plasma calcium.

Hypercalcaemia

The symptoms and signs are vague and non-specific but hypercalcaemia is common so you must have a high index of suspicion; measure serum calcium if there is anything to suggest the diagnosis. The signs affect a range of systems.

Renal: these are caused by hypercalcaemia-induced ADH insensitivity (nephrogenic diabetes insipidus):

- thirst, polyuria, nocturia
- symptoms and signs of volume depletion
- symptoms of renal stones/nephrocalcinosis.

Intestinal:

- nausea and vomiting
- constipation
- dyspeptic abdominal pain
- symptoms and signs of pancreatitis (acute pancreatitis is a sign of severe hypercalcaemia).

Neurological:

- lassitude
- mood disturbance, particularly depression
- confusion: sign of severe hypercalcaemia
- drowsiness: sign of severe hypercalcaemia

Ocular: corneal calcification; a visible band at the medial and lateral corneo-scleral junction. Corneal calcification, like renal stones, is evidence of longstanding hypercalcaemia. It is asymptomatic and best seen with a slit lamp.

Cardiovascular: hypertension.

Investigations

It follows from the basic physiology of calcium metabolism that you should measure calcium, phosphate and alkaline phosphatase as a triad. Alkaline phosphatase is raised if there is increased bone remodelling but may be normal in patients with abnormal serum calcium and phosphate (e.g. hyperparathyroidism without significant bone disease) and abnormal in patients with normal calcium and phosphate (Paget's disease and malignant bone destruction). The interpretation of calcium and phosphate is considered under the individual diseases. Once an abnormality of plasma calcium or phosphate has been established, these additional tests may be informative:

- 24-hour urinary calcium and phosphate excretion
- renal function (urea and creatinine)
- PTH and 25-hydroxyvitamin D
- urinary cyclic AMP, an index of PTH activity
- urinary hydroxyproline excretion (best measured as the hydroxyproline:creatinine ratio in an early morning urine sample), an index of bone remodelling.

Radiological investigations:

- plain radiology, which is not sensitive for early disease but may show specific abnormalities in Paget's disease, hyperparathyroidism, osteomalacia/rickets, renal bone disease, malignancy and osteoporosis
- densitometry (by photon-absorptiometry or quantitative computerised tomography), which is much more sensitive than plain radiology for a reduced bone mass
- radionuclide scanning, which is sensitive to increased bone remodelling, showing areas of increased vascularity as 'hot spots'
- CT and MR, used to investigate bone and joint structure in detail.

Bone biopsy. This provides detailed morphological information but is needed in only a small number of patients.

Hypercalcaemia

In its clinical presentations, hypercalcaemia ranges from a mild and asymptomatic biochemical abnormality to a medical emergency. The 'big two' causes are hyperparathyroidism and malignant hypercalcaemia. Vitamin D excess is less common but important to remember because it is steroid responsive. Immobilisation can worsen all causes of hypercalcaemia by increasing bone resorption. The causes you are most likely to encounter are shown bold in this list:

- hyperparathyroidism
  — **primary**
  — tertiary
- malignancy
  — **solid tumours**: breast, bronchus, thyroid, kidney, prostate
  — **haematological:** myeloma, leukaemias
- Vitamin D excess
  — excess intake, e.g. excessive consumption of vitamin tablets or cod liver oil
  — excess formation: granulomatous diseases including sarcoidosis and tuberculosis, glucocorticoid deficiency, lymphoma.

Hyperparathyroidism

Hyperparathyroidism and the resulting hypercalcaemia form a vicious circle where both are exacerbated by the metabolic disturbance. Hypercalcaemia results from increased delivery of calcium into the extracellular pool, which is enforced, in hyperparathyroid states, by increased renal reabsorption. As serum calcium rises, total urinary calcium excretion increases (though fractional excretion may not). Thus, hypercalcaemia can remain mild so long as glomerular filtration and flow are maintained and the patient experiences thirst and responds to it by drinking. Unfortunately, more severe hypercalcaemia causes anorexia, vomiting and drowsiness which, in the face of continued polyuria, lead to volume depletion and, ultimately, renal hypofiltration. When this occurs, the escape route for calcium is blocked and severe hypercalcaemia occurs (e.g. serum calcium > 3.5 mmol/l). The immediate management of severe hypercalcaemia follows from this:

- you should first assess blood volume and renal function: volume depletion and renal impairment (very high urea, high creatinine) are usually seen in severe hypercalcaemia
- if the patient is volume depleted, give intravenous saline, aiming for a urine output > 4 l/day; frusemide may help, once volume has been replaced, to increase calcium excretion.

Management is then directed at establishing the cause and achieving a cure. Appropriate steps include:

- careful history and physical examination for evidence of neoplasia, parathyroid disease, vitamin D excess, sarcoidosis, etc.
- measurement of PTH and 25-hydroxycholecalciferol
- steroid suppression test.

The definitive treatment depends upon the final diagnosis but emergency treatment with bisphosphonates (see below) should always be considered if rehydration fails to control hypercalcaemia.

Primary hyperparathyroidism

Primary hyperparathyroidism has a prevalence of 1 in 1,000 making it one of the commoner endocrine diseases: 80% of cases are caused by a parathyroid adenoma and 5% by multiple adenomata. The remaining 15% are caused by diffuse parathyroid hyperplasia and (least commonly) carcinoma. Rarely, hyperparathyroidism is part of the syndrome of multiple endocrine neoplasia. The prevalence of hyperparathyroidism increases with age. Modes of presentation in approximate order of frequency are:

- a chance biochemical finding
- thirst, polyuria or abdominal symptoms
- symptoms of bone disease, including pain, fractures and deformity
- renal stones

- hypercalcaemic crisis, particularly after periods of immobilisation
- hypertension.

The parathyroid glands are rarely palpable.

Investigation. The diagnostic features are:

- a raised serum calcium
- a low phosphate
- a raised or 'inappropriately normal' serum PTH
- hypercalciuria; this must always be checked to exclude 'familial hypocalciuric hypercalcaemia' caused by reduced calcium excretion, otherwise indistinguishable from primary hyperparathyroidism and unresponsive to parathyroidectomy.

Subperiosteal resorption of the phalanges is the commonest radiological sign; localised areas of bone resorption with fibrosis ('osteitis fibrosa et cystica') may also be seen on plain radiographs of the long bones and ribs. Plain radiographs and bone densitometry may show generalised osteopenia. Ultrasound, CT, MR and radionuclide scanning and venous catheterisation studies can be used to localise parathyroid adenomas, but exploration by an experienced surgeon is the most sensitive technique. Many clinicians proceed directly to surgery once the biochemical diagnosis has been made.

Management. Surgery is the only effective treatment and is indicated for:

- more severe hypercalcaemia; calcium > 3mmol/l
- symptoms
- complications, including renal stones, osteoporosis, pancreatitis and renal failure.

If surgery fails, treatment with a bisphosphonate may be needed to control hypercalcaemia. A 'wait and see' policy is appropriate for mild disease (serum calcium < 3 mmol/l), normal blood pressure and renal function and no evidence of osteoporosis. Many old people with hyperparathyroidism do not need surgery.

Malignant hypercalcaemia

There are four mechanisms by which malignant diseases cause hypercalcaemia:

- direct destruction of bone
- secretion of osteoclast-activating cytokines (as in multiple myeloma)
- secretion of PTH-rP (p. 316)
- overproduction of 1,25-dihydroxycholecalciferol (as may occur in lymphomas).

Malignant disease can cause extremely severe hypercalcaemia. This usually signifies widespread bone involvement. It has an aggressive course and patients may develop severe hypercalcaemia very rapidly because they are already anorexic as an effect of their underlying disease and get into a vicious circle. It has an extremely poor prognosis.

Investigation. Consider the possibility of malignancy, including myeloma, and arrange the following in every case of severe hypercalcamia:

- Hb and ESR
- liver function tests
- plain X-rays of the chest and pelvis
- plasma protein and urine electrophoresis to exclude myeloma.

A radionuclide bone scan may detect malignant deposits not seen on plain radiology.

Management. The importance of volume replacement has been considered earlier. Remember that severely hypercalcaemic patients may develop acute renal failure because of volume depletion or myeloma kidney so the neck veins and urine output must be carefully observed. Corticosteroids can lower calcium in myeloma and some other haematological malignancies but are otherwise ineffective. If these measures fail, the treatment is a parenteral bisphosphonate, such as pamidronate or clodronate, which prevents bone resorption by coating the hydroxyapatite crystals. This can normalise serum calcium within a few days.

States of vitamin D excess

These cause hypercalcaemia by increasing intestinal calcium absorption. Vitamin D intoxication is uncommon although it may occur inadvertently in the treatment of renal bone disease or hypocalcaemia (p. 159). Uncommon, but important, is the synthesis of 1,25-dihyroxycholecalciferol in the granulomata of sarcoidosis (p. 86) and tuberculosis, in which case the diagnosis may be made from a chest radiograph. Glucocorticoids antagonise the effect of vitamin D on calcium absorption so a trial of glucocorticoids can control hypercalcaemia and confirm the diagnosis.

Hypocalcaemia

Hypoparathyroidism is the main cause of severe hypocalcaemia because intact parathyroid glands can restore serum calcium to near normal in most other diseases. The causes of hypocalcaemia include:

- hypoparathyroidism
  — surgical
  — autoimmune
- resistance to PTH (pseudohypoparathyroidism)
- vitamin D deficiency (see osteomalacia/rickets, p. 319)
- renal failure (see renal bone disease, p. 159)
- binding of calcium (usually obvious from the clinical context)
  — acute pancreatitis
  — massive blood transfusion.

Clinical presentation

As in hypercalcaemia, the presentation of hypocalcaemia ranges from an asymptomatic biochemical finding to a life-threatening emergency (symptomatic and serum calcium < 1.8 mmol/l). Management is summarised in the emergency box.

Emergency treatment: management of severe hypocalcaemia

1. Establish venous access and quickly take blood for:
   - calcium, phosphate, alkaline phosphatase, PTH
   - urea and creatinine

2. Give intravenous 10% calcium gluconate, 10 ml over 10 minutes

3. Call for senior help

4. Give repeated doses or a slow infusion of calcium gluconate according to symptomatic response

---

Hypoparathyroidism

Hypoparathyroidism is most often a result of surgery for thyroid, parathyroid or pharyngeal disease and may present as a postoperative emergency. Less common is idiopathic hypoparathyroidism which:

- may be familial or sporadic
- is caused by autoimmunity
- is associated with other organ-specific autoimmune diseases such as Addison's disease and hypothyroidism
- may be associated with chronic mucocutaneous candidiasis and malabsorption syndrome.

With prolonged hypoparathyroidism, whatever its cause, calcification may be seen in the basal ganglia on a plain skull X-ray or CT scan. The biochemical signs of hypoparathyroidism are:

- hypocalcaemia
- a raised serum phosphate
- low serum PTH.

If PTH is unexpectedly high, the patient has pseudohypoparathyroidism (tissue PTH insensitivity).

Treatment. PTH is not available as a therapeutic agent so treatment is with a combination of oral calcium and a vitamin D metabolite or analogue (1,25-dihydroxycholecalciferol or 1α-dihydroxycholecalciferol) to increase its absorption.

Osteomalacia

The syndrome of vitamin D deficiency is termed rickets if it occurs in children and osteomalacia once growth has ceased. Failure of calcium absorption is compensated for by increased PTH secretion ('secondary hyperparathy-

roidism'), which reduces the bone mineral content and leaves osteoid unmineralised. The biochemical signs are:

- a low-normal or (uncommonly) low serum calcium
- a low phosphate, because of the phosphaturic effect of PTH.

Note that this low phosphate distinguishes rickets/osteomalacia from hypoparathyroidism. Alkaline phosphatase may be normal or raised if there is parathyroid bone disease. The serum 25-hydroxycholecalciferol level is low.

Osteomalacia is rarely caused by pure dietary deficiency, because vitamin D synthesis in skin can compensate; however, chronically ill or old people may lack sunlight exposure and an adequate diet and become vitamin D deficient. Asian people may have the same risk factors, compounded by a diet high in phytates (chapati), which bind calcium in the gut. Other causes include:

- malabsorption syndrome, reducing the absorption of fat-soluble vitamin D
- renal disease, in which there is impaired 1-hydroxylation of vitamin D
- liver disease, with impaired 25-hydroxylation of vitamin D
- anticonvulsant therapy, in which there is impaired 25-hydroxylation and tissue vitamin D resistance.

Clinical presentation. Adults with osteomalacia experience bone pain and may have weakness and a waddling gait. Radiological signs are:

- osteopenia
- Looser's zones: localised areas of decalcification on the concave surfaces of bones, particularly the femur and pelvis
- biconcave deformity of vertebrae.

Treatment. This is with calcium and vitamin D supplements.

Renal bone disease (renal osteodystrophy)

This is covered in Chapter 4 (p. 159).

Osteoporosis

Bone mass is determined by the relative activities of osteoblasts and osteoclasts. During growth, bone formation exceeds resorption. Bone mass peaks around age 25 and declines thereafter. A reduced bone mass, predisposing to fractures after relatively mild trauma, is termed osteoporosis. Unlike osteomalacia, the mass of osteoid as well as bone mineral is reduced. Trabecular bone is lost more than cortical bone, so fractures occur at sites composed mostly of trabecular bone.

Epidemiology and causes

Loss of bone mass is a feature of ageing. An individual is predisposed to osteoporosis by having a low peak bone mass, a rapid rate of loss thereafter or advanced age. Having reached a level of bone mass which predisposes to fractures, only a small further reduction greatly increases the fracture risk. Women differ from men in undergoing an abrupt and severe reduction in sex-steroid secretion at the menopause, which accelerates their rate of bone loss. As a result, they are more prone to osteoporosis. Osteoporosis is a major socio-economic problem. One in two women and one in six men will sustain a fracture related to osteoporosis by age 90. These fractures may cause permanent disability. Mortality is increased over the months after an osteoporotic fracture.

Osteoporosis may present at several stages of life:

- associated with the rapid loss of bone mass after the menopause
- associated with progressive bone loss into old age
- 'idiopathic' osteoporosis, caused by premature bone loss, presents in middle age.

Osteoporosis may be 'primary' or secondary to:

- endocrine/metabolic disease
  — glucocorticoid excess: Cushing's disease, steroid therapy
  — hyperthyroidism
  — hypogonadism
  — growth hormone deficiency (hypopituitarism)
  — hyperparathyroidism
  — diabetes mellitus
  — renal osteodystrophy
- neoplasia: multiple myeloma
- GI disease: malabsorption, gastrectomy, liver disease
- rheumatological disease: rheumatoid arthritis
- other: immobility, substance abuse, malnutrition, any chronic, debilitating disease.

Clinical presentation

Until fracture occurs, osteoporosis is asymptomatic. They are as painful as any other fracture. Typical sites are:

- distal radius
- femoral neck
- vertebral bodies.

Patients may lose height and develop increased spinal curvature and a protuberant abdomen.

Investigations

Radiologically, there may be generalised osteopenia, wedge collapse of vertebrae, 'codfish vertebrae' (caused by herniation of the discs into the centre of the vertebral body) and increased spinal curvature. Bone densitometry (p. 317) is used to confirm the diagnosis and estimate fracture risk. Plain radiology and bone scanning can be used to demonstrate fractures. Biochemistry is normal, apart from a raised alkaline phosphatase during fracture healing.

You should suspect secondary osteoporosis in young or middle-aged patients and investigate them for the diseases listed above.

Management

Patients with fractures need adequate analgesia; those with vertebral osteoporosis may have relentless pain. There are various treatments which reduce bone resorption and the risk of future fractures but do nothing for fractures which have already occurred. They include:

- oestrogen replacement, which reduces postmenopausal bone loss but can only be continued for 5–10 years because of an increased risk of breast cancer thereafter
- bisphosphonates (etidronate), which are proven to reduce the rate of vertebral fracturing
- a physiological dose of vitamin D with calcium, which may reduce fracture risk and is relatively safe.

Patients with osteoporosis should be physically active, take a high calcium diet and avoid the risk factors listed below. Their response to treatment can be monitored densitometrically.

Prevention

Risk factors for osteoporosis are:

- hypogonadism or an early menopause
- family history of osteoporosis
- substance abuse (alcohol and tobacco)
- inactivity
- corticosteroid therapy and the endocrine diseases listed above.

It is part of general health education to encourage weight-bearing exercise, a high calcium diet, a moderate alcohol intake and not smoking; this is particularly important in high-risk individuals. Hormone-replacement treatment for menopausal women is the most effective means of prevention. High-risk individuals can be selected for hormone replacement by densitometry. The value of densitometric screening of the general population is unproven.

Paget's disease of bone

Paget's disease affects 4% of the population over age 40 years, the prevalence increasing with age. It is more common in men than in women and most prevalent in Anglo-Saxons, particularly in the north-west of England. The primary abnormality is in the osteoclasts, which are enlarged, have more nuclei than normal and resorb bone excessively. This is thought to be the late effect of a virus infection. Osteoblast function is also increased. The bone is formed chaotically, expanded, poorly calcified and unusually vascular. It is soft and prone to deformity and fractures. Paget's disease affects the tibia, femur, vertebrae, pelvis and skull.

Clinical presentation

Increased osteoblast activity causes an increased plasma alkaline phosphatase and a characteristic radiographic appearance (see below). The disease is usually asymptomatic and found by chance radiographically or by measurement of alkaline phosphatase. It may, however, cause symptoms which can be disabling:

- pain, caused by bone expansion, deformity and fractures
- warmth, as a result of increased vascularity
- deformity, causing immobility and secondary osteoarthritis
- nerve root compression, typically deafness because of skull involvement; spinal compression may occur
- osteogenic sarcoma can rarely develop.

Investigations

Alkaline phosphatase and the hydroxyproline:creatinine ratio (p. 317) are high, reflecting increased osteoblast and osteoclast activity, respectively. Radionuclide bone scans show areas of increased uptake, caused by increased vascularity. Plain radiographs show:

- thickening of the cortex
- trabecular thickening and sclerosis
- areas of osteolysis
- deformity.

Management

The bisphosphonates bind to hydroxyapatite and increase the resistance of bone to osteoclasts. They are highly effective at relieving pain and can normalise the biochemical markers and prevent progression.

Self-assessment: questions

Multiple choice questions

1. The following are seen with NSAIDs:
   a. Improvement in renal function
   b. Increase in serum potassium
   c. Increased risk of peptic ulcer complications
   d. Improved long-term prognosis of rheumatoid arthritis
   e. Improvement in coexistent asthma

2. In giant cell arteritis:
   a. The ESR falls with steroid treatment
   b. Radiographs of MCP and IP joints are normal
   c. The patient often gains weight
   d. Muscle biopsy may be abnormal
   e. Pain may occur during mastication

3. The following are features of SLE:
   a. Raynaud's phenomenon
   b. Mononeuritis multiplex
   c. Thrombocytopenia
   d. Lymphopenia
   e. A very high C-reactive protein

4. Rheumatoid factor is:
   a. An antibody to sheep erythrocytes
   b. Present when rheumatoid nodules are present
   c. Diagnostic of rheumatoid arthritis
   d. Usually is of the IgA subtype
   e. Is not found in rheumatoid synovial, pleural or pericardial fluid

5. In primary osteoarthritis:
   a. The ESR is normal
   b. PIP joints are not usually affected
   c. Radiographs show characteristic erosions of articular margins
   d. Morning stiffness usually lasts over 1 hour
   e. First carpo-metacarpal joint involvement is a common finding

6. In gout:
   a. Tophi are an early sign
   b. Allopurinol is used to treat the acute attack
   c. Frusemide helps to increase urate excretion
   d. Large joints are not affected
   e. Raised serum urate makes the diagnosis certain

7. Clinical features characteristic of psoriatic polyarthritis include:
   a. DIP joint involvement
   b. Symmetrical small joint involvement
   c. Arthritis mutilans
   d. Sacroiliitis
   e. Temporomandibular joint involvement

8. Ankylosing spondylitis:
   a. Is more common in females
   b. May present as a severe oligoarthritis
   c. Is associated with the histocompatibility antigen HLA-DW3
   d. Is associated with pulmonary fibrosis
   e. Involves the PIP joints

9. The following statements are true of normal synovial fluid:
   a. The fluid is clear and colourless
   b. Calcium pyrophosphate crystals may be found
   c. The viscosity is low
   d. The fibrin content is high
   e. The predominant white cell is the lymphocyte

10. Presenting features of rheumatoid arthritis indicating a poor prognosis include:
    a. Rheumatoid factor in high titre
    b. Systemic features
    c. Rheumatoid nodules
    d. Erosive joint changes
    e. Hand involvement

11. The following are true:
    a. Three inflamed painful joints occurring together makes septic arthritis very unlikely
    b. If *Staphylococcus aureus* is cultured from an inflamed joint, oral flucloxacillin and bed rest are the primary treatments
    c. Viruses do not cause acutely inflamed, swollen joints
    d. Absence of fever rules out septic arthritis
    e. A chronic monoarthritis may be caused by *Mycobacterium tuberculosis*

12. Concerning osteomyelitis:
    a. Debridement of infected bone is essential for cure in chronic osteomyelitis
    b. It is usually accompanied by a very high ESR
    c. A distinctive feature of chronic osteomyelitis is a discharging sinus
    d. A positive culture from a sinus tract is a good indication of the bacterial cause of the chronic osteomyelitis
    e. Usually 2 or 3 weeks' antibiotic therapy is adequate for cure

13. The following autoantibody tests are matched with the relevant diseases:
    a. Antibasement membrane antibodies and Goodpasture's syndrome
    b. Intrinsic factor antibody and pernicious anaemia
    c. p-ANCA and polyarteritis

d. Antinuclear antibody and Raynaud's syndrome
e. Antimitochondrial antibodies and antiphospholipid syndrome

14. With regard to reactive arthritis:
   a. It may be caused by both *Salmonella* and *Campylobacter* spp.
   b. It is usually chronic and unremitting over 3–4 years
   c. Confidence in the diagnosis rests on growing a bacterium from stool or other sites
   d. NSAIDs are appropriate therapy
   e. Rheumatic fever should be excluded

15. The following are true:
   a. Plasma calcium and phosphate alter independently of one another
   b. Dietary calcium intake is the main determinant of plasma calcium
   c. Plasma alkaline phosphatase is a marker of the activity of osteoblasts
   d. Normal mineralisation of bone depends upon adequate intestinal calcium absorption
   e. Renal failure causes phosphate retention

16. The following are true:
   a. Osteoporosis is among the more common causes of hypercalcaemia
   b. Granulomatous diseases, whatever their aetiology, may cause hypercalcaemia
   c. A characteristic of PTH-mediated hypercalcaemia is a low serum phosphate
   d. Renal bone disease never causes hypercalcaemia
   e. A haematological malignancy should be considered as a possible diagnosis in a patient presenting with hypercalcaemia

17. The following are true:
   a. Osteoporosis is characterised by deficiency of osteoid and bone mineral
   b. Bone mass peaks at the age of 55 and declines thereafter
   c. Prolonged inactivity causes loss of bone mass
   d. An incidental effect of corticosteroid therapy is to increase bone mass
   e. Hypogonadism only causes osteoporosis in old age

18. The following are true:
   a. Hypocalcaemia may present as epilepsy
   b. Bedside examination is a highly sensitive way of detecting hypocalcaemia
   c. Calcitonin is an effective treatment for recurrent hypocalcaemia
   d. Cerebral calcification may occur in hypoparathyroidism
   e. Patients with hypoparathyroidism are treated with recombinant human PTH

Case history questions

History 1

A 28-year-old rugby player presents 2 days after a match in which he was not injured, other than a graze on the left shin, with a painful, swollen, red right knee and a slightly painful left elbow. He has a temperature of 38.6°C.

1. What is your initial differential diagnosis?
2. What further history should you seek?
3. List the four most appropriate immediate investigations.

History 2

A 65-year-old man presents to Casualty drowsy and vomiting. He has a short history of thirst, polyuria and weight loss and has complained to his wife of backache. He is drowsy and confused. A note from his GP states that a recent biochemical profile showed his serum calcium to be 3.9 mmol/l.

1. Name three other biochemical measurements which you would wish to know without delay.
2. Give two likely causes for the hypercalcaemia.
3. List two forms of treatment for his hypercalcaemia.

Data interpretation

Table 70 gives the biochemical results for six patients. Suggest an interpretation with reasons.

Table 70 Biochemical results for data interpretation question.

	1	2	3	4	5	6
Calcium (mmol/l)	3.5	3.9	2.0	1.2	2.3	2.05
Phosphate (mmol/l)	0.5	2.3	0.6	2.1	0.9	2.5
Alkaline phosphatase (IU/l)	230	190	200	120	280	320
Urea (mmol/l)	10	35	6	5.3	5.1	34
Creatinine (mo/l)	118	500	100	98	110	480

Reference ranges: as a final year student you should aim to know the reference ranges for all of these measurements (p. 5).

Picture questions

1. Picture 8.1 shows the hand of a 48-year-old man with rheumatoid disease, which he says has 'some bruises'.
   a. What is the problem?
   b. What does this mean in terms of the disease?
2. A 65-year-old man developed a very painful joint (Picture 8.2). He has had several attacks in the past affecting different joints and is supposed to be on treatment to reduce the frequency of the attacks but has not been taking it regularly.
   a. What is the diagnosis?
   b. What treatment should he have been taking?
   c. How should you treat this attack?
   d. What precipitating factors should you ask about?
   e. What treatment should be given?
3. Picture 8.3 is a CT scan of the lower chest on 'bone windows' to demonstrate bone and soft tissue defects. The descending aorta is seen just to the left of centre.
   a. Looking at it, what might you estimate of the patient's age to be?
   Just posterior to the aorta is some abnormal 'tissue' in front of the vertebrae with an outpouching slightly to the right of centre adjacent to this abnormal area:
   b. What do you think this might be?
   c. What is the correct term for this?
   The adjacent vertebra:
   d. Is it normal?
   e. What would you call this?
   f. Give a differential diagnosis
   g. State your plan of investigation knowing that the spine was not unstable and that there were no focal neurological signs but the patient was in great pain (requiring morphine).
4. Picture 8.4 is a radiograph of the lower leg of an 80-year-old man who has been admitted to an elderly care ward because of immobility. He complains of pain in the left knee.
   a. Describe the abnormalities.
   b. What is the diagnosis?

c. What biochemical tests would support the diagnosis?
d. What imaging investigation would you use to assess how extensively his bones are affected?
e. How could you treat him?

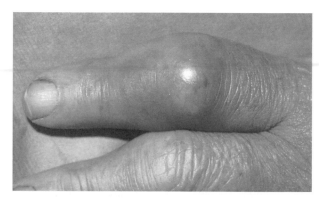

Picture 8.2

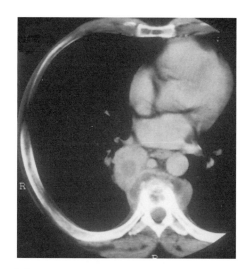

Picture 8.3

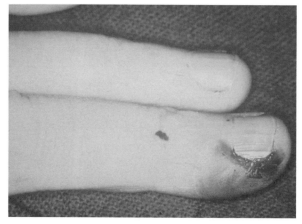

Picture 8.1

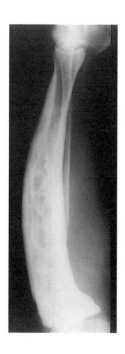

Picture 8.4

Short notes

1. In a patient with a symmetrical polyarthritis, what, apart from asking about joint problems, would you want to ask about and why?

2. In a patient suspected of having temporal arteritis, outline your immediate and, presuming the diagnosis is confirmed, long-term management plans.

3. Which investigations should you request in a person with an acute symmetrical polyarthritis? Given that the diagnosis is rheumatoid arthritis, what abnormalities might there be in the investigations that you ordered?

4. Outline how you would approach the management of a patient with rheumatoid arthritis.

5. You are asked to see a 77-year-old woman with known osteoarthritis in Casualty. She has been reasonably well but 3 days earlier she had noticed some pain in her calf which had progressed. Now her calf is swollen, indurated and tender with increased local warmth. What is the differential diagnosis and what investigations would you request?

6. A 45-year-old patient presents with right wrist drop. He has weakness of dorsiflexion of his left foot and he has also been complaining of some diplopia on looking to the right. Generally, he has not been very well for a few months with some weight loss and abdominal pain. What is the differential diagnosis? What is the basis for this? What investigations would you carry out and why?

7. Write short notes on:
   a. The symptoms of hypercalcaemia.
   b. The factors which predispose to osteoporosis.
   c. How you would manage a patient with severe hypercalcaemia?
   d. How you would manage a patient with severe hypocalcaemia?

Self-assessment: answers

Multiple choice answers

1. a. **False**. A consequence of cyclo-oxygenase blockade is a reduction in intrarenal generation of prostaglandins, which causes a deterioration in renal function.
   b. **True**. The change in renal function results in hyperkalaemia.
   c. **True**. There is a clear relationship between NSAID use and complications such as perforation, bleeding and death particularly in old people.
   d. **False**. NSAIDs relieve inflammation; they do not influence disease progression.
   e. **False**. A consequence of NSAID action is increased leucotriene production; these are powerful bronchoconstrictors.

2. a. **True**. Disease activity is monitored by measuring ESR or plasma viscosity.
   b. **False**. Some patients may have arthralgia but there is no damage to the joints.
   c. **False**. Weight loss is characteristic of polymyalgia rheumatica.
   d. **True**. A muscle biopsy may show patchy vasculitis; however, it is not a useful diagnostic test.
   e. **True**. Pain during mastication is a characteristic feature of temporal arteritis.

3. a. **True**.
   b. **True**.
   c. **True**. This is one of the typical blood dyscrasias seen.
   d. **True**. As with thrombocytopenia.
   e. **False**. Characteristically the C-reactive protein is normal; if high then another cause should be sought (e.g. infection).

4. a. **False**. They are directed against the Fc fragment of IgG.
   b. **True**. Nodules are associated with high titres of rheumatoid factor.
   c. **False**. It is not diagnostic of rheumatoid disease (for example, it can occur in endocarditis).
   d. **False**. The antibody is usually of the IgM class against normal IgG (sometimes it is IgG against IgG).
   e. **False**.

5. a. **True**. There are no haematological abnormalities.
   b. **False**. Bouchard's nodes are osteoarthritis of the PIP joints.
   c. **False**. Erosions are typical of rheumatoid disease.
   d. **False**. It should not last longer than 30 minutes.
   e. **True**. This is common, resulting in 'squaring' of the hand.

6. a. **False**. Tophi indicate chronic deposition of urate.
   b. **False**. Use of allopurinol would make an acute attack worse by stimulating the tissue mobilisation of water.
   c. **False**. Frusemide causes urate retention. Bumetanide is better
   d. **False**. After the big toe, the ankle and knees may be affected.
   e. **False**. Raised serum urate *supports* the diagnosis; you need to demonstrate crystals within the synovial fluid for a definitive diagnosis.

7. a. **True**. There is close correlation between nail psoriasis and DIP involvement.
   b. **False**. The joint involvement is characteristically *asymmetrical*.
   c. **True**. Joint involvement can be severe: 'mutilans'.
   d. **False**. Sacroiliitis occurs but only in about one-third of patients.
   e. **False**. Temporomandibular joint involvement is characteristic of *rheumatoid disease*.

8. a. **False**. It is three to four times more common in men.
   b. **True**. Commonly affects several joints and often presents with back pain.
   c. **False**. It is associated with HLA-B27.
   d. **True**. It is associated with upper lobe fibrosis and aortic incompetence.
   e. **False**. The hands and feet are not affected.

9. a. **True**. A clear viscous fluid.
   b. **False**. The presence of pyrophosphate crystals is indicative of gout.
   c. **False**. The viscosity is high.
   d. **False**. Fibrin is indicative of disease.
   e. **False**.

10. a. **True**.
    b. **True**. Systemic features are indicative of severe disease.
    c. **True**. Rheumatoid nodules are pathognomonic for the disease and are associated with high levels of rheumatoid factor.
    d. **True**. Erosions, particularly their early appearance, predict a poor prognosis.
    e. **False**.

11. a. **False**. It is less likely to be septic arthritis than a monoarthritis but septic oligoarthritis is quite common. It does rule out tuberculous arthritis, however. If joints are affected sequentially, consider rheumatic fever and Lyme disease (or reactive arthritis), if together consider gonococcus, rubella and parvovirus.

b. **False**. The keys to successful management and to preserve the joint cartilage are i.v. antibiotic treatment, joint aspiration to dryness, repeated at least daily and resting of the joint.

c. **False**. Rubella and parvovirus are common causes.

d. **False**. Although it would be unusual in a young, previously well person; it is more common with advancing age.

e. **True**. Not always with an acute presentation.

12. a. **True**. It is often difficult to remove all dead infected bone.

b. **True**. Virtually always and it is a useful marker of response to treatment and relapse.

c. **True**. Although there are other causes of a sinus including actinomycosis, implanted foreign body (such as shrapnel), mycetoma (fungal soft tissue and bony infection of the leg in the tropics).

d. **False**. If *S. aureus* is grown, this is helpful, but otherwise there is no relationship at all between bony cultures and sinus cultures.

e. **False**. Usually 3–6 weeks of i.v. therapy followed by 4–12 weeks of oral therapy is necessary and even then this often fails. Longer treatment is necessary for chronic osteomyelitis. It always fails if dead bone or metalwork remains.

13. a. **True**.
b. **True**.
c. **True**.
d. **False**.
e. **False**.

14. a. **True**. It usually occurs 3–12 weeks after the episode of diarrhoea.

b. **False**. It is self-limiting over several weeks or occasionally months.

c. **False**. It is helpful if it can be done but failure does not rule out the diagnosis.

d. **True**.

e. **True**. However, this is usually easy, as the flitting polyarthropathy seen in rheumatic fever is *not* characteristic of reactive arthritis, which usually afflicts large joints and does not 'move around'.

15. a. **False**. They are intimately interrelated.

b. **False**. Plasma calcium is regulated independently of dietary intake.

c. **True**. However, because osteoblasts and osteoclasts are 'coupled' as bone remodelling units, diseases which increase the activity of one will increase the activity of the other, and alkaline phosphatase may increase even in diseases which primarily activate osteoclasts (such as metastatic cancer).

d. **True**. It is secreted by osteoblasts.

e. **True**. This is one of the main pathophysiological processes in renal bone disease, lowering serum calcium and secondarily 'activating' parathyroid hormone secretion.

16. a. **False**. Osteoporosis rarely causes hypercalcaemia unless the patient is immobile.

b. **True**. Sarcoidosis, tuberculosis, berylliosis and other granulomatous diseases all cause increased vitamin D synthesis in the granulomata.

c. **True**. PTH increases renal phosphate excretion and lowers serum phosphate. The exception to this is renal bone disease in which the parathyroid glands may become autonomous (tertiary hyperparathyroidism) and cause hypercalcaemia with hyperphosphataemia, but this is very much the exception rather than the rule.

d. **False**. See the answer to (c).

e. **True**. Haematological malignancies are a close second to solid tumours as a cause of malignant hypercalcaemia.

17. a. **True**. Unlike osteomalacia where bone mineral only is reduced.

b. **False**. It peaks in early adult life, around age 25.

c. **True**. Weight-bearing exercise protects against bone loss and immobility exacerbates it; this can become a vicious circle for osteoporotic patients immobilised by fractures.

d. **False**. Steroids **reduce** bone mass.

e. **False**. Severe hypogonadism (as in hypopituitarism and some genetic disorders) can cause osteoporosis even in young adult life.

18. a. **True**. Both acute and chronic hypocalcaemia may present with epilepsy.

b. **False**. The bedside tests are insensitive and have been largely superseded by availability of calcium measurements as an emergency.

c. **False**. Calcitonin is used for treating *hyper*calcaemia.

d. **True**. In prolonged disease.

e. **False**. PTH is only available for diagnostic and research purposes. Hypocalcaemia, whatever its cause, is treated with vitamin D.

Case history answers

History 1

1. The differential diagnosis is:
   - staphylococcal septic arthritis (slightly less likely if two joints)
   - gonococcal arthritis (need sexual history)
   - Reiter's syndrome
   - reactive arthritis
   - parvovirus infection (less likely as knee inflamed)
   - mild haemophilia (fever against that diagnosis).

2. Sexual contact history and urethral discharge and any other symptoms now or recently, relevant to parvovirus or reactive arthritis (e.g. diarrhoea, rash, prodromal illness, etc.).
3. Investigations:
   - joint aspiration for cells and Gram stain and culture (including *N. gonorrhoeae)*
   - blood culture
   - white cell count
   - parvovirus serology (IgM).

History 2

Note the symptoms of hypercalcaemia and bone symptoms (backache). Apply the same principles as under the data interpretation questions.

1. Phosphate, urea, creatinine, alkaline phosphatase, sodium, potassium and bicarbonate are all needed. In a seriously ill patient, the immediate priority is to measure renal function and electrolytes to guide emergency management; assessment of acid/base status may also be needed if there is renal failure. Phosphate and alkaline phosphatase are needed to explore the differential diagnosis.
2. Malignant disease or hyperparathyroidism are the most likely diagnoses. Other causes are rare.
3. The first priority is to assess the patient's state of hydration; he is likely to be volume-depleted. Saline will increase renal perfusion and increase calcium excretion. If that alone fails to control hypercalcaemia rapidly, a bisphosphonate can be given, even if the diagnosis is not firmly established, because it reduces osteoclastic bone resorption. The remainder of the management plan will be to diagnose and treat the underlying disease.

Data interpretation

If this appears difficult, look first at the calcium (high, low, normal?), second at the phosphate (is it changed in the opposite direction from calcium, as might be expected if the primary problem was parathyroid over- or underactivity), then at urea and creatinine to see if there is renal failure (remember this could be the primary disease or a secondary effect of hypercalcaemia) and finally at the alkaline phosphatase (is there bone involvement?).

Patient 1. The main abnormalities are a raised calcium and lowered phosphate, characteristic of hyperparathyroidism. The raised alkaline phosphatase indicates parathyroid bone disease and the raised urea with normal serum creatinine suggests volume depletion, which could lead to renal failure.

Patient 2. Here, both phosphate and calcium are high. Both urea and creatinine are also high. There is phosphate retention and renal failure. One interpretation might be tertiary hyperparathyroidism in a patient with longstanding renal failure, but it would be surprising for alkaline phosphatase to be relatively nor-

mal. Malignancy such as myeloma is another possibility. An interesting feature of myeloma is that osteoblastic activity is 'paralysed' despite increased osteoclastic activity so alkaline phosphatase may be normal despite widespread bone disease.

Patient 3. Hypocalcaemia, but serum phosphate is low. This must mean that parathyroid function is intact and tending to correct hypocalcaemia caused by some other disease. A likely cause is vitamin D deficiency. Note that serum alkaline phosphatase is somewhat raised. This is evidence of secondary parathyroid bone disease. Longstanding osteomalacia would be a good explanation for these results.

Patient 4. Here serum calcium is low and phosphate is high. The diagnosis is hypoparathyroidism.

Patient 5. In this case, all parameters are normal except alkaline phosphatase. There is increased osteoblastic activity. This would be normal for a growing child or during fracture healing. In an otherwise asymptomatic adult, think of Paget's disease.

Patient 6. This patient is mildly hypocalcaemic, has moderate hyperphosphataemia, renal failure and a raised alkaline phosphatase. A likely diagnosis is renal bone disease.

Picture answers

1. a. He has a vasculitis with typical localised areas of infarction.
   b. The presence of a vasculitis indicates aggressive disease with a much poorer prognosis.
2. a. He has gout. The site is non-typical, but in a patient who has had multiple attacks, then joints other than the first MTP may be involved.
   b. Allopurinol.
   c. The diagnosis, given this history, can be made on clinical grounds. If in doubt, aspirate the joint looking for crystals.
   d. There are a number of causes which might precipitate gout (p. 313). In relation to common factors, ask about change in drug treatment (e.g. prescription of frusemide).
   e. The treatment would be to rest the joint and prescribe an NSAID such as naproxen. An alternative would be colchicine.
3. a. No calcification, therefore probably < 40 years.
   b. Abscess (not consistent with lymphadenopathy as variable intensity).
   c. Paraspinal abscess.
   d. No.
   e. Vertebral osteomyelitis.
   f. Most common organisms are *Staphylococcus aureus*, anaerobes and Gram-negative rods such as *Escherichia coli* and *Mycobacterium tuberculosis*.
   g. Aspiration of abscess contents or bone under CT guidance; blood cultures; 'work up' for cause of infection and tuberculosis, e.g. urine cultures and ultrasound search for dental sepsis, Heaf test, chest X-ray and sputum for acid-fast bacilli, etc.

In fact, this white patient from Salford of 37 years had an 18 month history of increasing back pain and turned out to have a tuberculous paraspinal abscess.

3. a. The tibia is bowed and widened, the cortex is thickened and the bone texture is irregular with patchy sclerosis. There is deformity of the knee joint.

   b. Paget's disease of bone.

   c. Raised alkaline phosphatase; raised urinary hydroxyproline:creatinine ratio.

   d. A radionuclide bone scan is the investigation of choice; plain radiography could also be used.

   e. Bisphosphonate therapy reduces bone remodelling and is likely to relieve pain, although the deformity and any secondary osteoarthrosis in the knee will not improve.

Short notes answers

1. You would need information about systemic features, including non-specific symptoms and those pointing to involvement of a particular system (e.g. mononeuritis). You should ask about the family history and any other possible aetiological factors (for example inflammatory bowel disease). Take great care and time (using the patient's notes and, in many instances, phoning the GP) to document previous drug treatment (see pp. 303–304).

2. A patient with suspected temporal arteritis is a medical emergency. The diagnosis is based on the history, examination and very high ESR. If these all fit together then high-dose steroids should be started *immediately*. The response within 24 hours can be regarded as a diagnostic test. The longer-term management is outlined on page 311.

3. The investigations should include: full and differential blood count, ESR (or plasma viscosity), C-reactive protein, urea, creatinine, rheumatoid factor, antinuclear antibodies, chest radiograph and radiographs of hands and feet. It may be necessary to exclude gout and septic arthritis if a single joint is particularly affected. Details of the abnormalities within these investigations are discussed on page 300.

4. The main concept is overall management of a person with a potentially disabling condition. Adequate opportunity for discussion of the disease and what it means are going to be very important. A team approach is essential and the expertise of the professions allied to medicine must be used. Aids for daily living and mobility may be required. The drug therapy will range from simple analgesia and NSAIDs to suppress inflammation to the introduction of disease-modifying agents (including low-dose corticosteroids). This would involve specialist care and careful monitoring of the disease and response to therapy (p. 304).

5. The history is consistent with a deep vein thrombosis, particularly as the patient may be immobile and inactive. Request a venogram and a chest radiograph (evidence of emboli). In a patient with osteoarthritis, it is very important to think of a **Baker's cyst** (see p. 314). This is best demonstrated using arthrography or ultrasound. The management of a ruptured cyst is rest and analgesia.

6. The history is diagnostic of a mononeuritis multiplex. He has involvement of the radial, lateral popliteal and sixth cranial nerve. This, together with the abdominal pain, malaise and weight loss is consistent with polyarteritis nodosa (p. 311), but it is a rare condition. The diagnosis can be confirmed by arteriography and biopsy.

   The more important aspect of this case is recognising the characteristic pattern of a mononeuritis: isolated nerves being 'picked off' which cannot be accounted for by a single lesion, whereas a metabolic (toxic) peripheral neuropathy would cause a symmetrical pattern.

   The differential diagnosis is the causes of mononeuritis multiplex; of which the most likely is a vasculitis. Diabetes mellitus can cause a mononeuritis and the general features would fit (e.g. malaise, weight loss) so a blood sugar level is needed. However, it would be most unusual for a diabetic patient to develop multiple nerve lesions simultaneously. Many of the connective tissue diseases such as SLE and rheumatoid arthritis may present with a vasculitis. The history, examination and investigations need to be tailored accordingly. A full blood count, ESR, urea and electrolytes (renal impairment), antinuclear antibodies and rheumatoid factor should be requested (p. 300).

7. a. See page 317. Think of volume depletion and 'stones, bones and abdominal moans':
   Renal
      Thirst, polyuria, nocturia, light-headedness (due to volume depletion); symptoms of stones in some cases
   Intestinal
      Nausea, vomiting, constipation, dyspepsia
   Neurological
      Lassitude, depression and confusion.

   b. See page 319. Approach this by thinking of the factors needed to attain and maintain a normal bone mass — normal sex-steroid levels, activity and adequate dietary calcium — and the factors, particularly hormonal, which can reduce bone mass:
      Hypogonadism or early menopause
      Immobility or chronic debilitating disease
      Endocrine excess: corticosteroid therapy, hyperparathyroidism, Cushing's or hyperthyroidism
      Neoplasia, particularly myeloma
      Malnutrition, malabsorption
      Rheumatological disease, particularly rheumatoid arthritis
      Alcohol abuse.

c. See page 317. This is covered in detail in the text. Priorities are:
   • Adequate volume replacement
   • Establishment of the diagnosis
   • Control of hypercalcaemia with bisphosphonate.
d. See page 318. You need to know this to the level of detail given in the emergency box, page 318. In summary:

• Establish venous access and take blood for diagnostic tests
• Give 10% calcium gluconate, 10 ml intravenously over 10 minutes
• Call for senior help
• Repeat intravenous calcium as needed.

Immunology and HIV infection

9.1 **Clinical aspects**

Introduction

The immune system is stupendously intricate and defies full understanding for the majority of practising doctors. Nonetheless it is vital for you to have a grasp of the fundamentals so as to recognise immunodeficiency and immune overactivity and then diagnose and treat your future patients effectively. It is possible to grasp and remember the principles with a few key facts and to use this knowledge effectively. In this chapter, the presentation of basic immunology is very clinically orientated to aid memory and understanding.

There are many parts to the normal immune system but all can be divided into non-specific defences and targeted defences (Table 71). The distinction is somewhat artificial as, for example, neutrophil activity (a non-specific defence) is substantially enhanced by the presence of antibody (a targeted defence mechanism). Therefore, although this division provides a starting point for learning, in reality there are substantial interactions between one defence system and another for most infections and in the pathogenesis of autoimmune disease.

Learning objectives

You need:
- to understand the major types of immunodeficiency
- to know the major categories of compromised patient
- to know the particular infectious problems they suffer from.

Terminology

The following terms are important to understand.

Immunodeficient refers to patients who have a clear immunological deficit, whether genetic, acquired or iatrogenic. Examples include neutropenia, AIDS, organ transplantation, corticosteroid treatment at more than replacement dose, etc.

Compromised refers to acutely or chronically ill patients who are at greater risk of infection by virtue of damaged barriers against infection, age, or relatively non-specific defects such as surgery. Examples are shown in Table 72.

Defects in humoral immunity

Patients may have complement deficiency (rarely) or immunoglobulin deficiency.

Complement deficiency

Complement refers to 19 plasma and about 10 membrane proteins. They range in size from 25 000 to 400 000 Da and the plasma complement is mostly produced by the liver. Therefore, severe liver disease or glomerulonephritis may lead to low circulating complement. Low complement levels may also be found in SLE and are a guide to the severity of disease.

The primary functions of complement are:

- killing of microorganisms, especially bacteria
- clearance of immune complexes.

The complement components form part of cascades leading to immune activation, just like coagulation. The cascades form two separate pathways — the **classical** and the **alternative** — which meet in a **common** third pathway. Deficiencies of the components of the classical pathway lead to both immune complex disease and/or recurrent infection, whereas deficiency of the alternative pathway leads only to recurrent infection. C3 is the anchor for the whole system and if deficient (which is rare) 70–80% of individuals suffer either or both of immune complex disease or recurrent infection. Immune complex disease in complement deficiency includes SLE, glomerulonephritis and vasculitis.

Isolated deficiency of components of the terminal attack complex, C5–C9, also leads to a predisposition to infection. These C5–C9 deficiencies can be screened for simply by measuring total haemolytic complement (CH50), which will be reduced. Infections are usually caused by *N. meningitidis* and typically manifest as meningitis (on multiple occasions) or a more chronic form known as chronic meningococcaemia (rash, fever and arthritis with positive blood cultures). Other encapsulated bacteria e.g. *S. pneumoniae* can also be a problem.

Table 71 Key components of the immune system

	Nonspecific defences	Targeted defences defences	Hypersensitivity
Cellular	Barriers against infection, e.g. skin	T lymphocytes B lymphocytes	Mast cells
	Neutrophils Macrophages Natural killer (NK) cells Cytotoxic T cells Eosinophils		
Humoral	Complement Interferons Cytokines	Antibodies	IgE antibodies

Table 72 Examples of 'non-immunological' immune deficiency states (compromised patients) and risks for specific infection

Underlying conditions	Infections found at higher frequency or in a more severe form
Old age	Pneumonia, urinary tract infection, skin and soft tissue infection, influenza
Pregnancy (2nd–3rd trimester)	Varicella pneumonia, pyelonephritis, serious bacterial infection
Alcoholic cirrhosis	Tuberculosis, pneumococcal and aspiration pneumonia, spontaneous bacterial peritonitis, invasive aspergillosis
Diabetes mellitus	Pyelonephritis, mucosal candidiasis, candidaemia, tuberculosis, cellulitis and osteomyelitis of feet, staphylococcal infection, invasive aspergillosis
Influenza	Staphylococcal pneumonia
Malnutrition	Pneumonia, skin sepsis, *Pneumocystis carinii* pneumonia
Chronic renal failure	Tuberculosis, bacteraemia, urinary tract infection, candidaemia
Iron overload/desferrioxamine therapy	*Yersinia* and *Listeria* infections and zygomycosis
Intensive care unit	Ventilator pneumonia, bacteraemia, especially *Staphylococcus*, *Enterococcus* spp. and candidaemia, sinusitis
GI surgery	Peritonitis, pelvic or subdiaphragmatic abscess, pneumonia, candidaemia
Pancreatitis	Peritonitis, candidaemia
Burns	Streptococcal, *Pseudomonas* and other bacterial infection, *Candida*, *Aspergillus* and *Zygomyces* spp. infection

Antibody deficiency

There are four major classes of antibody: IgA, IgE, IgG and IgM. Immunoglobulin deficiencies or dysfunction are relatively common.

IgA deficiency

There are three forms of IgA, IgA1, IgA2 and a dimer of two molecules, usually of IgA2, which together form secretory IgA. The first is the predominant form found in serum, making up 15–20% of the total immunoglobulin pool. Secretory IgA is produced by plasma cells in mucosal surfaces and binds microorganisms on the body's surface. Isolated IgA deficiency is found in 1 in 700 Caucasians and only rarely in other groups. IgA-deficient individuals are more prone to develop respiratory, GI tract and genitourinary tract bacterial infections but not viral infections. A higher incidence of cow's milk allergy, autoantibodies and autoimmune diseases has been noted. IgA-deficient patients are also much more prone to develop anaphylaxis. Complete absence of IgA through hypercatabolism also occurs in the rare **ataxia telangiectasia syndrome**.

IgG deficiency (hypogammaglobulinaemia)

IgG comprises the main circulating and extravascular antibody. There are four subtypes: IgG1, IgG2, IgG3 and IgG4. These are present in blood in a ratio approximately of 18:6:2:1, respectively. IgG1 and IgG3 are critically important for activation of complement after antigen binding. IgG2 is particularly important for defence against bacteria with capsules, such as *S. pneumoniae* and deficiency leads to recurrent invasive infections with these organisms. IgG binds efficiently to Gram-positive bacteria but less so to Gram-negative bacteria, which are better bound by IgM.

Clinical presentation

There are a number of immunoglobulin deficiency diseases, some inherited, some acquired and each of variable degree. Acquired hypogammaglobulinaemia (or common variable immunodeficiency) presents in adulthood with recurrent infections, usually of minor degree. However, unusual infections such as invasive *Campylobacter* or *Mycoplasma* spp. infections are a clue to the diagnosis. Usually these patients have a low total globulin. Ironically, they may also produce many autoantibodies and have a number of autoimmune diseases such as haemolytic anaemia, pernicious anaemia and alopecia areata. In women with hypogammaglobulinaemia, there is a 400-fold increase in lymphoma in middle age. All of these disorders require i.v. immunoglobulin replacement therapy and sometimes antibiotic prophylaxis. Infusions are given about every 3 weeks for life.

Cellular immune deficiency

The major defects in cellular immunity are neutropenia and T helper (T$_H$) cell deficiency (AIDS). However, none of these defects are pure as there are so many interdependent immune mechanisms. Neutropenia is described on page 239. The next sections covers the major cellular forms of immunodeficiency:

- immunodeficiency following splenectomy
- macrophage defects
- T4 (CD4) cell deficiency (HIV and AIDS)
- rejection and immunosuppression after transplantation.

Investigating immune deficiency

A careful synthesis of historical information from the patient and the medical notes is the first step in evaluating immune deficiency. You can then arrange appropriate investigations. There is no simple 'immune function screen' which acts like an investigative sieve. A guide to appropriate investigations in patients not already known to be immunodeficient is shown in Table 73. These tests should generally be done when the patient has improved from an episode of infection with the exception of T cell subsets and HIV antibody tests, which should be done as soon as HIV infection or AIDS is seriously considered. In most cases, these initial screening tests will be normal. You may need to refer the patient to a clinical immunologist or other specialist for further advice.

9.2 Cellular immune deficiency

Immunodeficiency following splenectomy

The largest lymphoid organ is the spleen, followed by the thymus and then lymph glands and the mucosal lymphoid system. The spleen has three major functions:

- removal of old platelets and red cells from the circulation
- lymphocyte processing and maturation
- phagocytosis of encapsulated bacteria and fungi.

There are several circumstances in which the spleen is completely or partially non-functional:

- removal after trauma or for treatment of ITP
- sickle cell disease
- coeliac disease.

The haematological features of splenic dysfunction are described on page 229. Patients with no spleen have a 50 times greater risk of developing overwhelming sepsis with encapsulated bacteria such as *S. pneumoniae*, *H. influenzae* and *N. meningitidis* or after a dog bite. Bacteraemia is so rapidly progressive in these patients that 50–80% die, usually within 3–5 days. Protection must be offered with vaccines and lifelong penicillin, even though not fully protective.

Monocytes and macrophage defects

Monocytes develop into tissue macrophages and, therefore, they can be considered together for clinical purposes. In the brain, microglial cells function partly as macrophages. Macrophages have several functions:

- cytokine production
- phagocytosis of bacteria and fungi
- antigen presentation to T cells.

Macrophage phagocytosis proceeds much as neutrophil phagocytosis does. One particular function that splenic macrophages normally fulfill admirably is the phagocytosis of antibody-coated bacteria. These bacteria are recognised by virtue of a receptor on macrophages (FCγ) An increased number of bacterial infections occurs if this receptor is functionally impaired as in:

- alcoholic cirrhosis
- end-stage renal disease
- SLE.

There are some organisms that are able to evade intracellular killing in macrophages. Examples include *Salmonella*, mycobacteria, *Histoplasma*, *Leishmania* spp. and *Mycobacterium leprae*. The adaptive mechanisms each organism has developed to achieve this are fascinating. However, the practical consequences of this include:

- carrier states (e.g. typhoid)

Table 73 Investigations in patients known to be immunodeficient

Problem	Investigation
Recurrent infection (e.g. pneumonia, sinusitis)	Igs (especially IgA) IgG subsets (especially IgG2) Neutrophil count, blood film (for features of lack of spleen)
Recurrent meningococcal infection	C3, C4 and CH50, Igs
Progressive (and relatively silent) staphylococcal or other infection (e.g. invasive aspergillosis)	Igs, neutrophil function tests
Oral candidiasis, 'pneumonia', other unusual infections with weight loss	T cell subsets, HIV antibody test, Igs
Chronic diarrhoea (? infection) with weight loss	Igs, T cell subsets, HIV antibody test
Unusually invasive or difficult infections	Igs, T cell subsets
Unexplained weight loss (≥ 10% body weight)	T cell subsets, HIV antibody test

Ig = immunoglobulin

- emergence of infection during immunosuppression (e.g. toxoplasmosis)
- long latency between infection and disease (e.g. tuberculosis, histoplasmosis, leprosy)
- need for drugs to penetrate and kill inside the macrophage phagosome.

Neutropenia caused by cytotoxic chemotherapy is also a marker for monocytopenia and, therefore, reduced tissue macrophage numbers. This combined cellular deficiency is partly what makes neutropenic patients so immuno-compromised. In addition, macrophage function is impaired by corticosteroids. Macrophage function is also grossly defective in AIDS, at least partly because of a lack of activation by T4 cells. Macrophage function is substantially improved after activation and, as with neutrophils, γ-interferon is a potent macrophage activator.

T4 cell deficiency

T cells are thymus-derived lymphocytes. There are many different types. Each type can be distinguished functionally and by cell surface (CD) markers. The main subtypes are:

- T helper cells (T4⁺ cells)
- T suppressor and cytotoxic cells (T8⁺ cells)
- TCR-1 cells (T cells carrying T cell receptor-1).

T4 cells have a number of critically important functions in the immune system. These include:

- recognition of processed antigens and clonal expansion
- detailed control of the cellular immune response
- generation of cytokines, which stimulate other cell types
- regulation of IgE production by plasma cells.

Several disease states cause a fall in T4 cells. The most profound is AIDS, but many severe illnesses will cause them to fall including, for example, measles. The cell counts are often slightly low in chronically ill patients and lower still in lymphoma and sarcoidosis patients.

9.3 HIV infection

Learning objectives

HIV infection, leading to AIDS, is now common throughout the world. AIDS was first recognised as a clinical entity in the early 1980s. Worldwide, over 30 million people are now infected. You must know how HIV and AIDS presents clinically and how to handle questions and concerns regarding HIV infection. To do this, you need a basic understanding of how HIV is transmitted and how it causes immune dysfunction. You need:

- to understand the basic elements of HIV reproduction and pathogenesis

- to know the important risk factors for HIV transmission
- to be cognisant of the major issues in counselling patients for HIV antibody testing
- to know how HIV disease progresses
- to know the important landmarks of T4 cell decline and action to be taken
- to know the clinical features of the common AIDS indicator diseases
- to grasp the importance of combination antiretroviral therapy.

Epidemiology

The retroviruses

Only four human retroviruses are known, human lymphotrophic viruses (HTLV) 1 and 2 and human immunodeficiency viruses (HIV) 1 and 2. It is likely that new human retroviruses will be discovered. They are all single-stranded RNA enveloped viruses. They are called *retro*viruses, i.e. backwards, because they carry an enzyme called reverse transcriptase which copies the RNA genes of the virus into DNA and this DNA is then integrated into the host cell's chromosomes.

HIV transmission

The primary modes of transmission of HIV are:

- unprotected sex
- blood transmission, e.g. drug addicts, infected blood products
- mother to child (vertical).

The risk of acquisition of HIV is lower than for hepatitis B following a needlestick exposure by a factor of approximately 1000-fold.

The modes of transmission in individual countries and different social groups within those countries is very variable. In the UK, the majority of HIV cases are in gay men, with a smaller number related to intravenous drug abuse. An increasing number of cases are in heterosexuals, some as a result of sexual exposures abroad. In contrast, in France there is a significant heterosexual component to HIV transmission and approximately one-third of French cases are related to heterosexual sex. In Italy, by contrast, the disease is spread primarily in drug addicts and among gay men, with a much smaller heterosexual component. In Africa, heterosexual sex has played the greatest role in transmission, resulting in much vertical transmission (mother to child) and some cases related to blood transmission and/or infected needles. In Thailand and north India, intravenous drug abuse is the primary culprit and in both cases there were explosive outbreaks resulting in several thousand infected individuals in a single year. Many of these individuals are from very poor communities and involved in the sex trade, and so transmission into the heterosexual population is assured.

High-risk behaviour

There are certain aspects of behaviour which increase the risk of transmission. Studies have shown, for example, that the risk of transmission of male to female is greater than female to male. Other factors are:

- higher risk of transmission
  — genital ulceration
  — not circumcised (men)
  — receptive anal intercourse (both sexes)
- lower risk of transmission
  — use of condom
  — vaginal intercourse
  — oral sex, kissing

'Safe sex' denotes stroking and massage, kissing and the use of condoms for any form of penetrative sex.

With respect to transmission by needles, the volume of blood that is exchanged is an important parameter. Most drug addicts using a syringe and needle draw back blood into the syringe before injecting their drug suspension. The drawing back and mixing of blood within the syringe and needle is a critical element in transmission between individuals. Needle exchange systems, which are in place in many cities in the world, are very important in the prevention of most epidemics of new HIV infections in these cities. There is some difficulty in provision of needles in the prison population and this certainly remains a potential reservoir of new infections. The US prison population has a 14-fold higher HIV seroprevalence rate than the general population.

Transmission in the health-care setting

For health-care workers who suffer a needlestick injury, the risk of HIV transmission related to solid needles (such as are used in surgery for sutures) is considerably reduced compared with hollow needles for taking blood or giving i.v. fluids. In addition, the (inadvertent) injection of blood at the same time as a needlestick injury imposes the greatest risk. The overall numerical risk of a health-care worker acquiring HIV following a needlestick infection is approximately 1 in 250 such incidents. The administration of anti-retroviral therapy immediately after a needlestick injury does partially protect individuals likely to acquire HIV infection. A mucosal splash with HIV-infected blood constitutes a negligible risk unless the skin is broken, for example by eczema.

HIV reproduction

Retroviruses reproduce by utilising the host cell's normal processes of transcription and translation to produce multiple virus particles. Reproduction of the virus proceeds in host cells at a variable pace. HIV may:

- be latent and not reproduce
- reproduce slowly with release of virus from the surface of the cell

- accelerate its own production with death of the host cell.

Understanding what controls the rate of HIV reproduction is central to an understanding of AIDS.

Entry of the virus into host cells requires cell receptors including the T4 surface molecule on lymphocytes, neural and other cells. About one in 10 Caucasians and one in 50 black people are resistant to HIV infection, despite exposure, because they lack an essential receptor protein. Once the virus has entered the cell and reverse transcriptase has transcribed the viral RNA into the host DNA, that cell is then infected for its life.

Initial infection, so-called primary HIV infection, is characterised by very high levels of circulating virus. As virus reproduction declines, the total viral burden falls and HIV antibody becomes detectable. At this stage, there is usually only one detectable strain of HIV. As the disease progresses, multiple mutants (strains) of the virus arise which have different biological properties, including preferences for different cell types (e.g. brain versus lymphocytes). These strains arise because there is no 'proof-reading capability' following RNA transcription during HIV reproduction so 1 to 40 DNA base errors are made during each reproduction cycle. Viral mutation has several important consequences:

- multiple related strains are present in a single person simultaneously
- different HIV strains are more or less pathogenic
- different HIV strains have a greater or less affinity for different tissues
- Resistance to antiretroviral therapy may occur quickly.

The amount of circulating HIV can be measured by precisely determining the viral RNA circulating in the blood (viral load). In the first few months after primary infection, determination of the viral load predicts how

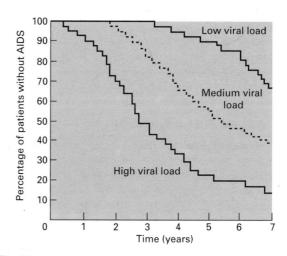

Fig. 64
Viral load shortly after primary HIV infection predicts the development of AIDS and survival. The first deaths in the high viral load group occur within a year of primary infection, whereas in the low viral load groups they start to occur nearly five years after primary infection.

fast that individual will progress to AIDS (Fig. 64). This has important consequences for when treatment should be started.

Control of HIV infection

For months or years after primary HIV infection, viral replication is partially controlled by mechanisms which are incompletely understood but include T8 cells. With time, the protective mechanisms slowly deteriorate and viral replication increases. The most clinically useful marker of increasing viral reproduction is the slow but inexorable decline in the T4 cell count in an initially asymptomatic patient. At the same time, there is gradual destruction of lymph node architecture, with increasing amounts of virus detectable in lymph nodes and peripheral blood, measured by viral load. Loss of cerebral matter and function is also detectable at lower T4 cell counts (e.g. $< 100 \times 10^6/l$).

Clinical stages of HIV infection

There are several stages of HIV infection (Table 74). Patients may present at any of the stages.

Primary HIV infection

Over 50% of those who acquire HIV infection suffer an illness shortly before seroconversion. This is known as primary HIV infection. The incubation period varies from 7–14 days. The clues to the diagnosis include neutropenia, thrombocytopenia, headache and diarrhoea (see Box 11). Oral, oesophageal or genital ulceration is also typical and the ulcers are highly infectious.

Diagnosis. At the time of a primary HIV infection, a person's HIV antibody test will be negative although their HIV p24 antigen test should be positive. A retest 2–4 weeks after the primary infection for HIV antibody will usually detect seroconversion, although there are rare instances of delayed seroconversion (retest after 6 months).

Prognosis. Patients who suffer an overt clinical illness of primary HIV infection progress to AIDS more rapidly than those with a silent primary HIV infection.

> **Box 11**
> **Clinical and laboratory features of primary HIV infection**
>
> | Clinical | Laboratory |
> |---|---|
> | Fever | Thrombocytopenia |
> | Sore throat | Leukopenia |
> | Myalgia | Lymphocytic CSF |
> | Headache | Reduced T4 cell count |
> | Diarrhoea | Negative HIV antibody |
> | Rash: macular, vesicular | Positive HIV antigen |
> | Oral, genital or | High-level HIV viral load |
> | oesophageal ulcers | |
> | Aseptic meningitis | |
> | Hepatomegaly | |
> | Splenomegaly | |
> | Facial palsy (Bell's) | |
> | Encephalopathy | |

Asymptomatic and early symptomatic HIV disease

The interval between primary HIV infection (whether overt or not) and development of AIDS is very variable. It varies in untreated patients from 9 months to greater than 12 years. One long-term study from San Francisco has shown that 11 years after seroconversion only 60% of the patients had developed AIDS. 20% had AIDS-related complex and 20% were still well. It is likely that a very small number of patients will never get AIDS and be long-term survivors, but further follow-up is necessary to establish this. These are the patients with very light viral loads.

During the asymptomatic phase of HIV infection, patients are clinically well and have low-grade viraemia and a positive HIV antibody test. They are able to function entirely normally and most do not know they are infected. In the majority of HIV-infected individuals, there is a gradual decline in T4 cell count from around $800 \times 10^6/l$ to $< 300 \times 10^6/l$, when symptomatic HIV disease appears. The falling T4 count is a marker, and only a marker, for a general decline in many aspects of immune function. As the T4 cell count falls below $300 \times 10^6/l$, opportunistic infections begin to appear.

Table 74 Centres for Disease Control classification of HIV infection and AIDS

CDC[a] group	Clinical category[b]	Disease stage	Synonym
Group I	A	Primary HIV infection	
Group II/III	A	Asymptomatic, persistent generalised lymphadenopathy (PGL)	
Group IV			
A	B	Symptomatic HIV infection	AIDS-related complex (ARC)
B	C	Neurological disease	AIDS
C	C	Opportunistic infection	AIDS
D	C	Malignancy	AIDS
E	C	Other conditions	

[a]Centers for Disease Control 1987 classification
[b]New classification

Symptoms of early HIV infection

Several minor problems herald the later development of AIDS. These include:

- superficial skin problems such as seborrhoeic dermatitis, recurrent staphylococcal skin infections or onychomycosis (fungal nail infection)
- low-grade fever
- diarrhoea
- unexplained weight loss
- fatigue
- loss of taste and oral discomfort (oral candidiasis).

Signs of early HIV infection

Several signs are highly suggestive of HIV infection. These include:

- hairy leukoplakia on the side of the tongue
- lymphadenopathy
- herpes zoster (shingles)
- severe mucosal herpes simplex infection
- oropharyngeal candidiasis (thrush).

Lymphadenopathy is a common feature in HIV infection but is by no means universal and may be found in any of the superficial groups of lymph nodes. Occasionally lymphadenopathy represents an opportunistic infection, such as tuberculosis, histoplasmosis or lymphoma, but this is unusual. A presentation of lymphadenopathy in an at-risk patient should prompt an HIV test.

Laboratory markers of early HIV infection

Clues to the diagnosis of HIV infection include:

- lymphopenia ($< 1000 \times 10^6/l$)
- thrombocytopenia
- reduced T4 cells
- elevated T8 cells.

Thrombocytopenia may be an early manifestation of HIV infection. Patients are frequently asymptomatic, having platelet counts in the $50 \times 10^9/l$ to $120 \times 10^9/l$ range. Occasionally, cases of symptomatic thrombocytopenia occur (p. 244).

There are several key T4 cell count landmarks that are used in the management of patients with HIV infection (Fig. 65). The normal count is 800–1200 ($\times 10^6/l$). Management approaches at different levels of T4 cell deficiency vary:

- four monthly checks if ≥ 500
- give antiretroviral therapy when < 350
- start *Pneumocystis carinii* prophylaxis when < 200
- many more opportunistic infections appear when < 50.

Patients with higher T4 cell counts but high viral load may also benefit from anti-retroviral therapy.

Clinical approach to a newly diagnosed HIV/AIDS patient

When you assess a new HIV/AIDS patient there are certain key aspects to your evaluation.

Examination of the mouth and skin is very important.

Your objectives include:

- diagnosis of the current complaint
- assessment of the stage of disease
- assessment of the risk of other (future) illnesses (e.g. from prior travel or risk behaviour)
- imparting of confidence to the patient who will need care for many years (e.g. sympathetic, knowledgeable attitude).

You should arrange the following investigations:

- confirmatory HIV test
- T4 cell count
- full blood count
- biochemistry especially liver function tests
- syphilis serology
- toxoplasma serology
- hepatitis B serology
- chest X-ray.

Treatment of HIV infection

There are two classes of antiretroviral agent — the reverse transcriptase inhibitors (such as zidovudine,

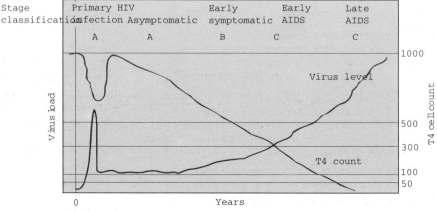

Fig. 65
The relationship between T4 cell counts and the disease stage in HIV infections.

didanosine, zalcitabine, lamivudine and others) and proteinase inhibitors (such as sequinavir, ritonavir and others). Resistance appears rapidly with monotherapy and so at least two drugs are now given concurrently. A typical starting combination would be zidovudine, didanosine and ritonavir. Combination therapy with zidovudine and didanosine reduces death by 40% compared with zidovudine alone.

AIDS

AIDS is characterised by being HIV positive and suffering infections or cancers typical of immunosuppressed patients. The presenting illnesses of AIDS in the UK are shown in Table 75. Each one of these specific diseases represents a marker diagnosis for AIDS and the incidence of many is an indicator of T4 cell levels (Fig. 66). The infections in AIDS are generally specific to AIDS, with the exceptions of cryptococcal meningitis, herpes zoster, tuberculosis and several bacterial infections such as salmonellosis. Some infections are more common in Africa (e.g. tuberculosis, pneumococcal pneumonia, salmonellosis) and others are less common (e.g. pneumocystis pneumonia, caused by *Pneumocystis carinii*). A clue to the diagnosis of AIDS is the presence of oral candidiasis or hairy leukoplakia.

Major infections in AIDS

Patients with AIDS suffer from many infections. Some of these occur at higher T4 cell counts, including pneu-

Table 75 Typical presenting illnesses of AIDS in the UK

Illnesses	Proportion presenting (%)
Pneumocystis pneumonia	37
Kaposi's sarcoma	14
Oesophageal candidosis	12
Weight loss (>10% body weight)	6
Lymphoma	4
HIV dementia	3
Cryptococcal meningitis	3
Other infections	21

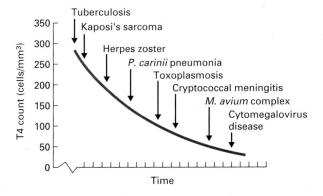

Fig. 66
Occurrence of AIDS-indicating conditions according to T4 cell count.

mocystis pneumonia, oesophageal candidiasis and others. Others occur later in the course of AIDS, including cytomegalovirus retinitis and *Mycobacterium avium intracellulare* (MAI) infection. The more common opportunistic infections are covered below; the less common are given in Table 76. Once patients get an infection it is almost always recurrent if treatment is stopped. Therefore, patients are usually placed on 'maintenance treatment' to prevent recurrence. As patients deteriorate so they tend to require more and more medication to prevent relapses of several infections.

Pneumocystis pneumonia (PCP). *P. carinii* (an airborne fungus) is a common cause of pneumonia in AIDS. It presents with

- dry cough for ≥ 2 weeks
- intermittent fever and/or night sweats
- recent weight loss
- dyspnoea out of proportion to physical signs
- 10% have a normal chest X-ray.

PCP is best diagnosed by bronchoalveolar lavage or lung biopsy. However the combination of a low T4 cell count, dyspnoea and cough, a bilaterally hazy infiltrate on the chest radiograph and hypoxaemia is sufficient to suggest the diagnosis. Treatment is with cotrimoxazole in high doses or i.v. pentamidine, with corticosteroids if markedly hypoxaemic ($pO_2 < 75$ mm Hg). The mortality is about 20%.

Oesophageal candidiasis. This affects about 25% of patients with AIDS. It may be asymptomatic but usually presents with

- dysphagia
- retrosternal discomfort or pain
- nausea and/or vomiting.

About 30% of patients have no associated oral candidiasis. Diagnosis is best made by endoscopy but a barium swallow is useful. Fluconazole is the best treatment.

Cytomegalovirus (CMV) retinitis. About 20% of patients with AIDS develop CMV retinitis and some get involvement of other organs, in particular colitis and encephalitis. The presentation of retinitis depends on which part of the retina is involved: central lesions present early with visual impairment, whereas peripheral lesions usually present with field deficits. The retina has a typical appearance of 'pizza' or 'cottage cheese and ketchup', showing haemorrhage and retinal necrosis together. The diagnosis is clinical as there is no diagnostic test. Treatment is with ganciclovir, foscarnet, or cidofovir and has to be continued for life or until the patient is blind. Retinal detachment is an infrequent complication.

MAI infection. This disseminated infection is thought to be waterborne and affects 30–50% of AIDS patients. Clinically it is insidious in onset and presents with:

- fever and/or night sweats
- cough
- diarrhoea
- anaemia
- weight loss.

Table 76 Opportunistic infections in AIDS (not covered in text)

Disease	T4 cell count (x 10^6/l)	Clinical features	Occasional features	Essential investigations	Treatment(s)
Early infections					
Tuberculosis	< 300	Cough, fever, weight loss Atypical CXR	Meningitis	Sputum for TB, bacteria, fungi; BAL for TB, fungi; blood culture for TB	Rifampicin, isoniazid, pyrazinamide and ethambutol
Salmonellosis	< 250	Fever, diarrhoea, dehydration	Septic shock	Blood culture, stool culture, stools for protozoa, electrolytes and urea	Quinolone or third-generation cephalosporin; rehydration
Mucocutaneous herpes simplex	< 250	Painful oral ulceration, pain in perianal area, 'cold sores'	Deep punched-out ulcers, oesophageal ulcers	None (biopsy/viral culture of blister fluid/lesion)	Acyclovir
Late infections					
Cryptococcal meningitis	< 200	Headache, fever, nausea, vomiting	Pneumonia, skin lesions	CT scan of brain, lumbar puncture with opening pressure (p. 188), fungal blood cultures, cryptococcal antigen	Amphotericin B and flucytosine initially
Toxoplasma encephalitis	< 200	Headache, focal neurology, fits	Myocarditis	CT (or MR) scan of brain, toxoplasma, serology	Pyrimethamine and sulphadiazine
Cryptosporidial diarrhoea	< 100	Diarrhoea, dehydration	Cholangitis	Stools for protozoa and culture, electrolytes and urea, albumin, liver function tests	Rehydration, experimental antiprotozoal therapy
PML	< 100	Focal neurology, fit, abnormal behaviour		CT/MR scan, brain, lumbar puncture	None
Invasive aspergillosis	< 50	Cough, fever, wheezing, haemoptysis	Tracheobronchitis	CXR, sputum for fungi, BAL for fungi, lung biopsy	Amphotericin B or itraconazole

BAL, bronchoalveolar lavage; PML, progressive multifocal leucoencephalopathy; CXR, chest x-ray/radiograph.

Diagnosis is by culturing MAI from blood, sputum, stool or tissue, or demonstrating its presence in bone marrow or liver. Treatment is with three or four unusual antituberculous agents as MAI is a multiresistant organism.

Cancers in AIDS

There are several cancers almost specific to AIDS or more common (Table 77). Kaposi's sarcoma is caused by a newly discovered herpes virus (HHV-8). Cerebral lymphoma is caused by Epstein–Barr virus (see p. 365).

Neurological problems in AIDS

About 5% of AIDS patients present with dementia as their AIDS-defining diagnosis. It becomes increasingly common in the later stages of AIDS. It is partially preventable with zidovudine therapy, even if multiple circulating HIV virus strains are resistant. Other problems include depression and peripheral neuropathy (Table 78).

Prognosis

Prior to the introduction of zidovudine and pneumocystis prophylaxis, most patients would survive 12–15 months following a diagnosis of AIDS. Drug addicts and children under the age of 2 tended to have shorter survival times compared with gay men, haemophiliacs

and older children. Certain diseases are associated with a good prognosis, e.g. Kaposi's sarcoma and PCP, whereas others such as CNS lymphoma or CMV retinitis have a poor prognosis. Since the introduction of combination antiretroviral therapy and PCP prophylaxis, HIV-positive patients will remain well for months or years longer than previously.

Terminal care

Given the multiple problems that occur in late-stage AIDS and the inevitable progression to death in all patients, once they reach this stage, questions of when to withdraw therapy are vexed. Most of the patients are in their 20s and 30s. Many of the treatments provide substantial symptomatic relief. Examples include antifungal therapy for oral and oesophageal candidiasis, corticosteroid replacement for adrenal dysfunction, antimycobacterial therapy to prevent fevers and cough, therapy for cytomegalovirus retinitis, etc. Most physicians caring for AIDS patients try to establish the patient's wishes in this regard early in their relationship with the patient and, in the case of gay patients, their partners may assist in the decision-making process. Many such patients have seen friends die of AIDS. Decision points for the termination of active treatment include advanced HIV dementia, a new life-threatening infectious episode, a stroke or major renal dysfunction.

Table 77 Common cancers in AIDS

	Kaposi's sarcoma	CNS lymphoma	Other lymphoma	Squamous cell carcinoma
Organs affected	Skin, gut, lungs	Brain	Lymph nodes, liver, bone marrow, skin	Rectum, uterus, cervix
Typical T4 count	< 350	< 100	< 200	< 200
Aetiological agent	HHV-8	Epstein–Barr virus	Epstein–Barr virus and others probably	Papilloma virus (?)
Presentation	Purple nodules/plaques on skin/mouth, cough, dyspnoea, peribronchial infiltrate	Focal signs, headache, papilloedema, single enhancing lesion (usually) on CT/MR scan with surrounding oedema	Adenopathy, anaemia, neutropenia, cutaneous abscess	Local pain, bleeding or lump
Treatment	Local radiotherapy, γ-interferon, chemotherapy	Radiotherapy, dexamethasone	Chemotherapy	Surgery, radiotherapy
Prognosis	Reasonable, one of the less aggressive presentations of AIDS; morbidity high because of unsightly nature of lesions (often on face)	Dismal, most patients die within 3 months	Variable, usually poor; patients tolerate chemotherapy badly because of poor bone marrow reserve	Variable, usually poor as locally invasive at presentation; cervical smears mandatory for HIV⁺ women at 6-monthly intervals

Sometimes toxicity forces therapy to be withdrawn, e.g. neutropenia or thrombocytopenia with ganciclovir therapy.

Larger AIDS units have a number of support staff including community nursing staff who are able to orchestrate community services in the final days of life to allow the patient to die at home if they so choose. As with the management of terminal illness of any other condition, symptomatic relief is paramount, which usually includes analgesia and sometimes fluids. It always necessitates a caring, supportive and empathetic attitude towards the patient and their loved ones. As AIDS patients' body fluids are potentially infectious, it also requires the provision of gloves and instruction for those caring for the dying (who are often incontinent or vomit) to prevent transmission of the virus. The relationship between patient and the doctor and nursing staff is often close, as the patients have usually been under their care for some years prior to death. It is emotionally taxing for all concerned.

HIV antibody testing

The indications for HIV testing in adults are shown in Box 12. Clearly the likelihood of a positive test is higher if your patient belongs to a risk group.

Table 78 Major neuropsychological manifestations of HIV infection/AIDS

Entity	Clinical features
HIV dementia complex	Slowly progressive dementia typically affecting memory and concentration initially, leading to severe dementia over a few months. A rapidly progressive confusional state is more likely to be caused by infection or a CNS lymphoma. CT scan shows cerebral atrophy
Depression	Depression is very common in AIDS as in other slowly progressive terminal diseases. Suicide occurs occasionally. Depression may be mistaken for dementia and vice versa
Peripheral neuropathy	Painful or non-painful distal peripheral neuropathy is common. Characteristic is painful soles of the feet with moderate sensory loss. Sometimes only one or two fingers are 'numb'. Tends to be progressive and refractory to therapy. May be caused by drugs

Box 12
Indications for HIV testing in adults

Patient request
Organ transplantation
Blood donation
Clinical features of AIDS including:

- opportunistic infection with no known immunosuppressing disease
- unusual lymphoma
- squamous cell carcinoma of anus or cervix
- early onset dementia or other unusual neurology
- unexplained weight loss

Suspicion of AIDS-related complex, e.g. oral candidiasis, night sweats and weight loss, thrombocytopenia
Unexplained lymphadenopathy
Suspicion of primary HIV infection[a]
Needlestick injury in health-care worker[a]
Rape victim[a]
Women with a child with HIV/AIDS

[a]May not be positive on first test.

There are a number of different parts of the virus to which antibodies are directed including surface protein gp120 and internal proteins p24 and p41. The presence of antibody is a marker of infection and is not protective, unlike in many other infectious diseases where the presence of antibody is both a marker of infection and protective against subsequent infection.

A number of different laboratory tests are used for HIV antibody testing. All reputable laboratories will do a second confirmatory test on all new positive sera to ensure that rare false-positive tests are excluded. The likelihood of two tests being false positive is now less than one in a million. The likelihood of a false-negative test is also extremely small and is most common after a primary infection and before seroconversion. This 'window period' is the reason that all at-risk persons are asked not to donate blood, as rare instances of HIV transmission have occurred from blood taken during this period.

HIV infection in neonates. Determining whether a baby is infected if the mother is HIV positive is more difficult as maternal HIV antibody is detectable in the baby for about 15 months after birth. At present, direct viral RNA detection by polymerase chain reaction (PCR) or viral culture can be used with reasonable reliability by 3 months of age.

Counselling

All patients to be tested for HIV antibody must be counselled. Performing an HIV test on a patient without their consent is regarded in many countries as an assault and in any case a positive test has profound implications for the patient. Therefore, it is now standard practice for all patients to be counselled before an HIV test and the counselling should be done by trained personnel if possible. Adequate time should be set aside for both the pre-test counselling and the post-test counselling. This is particularly important if the test comes back positive. The patient should not be informed of a positive result on a Friday without adequate counselling back-up.

The issues that need discussion before and after HIV testing include those listed in Box 13. The profound implications of a positive test, including life insurance and occupational implications, have spawned the development of anonymous testing clinics in areas. Despite this, around 20% of AIDS patients present without knowledge of their HIV status. Considerable denial among at-risk groups and the relative inefficacy of antiretroviral therapy (until recently) has prevented early testing and prevention of disease in these groups.

Infection control issues

Body fluids from all patients in risk groups and those who are HIV antibody positive should be handled carefully with gloves on. Gloves should be used for all invasive procedures, including venepuncture and most surgeons will use two pairs of gloves. Each hospital has detailed procedures for all aspects of handling body

---

Box 13
The major issues concerning HIV testing which should be raised during counseling

- Information needs and patient actions
  — Need to inform doctor and dentist of positive test result
  — Cannot donate blood if positive
  — Should be given advice about keeping healthy
  — May need to alter travel plans for holidays
  — Will need information in detail about HIV and AIDS

- Medical needs if positive
  — Will need medical supervision
  — Will need PCP prophylaxis pending T4 count
  — Other sexually transmitted diseases including hepatitis B may need to be excluded
  — Women will need 6-monthly cervical smears
  — Will be offered antiretroviral therapy depending on T4 count

- Insurance
  — May be denied life insurance if tested, despite result, unless done for occupational or travel reasons
  — Will certainly be denied life insurance if positive

- Personal issues
  — Will usually need discussion with partner and adoption of safe sex practices if partner not tested or negative
  — Question of where HIV infection acquired will need discussion and counselling, especially in monogamous relationships
  — Issues of pregnancy and transmission to children a major issue for women
  — Issues of terminal illness of major importance ('How much time have I got, doctor?')
  — Occupational issues, especially for health-care workers and overseas students
  — Institutional issues, especially for children and prisoners
  — Drug addicts' needs: needle acquisition, sharing and habit
  — Who to tell: family, friends, employer, and when

---

fluids including (usually) high-risk stickers for all samples and special sterilisation procedures for all endoscopes. These procedures enable *all* investigations and procedures to be carried out on patients with HIV. The only exception is autopsy, for which few hospitals are adequately equipped. This can pose problems for coroner's cases.

9.4 Transplantation

End-stage organ failure or untreatable cancer and leukaemia has led to the extensive use of solid organ or bone marrow transplantation. Different organs are more or less difficult to transplant, either for technical (surgical) reasons or because of problems of rejection and graft failure after transplantation. Relatively straightforward transplantation *procedures* are corneal, skin and bone transplantation. Other transplantation procedures such as pancreatic, small bowel and skeletal muscle are essentially experimental at present.

The two major problems with transplantation are organ rejection and infection (often with unusual pathogens).

Learning objective
- You need to have a working understanding of graft rejection and tolerance as it pertains to transplantation.

Bone marrow transplantation

Bone marrow transplantation (BMT) may be either allogeneic (someone else's marrow), autologous (own marrow previously collected) or peripheral stem cells (own circulating stem cells previously collected). Autologous bone marrow transplantation is increasingly used to allow increased chemotherapy for difficult-to-treat malignancy, such as breast cancer. Present indications are shown in Table 79.

Solid organ transplantation

Renal, heart, lung and liver transplantation are now well established for end-stage disease affecting these organs. When successful, which they increasingly are if performed in large experienced units, patients experience a whole new lease of life and a longer life. The best outcomes are in renal and heart transplantation, but substantial improvements in both survival and quality of life are now being seen in liver and lung transplant recipients. A young otherwise healthy recipient of a renal transplant can expect an 80–90% survival over 5 years, which is superior to dialysis. Unlike in other major organ transplants, the kidney can be lost (through rejection) but the patient survives. At 3 years, 80% of

kidneys are still functional. Survival for heart transplantation is lower but is still better than 60% at 5 years.

Rejection

Patients who develop rejection (which most do to variable degrees) receive additional immunosuppressive medication and are much more likely to develop serious infection. Some infections, in particular CMV, cause further immunosuppression because of cytokine release and also lead to additional infections.

Pathogenesis of rejection
The pathogenesis of organ rejection is well understood and reviewed extremely briefly here. Thirty years of research by some of the world's most talented scientists have unravelled the two sides of the same coin: rejection and immune tolerance. The central figures in the show are the MHC antigens, class I and class II. MHC antigens form two subsets of three antigens: A, B and C for class I and DR, DQ and DP for class II. There is enormous heterogeneity in both class I and class II antigens. Some varieties are rare, and finding a matching donor for bone marrow transplantation can require screening tens to hundreds of thousands of individuals. International databases have, therefore, been set up to facilitate matching of donors and recipients. Clearly HLA matching in solid organ transplantation from cadavers is necessarily less precise because of the limited time available before the transplanted organ has to be reperfused. Matching MHC class II antigens (DR, DQ and DP) is more important than class I.

When a transplant operation is done, the new organ is directly inserted into a recipient. Usually there is some degree of HLA mismatch. For example, three of the four HLA types may be identical and one different. This different HLA type is immediately recognised as different by T cells. T4 cells appear to be central in initiation of rejection. Once activated, several intracellular processes in the T4 cell follow, including cytokine release and activation of T8 cells. These cells cause direct cell-mediated cytotoxicity of transplanted tissue. B cells are activated and specific antibodies generated

Table 79 Indications for bone marrow transplantation

Disease	Autologous/peripheral stem cell BMT	Allogeneic BMT
Non-malignant disease		
Aplastic anaemia	Impossible	Yes, usually
Thalassaemia major	Impossible	Yes
Inherited immunodeficiencies	Impossible	Yes
Malignant disease		
Acute and chronic myeloid leukaemia	Possibly	Yes[a]
Multiple myeloma	Yes	Possibly
Non-Hodgkin's lymphoma	Probably	No
Hodgkin's disease after relapse	Yes	No

[a] in young adults

which bind to the transplanted organ and activate complement. Macrophages are also activated. All these events together lead to a typical inflammatory response.

The speed of these events depends on the mechanism and prior exposure to the transplanted antigens, usually from blood product transfusions. Prior blood transfusion from the donor has an 80% chance of reducing rejection episodes by inducing tolerance and a 20% chance of inducing hyperacute or accelerated rejection (Table 80).

Prophylaxis of rejection

Much attention has been paid by transplant units to the *prophylaxis* of rejection. All units give high immunosuppressive doses during and immediately after transplantation and then gradually reduce the doses according to a set schedule but modified by the patient's course and episodes of rejection. In the early years of transplantation, corticosteroids were the mainstay of immunosuppression. They suppress virtually all aspects of the immune response. Substantial reductions in both infection and rejection rates followed the introduction of cyclosporin and more recently tacrolimus, and many renal transplant units now reserve steroids for episodes of graft rejection. Cyclosporin works on T cells to prevent the cytokine cascade after stimulation by a new antigen. The major drawback of cyclosporin is toxicity, in particular nephrotoxocity but also hypertension and neurotoxicity. Serum levels must be monitored. Cyclosporin also has multiple drug interactions. Azathioprine is also used extensively as an immunosuppressant. It acts as an antiproliferative agent only.

Monitoring and diagnosing rejection

Monitoring for rejection is relatively simple in renal transplantation: urine output and serum creatinine (or clearance) are good indicators. Biopsy is necessary to confirm rejection. In cardiac transplantation and lung transplantation, sequential myocardial and lung biopsies are necessary as there are few simple markers of rejection to follow. Therefore, this necessitates an invasive procedure on each occasion. Monitoring of rejection in liver transplantation requires some liver biopsies and liver function tests. A biopsy is always necessary to confirm rejection and rule out viral infection.

Treatment of rejection

Drugs used for the treatment of episodes of rejection include methylprednisolone, OKT3 monoclonal antibody and antithymocyte globulin, in addition to increased doses of cyclosporin.

Graft versus host disease

Graft-versus-host disease (GVHD) is a form of 'organ rejection' but its manifestations spill over to other systems. The transplantation/transfusion procedures that give rise to GVHD are well recognised:

- allogeneic bone marrow transplantation (especially HLA mismatched grafts)
- small bowel transplants (because of lymphoid tissue in gut)
- transfusion of unirradiated blood products into immunocompromised patients.

The risk of GVHD following bone marrow transplantation depends on the HLA matching of the graft, whether GVHD prophylaxis is given and the patient's age. The incidence therefore varies from 10 to 80%.

Acute GVHD is manifest by:

- skin rash, itchy on palms, soles and ears
- intestinal dysfunction (especially small bowel)
- liver dysfunction.

The severity is graded I–IV. Grades III and IV carry a high mortality. Acute GVHD leads to profound immunosuppression in and of itself, and because the treatment of it with corticosteroids is immunosuppressive.

Infection

Patients given immunosuppressive therapy for transplantation (or who receive therapy for other reasons which has a secondary immunosuppressive effect, e.g. radiotherapy) are vulnerable to many of the opportunistic infections seen in HIV-positive patients (see above.

9.5 Hypersensitivity and allergy

There are several clinical manifestations of allergy. These include:

- anaphylaxis
- laryngeal oedema and/or bronchoconstriction
- asthma
- allergic rhinitis/hay fever
- gut allergy: vomiting and/or diarrhoea
- urticaria
- drug allergy manifest as rashes.

Table 80 Pattern of rejection of solid organ transplants

Pattern of rejection	Time	Mechanism
Hyperacute	Hours	Pre-existing specific antidonor antibodies and complement
Accelerated	Days	Reaction by previously sensitised T cells
Acute	Days/weeks	Activation of T cells
Chronic	Months/years	Multiple ill-defined mechanisms

Learning objective

- You need to understand the mechanisms, clinical presentation and treatment of anaphylaxis and other allergic phenomena.

Anaphylaxis

In this section, primarily for reasons of space, only immediate type I hypersensitivity will be covered: anaphylaxis, laryngeal oedema and acute bronchoconstriction.

Pathogenesis

Immediate hypersensitivity responses (Type 1), are mediated primarily by mast cells and IgE. Mast cells are derived from haematopoietic precursors and migrate to and mature in connective or mucosal tissue where they live for weeks or months. Mast cells have many granules which contain histamine, chymase, tryptase (both proteases which directly increase bronchial hyperresponsiveness and bronchial mucus production) and other substances. When released, these substances cause immediate local irritation (wheal and flare reaction) and a late-phase response characterised by infiltration of neutrophils and complement. The late-phase response is abolished if prostaglandin synthesis inhibitors (such as corticosteroids) are used explaining the potent effect of steroids on allergic asthma. Basophils probably contribute to the immediate hypersensitivity response.

IgE

The most potent stimulus for mast cell degranulation is IgE. IgE comprises less than 0.001% of total immunoglobulin and is produced by B cells. IgE production is stimulated by interleukin-4 and inhibited by γ-interferon and T8 cells. Higher total and specific levels of IgE are found in HLA types B8 and Dw3 and low levels with HLA type A2, emphasising a major genetic component to allergy and atopy. Specific IgE, for example to penicillin, can be detected in blood with a RAST test or doing a skin (prick) test. A patient with a positive RAST test to an antigen will have a positive prick test and vice versa. As exposure to an allergen is necessary to generate a population of B cells and specific IgE, so an allergic response cannot occur on first exposure to an allergen. Specific IgE then binds to mast cells without triggering degranulation. On further exposure to the antigen or other triggers, the mast cell degranulates leading to the clinical features of acute hypersensitivity. Triggers include complement C3a or C5a and carbohydrates found in some fruits, e.g. strawberries (Table 81).

Clinical features

Anaphylaxis is the most immediately life-threatening feature of type I hypersensitivity. It is characterised by:

- exposure to an allergen, e.g. bee sting, penicillin, etc.
- airway obstruction with stridor/wheezing
- hypotension
- cutaneous reactions, such as pruritus, flushing, urticaria
- GI symptoms, including vomiting and diarrhoea.

Treatment

Treatment of anaphylaxis *must* be immediate (see emergency box). All patients should be admitted to hospital for 24 hours after anaphylaxis to observe for relapse. The mortality is about 10% overall but is higher in patients out of hospital. Follow-up to prevent recurrence is essential.

Other allergic diseases

Other diseases mediated by type I responses include asthma, allergic rhinitis, hay fever and urticaria, and some forms of food allergy other than anaphylaxis. Common allergens include the house dust mite, pets, milk or milk products, eggs, and many other foods. In cases of urticaria, for example, identifying the trigger is often difficult and weeks and months of 'detective'

Table 81 Causes and mechanisms of anaphylaxis

Substance (example)	Mechanism
Venoms (bee sting, snake)	IgE mediated
Airborne allergens (moulds such as *Alternaria*, animal dander)	IgE mediated
Foods (e.g. peanuts, milk, seafood, egg)	IgE mediated
Proteins (streptokinase, insulin, tetanus antitoxin)	IgE mediated
Antibiotics (penicillins, sulphonamides)	IgE mediated
Blood transfusion in IgA-deficient individual	IgE antibodies to IgA
Intravenous solutions (contrast media, mannitol, dextran)	Direct activation of mast cells
Drugs (opiates, curare, vancomycin)	Direct activation of mast cells
Human proteins (gammaglobulin, blood products)	Complement activation
Dialysis (dialysis membrane)	Complement activation
Exercise (with food sometimes)	Unknown
Drugs (NSAIDs, lignocaine, steroids)	Unknown
Food preservatives (metabisulphites, benzoates)	Unknown

work is often unsuccessful. Some cases are caused by pressure and others result from autoimmunity (IgG antibodies to the mast cell IgE receptor).

Immunotherapy

There are various forms of immunotherapy now prescribable. Passive protection against infection relies on antibody. Immunisation is usually preferable if possible. Other forms of immunotherapy activate various arms of the immune system using cytokines.

Immunoglobulin

Intramuscular immunoglobulin (gammaglobulin) has several uses including:

- the prevention of hepatitis A in travellers
- prevention of hepatitis B in exposed health-care workers (if unimmunised) and newborns
- prevention of varicella in immunocompromised patients
- prevention of rabies after an animal bite in non-immune individuals
- treatment of severe cases of diphtheria and botulism
- prevention and treatment of tetanus.

Intravenous immunoglobulin is used to prevent infection in antibody-deficient individuals and for the specific therapy of a few diseases, including Kawasaki's disease.

Cytokines, interferons and colony-stimulating factors

To date, numerous cytokines have been described. The term cytokine means 'cellular signalling molecule' and as all are proteins (usually glycoproteins) there is little to distinguish a hormone from a cytokine. Initially all cytokines were described as having immunological functions. This is no longer true; for example, interleukin-1, which increases collagen synthesis and wound healing and neutrotrophic factor, which is a 'survival factor' for many types of neuron. Therefore, the distinction between a peptide hormone (such as gastrin or ACTH) and a cytokine (such as granulocyte-stimulating factor or tumour necrosis factor) is arbitrary. Some are 'renamed' growth factors or colony-stimulating factors, but the principles are the same.

Interferon

Alpha-interferon is composed of at least 22 subtypes whereas γ-interferon is essentially a single type. Interferons have several antiviral effects which include:

- increased expression of MHC receptors to allow for greater viral antigen recognition
- increased activation of natural killer cells and macrophages
- direct inhibition of viral replication and other viral processes, such as viral penetration of cells.

Treatment with cytokines. There are three cytokines and several growth factors that have proven to be therapeutically useful, after years of research work. Interferons have antiviral activity and are given subcutaneously. Colony-stimulating factors are given either intravenously or subcutaneously.

Alpha-interferon. Recombinant α-interferon is now available and marketed. There are now several indications for α-interferon:

- treatment of chronic hepatitis caused by hepatitis B or C virus
- eradication of hepatitis B surface antigen (and e antigen) carriage
- hairy cell leukaemia
- Kaposi's sarcoma in AIDS
- renal cell carcinoma.

Beta-interferon. This reduces the number of radiological exacerbations of multiple sclerosis.

Gamma-interferon. This cytokine is produced by activated T cells and natural killer cells and acts on lymphocytes, monocytes and some other cells such as microglial and endothelial cells. It increases macrophage and neutrophil activity. There is only one licensed indication for γ-IFN, which is the prophylaxis of infection in chronic granulomatous disease.

Granulocyte colony-stimulating factor. This is used primarily to shorten the period of neutropenia after cytotoxic chemotherapy, aplastic anaemia or in AIDS. It also improves neutrophil function.

Granulocyte macrophage colony-stimulating factor. This is similar to granulocyte colony-stimulating factor but also acts on the monocyte/macrophage arm to increase the production of cells from the marrow and to improve their function. Its role is less clearly defined.

Emergency treatment: management of anaphylaxis

Out of hospital

Think of quickest means of acquiring adrenaline and/or steroids (? local doctor, 999 call, direct transport to nearby hospital)

If in hospital act quickly

1. Stop infusions of any blood or drugs
2. Give oxygen by mask in high concentration
3. Measure blood pressure
4. Give adrenaline up to 0.5 ml (1 in 1000) slowly i.v. over 3–5 minutes (or i.m. if quicker)
5. If hypotensive, give 1–2 litres of colloid (e.g. Haemacell) quickly
6. Give hydrocortisone 100–300 mg i.v. over 1 minute (no immediate effect but will help prevent relapse)
7. If bronchoconstriction present, use nebulised β_2-antagonists such as salbutamol
8. Give antihistamine i.v. (to prevent relapse)
9. Depending on clinical status and response to treatment, transfer to ward or intensive care unit

Self-assessment: questions

Multiple choice questions

1. The following are true:
   a. Intravenous immunoglobulin therapy carries a substantial risk of hepatitis B
   b. Splenectomy has no substantial impact on susceptibility to infection
   c. *Neisseria* infections are more common in C3 complement deficiency
   d. Selective IgA deficiency is relatively common in oriental people
   e. Tetanus and diphtheria toxins are directly inactivated by antibody produced after immunisation

2. With respect to phagocytes:
   a. Once a phagocyte has ingested a pathogen (e.g. *Candida albicans*) progressive infection is arrested
   b. Macrophages directly kill viruses
   c. Gamma-interferon has no effect on neutrophil function
   d. Most neutrophils in the body are circulating in blood
   e. The respiratory burst in neutrophils is the primary mechanism for killing bacteria such as *Staphylococcus aureus*.

3. The following are true:
   a. Patients who have had anaphylaxis should wear a medic alert bracelet
   b. Hay fever is mediated mostly by switching of eosinophils
   c. High circulating IgE concentrations can be caused by *Aspergillus*
   d. RAST tests are useful for identifying causes of urticaria
   e. The first drug that should be administered to patients with anaphylaxis is an antihistamine

4. With respect to susceptibility to infection the following associations are true:
   a. Diabetes and *Staphylococcus aureus*
   b. Heart transplant recipient and cytomegalovirus
   c. Hodgkin's disease and herpes zoster
   d. Chronic renal failure and bacteraemia
   e. Pancreatitis and candidaemia

5. IgM antibodies:
   a. If present are useful in diagnosing recent hepatitis A
   b. Are useful in diagnosis of cytomegalovirus disease in AIDS
   c. Bind complement efficiently
   d. Because of their size are only found in blood and not at the site of infection or inflammation
   e. Are inefficient at binding Gram-negative organisms

6. The following are true:
   a. HIV-1 infection usually leads to AIDS within 4 years
   b. HIV infects T8 lymphocytes
   c. Macrophage dysfunction is a common feature of AIDS
   d. HIV may be transmitted by one episode of heterosexual intercourse
   e. Symptomatic HIV disease typically occurs when the T4 cell count falls just below $500 \times 10^6/l$

7. Delay in the onset of AIDS can be achieved with the following:
   a. Treatment of oral thrush for 7 days
   b. Prophylaxis of pneumocystis pneumonia
   c. Pneumococcal immunisation
   d. Influenza immunisation
   e. Combination antiretroviral therapy

8. Cutaneous manifestations of HIV infection include:
   a. Kaposi's sarcoma
   b. Seborrhoeic dermatitis
   c. Severe mucosal herpes simplex infection
   d. Herpes zoster (shingles)
   e. Onychomycosis

9. Concerning HIV infection and AIDS:
   a. Pneumocystis pneumonia is common in Africa
   b. Tuberculosis in AIDS presents like that in non-AIDS patients
   c. Oral thrush is a late feature of AIDS
   d. Toxoplasmosis is usually a cerebral disease
   e. Cytomegalovirus retinitis can be treated with acyclovir

10. Indications for an HIV test include:
    a. Recurrent cold sores on lips
    b. Tuberculosis in an ex-intravenous drug abuser
    c. Non-Hodgkin's lymphoma in a 62-year-old woman
    d. Parents of an adopted child from abroad
    e. Recurrent vaginal candidiasis

Case history questions

History 1

A 44-year-old man presents to Casualty with a 1-week history of breathlessness and cough. Over the last 3–4 weeks he has become increasingly tired, lost 5 kg in weight and had a troublesome boil on his left buttock. On examination, he is breathless talking, but not at rest, with a dry cough. Vital signs are a temperature of 38.3°C, respiratory rate 30/min, pulse 110 beats/min, BP 110/85. Examination of the chest is otherwise normal and there are no murmurs. Small lymph nodes are palpable in his neck and left groin. There is a small boil on his left buttock but no other skin lesions. There are no signs of i.v. drug abuse. Joints, nervous system and abdomen are normal. Blood sugar is normal.

1. What additional history should you seek?
2. What important part of the physical examination has been omitted and why might it be important?
3. Give a short differential diagnosis of his pulmonary problem.
4. List two essential investigations for which would need urgent results and why.

History 2

A 34-year-old woman is referred to you with tiredness and weight loss of 7 kg over 2 months. She has had a lot of stress at work (advertising) and attributes her symptoms to this and no time to cook for herself. There is no significant past medical history apart from pelvic inflammatory disease. She is separated.

Her vital signs were temperature 36.5°C, pulse 92 beats/min, BP 110/70, respiratory rate 18/min. Examination shows her to be thin with several small lymph nodes palpable in the neck and left groin. There are no signs in the mouth or elsewhere.

1. The following tests should be done immediately (True or False):
   a. Full blood count, differential white cell and platelet count
   b. Biochemistry panel
   c. Chest X-ray
   d. T4 cell count
   e. Thyroid function tests

She returns in 2 weeks and is no better. She describes a dull retrosternal chest pain and mild nausea. Her blood results were haemoglobin 11.7 g/dl, white cell count 3.9×10^9/l, neutrophils 2900×10^6/l, lymphocytes 650×10^6/l and platelets 93×10^9/l. She had normal biochemistry and chest X-ray. Her T4 cell count was 23%.

2. Now you should do the following (True or False):
   a. Examine her mouth
   b. Enquire more deeply into HIV risk factors
   c. Arrange an endoscopy urgently
   d. Counsel her (or arrange counselling) for an HIV test
   e. Treat her with omeprazole empirically

Seven days later, she has had a positive HIV antibody test and endoscopy shows extensive oesophageal candidiasis. She is at home.

3. Now you should do the following:
   a. Refer her to the local HIV/AIDS unit
   b. Start her on zidovudine therapy
   c. Start her on fluconazole therapy
   d. Arrange admission to hospital
   e. Phone her up to tell her the HIV test result as soon as you receive it.

Picture questions

1. Picture 9.1 is the appearance of the CSF from an HIV-positive man with a persistent headache and low-grade fever. His last T4 cell count was 123×10^6/l. The CSF showed 10 white cells, all lymphocytes, a protein of 0.6 g/l and a glucose of 3.5 mmol/l. There were < 100 red cells.
   a. What is shown?
   b. What test has been done to show the abnormality?
   c. What other piece of information do you need from the lumbar puncture to manage him properly?
   d. What other tests should be done (give four)?
   e. How should he be managed?

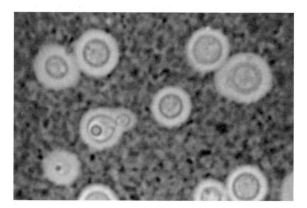

Picture 9.1

2. Picture 9.2 is the chest radiograph of a heart-transplant recipient with fever, shortness of breath and cough. He is 3 months post-transplant and doing reasonably well apart from two episodes of moderate rejection. He is taking antitoxoplasmal

prophylaxis as his donor had antibodies for toxoplasma and he did not.
a. Describe the abnormality.
b. Give a differential diagnosis.
c. What two investigations should be done urgently?
d. What empirical therapy you might start while waiting for a result?

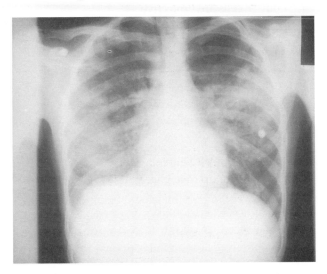

Picture 9.2

Short note/viva questions

1. A gay man (Tom) needs counselling about having an HIV test. He has come with his HIV-positive partner. They have been together for 9 months. Write a list of important issues you must cover today and when you give him the result in 2 days' time.
2. Write a list of headings you should cover and sketch out the details of the most important points for a discussion group of student nurses that you are leading about the risks of occupational acquisition of HIV.
3. Write short notes on the following:
   a. Indications for lymphocyte subset determination.
   b. Indications for measuring immunoglobulin levels.
   c. T4 cell counts in HIV/AIDS and the rationale for intervention.
   d. Why the development of an HIV vaccine might be difficult.

Self-assessment: answers

Multiple choice answers

1. a. **False**. Previous preparations carried a substantial risk of hepatitis C virus but this has been virtually eliminated from immunoglobulin preparations. There is also negligible to zero risk of transmission of HIV via this route.
   b. **False**. Splenectomised patients are at particular risk of overwhelming infection from capsulate organisms including *S. pneumoniae*. The problem is not only that patients are more likely to get infections with these organisms but that the infections are likely to be fatal. Splenectomised patients do not respond to pneumococcal vaccine very well. Patients going for elective splenectomy should be given pneumococcal vaccine at least 10 days prior to splenectomy to protect them against this fatal complication.
   c. **True**. C3 complement deficiency is rare but is associated with many infections especially Gram-positive infection. Deficiency of the complement components C5–C9 leads to either *N. meningitidis* infection or disseminated gonococcal infection.
   d. **False**. Selective IgA deficiency is common in Caucasians, occurring in 1 in 300–700 population. This means that any GP working in a

predominantly white neighbourhood will have between three and eight such patients on his list at any one time.
   e. **True**. This is the logic for giving not only tetanus toxoid, to induce the production of antitoxin, but also tetanus immunoglobulin following injury with soil-contaminated material.

2. a. **False**. Some organisms are essentially intracellular organisms (such as *Legionella pneumophila*) and, therefore, thrive intracellularly. Phagocytosis is only one step in the inactivation of an organism, intracellular killing is the next and there are many organisms which have evolved excellent defences for evading this.
   b. **False**. Important viruses may replicate inside macrophages (e.g. HIV) and macrophages may process viral antigens allowing the production of specific antibody and T cell responses to the viruses, but they do not kill viruses directly.
   c. **False**. Gamma-interferon upregulates and improves neutrophil function.
   d. **False**. Most neutrophils in the body are contained within the vascular space but exist mainly in what is called the marginating pool. These are 'resting' neutrophils loosely attached to

349

endothelium. A raised white cell count in response to infection reflects the release of neutrophils from the marginating pool. Left shift (or 'bands' in US journals) reflects the increased circulation of early neutrophils produced from the bone marrow.

e. **True**. The respiratory burst is a fundamental part of defence against infection and is deficient in chronic granulamatous disease which is why these patients suffer recurrent infection, particularly by *S. aureus*, *Candida* and *Aspergillus*.

3. a. **True**. If the patients know what they are allergic to. Some patients also carry a small phial of adrenaline with them, particularly if they are allergic to a common allergen such as peanuts or seafood to which they might be exposed to advertently.
 b. **False**. Eosinophils do not switch. However, nasal secretions in patients with hay fever contain increased numbers of eosinophils.
 c. **True**. But only in the context of allergic bronchopulmonary aspergillosis (ABPA), which occurs in asthmatic or cystic fibrosis patients.
 d. **False**. RAST tests are useful for identifying many causes of anaphylaxis and rarely urticaria.
 e. **False**. Adrenaline should be the first drug to be administered, followed by steroids and antihistamines.

4. a. **True**.
 b. **True**. CMV causes pneumonitis which is frequently fatal if not recognised and treated.
 c. **True**. The increased risk extends to 5 years after the diagnosis of Hodgkin's disease despite the lack of additional chemotherapy or steroids.
 d. **True**. Partly because of frequent use of i.v. catheters but also because of the reduced generalised defence against infection.
 e. **True**. Patients with pancreatitis and those who have had a perforated viscus in the abdomen repaired or removed surgically are at substantial risk for candidaemia.

5. a. **True**. They are also useful for diagnosing recent hepatitis B.
 b. **False**. Virtually all AIDS patients are seropositive for CMV and the development of disease (such as retinitis or colitis) is not reflected in an increase in the IgM. In addition, in immunocompromised patients, the IgM response may be either blunted or absent. It is also occasionally falsely positive.
 c. **True**.
 d. **False**. Increased concentrations of immunoglobulin and complement leave the blood space through the vascular endothelium to sites of inflammation and infection.
 e. **False**. IgM antibodies are particularly adept at

binding Gram-negative organisms, which is why immunoglobulin therapy for patients with recurrent Gram-negative sepsis is less effective than with patients with recurrent Gram-positive sepsis.

6. a. **False**. 60% progress to AIDS over 11 years.
 b. **False**. T4 cells and many other cells are infected but T8 cells are protective.
 c. **True**. AIDS-related infections include toxoplasmosis, salmonellosis, leishmaniasis and histoplasmosis (which are all intracellular pathogens of macrophages).
 d. **True**. Although the risk is not very high in the absence of genital ulceration.
 e. **False**. Typically below $200 \times 10^6/l$.

7. a. **False**. There is no evidence for this and prevention of thrush with continuous antifungal therapy may lead to resistance.
 b. **True**. Very important, should be introduced when T4 cell count falls below $200\text{-}250 \times 10^6/l$.
 c. **False**. A single episode of pneumococcal pneumonia is not an index disease for AIDS, but immunisation may prevent pneumococcal infection, which is about 100 times more common in AIDS although it may be less severe.
 d. **False**. There is no evidence that influenza is more severe in AIDS.
 e. **True**. Clearly shown in two double-blind controlled trials.

8. a. **True**. Purplish nodules on skin or in mouth.
 b. **True**. Common generally but more florid in HIV.
 c. **True**. Often rectal/anal and painful.
 d. **True**. An indication for an HIV test.
 e. **True**. Incidence in general population is 2–3% but in HIV may affect more nails and be recalcitrant to treatment.

9. a. **False**. Less than 10% of patients; pulmonary tuberculosis is much more common.
 b. **False**. Atypical chest X-ray without cavitation is common, less often smear positive in sputum.
 c. **False**. 90% of AIDS patients get oral thrush.
 d. **True**. Brain and heart. The CT/MR scan usually shows multiple ring-enhancing lesions, which are almost diagnostic of toxoplasmosis in AIDS. CNS lymphomas are usually single. Cardiac toxoplasmosis is usually diagnosed at autopsy.
 e. **False**. Only ganciclovir (i.v.), foscarnet (i.v.) and cidofovir are useful.

10. a. **False**. Recurrent cold sores are common and do not suggest immunodeficiency. Large and painful or prolonged HSV lesions, especially 'below the belt' would constitute an indication for HIV testing.
 b. **True**. Tuberculosis is rising throughout the

world and any risk factor in association with tuberculosis, or an atypical pattern of tuberculosis, would be an indication for HIV testing.

c. **False**. Non-Hodgkin's lymphoma occurs in AIDS but is more common in non-immunocompromised patients. Only if there is a risk factor would an HIV test be indicated.

d. **False**. Transmission of HIV from child to parents or from child to child is virtually unheard of. Many children from the USA, Romania, Africa and some south-east Asian countries are, however, HIV positive.

e. **True**. *Problematic recurrent* vaginal candidiasis is a clue to the diagnosis of HIV in women. However, in the UK at present, other causes are much more common, including antibiotics, pregnancy and for unknown reasons (p. 368).

Case history answers

History 1

1. His sexual history and possibly his travel history or history of any blood transfusions prior to 1985 in the developed world or more recently elsewhere.

2. The mouth. In particular, there might be oropharyngeal candidiasis, hairy leukoplakia and herpes simplex lesions. Also the genitals. If he is gay, he may have rectal herpes or warts which he has not declared.

3. PCP, pneumococcal pneumonia, other community-acquired pneumonia, pulmonary tuberculosis or pulmonary embolism.

4. Chest X-ray and arterial blood gases. The chest X-ray is abnormal in 85–90% of patients with PCP and > 95% in pneumococcal or other community-acquired pneumonias. Bilateral soft mid- or lower-zone shadows are typical of pneumocystis pneumonia but are only occasionally classical ground glass in appearance. Arterial blood gases usually show profound hypoxaemia and hypocapnia which is disproportionately abnormal compared with the patient's appearance. Corticosteroids are absolutely indicated as adjunctive therapy for any patient with pneumocystis pneumonia with a $PO_2 < 75$ mmHg on air.

History 2

1. a. **True**.
   b. **True**.
   c. **True**. She could have a mediastinal lymphoma, sarcoidosis or tuberculosis.
   d. **True**. There are enough clinical clues to suggest HIV infection to do either a T4 cell count or an HIV antibody test (or both).
   e. **True**. To rule out thyrotoxicosis (although if her

pulse rate was normal and there were no other features of thyroid hyperactivity, not necessary).

2. a. **True**. Key part of assessment: for oral thrush, hairy leukoplakia or Kaposi's sarcoma.
   b. **True**. But sensitively.
   c. **True**.
   d. **True**. After counselling.
   e. **False**. Oesophageal reflux or gastritis are unlikely diagnoses and may make oesophageal candidiasis worse.

3. a. **True**. As she needs their expertise.
   b. **False**. Combination therapy is the appropriate management and the use of zidovudine alone will lose her months or years of life.
   c. **True**.
   d. **False**. No need for admission, unless she cannot eat.
   e. **False**. The discussion of her result needs to be done with the HIV counsellor and not done on a Friday or in a rush. Set aside 30–40 minutes for the consultation.

Picture answers

1. a. Yeast cells with a capsule of *Cryptococcus neoformans*.
   b. India ink test.
   c. The CSF opening pressure. Patients with elevated pressure do badly unless the pressure is controlled.
   d. Cryptococcal antigen on CSF and serum, fungal blood culture, CT or MR scan of brain (mass-like lesions caused by *Cryptococcus* are rare, however).
   e. Amphotericin B and flucytosine followed by long-term fluconazole.

2. a. Bilateral midzone hazy shadowing.
   b. PCP, cytomegalovirus pneumonitis (check his and his donor's CMV status), invasive aspergillosis, pneumonitis caused by *Legionella pneumophilia*, or *Mycoplasma pneumoniae*, *Strongyloides stercoralis*, etc.
   c. Arterial blood gases and bronchoscopy.
   d. Broad-spectrum antibiotics to include cover for atypical agents, cotrimoxazole and possibly ganciclovir depending on the serostatus of the donor and patient.

Short note answers

1. The main issues are outlined in Box 13 (p. 342). The question of whether, if both are HIV positive, they should use safe sex is difficult to answer. If one has a much higher T4 count than the other, the one with the high count may acquire new pathogenic or resistant strains from his partner (speculation).

2. Risks include:

   - 1 in 250 for HIV needlestick, much higher for hepatitis B

- Higher risk for HIV if blood injected under skin, slightly higher risk if a hollow needle
- Other viruses, e.g. hepatitis C
- Very low risk for mucosal exposure (≈1 in 5000)
- No risk in touching patients or clothes/dishes/belongings.

Protection should involve

- use gloves if you handle any body fluids
- do not resheathe needles
- discard sharps in sharps containers only
- close and discard sharps containers before they are full.

If exposure occurs:

- *always* report the incident and see occupational health (no compensation possible otherwise)
- postexposure prophylaxis is proven (80% protection) but may need combination therapy
- administer antirectroviral therapy quickly (e.g. within one hour of exposure if possible).

3. a. AIDS/HIV infection, recurrent infection of undetermined aetiology, particularly suspected immunodeficiency in childhood and 'opportunistic' infection occurring in patients with no predisposing factors (e.g. cryptococcal meningitis). There are many causes of altered T cell subsets and reduced CD4 cell populations. Most of the changes in T subsets are not correlated specifically with clinical disease and are not diagnostically or therapeutically useful.
  b. Suspected immunoglobulin deficiency, e.g. recurrent pneumococcal infection, recurrent infection caused by unusual organisms or organisms in unusual sites (such as uveitis),

malabsorption syndrome eluding diagnosis of current sinusitis or pneumonia, alopecia areata, haemolytic anaemia, pernicious anaemia, anaphylaxis (for selective IgA deficiency), in the investigation of myeloma, Waldenström's macroglobulinaemia, and a few others.
  c. T4 cell counts ($\times 10^6$/l) can be divided into groups:
    800–1200. Normal in adults, higher in babies.
    500. Increase frequency of T4 cell counts and measure viral load to determine when to start antiretroviral therapy.
    350. Below this, tuberculosis, Kaposi's sarcoma, herpes zoster and other opportunistic infections start appearing. Patient needs more careful supervision. Start antiretroviral therapy as benefit is likely and toxicity small.
    ≤ 200–250. Start antipneumocystis prophylaxis with oral cotrimoxazole to prevent PCP
    ≤ 50. Most opportunistic infections are much more likely, especially cytomegalovirus retinitis (ask about eyesight regularly), MAI, azole-resistant candidosis, invasive aspergillosis, adrenal dysfunction, neurological problems.
  d. The main points are:
- difficult virus to work with as dangerous to staff
- mutates easily so may escape antigenic determinants selected for vaccine (e.g. influenza vaccine)
- immune response to HIV not protective
- vaccine should work at mucosal surfaces and in blood
- live vaccines fraught with uncertainty
- expensive, difficult animal model (chimpanzee and other primates)
- difficult to test in the field in humans against placebo, etc.

Infectious diseases

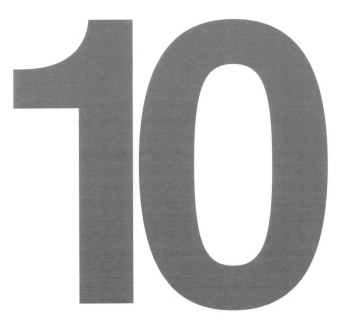

10.1 Clinical aspects

Introduction

Infections are common. Viral infections are substantially more common than bacterial infections, which are themselves more common than fungal infections, which, in the Western world, are more common than parasitic infections. In the developing world, parasitic infections are very common and may be chronic. For example, it is estimated that around four billion people worldwide are infected with roundworms.

In this book, the emphasis is on acute rather than chronic infections because it is acute infections that you as a house officer will be expected to manage. For reasons of space, large numbers of infectious illnesses are either completely omitted or dealt with in a cursory fashion and reference books should be used for further information particularly if knowledge of diseases rarely encountered in the UK is required.

Most infectious diseases are dealt with in this book in their respective organ-based chapters. Here, the focus is on your approach to the patient who may have a life-threatening infection, generalised infections, classical infectious diseases, genitourinary infections, skin and soft tissue infection and antibiotic therapy. Also described are the legal obligations you have with respect to infectious diseases.

Learning objectives

You must:

- be able to take a history relevant to infectious diseases
- be able to elicit and interpret important physical signs specific for the major infectious diseases.

Taking a history

Infection can arise from many sources. Often a clinical diagnosis can be made with confidence using only a combination of historical data together with findings on examination. In addition to the usual details that you should ask of the presenting complaint and the review of the systems, there are a few other factors which may be very important in evaluating a patient's illness. These are:

- immunisation history (including travel vaccines)
- travel history
- contact with animals, birds and reptiles
- whether anybody in the family, at work, or who has attended a recent social gathering is also ill
- the food or water the patient has consumed and how these were prepared
- prior prophylactic therapy or treatment (e.g. malaria prophylaxis)
- sexual history, particularly if the patient is gay
- history of i.v. drug or alcohol abuse
- immunocompromising factors in past medical history (see Chapter 9).

Sometimes the key elements of the history are rather subtle and require rather more questioning than might be apparent at first sight. Here is an example:

A 19-year-old male student was admitted with severe bloody diarrhoea and moderate fever of nine days' duration. Abdominal X-ray showed some dilatation of the colon. A diagnosis of ulcerative colitis with toxic megacolon was considered, as was colectomy. Detailed history revealed that he had recently moved away from home to student lodgings and was cooking for himself, having never done so previously. He had prepared a chicken by boiling it whole with vegetables in a pot which he served to some friends. The chicken was undercooked and some had been left over. The pot was too large for the refrigerator and was kept simply in the kitchen. He then finished the chicken off two days later on his own. A presumptive diagnosis of severe *Campylobacter* enteritis was made and he was treated with erythromycin and intravenous fluids and recovered.

Campylobacter was recovered from his stools three days after admission. He was given advice on how to prepare food safely.

Physical examination

A slightly different but complete physical examination is required for patients who may have an infection. This is because large numbers of infections have manifestations outside single organs and because there are many conditions with virtually pathognomonic physical signs. The presence of one of these signs allows a firm diagnosis and suitable treatment. A thorough systematic approach is particularly important.

The key elements of the examination include all parts of the mouth, the ears, the conjunctivae, the skin, a careful search for splenomegaly and, in any patient with neurological symptoms, a detailed neurological examination. Clearly examination of the respiratory system and a chest radiograph are important to diagnose many forms of pneumonia; auscultation of the heart, ECG and echocardiography are important in considering pericarditis and endocarditis; and abdominal examination and ultrasound are important for many reasons. In Table 82 are some examples of findings in the head and neck that may make or suggest a diagnosis which could easily be missed if not actively sought.

Fever, rigors and antipyretics

Learning objectives

You should:

- know how to record body temperature and interpret the value
- appreciate the significance of rigors and know how to act accordingly.

Body temperature

Body temperature is maintained by a balance between heat production from metabolic processes, particularly

Table 82 Contribution of the examination of the head and neck in the diagnosis of infectious disease (examples)

	Disease
Ears	
Auroscopy	Bullous myringitis of mycoplasma infection
	Otitis media
	Invasive (or malignant) otitis externa
External ear	Nodules on pinna of leprosy
	Bluish-red skin infiltrate of Lyme borreliosis
Nose and sinuses	Tenderness over the maxillae sinusitis
	Nasal escharin invasive fungal infections in neutropenia
Mouth	
Teeth and gingiva	Carious teeth consistent with lack of self-care, endocarditis and tooth abscess
	Gingivitis typical of HIV infection or HSV gingivostomatitis
Tongue	Hairy leukoplakia in HIV infection, bright red tongue of toxic shock syndrome, or Kawasaki disease
Tonsils and pharynx	Exudative tonsilitis of streptococcal pharyngitis, glandular fever or diphtheria
Mucous membranes	Koplick's spots of measles
	Oral candidiasis in HIV infection
	Kaposi's sarcoma in AIDS
	Ulcers in varicella, primary HIV or HSV infection
	Erythema in toxic shock syndrome
Eyes	
Conjunctiva	Non-purulent conjunctivitis in adenovirus infections, toxic shock syndrome, Kawasaki disease, measles
	Purpura consistent with meningococcal septicaemia
Neck	Tender lymphadenopathy at the angle of the jaw typical of streptococcal pharyngitis
	Non-tender bilateral lymphadenopathy consistent with glandular fever, toxoplasmosis and HIV infection
	Generally inflamed swollen neck bilaterally consistent with diphtheria
	Localised swelling on one side of the neck consistent with tuberculosis, Hodgkin's disease and streptococcal lymphadenitis

in the liver, muscle and brain, and heat loss through the skin. The control of this balance rests in the hypothalamus. There is a normal circadian rhythm of body temperature which varies by about 0.6°C (or 1°F) daily. The lowest body temperature is early in the morning and the high point is in the late afternoon. The implication is that early morning ward rounds may underestimate fever that day, delaying appropriate action. The normal body temperature in any given individual varies between 36.5°C and 37.3°C. All patients with a temperature of 37.5°C or above have a fever and some have fever with temperatures of 37°C.

The figures above refer to core body temperature as measured by oral readings. In many wards, axillary temperatures are taken and these are almost always a degree below oral readings. When patients are vasoconstricted, these may be 2 or 3°C below oral readings. You should know how temperature readings are recorded in the ward in order to interpret the charts appropriately.

Two groups of compounds stimulate fever:

Exogenous pyrogens. For example, Gram-negative endotoxin, enterotoxins of *Staphylococcus aureus*, toxic shock syndrome toxin 1, viruses, yeasts and some drugs (e.g. vancomycin and bleomycin).

The cytokines. Especially interleukin-1, tumour necrosis factor, interleukin-6 and γ-interferon. If these substances are released, particular neurons in the hypothalamus detect them and are stimulated to produce prostaglandin E_2. Other hypothalamic neurons 'reset' the target core temperature for the body. This results in peripheral vasoconstriction, muscle shivering and increased metabolic activity. A 1°C rise in body temperature above 37°C increases total oxygen consumption by 13%.

Hyperpyrexia

Occasionally, hyperpyrexia (> 40°C) can be produced because of a lack of heat loss. The causes include heatstroke and malignant hyperpyrexia, which is caused by certain anaesthetics and some neuroleptic drugs. In addition, the hypothalamic temperature set-point may be elevated following intracranial trauma or tumour or some other hypothalamic dysfunction, e.g. pontine haemorrhage. All of these syndromes are rare apart from the heatstroke, in which the history usually makes the diagnosis obvious. It is very important to reduce fever above 40°C because permanent brain damage can occur in patients whose temperatures remain sustained above 42°C.

Hypothermia

Occasionally severe infection is accompanied by hypothermia (< 36°C) rather than hyperthermia. This is uncommon but carries a poor prognosis if observed. Hypothermia is much more commonly related to excessive heat loss as in exposure, myxoedema or inadequate heating, particularly among the elderly.

Symptoms of fever

A common symptom of fever is chills. An exaggerated form of chills is rigors. The distinction between the two relates to the degree of shaking, which itself is usually related to both the rapidity of rise of pyrexia and its maximum height. Most patients with a significant temperature complain of being cold and wanting to get into bed with all their clothes on and with extra blankets. They may then lie there shivering, often with their teeth chattering. When this gets to the extent that the whole bed is shaking and their teeth are chattering uncontrollably for 3–10 minutes, that is termed a rigor. Shaking chills and in particular rigors are almost always caused by infection. High fever may occur with other diseases (such as Hodgkin's disease) but shaking chills and rigors rarely do.

Rigors are a distinctive clinic entity and are an absolute indication for admission of a patient to hospital. Common causes of rigors include:

- Gram-negative bacteraemia, especially pyelonephritis and cholangitis
- pneumococcal pneumonia or bacteraemia
- malaria.

Pyrexia makes most patients feel very uncomfortable. Common accompanying features include mild headache, fatigue, anorexia and irritability. Studies in ferrets and in vitro have shown that many immune responses are augmented by increased body temperature, suggesting that the febrile response is 'good'. However, there are few data suggesting that a *sustained* febrile response is good and so antipyretic therapy is appropriate for the relief of symptoms.

There are two approaches to reducing fever:

- the administration of prostaglandin synthase inhibitors, e.g. paracetamol or aspirin
- direct cooling of the patient by sponging down with cold water.

Naturally patients tend to prefer the former. Aspirin is not an appropriate choice in children with fever because of Reye's syndrome and, therefore, paracetamol (or acetaminophen) is preferred. Steroids should not be used simply for reducing fever. It should be noted, however, that patients taking steroids may have a blunted or absent temperature response to infection, which may mask serious infection and inflammation.

Serious sepsis and septic shock

Learning objectives

You must
- know how to distinguish patients with minor infections from those with life-threatening bacterial or fungal sepsis
- be able to diagnose meningococcaemia, serious staphylococcal infection, toxic shock syndrome and septic shock clinically.
- know the main complications of serious sepsis and be able to implement the basic management strategies.

Bacterial and invasive fungal infections are frequently life-threatening. Epitomised by bacteraemia and fungaemia they can lead to a cascade of interrelated pathogenetic mechanisms, culminating in hypotension, shock and multiorgan failure. The substances involved besides endotoxin and other products of the microorganisms include tumour necrosis factor, interleukin-1, complement C3 and C5 and several components in the coagulation cascade. In severe cases of sepsis, a cascade of ever worsening host responses is initiated by the above factors, which progresses over hours to days leading to a progressive downhill course. Probably the most dramatic examples are meningococcal septicaemia and toxic shock syndrome and the least dramatic examples

are older patients with bacteraemia from a urinary source or community-acquired pneumonia.

The old terms septicaemia and the sepsis syndrome have been replaced by four more explanatory terms embracing a spectrum of disease directly related to the magnitude of the host response to infection. The mildest form is the **systemic inflammatory response syndrome (SIRS)** and the worst is **septic shock** (Fig. 67). These terms are defined in Box 14. The older dogma is that the severity and mortality of infection are much more likely to be associated with *documented* infection than not, but this is now known to be false. The body's response to infection can occur in the absence of *documented* infection, although it is relatively rare to have patients present with these features and have no focus of infection apparent at all. The major exception to this is toxic shock syndrome.

Complications of sepsis

Complications of sepsis include:

- septic shock (see below)
- acute respiratory distress syndrome (ARDS) (see below)
- acute renal failure (p. 155)
- disseminated intravascular coagulation (DIC) (p. 248)
- peripheral symmetrical gangrene (see below).

Septic shock

Septic shock occurs as two relatively distinct syndromes.

Warm septic shock. This is manifest by patients with hypotension and a bounding pulse, often with warm but cyanosed peripheries. These patients are alert, anxious, hyperventilating with a substantial tachycardia.

Cold septic shock. This has a much worse prognosis and is manifest by cold, peripherally cyanosed

---

Box 14
Sepsis and septic shock: definitions

Systemic inflammatory response syndrome (SIRS): at least two of the following:

- temperature > 38°C or < 36°C
- heart rate > 90/minute
- respiratory rate > 20/minute or pCO_2 < 32 mmHg
- white blood cell count > 12 or < 4.0×10^9/l or immature neutrophils (left shift or band) > 0.1×10^9/l

Sepsis: SIRS with a confirmed infectious process, e.g. positive blood culture, abnormal chest X-ray, cellulitis, etc.

Severe sepsis: sepsis + organ dysfunction, hypoperfusion abnormalities (e.g. lactic acidosis, oliguria, mental status alteration) or hypotension

Septic shock: sepsis-induced hypotension (< 90 mmHg systolic) despite i.v. fluids, with hypoperfusion abnormalities

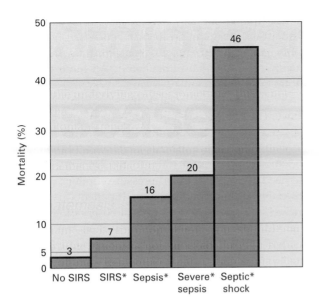

Fig. 67
Mortality in relation to infection with SIRS, sepsis and septic shock.

Acute respiratory distress syndrome

ARDS is preceded by acute lung injury. There are many causes of acute lung injury, primarily infection, but including hypotension, smoke inhalation and other systemic diseases. The definition of ARDS is:

- ratio of arterial oxygen (PaO_2) to inspired oxygen (F_iO_2) of ≤ 200 whether or not positive end-expiratory pressure (PEEP) is used
- bilateral pulmonary infiltrates
- normal or low left atrial pressure (or wedge pressure ≤ 18 mmHg).

In the early hours after the precipitating event causing ARDS, the chest X-ray may be normal, but diffuse bilateral alveolar infiltrates usually appear within 4–24 hours. The risk of ARDS with some insults is higher than with others. For example, it occurs in 30–40% of patients who aspirate gastric contents but is much less common with cellulitis or mycoplasma pneumonia.

All patients with established ARDS can only be managed in the intensive care unit with assisted ventilation. Patients with mild but acute lung injury may be managed with other forms of oxygen supplementation initially but usually will require mechanical ventilation at some stage. Fluid should be restricted, if possible, to prevent excessive alveolar accumulation of fluid, as there is increased vascular permeability and usually a low serum albumin. The position of the patient should be taken into account, as some patients may not have equal lung injury on both sides and certain positions will allow better ventilation than others.

Most patients with ARDS require 10–20 days of ventilatory support. A tracheostomy is warranted if patients will require more than 10 days of ventilation, to prevent late strictures of the trachea. Patients who survive ARDS have a good outlook with virtually complete recovery of lung function.

Peripheral symmetrical gangrene

Peripheral symmetrical gangrene is an unusual complication of septic shock, but it is devastating. The patient's fingers, toes and, sometimes, hands and feet, become dusky and cold initially. Then gradually over the next 3–7 days they become obviously gangrenous with a clear demarcation line (dry gangrene). All these patients have DIC. Eventually surgery is required to remove the devitalised digits if the patient survives.

Management of severe sepsis

The key to the successful management of patients with severe sepsis with or without shock is appropriate antibiotic therapy and excellent supportive care.

Supportive care may mean simply the judicious administration of fluids and oxygen until the septic episode resolves. Alternatively, it may mean full intensive care management requiring mechanical ventilation, blood pressure support with pressor agents and haemodialysis or haemofiltration. Clearly, early recog-

peripheries, an ill and quiet patient who is grey and sweaty, hypotensive, hypoventilating and usually non-communicative.

Patients may progress from the warm phase to the cold phase and this is a bad prognostic feature.

There are two major derangements in the cardiovascular system in septic shock:

- reduced peripheral resistance, leading to a low blood pressure and inappropriate distribution of blood
- myocardial depression leading to a low cardiac output.

In warm septic shock, the first of these is operative and cardiac output is often increased. In cold septic shock, both are operative and the patient is often substantially fluid-depleted and oxygen-deficient in addition.

All patients with septic shock should be monitored extremely closely for respiratory rate, pulse rate, blood pressure, temperature and urine output (e.g. hourly). Arterial blood gases are essential to assess the degree of metabolic acidosis (p. 172) and hypoxia (p. 65). Oxygen should be administered in large quantities as further organ dysfunction can be exacerbated by hypoxia. In addition, ARDS is a common complication and serial monitoring of arterial blood gases will give an early indication of the development of ARDS and, therefore, the need for assisted ventilation. A raised respiratory rate reflects not only hypoxia but also acidosis and you cannot use it as a guide to the need for ventilation in patients with serious sepsis.

Renal dysfunction and in particular acute renal failure (p. 155) is common but not universal. Serum creatinine and electrolytes should be measured at least daily in these patients. A fall in the platelet count will give an early indication of DIC, which should prompt the measurement of fibrin degradation products or D-dimers.

nition of sepsis and the prompt administration of appropriate antibiotics can reduce the need for intensive care management.

There is a large number of different organisms that can invade the blood or cause sepsis. What follows, in this section, are four examples: one Gram-negative, one Gram-positive, one toxin-mediated and one fungal. The first three are clinically distinctive, the last not so. All carry a high mortality despite therapy: 10–60%.

Meningococcaemia

Neisseria meningitidis is a common Gram-negative coccus that resides in the nasopharynx in up to 20% of the population. Transmission is greatest between members of the family and can also occur in other closed groups such as school classrooms, military recruits, etc.

There are two major manifestations of severe meningococcal disease:
- meningitis with or without bacteraemia (p. 189)
- meningococcaemia without meningitis.

Clinical features
The features of meningococcaemia are variable initially. Early clinical features are:

- fever
- macular rash on the trunk.

As the disease progresses the macular rash, if present, fades (within the first 12–24 hours) and the patient becomes acutely and obviously unwell. Vomiting, pallor, high fever, drowsiness and hypotension are characteristic. There are three clinical features which help to distinguish this infection from other causes of septic shock. These are:

- petechiae and purpuric lesions on the skin and conjunctivae
- rapid onset
- relatively young age of the patient, e.g. child or young adult.

When you are presented with such a very ill patient, it is important to undress them completely to look for petechiae. They are typically 1–2 mm in diameter and found on the trunk, ankles and wrists. They are more likely to be found in clusters where there are areas of pressure applied to the skin by socks or underwear. As the lesions progress, they may coalesce and form large ecchymoses. The lesions may also be found in the conjunctivae. Although difficult to see in black skins, they are usually visible on brown-skinned people.

Investigations
Specific investigations on admission should include a blood culture, a nasal culture, arterial blood gases, urea, electrolytes, full blood count, platelet count and coagulation studies. DIC and thrombocytopenia are common.

Management
The rapid progression of disease is striking and patients may go from first symptoms to death in less than 36 hours. If such a patient presents in general practice, you should give them i.m. or i.v. penicillin (assuming the patient is not allergic) immediately. All these patients require hospitalisation.

All *N. meningitidis* isolates are susceptible to penicillin and to second- and third-generation cephalosporins (e.g. cefuroxime or cefotaxime). Early administration of antibiotics will reduce the case fatality rate of meningococcaemia from around 100% to around 50%. Patients also need appropriate blood pressure support, possibly artificial ventilation and isolation. If patients are not yet shocked, very frequent and careful observation should be made for the development of shock as this is common and very rapid in onset. Steroids are not indicated.

Prevention of disease
All cases of disease produced by *N. meningitidis* are notifiable (p. 375) and this should be done by telephone as soon as the diagnosis is made. If two cases occur that are epidemiologically linked, the episode will be defined as an epidemic. Usually this occurs in the context of a school classroom. In this case, all should receive chemoprophylaxis and possibly immunisation (see below). This will be done by the Consultant for Communicable Disease Control. In addition, all household members of the patient should be given chemoprophylaxis and any other close family contacts who spend a lot of time in the same household. The only health-care staff who require chemoprophylaxis are those who have given mouth-to-mouth resuscitation.

In the UK, most cases of meningococcal disease are caused by groups B or C strains. If the outbreak is caused by group C, immunisation with meningococcal vaccine is appropriate; therefore, it is vital to isolate and group the organism from nasal or blood cultures rapidly to prevent other cases.

Staphylococcal bacteraemia

S. aureus and coagulase-negative staphylococcus (including *S. epidermidis*) infections are increasing in frequency. Both are major hospital pathogens and *S. aureus* is also a major community pathogen. Both are related to intravascular catheter use. Although *S. aureus* causes many types of infection, this section will focus on bacteraemia.

S. aureus bacteraemia

Clinical features
S. aureus bacteraemia presents in a relatively non-specific way although some features are distinctive. Virtually all patients look unwell and have fever, usually with chills and/or rigors. Tachycardia, a gallop rhythm murmur and pleural rubs are common. The distinctive clinical features are:

- diarrhoea
- joint pain or pleuritic pain

- cutaneous petechiae or subconjunctival haemorrhage
- confusion (related to 'staphylococcal cerebritis')
- external focus of infection, e.g. infected intravascular catheter site, cellulitis, marks of i.v. drug abuse
- Roth spots in fundi
- *normal* or raised total white cell count (with marked neutrophilia).

Investigations

The blood culture usually becomes positive within 24 hours, sometimes less. Given that many of the patients have murmurs, it is often difficult to decide whether the patient has endocarditis. Echocardiography is essential for evaluation. If the patient has a prosthetic heart valve, you should assume that the valve is infected (antibiotics and *urgent* surgery) (p. 36).

Treatment

Flucloxacillin (at least 2 g 6-hourly) is the standard necessary treatment for *S. aureus* bacteraemia. A repeat blood culture should be done on day 3 of therapy. If this culture is negative *and* the patient has no focal features of disease (e.g. osteomyelitis) a 2-week course of therapy is adequate. If the day 3 culture is positive or focal disease is present, 6 weeks of therapy (at least half intravenously) is necessary. Longer therapy is also necessary in some immunocompromised patients. Some isolates such as multiply resistant *S. aureus* (MRSA) are resistant to flucloxacillin, so vancomycin or teicoplanin are required. Other antibiotics in combination, e.g. rifampin, gentamicin or fusidic acid, are often used for the more difficult forms of staphylococcal infection.

Coagulase-negative staphylococcal bacteraemia

Clinical features

In contrast, patients with coagulase-negative staphylococcal bacteraemia are usually not as ill and virtually always have one of the following:

- immunocompromised status (e.g. neutropenia)
- indwelling intravascular catheters
- prosthetic intravascular devices, e.g. pacemakers, cardiac valves.

By no means all positive blood cultures for coagulase-negative staphylococci reflect disease. The organism is a normal inhabitant of the skin and improper skin cleaning or a break in aseptic techniques in the laboratory may lead to contamination. However, nowadays, isolates represent real disease more often than previously and should be managed as such.

Management

The principles of management are:

- to remove any infected device or catheter; occasionally cure can be effected with high doses of i.v. antibiotics without removal of a device, but this is rare
- to give appropriate antibiotics.

Like MRSA, coagulase-negative staphylococci are often resistant to flucloxacillin, so vancomycin or teicoplanin are usually used. The duration of therapy is usually much shorter than with *S. aureus* infection, depending on the status of the patient. If longer-term oral therapy is required, this can be quite a problem because of resistance, and it requires detailed microbiological advice.

Toxic shock syndrome

First described in 1978, toxic shock syndrome (TSS) is the archetypal superantigen disease. Around 100 cases occur in the UK each year.

Antigens and antigen-presenting cells

Most antigens are protein molecules that evoke a specific immune response. Sometimes nucleic acids (as in SLE), glycolipids or small molecules such as metal ions (in combination with protein) act as antigens. Some antigens are more potent than others. Protein antigens can be recognised in either of two ways: as a sequence of 4–6 amino acids or as a small surface site on a globular protein. In the latter case, the components of the antigenic site may be 3–8 amino acid residues separated in terms of sequence but which happen to be together on the surface of the protein as a result of folding.

The majority of protein antigens are not directly recognised by T cells. Instead the protein is taken up by an antigen-presenting cell.

Most antigen presentation is done by three cell types:

- macrophages
- B cells
- Langerhan's (skin) and dendritic (lymphoid tissue) cells.

Antigen-presenting cells partially digest the antigen and shift the antigenic fragments to the cell surface, adjacent to an MHC molecule (p. 343). The combination of a foreign protein next to an MHC molecule activates T helper cells. A positive feedback loop between the T and B cells is then set up and specific antibody and cellular responses follow. T4 cells can only recognise antigens presented with MHC class II molecules and T8 cells only those presented with MHC class I.

Superantigens

A few proteins are able to join up the MHC receptors on antigen-presenting cells with T cells, without being processed (Fig. 68). These are superantigens. The best example is in TSS. Ordinarily, antigen presentation is the rate-limiting step in immune responses. However superantigens bypass this by activating up to 10% of all T cells and in this way a vast array of immune responses are set in motion rapidly, which is the main reason these patients get so ill so quickly.

TSS is usually produced by a staphylococcal toxin (TSST-1) produced by *S. aureus*. Occasionally TSS is

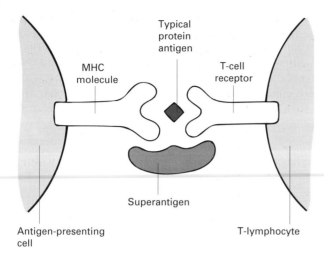

Fig. 68
Toxic shock syndrome: toxin (superantigen) bridges antigen recognition sites of T-cells and antigen-presenting cells to switch on massive T cell proliferation and cytokine release.

caused by toxins of *Streptococcus pyogenes*. TSST-1 is a protein produced in the body under favourable conditions (e.g. around a tampon in the vagina during menstruation). Ordinarily antibody is protective but many teenagers have none and so they are at greater risk of disease.

In most cases in women, there is no focus of staphylococcal infection and the organism is a 'commensal' that produces toxin. In a few cases (10% in women and > 90% in men) the patients have a focus of infection, such as a wound infection, sinusitis, etc.

Clinical features
The onset is usually rapid. Feeling like 'I'm getting flu' rapidly progresses to severe illness over 12–24 hours. The key presenting features are:

- diarrhoea
- fainting, near fainting or postural hypotension
- high fever with chills and/or rigors
- faint body rash
- drowsiness and/or confusion.

On examination you will see the following features:

- fever > 38.5°C
- hypotension or postural hypotension
- macular body rash usually with red cheeks
- erythema of buccal and/or vaginal mucosa
- conjunctivitis.

Investigations show multisystem disease, such as renal dysfunction, raised CPK (myositis), thrombocytopenia, etc.

The mortality is about 10%. Treatment is supportive. After 2 weeks of illness, if the patient survives, desquamation of the skin of the hands, soles and body occurs. There is no diagnostic test for this disease and the diag-nosis is entirely clinical. Sometimes TSST-1-producing *S. aureus* can be isolated from the vagina or wound.

Candidaemia

Candidaemia is increasingly common, particularly in cancer and intensive care unit patients (p. 356). Unfortunately, only half the patients with documented invasive candidiasis at autopsy have a positive blood culture before death and, therefore, empiric therapy is frequently justified. There are probably over 2000 cases of invasive candidiasis in the UK each year, although less than half of these are confirmed. The major risk factors for candidaemia are:

- Perforated GI tract (e.g. faecal peritonitis)
- pancreatitis
- intensive care with central venous catheter
- multiple i.v. antibiotics
- diabetes mellitus
- renal failure or renal replacement therapy.

Clinical features
The clinical presentation of candidaemia is very variable. Some patients are acutely ill, others only mildly so. Not all have fever although most do. The following are typical presentations:

- severe sepsis progressing to septic shock (indistinguishable from bacteraemia, but in an at-risk group)
- low-grade fever and leucocytosis in an at-risk patient
- high fever with skin lesions (typically *Candida tropicalis* infection)
- general lack of improvement or deterioration in an intensive care unit patient.

Management and outcome
Some patients have one positive blood culture, others multiple positives; all require therapy. Some species of *Candida* are fluconazole-resistant, others amphotericin B-resistant (rare). The two best drugs are still fluconazole and amphotericin B.

The mortality from candidaemia is approximately 65% even if treatment is given early. Half of the deaths are attributable to underlying disease rather than directly caused by the candidaemia.

10.2 Skin infections

Learning objectives

You should:
- know the major forms of skin infection, their microbiology and their treatment
- be able to recognise cellulitis and erysipelas and distinguish these from gas gangrene and necrotising fasciitis.

Types of skin infection

There are a number of different skin infections, varying from the trivial, e.g. impetigo, to the life-threatening.

Impetigo and localised skin sepsis

Impetigo is a very superficial infection usually caused by *S. aureus* or streptococci and common in children. Topical or oral antibiotics are usually successful. *S. aureus* also causes a number of localised infections such as boils, carbuncles and folliculitis, which can be appropriately treated with drainage if large and anti-staphylococcal antibiotics.

Erysipelas

Erysipelas is a distinctive type of superficial cellulitis caused by group A streptococci. The most common site is on the lower limbs but the face may be involved. Clinically the skin is somewhat painful, bright red, oedematous and indurated in appearance *with a sharply demarcated border* (Table 83). Virtually all the patients have fever. Only rarely is the organism grown from a blood culture or from aspiration of skin in the infected area. Therefore, the combination of fever, typical skin lesions and a leucocytosis makes the diagnosis of erysipelas. Treatment is with penicillin, initially i.v. or i.m. and subsequently orally, or with erythromycin or cefuroxime.

Cellulitis

Cellulitis is also an acute infective condition of the skin but extends more deeply to involve subcutaneous tissues. Group A streptococci or *S. aureus* are the most frequent causes, but occasionally Gram-negative bacteria or fungi may cause this disease in immunocompromised patients. Unlike erysipelas, the borders of an area of cellulitis are *not* sharply demarcated. Regional lymphadenopathy and fever are usual (Table 83). 'Blood cultures are occasionally positive. The diagnosis is a clinical one based on fever, typical appearance of the skin and leucocytosis. Treatment with penicillin i.v. and flucloxacillin or cefuroxime alone is appropriate.

Streptococcal gangrene, gas gangrene and necrotising fasciitis

Life-threatening skin infections include gas gangrene and necrotising fasciitis. Most are caused by *Clostridia* or Group A stretococci alone. A few are caused by a mixture of aerobic and anaerobic organisms and the term synergistic necrotising cellulitis is preferred. These include, for example, Fournier's gangrene, occurring in the perineal area in elderly patients, often with diabetes.

Clinical features. Characteristic clinical features are:

- local pain which is often severe (Table 83)
- localised oedema
- brown or black discoloration of the skin
- crepitus of the skin
- foul odour.

Treatment. There are two major aspects of management:

- antibiotics
- surgical debridement.

The antibiotics of choice are i.v. penicillin, metronidazole and a broad-spectrum Gram-negative antibiotic such as ceftazidime. Resection of infected areas is critically important even if mutilating surgery is necessary to save the patient's life. In instances where surgery cannot be completely undertaken without removing vital structures there may be a role for hyperbaric oxygen therapy.

10.3 Classical infectious diseases

In the developed world, most of the major infectious diseases of the last century have now virtually been eradicated. This is, however, not true of the developing world, where these diseases are still common major killers. Measles, in particular, has a major impact on mortality in children in the developing world. This section, therefore, focuses on some of the classical infectious diseases that either are common in the UK or are immunised against. Rabies and tetanus are dealt with on pages 193 and 194 respectively.

Learning objectives

You should:

- know how to diagnose the major classical infectious diseases that occur in adults, including varicella,

Table 83 Life-threatening skin infections

	Fever	Local pain	Crepitus	Erythema	Dusky/black areas	Systemic toxicity
Erysipelas	++	+	−	+++	−	+
Cellulitis	++	+	−	+++	−	++
Streptococcal gangrene/necrotising fasciitis	+++	+++	+/−	+/++	++	+++
Gas gangrene	++	+++	++	+	+++	+++

herpes zoster, rubella, parvovirus and glandular fever

- know the key clinical manifestations of rarer infectious diseases such as mumps, diphtheria, whooping cough, Lyme disease and leptospirosis
- know how to approach the investigation and management of patients complaining of fatigue
- know which classical infectious diseases are preventable by immunisation.

Diphtheria

Diphtheria is caused by *Corynebacterium diphtheriae*. The manifestations of disease are produced by an exotoxin which is carried on a bacteriophage within the bacterial cell. Therefore, not all strains of *C. diphtheriae* are pathogenic. In the early 1700s, a major epidemic of diphtheria occurred in New England which killed an estimated 2.5% of the population and approximately one-third of all the children. It is for this reason that immunisation programmes are maintained. Immunisation is with a modified toxin (toxoid) and is highly effective.

Clinical features

There are several forms of diphtheria. In all cases, *C. diphtheriae* remains superficial (i.e. not invasive) and the organism can be grown from skin, throat or nasal cultures. There are two common forms.

Pharyngeal diphtheria. Symptoms are low-grade fever, sore throat and the development of a 'membrane' on one or both tonsils. It may be mistaken for glandular fever. Cervical adenopathy and local tissue swelling of the neck is common. The membrane can descend to involve the larynx and cause respiratory obstruction.

Cutaneous diphtheria. Indolent skin ulcers sometimes occur with an overlying membrane and are coinfected with other bacteria. Cutaneous ulcers are the major means of disseminating the organism. Chronic skin ulcers in recent immigrants are the most common manifestation of diphtheria in the UK.

Management

Strict isolation in an infectious disease unit is necessary for all patients with possible or confirmed diphtheria (as required by law). Management of acute disease involves administration of diphtheria antitoxin and antibiotics. Antiserum is produced in horses and occasionally produces life-threatening toxic reactions. The best antibiotics appear to be penicillin, erythromycin and clindamycin. Diphtheria is a notifiable disease.

Varicella (chickenpox)

Varicella is caused by herpes zoster virus (VZV). It is a common infection. Over 60% of the UK population have evidence of prior infection. It is acquired by inhalation of virus particles and is among the most communicable of infectious diseases. If a susceptible individual is exposed to someone infected, they have an 80% chance of catching varicella. The incubation period is long, 10–21 days.

Clinical features

The hallmarks of varicella are fever and a vesicular rash on the trunk.

Fever precedes the rash by 1–3 days and lasts from 5–8 days. There is a wide spectrum of severity, particularly in children, in which the number of skin lesions may range from only one or two lesions to complete covering of the patient with lesions. The disease tends to be worse in adults. At least one of the reasons for this is that most adults are secondary cases. This means that the disease is brought home by one of their children who has caught it at school or at a friend's house and was exposed to a low inoculum. The child is only mildly ill. However, because the parent is exposed over several days to the infected child, the parent's inoculum is much larger and as a result he/she gets much more severe disease. The same is true for other siblings at home, particularly pre-school children or infants.

Skin lesions
The skin lesions start as small red papules, about 3–5 mm across, and quickly evolve into vesicles containing clear fluid. They are pruritic. Over the next 2–3 days the vesicles rupture and after 4–6 days, the lesions crust over. Eventually the crust falls off leaving a slight scar at the site. Lesions are most pronounced on the trunk and head with few lesions on the limbs. In addition, there are usually small ulcers inside the mouth. These ulcers may be profuse and painful, preventing the patient from eating and drinking.

Immunocompromised patients
The illness is much more severe in immunocompromised patients, particularly those with defective T cell immunity, including patients taking steroids. In these patients, fever and back pain are the typical presenting features and the rash may either not be present or be atypical. The mortality of varicella in immunocompromised patients is high.

Management

In hospital, *all* patients need respiratory isolation and should be managed in an infectious disease unit. Transmission from patients to staff and then to immunocompromised patients with a fatal outcome is well documented.

Patients with mild varicella need no treatment other than antipyretics and antipruritics. Immunocompromised patients, secondary cases and those with severe disease should be treated. The drug of choice at present is acyclovir given at high dose i.v. or orally. Acyclovir probably reduces the period of infectivity by 1 or 2 days.

Complications

Complications of varicella are common with severe disease. They include:

- secondary bacterial skin infection
- difficulty swallowing
- pneumonitis (6% of adults, severe in pregnancy)
- haemorrhagic varicella with or without thrombocytopenia
- congenital varicella syndrome ($\approx 2\%$ risk) if the mother is affected in the second or third trimester of pregnancy
- neurological complications including postinfectious encephalitis, transverse myelitis and cerebral infarction.

Herpes zoster (shingles)

VZV is a lifelong inhabitant of the body following primary infection. Reactivation occurs from dorsal root ganglia to produce a skin eruption, usually in a single dermatome. Precipitating factors for herpes zoster include immunosuppression and stressful life events, but in most cases none are found. Herpes zoster may be a presentation of AIDS and it is common following the treatment of lymphoma.

Clinical features

The earliest sign of herpes zoster is pain or discomfort in the area infected. This may be present for up to 36 hours before any rash is visible, which makes diagnosis difficult. The rash appears as a vesicular eruption, much like chickenpox, with lesions appearing in the first 2–5 days of the episode. One of the characteristic features of shingles which distinguishes it from other rashes is the sharp demarcation seen at the midline. Usually there are up to 10 additional lesions typical of chickenpox in other parts of the body. If there are more than ten you should consider that the virus has disseminated, which is an indication for hospitalisation and i.v. acyclovir therapy.

As the rash progresses it starts to crust and requires careful dressing if it is extensive. Typically the whole episode is over in about 10–14 days (apart from post-herpetic neuralgia).

Cranial zoster

Occasionally herpes zoster will occur over the cranium in dermatomes C1 to C4 or in the distribution of the trigeminal nerve. Some of these patients develop a mild and self-limited form of encephalitis. In patients with infection of the superior branch of the trigeminal nerve (e.g. the forehead) or the maxillary branch, there is a possibility of corneal involvement as a result of infection of the nasolabial branch of the trigeminal nerve. As you recall, the nasolabial branch supplies a small area of sensation at the lateral side of the nose and the cornea.

Corneal zoster

Herpes zoster of the cornea is a destructive keratitis that requires acyclovir eye drops for treatment. These patients also get substantial oedema around the eyes, which may be bilateral even though there is unilateral involvement.

Ramsay–Hunt syndrome

The involvement of the facial nerve can lead to a condition known as the Ramsay–Hunt syndrome (p. 186) in which skin lesions and pain occur on the pinna and external canal of the ear and there is ipsilateral facial paralysis which rarely recovers.

Treatment

Non-immunocompromised patients with mild herpes zoster do not require therapy. Immunocompromised patients always require therapy. Patients with extensive involvement may justify therapy although it is sometimes difficult to ascertain the extent of involvement early enough in the illness for therapy to have any impact. At present acyclovir or one of its new prodrugs are the only agents useful for the treatment of shingles. The impact of treatment is to reduce viral excretion and dry up the lesions a couple of days earlier than would be the case without treatment. In the immunocompromised patient, however, varicella zoster can disseminate and cause extensive local disease leading to scar formation. Treatment will prevent this.

Post-herpetic neuralgia

Post-herpetic neuralgia is defined as the persistence of localised pain 4 or more weeks after the rash disappears. The pain can last for months or years and is often severe and resistant to treatment. It is a disease of the elderly patient; there is virtually no risk under the age of 60 but approximately 50% of patients over 60 suffer from it. The cause of post-herpetic neuralgia is not known but it is likely to reflect continuing inflammation in the ganglia. This is supported by finding circulating herpes zoster virus in mononuclear cells months after the rash has resolved in those with post-hepatic neuralgia but not in those without it. However, continued antiviral therapy with acyclovir does not seem to diminish the problem.

Treatment of the pain of post-herpetic neuralgia differs from the treatment of most other forms of pain. Conventional analgesics are usually ineffective. Tricyclic antidepressants are of some benefit. When there is dysaesthesia or lancinating pain, then an anticonvulsant such as carbamazepine may be helpful. Local cutaneous treatments include ethyl chloride spray, transcutaneous nerve stimulation, topical capsaicin (a substance P antagonist). Local anaesthetic cream under cling film may also be of benefit.

Older textbooks will often cite the use of steroids during herpes zoster, but these have been shown to be ineffective in preventing post-herpetic neuralgia.

Measles

Measles is caused by an RNA virus for which there is no specific treatment. The success of childhood immunisation has left a large number of susceptible teenagers and adults at risk because of individual vaccine failure and waning of incomplete immunity. There is a resurgence of measles cases in young adults in the USA and this was one of the reasons that led the UK Department of Health to reimmunise all schoolchildren in the UK in late 1994.

Measles can be clinically suspected in adults with five features:

- high fever (100%)
- cough (98%)
- conjunctivitis (96%)
- maculopapular rash on trunk on days 3–5 (100%)
- coryza (84%).

Adults with the disease are often febrile for 10 days or so and are quite ill. Secondary pneumonia and/or otitis media are common. The incubation period is typically 10 days. Patients require respiratory isolation to prevent airborne transmission. Measles is a notifiable disease.

Mumps

Mumps can be a mild disease with low-grade fever and malaise its only manifestation. Complications include meningitis (p. 189), encephalitis (p. 192), orchitis, parotitis and pancreatitis. You should consider the diagnosis in a patient with any of these problems. Immunisation is effective but there is no specific treatment. Mumps is a notifiable disease.

Rubella (German measles)

Without immunisation against rubella, 15–20% of women are at risk of acquiring it in pregnancy. This figure has fallen to below 3% in the 1990s with the success of the MMR vaccine. The recent reimmunisation of all schoolchildren against measles and rubella is likely to reduce this figure further.

Rubella is an RNA virus and the incubation period is long like varicella, e.g. 10–21 days. There is no specific treatment.

Most patients with rubella have a mild illness, with or without fever but with a rash. The rash is macular, particularly apparent on the trunk and face and is typically associated with conjunctivitis. Other clues to the diagnosis include lymphadenopathy, especially if suboccipital, and arthritis and arthralgia.

It can be difficult to distinguish rubella from a parvovirus infection clinically if there are joint symptoms.

The diagnosis can be made serologically. This is of critical importance in pregnancy because the risk of fetal infection is 80–90% if rubella is contracted in the first 12 weeks of pregnancy. About 85% of infected infants are damaged. Rubella must be notified.

Parvovirus infection (fifth disease)

Parvoviruses are small single-stranded DNA viruses which cause erythema infectiosum (fifth disease). In the UK, 50% of adults have evidence of exposure to the virus, mostly in childhood. However, the virus has a number of important properties if infection occurs in adulthood.

Approximately 20% of infections are asymptomatic. Symptomatic patients typically have:

- low-grade fever
- a facial rash (slapped cheek appearance)
- a reticulated or lace-like rash on the trunk and extremities
- symmetrical, peripheral polyarthropathy or arthralgia.

Symptoms are usually self-limited but may persist for months. Joint symptoms may be the only manifestation of disease.

Complications

In patients with any chronic haemolytic anaemia (e.g. sickle cell disease) and AIDS, parvovirus can cause severe anaemia. In pregnancy, parvovirus may cause fetal loss (15–20%), particularly if infection occurs in the first and second trimesters of pregnancy. As the presentation of parvovirus is similar to that of rubella in pregnancy, blood should be tested for both these viruses in pregnant patients presenting with a fever and/or a rash, particularly if there are any joint symptoms.

Management

The diagnosis of parvovirus infection can be made either by direct detection of viral DNA in blood or by serology. There is no known treatment, although the chronic anaemia may be successfully treated with immunoglobulin therapy.

Glandular fever (infectious mononucleosis)

Glandular fever is caused by the Epstein–Barr virus. It is one particular clinical manifestation of a whole range of diseases caused by the same virus.

Clinical features

Glandular fever typically presents over several days with mild chills, sweats, anorexia and, in particular, sore throat (Box 15). Examination reveals non-tender, bilateral and often generalised lymphadenopathy which is particularly characteristic at the root of the neck. In florid cases, the tonsils or posterior pharynx may be coated with a white membrane, which is often more marked than that seen in streptococcal sore throat and is akin to that seen in diphtheria. However, the presence of splenomegaly and atypical lymphocytosis are features found frequently in glandular fever but virtually never in diphtheria. Most patients, however, have elevated liver function test results. About 5% of the patients are jaundiced and hepatomegaly is found in about 10%. Virtually all patients have an abnormal lymphocytosis of > 10% when ill. More specific tests include the monospot and Paul Bunnell tests.

Outcome

The majority of cases of glandular fever resolve over 2–3 weeks. Often, however, patients feel tired and unable to concentrate for a much longer period. Occasionally this leads on to typical features of the chronic fatigue syndrome (p. 366). Treatment is usually symptomatic. If amoxycillin or ampicillin is given, this results in a maculopapular eruption in almost all patients. This should not be mistaken as an allergy to these drugs; the mechanism is unclear.

Complications

There are a number of rare complications of glandular fever including:

- splenic rupture (advise no contact sports until the spleen is no longer palpable)
- encephalitis and meningitis
- neurological problems, e.g. peripheral neuropathy
- pericarditis and myocarditis.

Oncogenic potential

The Epstein–Barr virus infects a number of different cell types in the body including B cells, nasopharyngeal epithelial cells and probably other cell types as well. It is a transforming virus which has now been clearly associated with a number of different tumours including nasopharyngeal cancer, Burkitt's lymphoma, Hodgkin's disease, non-Hodgkin's lymphoma in patients with AIDS, a rare form of thymic tumour and smooth muscle tumours. It is also responsible for an unusual form of post-transplantation lymphoproliferative disease which is often rapidly fatal. Hairy leukoplakia in the context of AIDS is probably a form of cell transformation related to Epstein–Barr virus as well. Therefore, it is a virus with remarkable oncogenic potential. However, the risk of any of these tumours in a given individual seems to be low.

Leptospirosis

Leptospirosis is caused by a number of different varieties (serovars) of *Leptospira*. It is a zoonosis occurring all over the world including in the UK. It is particularly associated with contact with infected water. It is an occupational hazard of sewer workers and canoeists. The most severe form of the disease with jaundice and renal failure is called Weil's disease, but the majority of infections are mild and undiagnosed. It is a cause of aseptic meningitis.

Clinical features

The clinical manifestations are not usually specific but if severe the initial phase of the illness is like that of dengue fever. It has a sudden onset with headache and myalgia. Usually patients have non-purulent conjunctivitis as well.

Management

The diagnosis can be made by isolation of the organism in the urine but very few laboratories are capable of doing this so a clinical diagnosis is usually appropriate. Serology is available. Patients should be treated with i.v. penicillin for 7–10 days because this causes a more rapid resolution of disease and reduces mortality. Untreated, jaundiced patients have a mortality of 5–30% usually as a result of renal failure but sometimes through haemorrhagic manifestations.

Rheumatic fever

A scourge of children in the pre-antibiotic era, rheumatic fever would confine children to bed, at home or more likely in sanatoria, for months. It is still common in the developing world. Lack of antibiotics, relative crowding and the prevalence of particular strains of *Streptococcus pyogenes* are responsible for occasional resurgences of disease. Strains such as mucoid M18 seem to be particularly 'rheumatogenic'.

Rheumatic fever, like poststreptococcal glomerulonephritis, is a result of cross-reaction of the patient's tissues with parts of the streptococcus. The sequence of events is as follows. A person has a pharyngitis or tonsillitis caused by one of these unusual streptococci. An antibody response follows, particularly if antibiotic treatment is delayed or inadequate. These antibodies cross-react with the relevant tissues to produce the manifestations of rheumatic fever (or glomerulonephritis).

As rheumatic fever is a clinical diagnosis, with little support from the laboratory (positive antistreptolysin 0 antibody test only), clinical criteria (the Duckett–Jones criteria) were developed and refined. Major textbooks have a complete list of these. The five major criteria, the presence of any two of which makes the diagnosis, are:

- evidence of heart disease, e.g. new murmur, prolonged PR interval
- polyarthropathy which affects different joints at different times
- subcutaneous nodules
- chorea (abnormal athetoid movements) (St Vitus' dance) (later manifestation)
- erythema marginatum: a rapidly expanding circularised rash on the trunk or proximal limbs.

Patients with rheumatic fever need penicillin to eradicate any residual streptococci and anti-inflammatory agents for arthritis. To prevent relapses, which are common when reinfection with other streptococci occurs, long-term penicillin is advised in those with carditis.

Lyme borreliosis

Lyme borreliosis is a multisystem infection caused by the spirochaete *Borrelia burgdorferi*. It is transmitted by tick bites. It has been reported from most of the North American states, nearly all European countries and throughout Asia. The reservoirs of infection are various small mammals; in addition, birds help to distribute infected ticks during migratory flights. The organism is transmitted by the salivary gland of the tick in the latter part of the 72 hours that the tick is adherent to the skin. Therefore, early removal of the tick is an important part of prevention of the disease. The chance of a person becoming ill after a tick bite in an endemic area is less than 1% in Europe. For this reason, antibiotics are not routinely indicated to prevent Lyme borreliosis after a tick bite.

Clinical features and treatment

There are three clinical stages of disease in Lyme borreliosis and not all of these may appear. Stages 1 and 2 appear within a few weeks or months after infection, Stage 3 several months or years later.

Stage 1

Erythema chronicum migrans (ECM) represents stage 1. This is a rash that spreads over some days or weeks and gradually spreads centrifugally. The border of the rash is not usually raised or hot but it does migrate slowly, increasing in size. It will resolve spontaneously in a few weeks or months but more quickly if antibiotic therapy is given. Many antibiotics are effective for ECM including doxycycline, cefuroxime, amoxycillin or azithromycin. Erythromycin is less effective.

Stage 2

Stage 2 disease represents early disseminated infection. The common clinical features include:

- neurological features, e.g. meningoradiculitis, neuritis, meningitis, facial nerve paralysis, etc.
- Lyme carditis, including transient atrio-ventricular block, rhythm disturbance and myo(peri)carditis
- *Borrelia* lymphocytoma, which is a bluish-red tumour-like skin infiltrate commonly observed in the earlobe or nipples
- arthralgia, myalgia and regional lymphadenopathy.

Effective antibiotics include high-dose i.v. penicillin, ceftriaxone or cefotaxime. Supportive therapy for carditis is appropriate and rarely a permanent pacemaker is required.

Stage 3

Stage 3 disease represents chronic organ involvement, which has a number of clinical manifestations, the commonest of which are:

- arthritis, monoarthritis or oligoarthritis
- acrodermatitis chronica atrophicans, which is a bluish-red discoloration and swelling of the extensor surfaces of the limb (rare)
- Lyme encephalitis and encephalomyelitis, presenting as a spastic paresis and ataxia (rare).

Successful treatment of stage 3 disease is difficult and the resolution of disease is slow. Doxycycline, amoxycillin or cefuroxime are appropriate for cutaneous and joint disease. Neurological involvement requires i.v. penicillin, ceftriaxone or cefotaxime. Failure of therapy or relapse after therapy is frequent and these patients require continued surveillance.

Diagnosis

The diagnosis of Lyme borreliosis can be made in part clinically, as the cutaneous manifestations are extremely distinctive. Diagnosis of cardiac, joint or neurological involvement requires serology. Unfortunately serology does not distinguish prior infection (without disease) from current active infection. False-positive results occur with positive rheumatoid factor and Epstein–Barr virus infection. There are also rare false-negative results.

Chronic fatigue syndrome

Many viral infections lead to malaise and fatigue as part of the manifestations. Usually these features resolve in 2–4 weeks but occasionally it takes as long as 2–3 months for such symptoms to resolve. Since the early 1970s, there has been growing recognition of an entity variously termed myasthenia, Royal Free disease, myalgic encephalomyelitis, and, most recently, the chronic fatigue syndrome. The diagnosis is a clinical one and should not be made lightly. You should not make it, for example, simply on the basis of a possible viral infection and a patient who complains of being tired. The reasons for this are two-fold. First, the patient may have a treatable medical condition such as hypothyroidism, HIV infection, endogenous depression and many others. In particular, fatigue is highly correlated with other emotional stress arising from many different causes. The second reason for not making the diagnosis lightly is that the label chronic fatigue syndrome often sends patients searching medical textbooks and to societies which may serve to reinforce symptomatology without clear positive benefit to the patient other than being confirmed in their sick role.

Criteria to make the diagnosis are:

1. Disabling fatigue for at least 6 months
2. Exclusion of other medical conditions.

The latter requires complete detailed physical examination, exclusion of endocrine disease, neuromuscular disorders such as myasthenia, HIV infection and other chronic infections such as tuberculosis. In particular, patients with associated weight loss need to be very carefully evaluated, even though weight loss is a common manifestation of depression.

In those in whom an underlying treatable medical condition is not found, a detailed psychological or psychiatric evaluation is usually beneficial. Depression is common in these patients and they often improve with antidepressant therapy. Cognitive psychotherapy can be valuable. Other psychological morbidity as determined by a detailed psychological assessment is a predictor of a low likelihood of improvement. Recent work has shown that only 6% of patients are fully recovered at 3 years and the majority of patients are substantially disabled either socially or physically. In addition, many patients have substantial difficulties in concentration and many jobs are frequently beyond them.

10.4 Sexually transmitted disease and vaginal infection

Sexually transmitted diseases are common. Certain patient groups are at high risk: these include gay men, sex workers and young, particularly single, sexually active men and women. Rates of gonorrhoea and syphilis are a useful quantitative guide to unprotected sexual activity and, therefore, are a surrogate marker for HIV transmission rates in populations where HIV exists. Transmission of all sexually transmitted diseases would fall to near zero if condoms were used for all episodes of penetrative sex. However, there are several major factors preventing their use, including lack of availability in many poor, rural parts of the world and inadequate education and protection of teenagers prior to first sexual exposure. In the UK, a recent large survey of sexual activity showed a much higher (about 50%) usage of a condom during the first sexual experience than previously (about 20%). Fear of AIDS and education are the probable reasons for improvement.

Learning objectives

You should:

- know the causes of vaginal discharges and how to treat them
- know the principles of management of penile discharges and urethritis in men
- know the major causes of genital ulcers and the principles of management.

Most sexually transmitted diseases fall into two groups:

- discharges
- ulcers.

The approach taken here, for your ease of learning, is syndromic rather than organism-based. However, control of sexually transmitted diseases is heavily dependent on efficient screening as many are asymptomatic, especially in women.

Discharges

Urethritis (male) and cervicitis (female)

Male urethritis. In men, a discharge from the penis is the most common complaint in genitourinary medical practice. The most common symptoms are:

- discharge from urethra, on underpants or by expressing pus along the urethra
- a stinging or burning sensation on passing urine.

However, you should not take these complaints simply at face value. You should carefully examine the penis and genitals as there is often more than one diagnosis. Skin rash and joint pain should be carefully sought and you should check the conjunctiva and mouth for features of Reiter's syndrome (p. 309).

Cervicitis in women. In women, the equivalent to urethral discharge is cervicitis. It is commonly asymptomatic or may present with vaginal discharge. The symptoms associated with a vaginal discharge include:

- increased non-menstrual flow
- altered smell or texture of non-menstrual flow.

A significant proportion (about 10%) of women with cervicitis have associated pelvic inflammatory disease. Urethritis in women or the acute urethral syndrome (p. 163) is more commonly caused by the ordinary bacteria that cause bladder infection than by sexually transmitted organisms.

Causes and diagnosis

The common causes of urethral discharge and cervicitis with their pertinent features are shown in Table 84. For the diagnosis of sexually transmitted disease, high vagi-

Table 84 Major sexually transmitted causes of male urethritis and female cervicitis

Cause	Comment
Neisseria gonorrhoea	Incubation period 2–5 days, 10% have no symptoms. Also found in rectum and throat. Penicillin-resistant isolates now common outside the UK
Chlamydia trachomatis	Common cause of urethritis and cervicitis; incubation period 7–14 days, can be cultured or diagnosed by antigen detection
Mycoplasma hominis	Not a cause of urethritis but does cause pelvic inflammatory disease and postpartum fever (15%). Increasing tetracycline resistance
Ureaplasma urealyticum	A relatively common cause of urethritis but may be asymptomatic. Sensitive to erythromycin. A cause of postpartum fever (10%)

nal swabs alone are useless. You should take special *Chlamydia* and *N. gonorrhoae* cultures directly from the urethra in men, from the cervix and urethra in women, and from the anus if anal intercourse has taken place. Microscopy with Gram stain is desirable for the immediate diagnosis of gonorrhoea.

In about 10–30% of cases of urethral discharge, microscopy and culture fails to make a specific diagnosis. Cases without a microbiological diagnosis are termed non-specific urethritis (NSU). It is likely that the vast majority of such cases are infectious but either the sensitivity of the present diagnostic methods is inadequate or new organisms remain to be discovered.

Treatment

Treatment regimens are changing for urethritis and cervicitis. Penicillin G (i.m.) or oral amoxycillin is still the standard treatment for gonorrhoea acquired in the UK, but abroad resistance is frequent. The introduction of the quinolones (e.g. ciprofloxacin) and the new macrolides (e.g. azithromycin) will drastically alter present approaches to therapy. For example, a single 1 g dose of azithromycin is as effective for chlamydial infection as 10 days of doxycycline and a 2 g single dose presently has a 99% response rate for gonorrhoea.

Vaginal discharge

If a woman presents with a vaginal discharge, it is important that you ascertain whether she has had a new partner recently or any other reason to suspect a sexually transmitted disease. However, increased vaginal discharge alone may be physiological.

Clinical approach to vaginal discharge

There are several causes of vaginal discharge which you can partly distinguish by history.

Vaginal candidosis. Vaginal candidosis is very common. At least 75% of women suffer it at least once in their lives and about 30% suffer recurrent episodes. Diabetes, pregnancy, antibiotic therapy, cystic fibrosis and HIV infection increase the number of episodes. Some women without the above factors have intractable or frequently recurring vaginal candidosis for reasons that are not clear. Suspect vaginal candidosis if a woman complains of pruritus *and* a non-offensive discharge.

Treatment. In the general practice setting, you can treat with local or oral antifungals without culture or examination on the first occasion. If symptoms do not resolve or recur quickly then a full genital examination and microbiological tests are necessary. If a woman complains of discharge without pruritus, do an examination and culture directly.

Bacterial vaginosis

Bacterial vaginosis is a polymicrobial bacterial infection that is sometimes chronic and apparently refractory to therapy. Patients complain of a vaginal discharge which may be offensive.

The characteristics of bacterial vaginosis are a rise in vaginal pH (to ≥ 4.7), a fall in the numbers of aerobic *Lactobacillus* and a rise in *Gardnerella vaginalis* and 'clue' cells. Clue cells are exfoliated vaginal epithelial cells with a granular appearance because of adherent bacteria. Treat with an anti-anaerobic antibiotic, such as metronidazole.

Trichomonas infection

Trichomonas infection is a sexually transmitted infection of the vagina caused by *Trichomonas vaginalis*, a protozoan. It usually causes a mildly offensive yellow/green, frothy discharge. It is commonly associated with vulval irritation and sometimes dysuria. Organisms can be seen by microscopy in discharge. A single dose of metronidazole is curative. Partners need treatment to prevent re-infection.

Genital ulcers

Ulcers of the penis, scrotum, vulva or perineal area are common. Their presence substantially increases the risk of HIV transmission both through heterosexual and homosexual intercourse. Most causes are infectious but there are unusual causes such as Behçet's syndrome, Crohn's disease, Stevens–Johnson syndrome and others.

Ulceration can be divided into multiple painful or solitary non-painful ulcers. In the UK, the most common painful cause is genital herpes and non-painful cause is primary syphilis.

Genital herpes

In a primary attack, patients have multiple, painful ulcers in the vulva, with low-grade fever. They can be so painful in women that walking is impaired or retention of urine follows. The incubation period is 7–14 days. Subsequent episodes are usually less severe than primary attacks and localised to one site, with a characteristic itching sensation preceding appearance of small, clear vesicles. About one-third of those with genital herpes get recurrent attacks, but asymptomatic shedding of virus is common (30%). If the episode is severe, prolonged or in an unusual site, consider an HIV test.

Genital herpes is a cause of erythema multiforme.

Treatment

Genital herpes can be treated with acyclovir orally if started within 48 hours of the lesions appearing. As very frequent recurrences are uncommon, patients are usually treated with intermittent therapy rather than continuously.

Syphilis

Syphilis is one of the oldest diseases known and has a number of diverse clinical manifestations. It is transmitted exclusively by sexual contact, vertically from mother to child or, extremely rarely, by transfusion. Syphilis is caused by *Treponema pallidum*. *T. pallidum* is both a spirochaete and a bacterium. It is not possible to grow it in the clinical microbiology laboratory, although it can be cultured in rabbit testicles.

The disease has four stages although frequently in a given patient only one or two of these will be manifest. The stages are:

1. Primary syphilis (e.g. primary chancre)
2. Secondary syphilis (e.g. rash on the palms and soles and oral lesions)
3. Latent syphilis (e.g. positive serology)
4. Tertiary syphilis (e.g. general paralysis of the insane, syphilitic aortitis, tabes dorsalis or gummas).

It is important to be able to interpret positive serology for syphilis and to formulate a management plan.

Primary syphilis

A primary chancre is a non-painful ulcer up to 1 cm across. The primary chancre in women may be in the vagina or the cervix and as it is painless it is easy to overlook. In men, it is frequently concealed by the foreskin, and in gay men the lesion may be on the anal margin. If the genitals are involved, there is usually painless inguinal lymphadenopathy, which may be the presenting complaint. The incubation period is from 9–90 days. Primary syphilis can only be reliably diagnosed by dark ground microscopy or detection of FTA IgM in the serum, as standard serological tests are not positive until 2 weeks after appearance of the chancre.

Secondary syphilis

Secondary syphilis occurs 2–10 weeks after the primary chancre; occasionally both are coexistent. Clinical features are:

- fever and headache
- sore throat
- generalised lymphadenopathy

- a rash that is non-pruritic and often involves the palms and soles
- snail track ulcers on mucous membranes
- condylomata lata, which are fleshy masses around the anus and vagina similar to soft warts.

Both condylomata lata and mucous membrane lesions are highly infectious. Patients with secondary syphilis may have other organ system involvement, such as hepatitis, meningitis or optic neuritis. The disease of secondary syphilis waxes and wanes over a period of some weeks. The diagnosis is usually made by serology.

Latent syphilis

Latent syphilis has no clinical features and is diagnosed by serology. Many patients in whom primary or secondary syphilis is not diagnosed will in fact have the disease successfully treated inadvertently by a course of antibiotics given for another problem.

Tertiary syphilis

Tertiary syphilis follows primary/secondary syphilis 3–20 years later. The serological tests for syphilis are positive in all forms of tertiary syphilis.

Serological diagnosis

The frequency of positivity of serological tests for syphilis are shown in Table 85. The TPHA test once positive stays positive for life. A rise in titre might occur with reinfection. VDRL tests will rise and fall with infection and treatment, respectively, but slowly. There are occasional false negatives. FTA-IgG is more sensitive than TPHA initially but is then similar to the TPHA. The FTA-IgM is useful as it reflects acute infection and will often rise and fall with each episode of syphilis. It is, however, rather subjective to read in the laboratory and both over-reading and under-reading errors occasionally occur. Occasionally there are false-positive tests in, for example, SLE, but in most cases the disease causing the false positive is apparent.

Treatment

Syphilis is best treated with penicillin. There is still dispute about the best dose, formulation and duration of therapy. The Jarisch–Herxheimer reaction is a reaction to treatment and is manifest as fever and 'flu-like' symptoms 3–12 hours after a dose of penicillin. It occurs

Table 85 The frequency of positive serological results in testing for syphilis

	Frequency of positivity (%)			
	Primary	Secondary	Latent	Tertiary
VDRL	75	100	75	75
TPHA	60	100	97	100
FTA-IgG	90	100	97	100
FTA-IgM	90+	100	< 10	< 10

following therapy for primary (50% of treatment courses) and secondary syphilis (70–90% of treatment courses). It can usually be managed symptomatically; occasionally steroids are required.

Genital warts

Genital warts are common. They usually present as small (2–5 mm) fleshy protuberances on the skin surfaces of the genitals. They may also appear as flat and slightly pigmented areas of skin. They also occur on the mucosal surfaces but are much harder to visualise and may be 'silent'. Caused by many varieties of papilloma viruses, they constitute a large part of the workload of all genitourinary medicine clinics because they are resistant to treatment.

Papilloma viruses have also been implicated as a predisposing factor leading to carcinoma of the cervix and anus, especially in AIDS patients.

Treatment

Topical podophyllin or podophyllotoxin and cryotherapy with liquid nitrogen are the commonest modes of treatment. The former does not work well for established and keratinised warts, and many applications of liquid nitrogen are often necessary for cure of large warts. Other treatments are available but none are very effective.

Other aspects of genitourinary medicine practice

There are several other major functions besides the diagnosis and treatment of sexually transmitted disease that clinics undertake. These are:

- HIV counselling, pre- and post-test (p. 342)
- contact tracing
- dealing with psychosexual problems
- health promotion and sexual health education
- family planning advice and provision
- screening for cervical precancer and management of abnormal smears in high-risk patients.

All genitourinary clinics hold an independent set of confidential clinic records, as required by law. Names of contacts are recorded if the patient provides details. Staff then may contact them discreetly for screening for sexually transmitted infections.

Psychosexual problems accompanying sexually transmitted disease are common. Examples include:

- concern about repeated transmission of *Candida* (which is not the case), or herpes and warts (which is)
- in the context of a stable relationship, where the infection came from
- feelings of being 'dirty' or 'defiled' leading to a lack of libido and low self-esteem.

Considerable patience, time and skill are required to help affected individuals resume normal sexual relations.

10.5 **Imported diseases**

There are a large number of tropical diseases. Space permits coverage of only a tiny selection. A few others are dealt with in the systems chapters. Consult reference books or knowledgeable clinicians if faced with a diagnostic problem.

Learning objectives

You must:

- know in detail about the different types of malaria, how it presents, how to diagnose it and what the management should be
- be able to suspect viral haemorrhagic fever and know what to do if you suspect it
- have a clinical approach for the main differential diagnoses of a returning traveller with fever or other manifestations of infection.

Malaria

Malaria is a parasitic disease transmitted by the female *Anopheles* mosquito in most sub-tropical and tropical countries of the world. There are 100–200 million cases and 1.5–3 million deaths annually from malaria worldwide. There are four species of parasites infecting humans. *Plasmodium falciparum* is the only one that regularly causes death and the only one that does *not* cause delayed disease months or years after leaving an area endemic for malaria. *P. vivax* and *P. ovale* both have liver and red cell cycles and cause milder infections than *P. falciparum*. *P. malariae* is rare in the UK but may occur decades after leaving an endemic area.

Geography

P. falciparum is found virtually wherever the other three species of *Plasmodium* are found. Areas that are malaria-free include western and eastern Europe, the parts of North Africa that adjoin the Mediterranean, the Middle East, Canada and the USA, Japan, Australia, New Zealand and the southernmost parts of South Africa. Sixty per cent of the world's population live in malaria-free areas. The likelihood of getting infected with malaria in the centre of major cities in Asia and Central America is relatively small even if malaria occurs in these countries. Therefore, malaria prophylaxis is not indicated for a trip to Bangkok or Singapore, for example.

Incubation period

In countries free of malaria, all cases are imported. *P. falciparum* infection usually presents within a month of returning from an endemic area, but at least 10% of cases occur up to 4 months after leaving an endemic area. Cases involving the other three species of parasites can occur months or years after leaving an endemic area, although most cases of *P. vivax* or *P. ovale* present within 3 years.

Clinical features

The clinical diagnosis of malaria can be difficult. Characteristic features include:
• fever and shaking chills and/or rigors
• headache and myalgia
• vomiting and diarrhoea.

The first 1–3 days of a malarial illness are often hard to separate from many other infectious illnesses. After this, the patient typically has paroxysms of fever. These paroxysms comprise three stages, together lasting about 6 hours:

• the cold stage (rigors/chills)
• the hot stage (high fever)
• the sweating stage (defervescence).

After several days of illness in *P. vivax* and *P. ovale* infections, the pattern of paroxysms may develop into the well-described **tertian pattern**, when paroxysms occur every second day. Such characteristic synchrony of fever is uncommon in *P. falciparum* infections, when a more chaotic temperature chart is typical.

Prognostic features
In falciparum malaria, the following are poor prognostic features:

• coma
• increased respiratory rate
• oliguria
• high parasitaemia (e.g. ≥ 10%).

Investigation

All patients who return from the tropics with fever should have a blood culture (for typhoid, etc.) and malaria film taken. You should adopt this rule whether you are working as a GP, in Accident and Emergency, as a medical house officer or working abroad. Without this, you can miss cases of malaria and typhoid (p. 372). Every year there are three to five deaths from malaria in the UK because the diagnosis is considered late or not at all, and instead a viral disease is diagnosed. Do not make this mistake; whenever you see a patient with fever always ask if they have been abroad.

Patients with falciparum malaria are likely to have a normocytic normochromic anaemia, an elevated reticulocyte count (or polychromasia), a normal white cell count and a reduced platelet count. Careful inspection of the blood film will show parasites in the vast majority of patients on the first blood film. If parasites are not found but symptoms continue, together with anaemia

and/or thrombocytopenia, additional films should be sent to the laboratory. In patients taking malaria prophylaxis, it can take 3–5 films over the same number of days to make the diagnosis.

The diagnosis of *P. malariae*, *P. vivax* and *P. ovale* infections can be more difficult and films should be done around the time of fever if the first couple of films are negative and the diagnosis is still suspected.

Management

Falciparum malaria
All patients with falciparum malaria should be admitted to hospital immediately. You should contact the local infectious disease consultant and it is usual to transfer the patient to the local infectious disease unit for management. The management of falciparum malaria is difficult and, improperly managed, it carries a high mortality related to ARDS, renal failure, hypoglycaemia, cardiac arrhythmias and cerebral malaria. Ten per cent of adults suffer cerebral damage after cerebral malaria.

Standard therapy for falciparum malaria is oral or i.v. quinine. The vast majority of isolates worldwide are resistant to chloroquine, which is why this is no longer used for falciparum malaria. Alternative drugs include mefloquine (oral), halofantrine and artemether. Mefloquine and quinine cannot be combined because of neurotoxicity. *P. falciparum* in Northern Thailand and Burma (1994/5) is now resistant to both quinine and mefloquine. Mefloquine resistance is spreading. Strategies for the management of these patients are presently being evolved.

Patients with parasitaemia above 5% should be actively considered for exchange transfusion depending on how ill the patient is.

Non-falciparum malaria
Patients with *P. vivax*, and *P. ovale* and *P. malariae* infections may need admission to hospital for 1–2 days depending on their clinical status but many can be managed as outpatients. They can be treated with oral chloroquine given for 3 days. Patients with *P. vivax* and *P. ovale* infection should then have their glucose 6-phosphate dehydrogenase levels checked. If these are normal, they should then be given 2 weeks of primaquine to eradicate the liver cycle. There are substantial difficulties in the management of pregnant patients with malaria. All forms of malaria are notifiable diseases.

Prevention of infection and prophylaxis

Most *Anopheles* mosquitoes bite at dawn or dusk. If it is possible not to go out at these times, the risk of acquisition of disease is reduced. Long sleeves, socks and long trousers will also reduce the likelihood of being bitten. Insect repellants are useful and should be liberally applied. Travellers should sleep under bed nets, preferably treated with insecticide.

Advice on malaria prophylaxis changes at least 6-monthly so check frequently. The choices for prophylaxis are (i) mefloquine or (ii) chloroquine and proguanil. All forms of prophylaxis should be taken before leaving the home country for two reasons: (i) to make sure that the tablets are tolerated and if they are not then an alternative regimen can be provided, and (ii) to build up tissue levels prior to departure. In addition, drugs should be continued after return home to prevent late infections.

Typhoid and paratyphoid fever

Typhoid fever is caused by *Salmonella typhi* and paratyphoid fever by *S. paratyphi* A, B or C. These four infections constitute enteric fever. They are usually acquired abroad: most cases of typhoid are from the Indian sub-continent, whereas most paratyphoid fever comes from the Mediterranean basin. All are notifiable diseases.

Clinical features

The early features of typhoid or paratyphoid fever are relatively non-specific:

- fever and chills
- headache
- lethargy
- mild cough
- low white cell count.

Examination initially reveals only abdominal tenderness. After 7–10 days, rose spots may become apparent on the skin and are particularly common in paratyphoid fever. Diarrhoea or constipation, and delirium, splenomegaly and hepatomegaly also become detectable. Few patients in the UK enter the third week of disease (with the complications of intestinal bleeding, perforation and shock) although this is not uncommon in the developing world.

The diagnosis is established by blood culture although occasionally this is falsely negative when antibiotics have been taken empirically. In such patients, a clinical diagnosis has to be made and sometimes positive cultures can be obtained from bone marrow or stool. Antibiotic resistance is common. Ciprofloxacin or a third-generation cephalosporin such as cefotaxime are appropriate. Intravenous therapy should be given initially in all but the most mildly ill patients. Ten day's therapy is appropriate. Untreated disease has a 30% mortality. Convalescence in survivors is prolonged.

Chronic carriage

Patients with typhoid require isolation during hospitalisation. All family members should also be screened for stool carriage. After therapy has finished, stool cultures should be checked to ensure that the patient has not become a carrier. This is particularly important in professional food handlers (including those preparing food at home). Sometimes the gall bladder acts as a source of infection for chronic carriers and has to be removed.

Immunisation

The long-established heat-killed whole cell vaccine, the Vi capsular polysaccharide vaccine and, most recently, an oral live attenuated vaccine are useful in prevention. The first two have to be given parenterally as single doses. The oral vaccine is given as a three-dose schedule. The efficacy is around 70% for the parenteral vaccines and probably slightly lower for the oral attenuated vaccine. Only those visiting the Indian sub-continent or long-term holidaymakers to the Mediterranean basin, Kenya, Far East and South America require immunisation.

Viral fevers

Dengue fever

Dengue fever (breakbone fever) is caused by one of four viruses transmitted by mosquito bite. It occurs in Central and South America, much of Africa, India and South-East Asia. It is one of the most common causes of imported fever in the UK (465 proven cases in 1994) and has an incubation period of 2–14 days. The diagnosis is made by acute and convalescent serology. Treatment is supportive.

Clinical features
In older children and adults, dengue produces a characteristic clinical syndrome, the first manifestation of which is the sudden onset of high fever. Dengue causes:

- sudden high fever
- frontal headache
- nausea and vomiting
- backache, severe muscle and joint pains
- flushing of the face
- non-purulent conjunctivitis
- initial transient macular generalised rash (like sunburn) then a generalised morbilliform rash.

Viral haemorrhagic fever

There are a number of other viral haemorrhagic fevers (VHF) which are acquired abroad. The major VHFs are **Lassa fever** and **Ebola fever** which occur in Africa. They carry a major risk of transmission to health-care workers and especially laboratory staff. Patients with suspected viral haemorrhagic fever must be managed in an infectious disease unit with the appropriate containment facilities. You have a legal obligation to consult an infectious disease physician if you suspect any VHF.

The maximum incubation period for all viral haemorrhagic fevers is 20 days. Suspect the diagnosis in anyone with:

- fever following a recent trip abroad
- haemorrhagic manifestations, or coagulopathy without a bacterial cause.

Prognosis

The case fatality is lowest for haemorrhagic fever with renal syndrome and dengue fever (1–5%) and highest for Congo Crimean haemorrhagic fever (55–88%). Lassa fever, and possibly others, can be successfully treated with ribivirin.

Leishmaniasis

Leishmaniasis is an overall term to describe any disease caused by the protozoan *Leishmania*. Visceral leishmaniasis (**Kala-azar**) is a common cause of splenomegaly and fever, whereas the cutaneous and mucosal syndromes are chronic and are effectively dealt with by tropical medicine specialists. Visceral leishmaniasis is occasionally seen in AIDS.

There are a number of different species of *Leishmania* that cause visceral leishmaniasis, particularly *L. donovani*, which can be acquired in the Indian subcontinent, China, Middle East and around the Mediterranean basin, sub-Saharan Africa, Kenya and Ethiopia, Latin America and Brazil.

The incubation period for visceral leishmaniasis is 3–8 months but may be longer. The key manifestations of visceral leishmaniasis are:

- hepatosplenomegaly (sometimes massive)
- fever
- weight loss.

Usually symptoms appear gradually, with a vague abdominal discomfort related to splenomegaly, fever, weakness, weight loss and then the symptoms of anaemia. The fever is low grade initially but may become high later. Occasionally the symptoms are much more acute, in which case high fever and chills are typical. Hepatosplenomegaly is virtually always found, with the spleen being larger than the liver. In chronic cases, splenomegaly may be massive.

Diagnosis. A profound normocytic, normochromic anaemia is typical together with leucopenia and sometimes thrombocytopenia. A bone marrow exami-

nation, splenic aspirate or liver biopsy will establish the diagnosis.

Treatment. Treatment is now given usually with liposomal amphotericin B, or conventional amphotericin B or pentavalent antimony compounds.

10.6 Pyrexia of unknown origin

Pyrexia of unknown origin (PUO) is defined as a fever > 38°C (or > 1°C above patient's normal temperature) over at least 3 weeks and defying standard diagnostic evaluation (e.g. blood culture, urine culture, chest X-ray, etc). In many cases, the fever has been present for months, perhaps intermittently. The differential diagnosis is extremely wide and the topic is introduced only briefly here.

Learning objectives

You should:

- know how to construct a differential diagnosis
- be able to develop a rational approach to investigation in patients with PUO.

Clinical features

The causes of PUO include those in Table 86. This list is not exhaustive but as you can see it is already long.

There are several key points that you need to know about the evaluation of this type of patient:

- confirm the elevated temperature, if necessary by admitting the patient to hospital; some 'cases' are merely exaggerated circadian rhythms
- repeatedly examine the patient seeking splenomegaly, dental or sinus problems, changing heart murmurs and lymphadenopathy in particular
- consider a drug cause early in the evaluation, to avoid multiple tests and invasive procedures

Table 86 An incomplete list of the causes of PUO

	Infections	Neoplasms	Other
Common causes

vancomycin, | Tuberculosis
Occult abscesses (e.g. liver,

epidural)
Invasive candidiasis
AIDS | Hodgkin's disease
Non-Hodgkin's lymphoma | Sarcoidosis
Drug fever (e.g.

bleomycin)
SLE
Vasculitis |
| Uncommon causes | Subacute bacterial endocarditis
Osteomyelitis
Brucellosis
Psittacosis
Relapsing fever
Histoplasmosis

Trypanosomiasis | Leukaemia
Renal cell carcinoma
Hepatoma
Atrial myxoma | Still's disease
Polymyalgia rheumatica
Temporal arteritis
Granulomatous hepatitis
Inflammatory bowel disease
Familial Mediterranean fever
Fabry's disease
Factitious fever |

- do a Mantoux/Heaf test and consider antituberculous treatment early, as up to one-third of PUO cases are caused by tuberculosis
- ask for relevant consultant opinions early, particularly if there are abnormalities in one or other body systems
- if patients are not too ill, avoid major invasive procedures (such as laparotomy); rather take a watching brief: 'first do no harm' as a tenet of medical practice applies here, perhaps more than in most other situations.

Important causes of PUO not discussed elsewhere in this book include brucellosis, amoebic liver abscess and factitious fever. These are discussed briefly below. About 10–15% of genuine cases of PUO are never diagnosed, despite multiple investigations over months or years.

Investigations

Most investigations for PUO are covered elsewhere in this book, e.g. Mantoux tests for tuberculosis. However, two additional tests may be valuable if occult abscesses are considered likely. These are white cell and gallium scans.

White cell scans

White cell scans detect recent large collections of neutrophils. It is particularly useful for intra-abdominal, bone and soft tissue infections. The patient's cells are collected by venepuncture, labelled with indium-111 and reinfused. Patients are scanned 18–24 hours later. Very chronic infections are likely to be falsely negative.

Gallium scans

Gallium-67 is used to label transferrin and lactoferrin at the site of infection. It is more useful for chronic inflammatory, especially granulomatous, disease, in identifying either the site of disease or its activity, as the scan abnormality returns to baseline quickly after resolution of disease. Scanning is done daily for 3 days.

Brucellosis

The incubation period of brucellosis varies from 1 week to several months. Most patients get a mild influenza-like illness without complications. The characteristic features of brucellosis include:

- drenching sweats
- chills and fever
- weakness
- myalgia
- back pain.

On examination, lymphadenopathy and splenomegaly are found in up to one-third of patients. Usually the disease resolves spontaneously, although in some instances relapses may occur. Relapse is very unusual if the disease is appropriately treated. The diagnosis can sometimes be made by doing special blood cultures (ask a microbiologist) but is more commonly made by serology.

Complications of brucellosis include sacroiliitis or arthritis, meningoencephalitis and psychiatric problems, epididymo-orchitis and endocarditis. Brucellosis is also more severe in immunocompromised patients.

Treatment consists of doxycycline plus rifampicin for a minimum of six weeks.

Amoebic liver abscess

Liver abscess is a relatively frequent cause of PUO. Bacterial liver abscesses are discussed on page 124. Amoebic liver abscesses occur in returned travellers. Most patients present within 2–5 months after leaving the endemic area, although the presentation can be delayed for years. There are two presentations of amoebic liver abscess:

1. abdominal pain and fever
2. weight loss, low-grade fever and mild or absent abdominal pain.

Diarrhoea is common in both.

Physical examination reveals exquisite point tenderness over the liver. Signs of pleural effusion or infection in the right lung base are common.

Diagnosis

Virtually all the patients have a peripheral leucocytosis and abnormal liver function tests, in particular a raised alkaline phosphatase. The diagnosis initially should be considered on the basis of travel to any part of the world with poor sanitation, together with tenderness in the right upper quadrant on examination.

A differential diagnosis includes cholecystitis, acute viral hepatitis and a bacterial liver abscess. However, leucocytosis is essentially never found in patients with viral hepatitis and imaging of the liver helps to differentiate cholecystitis from liver abscesses. Travel history will suggest amoebic liver abscess, whereas the absence of a travel history would suggest a bacterial liver abscess.

Aspiration of very large abscesses is appropriate, to yield the classical pus (anchovy paste). Cultures of the pus are negative. Amoebic serology is positive in approximately 95% of patients. Stools are usually negative for amoebic cysts.

Treatment with metronidazole is curative and this should be given for at least 10 days. Occasionally, amoebiasis affects other organs of the body, including the brain, skin and genitals.

Factitious fever

Occasionally Munchausen's syndrome manifests as factitious fever. Usually the reading on the thermometer is falsely elevated by rubbing the thermometer or holding it next to a light or hair dryer. To diagnose factitious fever, it is essential to ensure that all temperature readings are directly supervised by the nursing staff. Sometimes patients inject bacteria or yeast into themselves causing genuine infection.

10.7 Notifiable diseases

There are a number of diseases that are notifiable to the local Consultant for Communicable Disease Control (CCDC). It is important that these are notified (you have a ᵔrms are provided ᵔospital and in the ᵔat should be noti-ᵔtain 24-hour cover ᵔhese are:

clinical diagnosis culture confirma-made in writing, it is important to ᵔfidential notifica-ᵔe Communicable ᵔe, London.

ᵔerapy

ᵔvailable and this is ᵔmicrobiology and ᵔhis short section is ᵔl help you to make ᵔhoices for most of

• understand the main uses and limitations of each main antibiotic class
• know key members of each class.

Hospital prescribing

In the hospital setting, antibiotic policies are designed to achieve three objectives:

1. The use of appropriate antibiotics and doses for common indications
2. Use that reflects the local prevalence of antibiotic resistance in the usage of antibiotic for common conditions to prevent the emergence of resistance
3. To give the pharmacy sufficient buying power to negotiate lower prices for the antibiotics that are used in large volumes.

Endeavour to stick to the antibiotic policy in a hospital as much as possible. However, advice from the consultant microbiologists may suggest a deviation from the policy, especially with very ill patients or unusual problems. Allergy to antibiotics is common, but most cases are not true allergy but merely common side-effects such as nausea. Skin rash, anaphylaxis, angio-oedema and bronchoconstriction are legitimate reasons to use an alternative, although a skin rash many years ago could reflect a coexistent viral infection then or a mild allergy that is no longer present.

Do not prescribe unless there is good evidence for bacterial infection; do not use antibiotics as placebos.

The following and Table 87 are summaries of some of the more common antibiotics and their particular uses.

Individual antibiotics

Penicillin. Poorly absorbed orally, the only use of penicillin given by mouth is continuation after i.v. or i.m. therapy for streptococcal sore throat, and for prophylaxis in patients without spleens and after

---

Box 16
Notifiable diseases by law

Neurological infections
Meningitis
Encephalitis
Leprosy

GI infection or intoxication
Food or water poisoning (including *Salmonella*, *Campylobacter* spp., etc.)
Dysentery (*Shigella* or amoebic)
Viral hepatitis

Classical infectious diseases
Scarlet fever (not covered in this book)
Rubella
Measles
Mumps
Diphtheria
Whooping cough (not covered in this book)
Poliomyelitis
AIDS (special confidential reporting)
Anthrax (not covered in this book)
Leptospirosis
Meningococcal septicaemia

Imported acute diseases
Cholera
Plague (not covered in this book)
Malaria
Typhoid fever
Paratyphoid fever
Typhus and relapsing fever (not covered in this book)
Viral haemorrhagic fever

Table 87 A simplified guide to antibiotic use for some important common organisms

	Susceptibility to listed antibiotics		
	Predictable	Intermediate predictability	Unpredictable (and/or unresponsive to common antibiotics, but responsive to listed antibiotics)
Gram-positive	Streptococcus Enterococcus	Staphylococcus aureus	Staphylococcus epidermidis
Gram-negative	Neisseria gonorrhoeae	Haemophilus influenzae Escherichia coli Klebsiella sp. Proteus sp.	Other Gram-negative rods, e.g. Pseudomonas aeruginosa, Enterobacter cloacae
Useful antibiotics	Penicillin, ampicillin/amoxycillin	Cefuroxime, cefotaxime, ceftriaxone, co-amoxyclav, gentamicin and other aminoglycosides, quinolones, flucloxicillin for S. aureus	Special antibiotics because of resistance, e.g. vancomycin for S. epidermidis, piperacillin or ceftazidime for Pseudomonas, gentamicin or tobramycin for Enterobacter

rheumatic fever. Intravenously, it is useful for streptococcal, meningococcal, clostridial and skin infections and lobar pneumonia. For meningitis now it is superseded by third-generation cephalosporins because resistance in *Streptococcus pneumoniae* is now a problem (5–40%). The maximum dose is 20 million units daily, which should be reduced in renal failure. For the last 5 years penicillin resistance in *S. pneumonia* (which causes pneumonia and meningitis) has been increasing and penicillin has been dropped. Recent studies show that despite resistance penicillin works for pneumonia if given i.v. but not meningitis.

Ampicillin/amoxycillin. Previously a very useful antibiotic, now of less value. Key agent for endocarditis and enterococcal infections, liver and brain abscesses and *Listeria* infections. When combined with clavulanic acid, *co-amoxiclav* (Augmentin) is a useful antibiotic for upper respiratory tract infections including otitis media, sinusitis and bronchitis.

Flucloxacillin. Used only for staphylococcal infections, although it has some efficacy against streptococci. Oral doses are adequate for skin sepsis and continuation after i.v. therapy. Staphylococcal bacteraemia, osteomyelitis, endocarditis and other deep focal manifestations require large i.v. doses (e.g. 8–12 g/day). Activity is enhanced by combination with gentamicin or rifampicin. It is not active against multiply-resistant *Staphylococcus aureus* (MRSA).

Extended-spectrum penicillins. For example, *ticarcillin, mezlocillin, azlocillin, piperacillin*. These drugs offer a greater Gram-negative spectrum, including antipseudomonal activity, but none of them have any antistaphylococcal activity. They do, however, have enterococcal activity, unlike the extended-spectrum cephalosporins. They are used exclusively for patients with hospital-acquired infections, especially with neutropenia or in intensive care. Some agents are combined with β-lactamase inhibitors (e.g. Timentin and Tazobactam) to give even more broad-spectrum activity.

Oral cephalosporins. These drugs (e.g. *cephalexin, cephradine and cefaclor*) have reasonable Gram-positive activity with a limited Gram-negative spectrum (e.g. *E. coli* and most *H. influenzae* isolates). They are, therefore, a useful alternative for mild skin sepsis, respiratory tract infections and urinary tract infections. However, resistant rates among urinary pathogens exceed 50%.

Second-generation cephalosporins. These drugs (e.g. *cefuroxime*) have good Gram-positive and moderate Gram-negative activity. Cefuroxime is a useful antibiotic for moderate to severe skin sepsis and urinary tract infections requiring hospital admission. It has no activity against *Pseudomonas*, other resistant Gram-negatives, or *Enterococcus* spp.

Third-generation cephalosporins. These drugs (e.g. *cefotaxime, ceftriaxone* and *ceftazidime*) have become workhorse antibiotics in the hospital setting. They can only be given intravenously but have a broad spectrum of activity for both Gram-positive and Gram-negative pathogens. They have good activity against streptococci but only moderate activity against *S. pneumonia* and should not be used alone for a staphylococcal infection. They have no enterococcal activity and their frequent use has led to the emergence of *Enterococcus* as a major hospital pathogen worldwide. They have little anti-anaerobe activity. Ceftriaxone or cefotaxime are now the agents of choice for meningitis, however they have no anti-*Listeria* activity.

Pseudomonal infection. Cefotaxime and ceftriaxone have no antipseudomonal activity whereas ceftazidime is an excellent antibiotic for *Pseudomonas* infections. *Pseudomonas* sp. is particularly common as a urinary pathogen in the intensive care unit, in renal patients and in neutropenia. However, ceftazidime has slightly less Gram-positive activity and that is the reason for preferring ceftriaxone or cefotaxime in the majority of hospital settings.

Quinolones. *Norfloxacin* is only useful for urinary tract infections. Both *ofloxacin* and *ciprofloxacin* have a broad spectrum. Neither has good activity against *S.*

pneumoniae and, therefore, they are not good agents alone for the treatment of pneumonia. Ciprofloxacin has slightly greater activity against *Pseudomonas* and some difficult Gram-negative species compared with ofloxacin, but otherwise the spectrum between the two agents is similar. Ciprofloxacin is the agent of choice for typhoid fever and other infectious diarrhoeas. In addition, it also has antituberculous activity against both *Mycobacterium tuberculosis* and atypical mycobacteria.

Macrolides. *Erythromycin* is the agent of choice for most atypical pneumonias. It is likely that *clarithromycin* and *azithromycin* are equally effective for these. Erythromycin has good activity against streptococci and staphylococci and is, therefore, a useful agent for the treatment of mild skin sepsis, sore throat, some cases of sinusitis and some staphylococcal infections (but not bacteraemia). Erythromycin has no useful activity against the majority of *Haemophilus influenzae* isolates and is, therefore, not a good choice for exacerbations of chronic bronchitis or serious pneumonia unless accompanied by another agent. This is one of the advantages of clarithromycin and azithromycin, in that they have better *Haemophilus* activity. *Clindamycin* has better antianaerobe activity and penetrates well into bone; it is, therefore, a useful antibiotic for the treatment of bone infection caused by staphylococci. Both clarithromycin and azithromycin have antituberculous activity and are now used commonly for *Mycobacterium avium* infections in AIDS.

Glycopeptides. Both *vancomycin* and *teicoplanin* have only Gram-positive activity but they cover virtually everything in the Gram-positive spectrum, including enterococci. There is slightly more resistance in *Staphylococcus epidermidis* to teicoplanin than vancomycin but teicoplanin can be given intramuscularly which vancomycin cannot. Primary uses are the treatment of MRSA, *S. epidermidis* and enterococcal infections.

Folate antagonists. *Trimethroprim* only has a use as a urinary tract antibiotic, with efficacy rates of approximately 75% in uncomplicated cases. *Cotrimoxazole* has a much broader spectrum of activity, including most common Gram-negative pathogens (but not *P. aeruginosa*). It is, therefore, useful for urinary tract infection and also for hospital-acquired Gram-negative pneumonia. It is also the treatment of first choice, in very large doses, for *P. carinii* pneumonia (p. 339). It has reasonable Gram-positive activity although a considerable number (> 10%) of *S. pneumoniae* isolates are now resistant. Toxicity may be a problem.

Aminoglycosides. The aminoglycosides (e.g. *gentamicin, netilmicin, tobramycin* and *amikacin*) have an excellent Gram-negative spectrum and good activity against *Staphylococcus*. There has been a substantial change in their dosage levels over the last few years, so that they are now generally used in once a day dosing regimens (4–7 mg/kg). This produces higher peak concentrations, which may be more clinically effective, and low trough concentrations, which reduces the risk of toxicity. If once a day dosing is used, levels do not need to be measured unless the patient has impaired renal function, is over 65 years or the course of therapy exceeds 5 days. They also have a particular role as synergistic agents in the treatment of endocarditis caused by streptococcal, enterococcal and staphylococcal organisms, or indeed for other deep-seated, difficult-to-treat infections with these organisms. Resistance is infrequent.

Carbapenems. These antibotics (e.g. *imipenem* and *meropenem*) are only given intravenously and are extremely broad spectrum. In the mid-1990s they are primarily used as reserve antibiotics for difficult-to-treat cases of hospital sepsis.

Amphotericin B. This is a useful agent for the treatment of most systemic fungal infections, except *Pneumocystis carinii*. It also is effective for leishmaniasis. There are a number of new lipid-associated formulations of *amphotericin B* which are generally less toxic but larger doses have to be given.

Flucytosine. *Flucytosine* should only be used in combination with *amphotericin B* or *fluconazole* for the treatment of cryptococcal meningitis or serious forms of candidiasis. It is potentially toxic (bone marrow toxicity) and it is essential that levels are monitored in all patients.

Fluconazole. Fluconazole is a useful drug for the treatment of superficial and deep infection caused by *Candida* and *Cryptococcus* spp. It has no activity against *Aspergillus* or many of the other rarer fungal infections such as mucormycosis. Some species of *Candida* are resistant to fluconazole including *Candida krusei*, *Candida glabrata* and some isolates of *Candida tropicalis*. In AIDS, there is increasing resistance among isolates of *Candida albicans*.

Itraconazole. This is the only other agent (besides amphotericin B) which is useful for *Aspergillus* infections. At present, it can only be given orally, whereas amphotericin B can only be given intravenously. It is also effective against most other fungi and is second only to amphotericin B in its breadth of activity.

Acyclovir. Acyclovir is a useful antiviral agent for the treatment of herpes simplex and, to a lesser extent, herpes zoster infections. It is the treatment of choice for herpes simplex encephalitis and other disseminated viral infections caused by these viruses. Resistance is rare except in the context of late-stage AIDS. Two new analogues of acyclovir, *famciclovir* and *valciclovir*, are more bioavailable than acyclovir for the treatment of herpes zoster and may be preferable. It has no useful clinical activity against cytomegalovirus or Epstein–Barr virus infections.

Ribivirin. Ribivirin has two clinical uses. First, it is useful given in aerosolised fashion for the treatment of life-threatening respiratory syncytial virus pneumonia in immunocompromised patients, and, second, it is useful for the treatment of Lassa fever and possibly other viral haemorrhagic fevers.

Self-assessment: questions

Multiple choice questions

1. Penicillin is a good therapeutic choice for the following diseases:
   a. Syphilis
   b. *Escherichia coli* urinary tract infection
   c. Group A streptococcal necrotising fasciitis
   d. *Clostridium* spp. infection, such as tetanus
   e. *Clostridium difficile* causing antibiotic-associated diarrhoea

2. Ampicillin is active against ≥ 50% of the following pathogens:
   a. *Pseudomonas aeruginosa*
   b. *Haemophilus influenzae*
   c. *Staphylococcus aureus*
   d. *Staphylococcus epidermidis*
   e. *Listeria monocytogenes*

3. Flucloxacillin would be a reasonable choice for treating the following:
   a. *Staphylococcus aureus* endocarditis
   b. Impetigo
   c. Central line infection in an intensive care unit patient with Gram-positive cocci in blood cultures
   d. Osteomyelitis
   e. Gonorrhoea

4. Extended-spectrum penicillins (such as ticarcillin or piperacillin) are generally effective for the following:
   a. *Enterobacter* bacteraemia
   b. Enterococcal endocarditis (e.g. *Streptococcus faecalis*)
   c. Staphylococcal osteomyelitis
   d. *Pseudomonas aeruginosa* urinary tract infections
   e. *Klebsiella* bacteraemia

5. The following would be appropriate indications for vancomycin:
   a. *Staphylococcus epidermidis* central venous line infection
   b. Multiply resistant *Staphylococcus aureus* (MRSA) deep wound infection
   c. Prosthetic hip infection
   d. Endocarditis caused by *Enterococcus* (*Streptococcus*) *faecalis* in a penicillin-allergic patient
   e. Candidaemia

6. Differences between cefuroxime and cefotaxime (or ceftriaxone) are:
   a. Cefuroxime has better *Staphylococcus aureus* activity
   b. Cefotaxime is much more likely to be active against *Pseudomonas* spp. than cefuroxime
   c. Cefuroxime is more active than cefotaxime against *Streptococcus faecalis* and *Listeria monocytogenes*
   d. With respect to *Streptococcus pneumoniae*, both are equally active.
   e. For an *E. coli* infection caused by a fully sensitive organism, cefotaxime is preferred over cefuroxime

7. In treating *Pseudomonas aeruginosa* infections, the following are true:
   a. Ciprofloxacin is more active than ofloxacin
   b. Ceftazidime is more active than cefotaxime
   c. Gentamicin is no longer useful because of resistance
   d. Imipenem and meropenem are 'last resort' antibiotics
   e. Two agents are better than one

8. The following antibiotics have reasonable anaerobic activity (especially against *Bacteroides* spp.)
   a. Ciprofloxacin
   b. Imipenem
   c. Metronidazole
   d. Erythromycin
   e. Cefotaxime

9. The following is true of ciprofloxacin:
   a. It is not active against *Streptococcus pneumoniae*
   b. Blood levels following 200 mg i.v. are lower than following 750 mg orally
   c. It is a reasonable alternative therapy for serious staphylococcal infection on its own
   d. It is active against *Mycobacterium* spp.
   e. It is the treatment of choice for typhoid fever

10. With respect to erythromycin and clarithromycin:
    a. Their activity against *Haemophilus influenzae* (and, therefore, for exacerbations of chronic obstructive airways disease) is equivalent
    b. Both are useful for *Legionella* pneumonia
    c. Erythromycin would make a better choice for pharyngitis
    d. Both will be effective for *Mycoplasma* pneumonitis
    e. Clarithromycin is more active against *Mycobacterium avium intracellulare* infection in AIDS

11. The following would be appropriate indications for acyclovir:
    a. Viral encephalitis
    b. Shingles
    c. Chickenpox
    d. Prevention of cytomegalovirus infection post-transplant
    e. Chronic fatigue syndrome

12. There is no treatment for the following viral diseases:
    a. Influenza
    b. Lassa fever
    c. Chronic hepatitis B infection of the liver
    d. Respiratory syncytial virus pneumonia
    e. Rubella

13. With respect to treating fungal disease, the following are true:
    a. In oral candidiasis, topical therapy is just as good as systemic therapy
    b. Fluconazole is active against *Cryptococcus* sp.
    c. Fluconazole is active against *Aspergillus* sp.
    d. Amphotericin B is so toxic, treatment should generally only be given if the diagnosis is confirmed
    e. Amphotericin B is well absorbed from the GI tract

14. The following statements are true:
    a. There is no resistance to quinine in falciparum malaria
    b. Mebendazole is effective treatment for all types of GI worm
    c. Cryptosporidium is as easily treated with metronidazole as is giardiasis
    d. Leishmaniasis is best treated with single doses of ivermectin
    e. Visceral leishmaniasis is best treated with antimonial compounds

15. The following statements are true:
    a. It is important to measure trough gentamicin levels to avoid toxicity
    b. In endocarditis, antibiotic levels should be measured to ensure efficacy
    c. Deafness (usually temporary) is associated with high doses of erythromycin
    d. Nausea is a common dose-limiting side-effect of cotrimoxazole when used for treating pneumocystis pneumonia
    e. Itraconazole levels need to be measured when it is used for treating life-threatening fungal disease (e.g. invasive aspergillosis)

16. The following are notifiable diseases:
    a. Legionnaire's disease by telephone
    b. Only bacterial meningitis is notifiable
    c. Typhoid fever by telephone
    d. Measles
    e. Chicken pox (varicella)

17. In genitourinary infections:
    a. Vaginal candidosis is usually transmitted sexually
    b. External anal warts that have just appeared should prompt tests for syphilis
    c. Herpes simplex virus is fast becoming resistant to acyclovir

    d. Chlamydial infections may be asymptomatic
    e. Small multiple painful genital ulcers may be a feature of primary HIV

Case history questions

History 1

A 35-year-old Nigerian man presents to Casualty with fever of 2 days' duration, rigors and myalgia. He is a businessman based in Lagos who is visiting the UK for the third time in his life. He arrived 6 days ago. Apart from a fever of 38.9°C and a tachycardia, he has no abnormal physical signs. His urine contains blood (++) and protein (++) on dipstick testing.

1. What is the differential diagnosis?
2. List four essential urgent investigations
3. How should you treat him?
4. What advice (if any) should you give him with respect to his return home?

History 2

A 28-year-old Liverpudlian with high fever, pain in his toes and left wrist and sweating is admitted to hospital by his GP. He has a fever of 39.3°C, tachycardia of 152 beats/min, blood pressure 78/53 and a respiratory rate of 28/min. He has a moderately quiet systolic murmur at the left and right sternal borders, no chest, abdominal or neurological signs and a tender, swollen and red left wrist. Two of his toes show small painful red spots in the pulp of the toe.

1. Give a differential diagnosis
2. List your immediate three most useful investigations
3. List three investigations for the next morning
4. Suggest a straightforward management plan

History 3

A 29-year-old Glaswegian artist presents with increasing fever of 5 days' duration. She has lost her appetite and is slightly nauseated. She has a mild cough and her muscles ache slightly. Her travel history reveals a 2-month trip to India, Nepal and Bangkok, which finished about 10 weeks ago. She took mefloquine prophylaxis correctly and was immunised against yellow fever, hepatitis A, rabies, meningococcus, typhoid and Japanese B encephalitis. She had one mild bout of diarrhoea when she was away that resolved spontaneously after 3 days.

1. Give a differential diagnosis
2. Name five key investigations

History 4

The nursing staff in an elderly care ward call you to see an 82-year-old lady admitted with a fall 3 days previously. Before admission, she was well and living independently. The notes indicate that a cardiac cause for the fall is likely, possibly a Stokes–Adams attack. A 24-hour ECG recording has been arranged for the following week. The night sister is concerned because she appears to be drowsy and 'not her usual self'. The pulse rate is 100/min and other observations are unremarkable. When examined she is peripherally shut down, definitely drowsy and orientated only in person.

1. The following would be appropriate immediate actions:
   a. Reassure the nursing staff and leave it to her own medical team to sort out in the morning
   b. Take an oral or rectal temperature yourself
   c. Examine her chest carefully
   d. Take a blood culture and full blood count
   e. Do an ECG

In 40 minutes' time, the following data are available: rectal temperature is 37.8°C, blood pressure 85/40, white cell count 11.8 × 10⁹/l, 88% neutrophils, ECG showing sinus tachycardia and no additional physical signs.

2. Now the following actions would be appropriate:
   a. Pass a urinary catheter and send urine for culture and leave the catheter on free drainage
   b. Arrange a CT scan of the head
   c. Do a lumbar puncture
   d. Prescribe oral antibiotics, e.g. amoxycillin
   e. Write out blood request forms for the morning for autoantibodies and complement levels

History 5

A 58-year-old hospital patient complains of severe abdominal pain 5 days after a laparotomy and right hemicolectomy. The patient is a known insulin-dependent diabetic on twice daily insulin sub-cutaneously and his blood glucose values (by BM stix) are in the 15–23 mmol/l range despite an increase in insulin yesterday. He is flushed and unwell with a temperature of 37.8°C, pulse 110/min, blood pressure 150/80 and respiratory rate of 28/min. His chest has a few crackles that clear on coughing (he is a smoker). His abdomen is not diffusely tender and a few bowel sounds are present. His wound is covered with bandages.

1. Give four differential diagnoses

2. Give five actions that are immediately appropriate to his abdominal pain and fever
3. Why are his blood sugars elevated?

History 6

A bisexual man, who has visited the genitourinary clinic before, attends Casualty after a 9-month interval. He is complaining of penile discharge. He seems rather anxious. On examination there are no abnormalities other than discharge. Gram stain of the discharge shows Gram-negative cocci and white cells.

1. The following are appropriate courses of action:
   a. A prescription for a 10-day course of doxycycline
   b. A blood sample for syphilis serology
   c. Discussion about HIV risk and an HIV test
   d. Refer to GU clinic for contact tracing
   e. Admission to hospital for i.v. antibiotics

You treat him and ask him to come back in 7 days for the results of tests. On return to clinic, the discharge is a little better but not gone. Culture results confirm the diagnosis of gonorrhoea fully sensitive to antibiotics. One of his male sexual contacts is known to the clinic as a highly promiscuous exclusively gay man who was HIV negative 9 months before.

2. At this stage the following management is appropriate:
   a. Reculture for gonorrhoea
   b. Take samples for chlamydia, mycoplasma and ureaplasma
   c. Treat empirically for syphilis
   d. Refer to urologist for cystoscopy
   e. Encourage him to have an HIV test

He declines an HIV test but takes the course of treatment you prescribed. His most recent female partner is found to have both gonorrhoea and chlamydial cervicitis. They had intercourse again after you treated him but before she was seen. He returns to the clinic 2 weeks later with no discharge. His VDRL is 1:8, TPHA positive (both the same as 9 months ago) and FTA-IgM weakly positive.

3. At this point:
   a. There is no need to examine him again
   b. He should be retreated for gonorrhoea
   c. He should be treated for syphilis again
   d. He should have a lumbar puncture done to exclude neurosyphilis
   e. Your enthusiasm for him to have an HIV test is related to whether he was practising safe sex

Data interpretation

Choose the best antibiotic regimen from those given for each of the conditions listed (the route for administration is given if more than one route is possible).

1. Endocarditis, no organism yet isolated, in a patient with a rheumatic mitral valve:
   a. piperacillin and i.v. gentamicin
   b. flucloxacillin (i.v.) and oral rifampicin
   c. ampicillin and netilmicin (both i.v.)
2. A 60-year-old with severe left leg cellulitis, blood cultures pending:
   a. oral ciprofloxacin and i.v. gentamicin
   b. ceftazidime
   c. cefuroxime (i.v.)
3. A 19-year-old with hypotension, vomiting and purpuric rash
   a. high-dose i.v. penicillin
   b. erythromycin (i.v.)
   c. cefuroxime (i.v.)
4. A 78-year-old man with 3 days of severe diarrhoea and dehydration during convalescence after treatment for pneumonia, stool cultures pending:
   a. piperacillin and gentamicin (both i.v.)
   b. oral and i.v. vancomycin
   c. oral and i.v. metronidazole
5. Intensive care unit patient on renal replacement following a previous episode of septic shock, now with fever and Gram-positive cocci in blood culture:
   a. cefotaxime
   b. vancomycin (i.v.)
   c. flucloxacillin (i.v.)
6. Intensive care unit patient on renal replacement following a prior episode of septic shock, now with fever, raised peripheral white cell count and yeasts in the urine
   a. cefotaxime
   b. amphotericin B
   c. fluconazole (i.v.)
7. Cystic fibrosis patient with *Pseudomonas aeruginosa* in sputum and increasing breathlessness and sputum production, sensitivities pending:
   a. cefotaxime
   b. oral ciprofloxacin
   c. imipenem
8. Severe sore throat in a 17-year-old who also has tender cervical lymphadenopathy and fever:
   a. oral erythromycin
   b. flucloxicillin (i.v.)
   c. penicillin (i.v.)
9. A 38-year-old gamekeeper from Scotland with chronic monoarthritis of his left knee:
   a. oral doxycycline
   b. oral penicillin
   c. oral erythromycin
10. A 31-year-old with green discharge from one nostril, mild headache and feeling 'off colour':
    a. oral co-amoxiclav
    b. cefotaxime
    c. oral erythromycin

Short note questions

Write short notes on:
1. Management of the febrile shocked patient.
2. Fever in a recent traveller from Africa.
3. Appropriate investigations for PUO.

Self-assessment: answers

Multiple choice answers

1. a. **True**. The treatment of choice, unless allergic.
    b. **False**. *E. coli* are intrinsically resistant.
    c. **True**. Intravenously in large doses, together with surgery.
    d. **True**. Except for *Clostridium difficile*. Metronidazole is also very effective against *Clostridium* infections.
    e. **False**. Oral vancomycin or metronidazole are effective, with a 15% relapse rate.

2. a. **False**. *P. aeruginosa* is intrinsically resistant to ampicillin.
    b. **True**. Approximately 5% resistance in the UK.
    c. **False**. Virtually all staphylococci are resistant to ampicillin. Approximately 5% of *S. aureus* isolates are, however, sensitive to penicillin; if they are sensitive, penicillin is a better choice than flucloxacillin because it is more active.
    d. **False**.
    e. **True**. Ampicillin is a treatment of choice with *Listeria* infections given in large doses.

3. a. **True**. Given with aminoglycoside or rifampicin.
    b. **True**. Although erythromycin or topical mupirocin would be reasonable alternatives.
    c. **False**. This infection is most likely caused by coagulase-negative staphylococci (e.g. *Staphylococcus epidermidis*) and vancomycin (or teicoplanin) would be the best first choice.
    d. **True**. Although some cases of osteomyelitis are not caused by *Staphylococcus aureus*.
    e. **False**.

4. a. **True**. *Enterobacter* tends to be multiresistant and sensitivity testing is essential to determine the right treatment.
    b. **True**. But only if given with an aminoglycoside. In fact, ampicillin and gentamicin would represent the first choice here.
    c. **False**. All the extended-spectrum penicillins are not active against *Staphylococcus aureus* unless combined with a β-lactamase inhibitor such as sulbactam (Tazobactam or clavulanic acid (Timentin). In that case, the combination may be active but it would not be the first choice.
    d. **True**. Slightly more isolates are sensitive to piperacillin than they are to ticarcillin but sensitivity testing will determine this quickly.
    e. **True**.

5. a. **True**. And the treatment of choice. Teicoplanin is also effective. Removal of the line is essential except in the exceptional circumstances in which it cannot be removed.

    b. **True**. MRSA stands for both multiply resistant *S. aureus* and methicillin-resistant *S. aureus*. From your point of view these are the same and none of them are resistant to vancomycin.
    c. **True**. These infections are most often caused by coagulase-negative staphylococci.
    d. **True**. But only if combined with an aminoglycoside. Given that enterococcal endocarditis has to be treated for 6 weeks, this means treating a patient with two potentially nephrotoxic antibiotics that both need to be assayed for 6 weeks, which is quite a challenge.
    e. **False**.

6. a. **True**. Although the differences are small.
    b. **False**. *Pseudomonas* spp. are resistant to both cefuroxime and cefotaxime.
    c. **False**. All the cephalosporins have no activity at all against *S. faecalis* or *L. monocytogenes*.
    d. **True**. For almost all clinical purposes. However, cefotaxime is preferred over cefuroxime for meningitis because of better ratio between CSF concentrations and the MIC (minimum inhibitory concentration) of the organism.
    e. **False**. There is no advantage in giving a more broad-spectrum agent for a simple infection when a more narrow spectrum (e.g. cefuroxime, ampicillin or trimethoprine) can be given.

7. a. **True**. Ofloxacin has very limited activity against *Pseudomonas aeruginosa*.
    b. **True**. Ceftazidime is one of the most useful drugs in treating *Pseudomonas* infections. Cefotaxime has no activity.
    c. **False**. The prevalence of resistance in *Pseudomonas* spp. depends very much on how frequently drugs are used. In many hospitals in the UK, the aminoglycosides such as gentamicin are used infrequently and so most isolates (e.g. more than 80%) are susceptible.
    d. **False**. Both imipenem and meropenem are highly active against *Pseudomonas aeruginosa* but most hospital formularies do not include them. There are three indications for imipenem which fit within most British hospital formularies. These are (i) resistant organisms susceptible to imipenem; (ii) polymicrobial infection when imipenem alone will be as efficacious as three or four antibiotics together; and (iii) in patients who are deteriorating with sepsis with no organism identified and who are already on broad-spectrum antibiotics.
    e. **True**. *Pseudomonas* is notorious for developing resistance on therapy. This is not usually a problem for short courses of therapy for urinary

tract infections, etc., but in patients with a difficult infection (e.g. ventilator pneumonia, *Pseudomonas* bacteraemia during neutropenia, etc.) two agents are preferred in the likelihood that the development of resistance will be substantially reduced and activity is slightly enhanced.

8. a. **False.** Ciprofloxacin has no anti-anaerobe activities at all, which is one of its virtues because it disrupts bowel flora less.
   b. **True.** Excellent broad-spectrum anti-anaerobe coverage.
   c. **True.** Excellent broad-spectrum anti-anaerobe coverage with very little resistance identified. Metronidazole also penetrates very well into abscesses in which anaerobic organisms are often found.
   d. **False.**
   e. **False.** Some activity against anaerobic streptococci but very little for other organisms.

9. a. **True.** One of the substantial defects of the present quinolones is inadequate activity against *S. pneumoniae*.
   b. **True.** Oral therapy is preferred for reasons of convenience and cost.
   c. **False.** Ciprofloxacin does have reasonable antistaphylococcal activity but it is not a mainstream antibiotic for this organism because it is best used for other indications where its breadth of spectrum is more valuable.
   d. **True.** Useful for the treatment of resistant mycobacterium infection including *M. avium intracellulare* in AIDS. Its use can obscure positive cultures of *M. tuberculosis*, particularly if used for respiratory infections.
   e. **True.** *Salmonella typhi* from the Indian subcontinent is now frequently resistant to almost all other drugs apart from the third-generation cephalosporins and ciprofloxacin.

10. a. **False.** Erythromycin has marginal activity against *H. influenzae* and both clarithromycin and azithromycin are superior in this regard.
    b. **True.** Although the clinical data with clarithromycin are scant.
    c. **False.** Probably equivalent.
    d. **True.** Although the clinical data for clarithromycin against *Mycoplasma* are limited.
    e. **True.** As erythromycin has no activity against mycobacteria.

11. a. **True.** For all cases, in large i.v. doses.
    b. **True.** Of marginal benefit and only indicated if given in the first 48 hours of pain or in an immunocompromised patient.
    c. **True.** But only for secondary cases in a household or for immunocompromised patients.
    d. **True.** For reasons that are not entirely clear,

acyclovir (which has little activity against cytomegalovirus) does seem to prevent or postpone many cytomegalovirus infections after transplantation.
    e. **False.**

12. a. **True.** Although amantidine is effective prophylaxis if given before symptoms appear in exposed patients. This is difficult as the incubation time for influenza is about 3 days and it clearly requires taking samples from patients first affected to prove the diagnosis and in getting a very rapid result.
    b. **False.** Ribivirin is effective.
    c. **False.** Alpha-interferon is often effective (around 30%).
    d. **False.** Ribivirin is effective.
    e. **True.**

13. a. **True.** For many groups of patients, e.g. neonates, those who get thrush following antibiotics and patients with AIDS-related complaints. However, in neutropenic patients, patients with candidiasis following radiotherapy to the head and neck and late stage AIDS patients, systemic therapy is superior.
    b. **True.** Fluconazole is the maintenance therapy of choice for cryptococcal meningitis in AIDS.
    c. **False.** Itraconazole and amphotericin are the only agents useful for *Aspergillus* infections.
    d. **False.** This statement was true in the early 1980s, but with the substantial rise in both the incidence and mortality of fungal disease, therapy should not be delayed until the diagnosis is confirmed, partly because it is very difficult to confirm the diagnosis.
    e. **False.** Amphotericin B is not absorbed at all from the GI tract.

14. a. **False.** Resistance to quinine is rare but does occur around the Cambodian, Thai and Burmese borders. Resistance may be partial.
    b. **False.** Although mebendazole is a good drug for many intestinal parasites.
    c. **False.** Aside from experimental therapy, there is no treatment at all for *Cryptosporidium*, whereas the response of giardiasis to metronidazole exceeds 90%.
    d. **False.**
    e. **False.** This is the old teaching and these compounds are somewhat effective. However, i.v. liposomal amphotericin B such as AmBisome or Amphocil are highly effective and are now first-line therapies in the UK.

15. a. **True.** Trough concentrations of gentamicin above 1 µg/ml and particularly above 2 µg/ml have a much higher incidence of renal or ototoxicity.

b. **True.** These can be measured directly, as in the case of gentamicin and vancomycin, or indirectly using serum killing levels.

c. **True.** But the dose should not be reduced if you are treating Legionnaire's disease.

d. **True.** And a reduction in dose to 75% may help and be just as efficacious.

e. **True.** Low or undetectable levels are associated with a high incidence of failure and intestinal absorption is somewhat unpredictable. Therefore, in all patients with life-threatening fungal disease treated with itraconazole, levels should be measured.

16. a. **False.** Not notifiable at all although you should tell your microbiologist if you suspect the diagnosis in case it is a hospital outbreak.

b. **False.** *All* forms of meningitis are notifiable.

c. **True.** As other cases could present from the same locality.

d. **True.**

e. **False.** One of the few non-notifiable classical infectious diseases.

17. a. **False.** *Candida* resides in the vagina in many women. Occasionally disease appears to follow intercourse, but this reflects a changed vaginal environment rather than transmission.

b. **True.** Condylomata lata of secondary syphilis can be mistaken for warts.

c. **False.** A few cases of resistance are reported in AIDS only.

d. **True.** And lead to infertility in women.

e. **True.** Oral, oesophageal and genital ulceration is one presentation (usually with fever) of primary HIV infection (p. 337).

Case history answers

History 1

1. Falciparum malaria, pyelonephritis, community-acquired bacteraemia, e.g. *Pneumococcus*, *Staphylococcus* spp., infection with hypertension or glomerulonephritis.

2. Key investigations: malaria film, blood count, urea, and blood culture. Other investigations: differential white cell count, electrolytes, urine microscopy (urgent) and culture.

3. With i.v. quinine for malaria (the diagnosis in this case). If he has a neutrophilia, broad-spectrum antibiotics to include Gram-negative antibiotics and pneumococcal coverage, e.g. third-generation cephalosporin such as cefotaxime.

4. There is no point giving him prophylaxis against malaria if he intends spending most of his time in Lagos for two reasons: (i) he will have partial immunity to malaria and be in less danger of dying from an acute attack, although he is still likely to get ill with it; (ii) he will get constantly reinfected in

Nigeria and lifelong prophylaxis is not really a tenable option for people living in these countries.

History 2

1. Staphylococcal tricuspid valve endocarditis (common in i.v. drug abusers), staphylococcal septicaemia, group A streptococcal sepsis, gonococcal bacteraemia, Henoch–Schönlein purpura. The key factor to elicit on the history is whether he is an i.v. drug abuser or not. If he is, tricuspid endocarditis is more likely; if he is not then other diagnostic possibilities are more likely.

2. Blood culture, aspiration of the left wrist (if possible) and full blood count. Others are differential blood count, ECG, urethral swab for *N. gonorrhoeae*, chest x-ray, blood gases.

3. Echocardiogram, hepatitis B and C antibodies (possibly HIV antibodies) if he is an i.v. drug abuser and ASO titre.

4. Assuming he is a drug abuser, the following steps should be taken.

a. Ascertain how much heroin he takes and prescribe methadone to prevent withdrawal symptoms.

b. Prescribe flucloxacillin in large doses, e.g. 2 g 4-hourly, and a broad-spectrum agent such as cefotaxime to cover diagnoses above. If there is any evidence of a localised abscess, also prescribe metronidazole.

c. Arrange for the HIV counsellor to see him with respect to HIV testing.

d. Make provisional plans for central venous line insertion if he has very poor peripheral veins, which is likely.

e. Send all blood tests to the lab with a 'high-risk' sticker and then warn the laboratory staff on call that he is at risk for blood-borne viruses. (e.g. hepatitis B, C and HIV).

If he is not a drug abuser, he would be treated as above but there would be less concern about hepatitis B and C, HIV, etc. Veins should not be a problem.

History 3

1. The most likely diagnosis is amoebic liver abscess. Other possibilities include hepatitis B (unlikely in view of fever), community-acquired infection acquired locally (e.g. mycoplasma), malaria (especially *Plasmodium vivax*), brucellosis and tuberculosis.

2. Blood film for malaria, blood culture, liver function tests, serology for amoebiasis and brucellosis, ultrasound of the liver, chest radiograph.

History 4

1. a. **False.** She has clearly had a sudden deterioration and it needs action tonight, not in the morning.

b. **True.** In many wards axillary temperatures only are measured and when patients are peripherally shut down a pyrexia may fail to be recorded.

c. **True.** The most common causes of sudden deterioration and fever in elderly people is pneumonia or urinary tract infection. Physical examination is likely to be as sensitive as chest X-ray in the early phases of the disease.

d. **True.** Although if she has a fever, the full blood count tonight is unlikely to help very much.

e. **True.** If you did not demonstrate any pyrexia and it appeared that her heart rhythm was abnormal or very fast and the blood pressure was reduced, then an ECG might be as appropriate as a blood culture because she could be in fast atrial fibrillation or some other tachyarrhythmia. Also consider drugs as a cause of her drowsiness.

2. a. **True.** A disorientated patient on an elderly care ward is highly likely to be incontinent of urine. The catheter allows accurate measurement of urine output and if this falls it alerts you to impending renal failure or the need for i.v. fluids. Also she may well be moved less frequently than is desirable and is, therefore, at moderate to high risk of development of pressure sores. The passage of a urinary catheter will reduce the risk of this to some extent, although the nurses should be encouraged to use prophylactic measures to prevent pressure sores as part of a change in the original nursing care plan.

   b. **False.** Unless there are localising neurological signs.

   c. **False.** Unless there is neck stiffness or no other focus of fever is found.

   d. **False.** Given that this rapid deterioration in association with low blood pressure in this patient represents severe sepsis, she requires i.v. antibiotics, not oral antibiotics. In addition, oral amoxycillin will only cover a small number of the appropriate pathogens because resistance is now common in hospital pathogens.

   e. **False.** The acute onset of SLE or another connective tissue disease leading to fever and features of sepsis is so unlikely as to be an untenable differential diagnosis. She is so much more likely to have a bacterial infection that these and/or antibody tests do not need to be ordered out of hours or, except in exceptional circumstances, ever.

History 5

1. (i) Peritonitis (but you may not expect bowel sounds and he would probably have generalised tenderness). (ii) Wound infection with or without bacteraemia (likely, but severe pain unusual for standard pathogens (e.g. *S. aureus*). (iii) Postoperative pneumonia (certainly possible, but again severe abdominal pain unlikely). (iv)

Necrotising fasciitis of the abdominal wall (the diagnosis in this case, the clue to which was the severe pain. Failure to take off the wound dressing (which revealed black necrotic areas adjacent to the wound) would have allowed you to miss the diagnosis.

2. (i) Take the bandages off, inspect the wound and take a wound swab; (ii) arterial blood gases (to check for hypoxia/acidosis); (iii) blood culture (probably infected and may be bacteraemic); (iv) blood count and differential white cell count (to check for raised white cell count and anaemia); (v) chest X-ray (as he may have pneumonia); (vi) urea and electrolytes and blood sugar (for management of raised blood sugar and because he is at risk of renal failure); (vii) urine culture.

3. He has temporary 'insulin resistance' caused by an infection.

History 6

1. a. **False.** You have made a diagnosis of gonorrhoea, treat that but not with doxycycline. (If the other tests you have done (or future tests) show chlamydia then doxycycline would be effective.)

   b. **True.** For all new presentations, even old patients.

   c. **True.** Clearly an at-risk patient.

   d. **True.**

   e. **False.** Virtually no sexually transmitted diseases require admission to hospital, except HIV and AIDS and investigations and treatment of latent or tertiary syphilis.

2. a. **True.** Although it is unlikely to be culture positive. From a quarter to half of patients have continuing discharge despite 'cure', representing another pathogen.

   b. **True.** You did this before, of course, but as the incubation period for these organisms is longer, the results were negative (? falsely negative). Most laboratories only do tests for chlamydia.

   c. **False.** Syphilis does not cause a discharge: await serology.

   d. **False.** Unhelpful in almost all cases of discharge. No bladder symptoms described.

   e. **True.** As before, especially knowing his contact.

3. a. **False.** Syphilis has a longer incubation period and now is the time when you would expect to see a chancre. You also want to reculture his urethral secretions for *N. gonorrhoeae*.

   b. **True.** Clearly history of contact after treatment for chlamydia; however, some drugs such as azithromycin will often also treat gonorrhoea.

   c. **False.** The VDRL and TPHA titres are stable. The FTA test is read visually and is somewhat subjective. It is only weakly positive. However, he does need follow-up serology in, say, 2 months.

   d. **False.** This is standard practice for new, untreated cases of latent syphilis, but he has been treated before by you.

e. **False.** Possibly true in general, but you know he was not practising safe sex because he caught gonorrhoea. Patients are not always entirely straight about this.

Data interpretation

1. c. The combination of ampicillin and an aminoglycoside covers all of the streptococci, enterococci and unusual causes of endocarditis, such as the HACEK organisms. In addition, the aminoglycoside has some activity against *S. aureus* and about 50% of *S. epidermidis* infections. Aminoglycosides are also active against a number of Gram-negative organisms which are occasional causes of endocarditis. It does not matter from the point of view of activity which aminoglycoside is used and gentamicin, netilmicin, streptomycin or tobramycin would all be equivalent, but all of them would require blood levels to be measured.

2. c. The most likely pathogen is a group A or G Streptococcus or *S. aureus*. Intravenous cefuroxime would treat this well. Ciprofloxacin is not sufficiently active against the streptococci (in particular *S. pneumoniae*) to be useful. Ceftazidime has some streptococcal and staphyloccal activity, but this is less than that of cefuroxime.

3. a. This young man probably has meningococcal septicaemia. Penicillin is the drug of choice, although cefuroxime would be equally good as would any third-generation cephalosporin. Note that all choices are for i.v. therapy. If you saw this young man at home as his GP, it would be appropriate to give him i.m. or i.v. penicillin.

4. c. The likely diagnosis is *C. difficile* diarrhoea. Piperacillin and gentamicin have no activity against these pathogens. *C. difficile* is not an invasive organism at all and the disease is caused by toxin production. Oral vancomycin is active but only in the lumen of the bowel. Intravenous vancomycin does not penetrate into the bowel at all and, therefore, is not a useful drug. Vancomycin is expensive for this indication. Metronidazole orally is given for mild cases and in severe cases i.v. metronidazole can also be given, which penetrates extremely well into the wall and lumen of the bowel.

5. b. The most likely pathogen is *S. epidermidis* or another coagulase-negative *Staphylococcus*. Vancomycin is active against 100% of these organisms, whereas flucloxacillin will only be active against 20–50%. Cephalosporins are not clinically active for *S. epidermidis* infection and, therefore, (a) is positively the wrong choice.

6. b. As the patient had received multiple antibiotics previously for septic shock, he/she is at risk for candidaemia, particularly as the patient is on haemodialysis and, therefore, has multiple i.v. lines. Fungal blood cultures should be done in this patient but, unfortunately, approximately 50% are negative even in patients with documented candidaemia at autopsy. An excellent surrogate marker for candidaemia is candiduria, as in this case. Cefotaxime is clearly the wrong choice. Intravenous fluconazole would be a reasonable alternative and might be preferred because there is no nephrotoxicity associated with it. However, some species of yeast are resistant to fluconazole and until you know whether it is or is not resistant it is wise to use amphotericin B. All intensive care unit patients with candiduria and any sign of infection or deteriorating status require antifungal therapy.

7. b. If these patients can be treated orally this is preferable, although this does depend on the status of the patient. Cefotaxime is not active against *P. aeruginosa*. Imipenen and ciprofloxacin would be reasonable choices. Check previous sensitivities in the notes because if the organism has been found before and is known to be resistant to either ciprofloxacillin or imipenem this would influence your choice.

8. c. This patient almost certainly has a bad streptococcal sore throat. Intravenous (or i.m.) penicillin is preferred because the symptoms resolve much more quickly than they do by giving oral therapy. The vast majority of isolates are susceptible to erythromycin, although perhaps 5% are resistant. Intravenous flucloxacillin is not as active as penicillin and, therefore, this is an inferior choice. In mild cases, oral therapy alone suffices. Treatment should be continued for 10 days or recurrence and possible transmission to the family is likely. The switch from i.v. to oral therapy can be made usually after 1 to 2 days but probably should be made to amoxycillin or coamoxiclav as penicillin is so poorly absorbed. There is also some evidence for persistence of streptococci despite therapy because the tonsillar concentrations of antibiotics are relatively low and further reduced by anaerobic organisms living in the crypts of the tonsils, which produce β-lactamase and inactivate the penicillin or amoxycillin in situ, allowing local persistence and subsequent recurrence. Co-amoxiclav or a drug such as erythromycin or clindamycin or the new macrolides (e.g. azithromycin or clarithromycin) may, therefore, be preferable to simple penicillin V or amoxycillin.

9. a. This patient probably has Lyme borreliosis stage 3. Other considerations included tuberculosis or injury-related osteoarthritis. Doxycycline is one of the treatments of choice for Lyme borreliosis. Oral penicillin is inadequately absorbed,

although i.v. penicillin might be adequate. Erythromycin is less active (p. 366).

10. a. This patient probably has sinusitis. The common causes of sinusitis include *Streptococcus pneumoniae*, *Haemophilus influenzae*, *Staphylococcus aureus* and, in 30% of cases, anaerobic organisms such as oral *Bacteroides* are also found. Therapy should be directed at these pathogens. Oral co-amoxiclav is a good choice because it will cover all of these commonly occurring organisms. Larger doses are required for sinusitis than for many other indications, because the sinus represents quite a large volume of pus and penetration of the antibiotic into the centre of that pus requires good concentrations. Cefotaxime would be a good choice if the patient was admitted to hospital but it should be given with metronidazole. Although erythromycin may be active against some of the pathogens, it is an inferior choice. Consideration should be given to sinus X-rays and to decongestant therapy.

Short note answers

1. **Initially**. Resuscitate the patient: high oxygen concentrations, i.v. fluids (N/saline and colloid).

   Appropriate key investigations:
   - blood culture
   - FBP, urea and electrolytes, liver function tests, creatine phosphokinase, clotting tests
   - urine culture
   - throat culture if ?meningococcal
   - respiratory tract culture
   - arterial blood gases
   - chest X-ray.

   Therapy. Choose appropriate antibiotic therapy depending on clinical features. These can be obtained by collecting a history from patient, relatives, notes, nursing staff, etc. and by examining the patient carefully, especially skin, chest, abdomen, joints, etc. Choose a broad-spectrum agent with an additional agent if there is an apparent focus, e.g. cefotaxime plus (i) erythromycin if pneumonia; (ii) flucloxacillin 2 g 6-hourly if features of staphylococcal sepsis (p. 358), (iii) metronidazole if an intra-abdominal focus. If an intensive care or renal patient use ceftazidime ± vancomycin.

   Management. Consider the best care options over the next 12–24 hours:
   A. *Anticipate complications:* hypoxia (ARDS), DIC,. acute renal failure (p. 155), etc.
   B. *Nursing area.* Transfer to intensive care unit, high dependency or allow to remain on the ward: depends on age, severity of sepsis, underlying disease, patients, and relatives, wishes, response to initial therapy with oxygenated fluids and decision to resuscitate.
   C. *Consult.* Who to advise and seek advice from: your consultant/registrar, microbiologist, intensive care consultant, etc.

2. Must exclude malaria and typhoid; also consider dengue fever, viral haemorrhagic fever, tick typhus, HIV, tuberculosis, other viral infections, standard bacterial infections (e.g. pneumonia, urinary tract infection, infectious diarrhoea, etc.).

3. Do investigations depending on clinical findings and differential diagnosis, e.g.
   - TB: Heaf test, cultures of sputum, CSF, urine, peritoneal fluid, etc.
   - brucellosis: special blood culture for *Brucella*, brucella serology
   - occult abscess: imaging of liver, spleen and kidney, ultrasound, CT of abdomen, MR of spine for osteomyelitis and epidermal abscess, pelvic ultrasound, white cell and gallium scan
   - AIDS: HIV test and T4 count
   - hypogammaglobulinaemia: immunoglobulins
   - autoimmune disease: autoantibodies, ESR, plasma viscosity
   - endocarditis: blood culture, serology for Q fever, *Candida*, etc.
   - tropical diseases: eosinophil count and get advice
   - tumours: CT scan, bone marrow, α-fetoprotein
   - sarcoidosis: Kveim test
   - drug fever: eosinophil count, stop drug, etc.
   - seek advice earlier rather than later.

Index

Note: Question and Answer Sections are indicated in the form 14Q/16A

Lumbar puncture, 187, 215Q/220A
  meningitis, 189, 190
Lung function tests, 66–67, 91Q/96A,
      92Q/97A, 94Q/99A:100A
  asthma, 83
  chronic bronchitis and emphysema, 79
Lungs
  abscess, 72
  anatomy, 64
  cancer, 74–77, 90Q/95A
    metastatic, 77
  functions, 64–66
  rheumatoid disease, 308
  sepsis, 74
  solitary nodules, 77
  transplantation, 25, 343, 344
Luteinising hormone (LH), 256
Lyme borreliosis, 366
Lymph node biopsy, 231
Lymphadenopathy
  HIV infection, 338
  infectious diseases, 303
  white cell disorders, 229
Lymphangitis carcinomatosis, 64, 77
Lymphatics, respiratory system, 64
Lymphocytes, 239
  normal values, 4
  see also B cells; T cells
Lymphocytoma, Borrelia, 366
Lymphomas, 240, 242–243, 249Q/252A
  AIDS, 339, 340, 341
  central nervous system, 195
  gastric, 110
  lung, 77
  non-Hodgkin's, 242–243, 250Q/253A
  signs, 229
  thyroid, 262
Lymphopenia, 239, 300

M

Macrocytosis, 230, 233
Macroglobulinaemia, Waldenström's, 243
Macrolides, 377
Macrophages, 334
  defects, 334–335
Maculopathy, 280
Magnetic resonance imaging (MRI)
  endocrine diseases, 257
  metabolic bone disease, 317
  neurological disease, 187–188
  respiratory disease, 66
MAI infection, 340, 341
Major histocompatibility complex, 343,
      359
Malabsorption, 111–112, 142Q/147A
Malaria, 370–372
Mallory-Weiss tear, 103
Mantoux test, 73
Marfan's syndrome, 48
Mast cells, 345
Mean cell volume (MCV), 230, 231
  normal values, 4
Measles, 364
Median nerve, 211
  damage, 210–211
Medulla oblongata, damage, 187
Mefloquine, 371, 372
Melaena, 103
Meningioma, 194
Meningitis
  bacterial, 188, 189–190, 215Q/220–221A
  fungal, 188, 191, 339, 340
  lymphocytic, 192, 215Q/220A
  tuberculous, 188, 191
  viral, 188, 191–192
Meningococcaemia, 358
  chronic, 332
Meningococcus (Neisseria meningitidis),
      189, 190, 332, 358

Mesalazine, 120
Mesothelioma, pleura, 89, 90Q/95A
Metformin, 277
Methotrexate, 304
MHC antigens, 343, 359
Microcytosis, 230, 232, 234, 236
Mineralocorticoid deficiency, 268, 269
Misoprostol, 108, 303
Mitral valve disease, 31–33
  floppy valve, 33
  prolapse, 32, 33
  regurgitation, 32–33
  stenosis, 31–32, 50Q/58A
Monocytes, 239, 334
  normal values, 4
Mononeuritis/mononeuritis multiplex,
      211, 308
  diabetic, 281
Motor neurone disease, 189, 204–205
Mouth, infectious diseases, 355
Multiple myeloma, 243–244
Multiple sclerosis, 188, 207–208,
      214Q/220A
Mumps, 364
Muscle
  disease, 212–213
  structure, 212
  symptoms in musculoskeletal disease,
      300
Musculoskeletal disease
  clinical aspects, 298–304
  infection, 304–306
  investigations, 300–302,
      323:324Q/328–329A
  management, 302–304
  symptoms, 298–300,
      323:324Q/327–328A
  see also specific diseases
Myalgic encephalomyelitis, 366–367
Myasthenia, 366–367
Myasthenia gravis, 189, 212–213,
      214Q/219A, 218Q/224A
Mycobacteria, atypical, 72
Mycobacterium avium intracellulare (MAI)
      infection, 340, 341
Mycobacterium tuberculosis, 72–73, 304
Mycoplasma hominis, 368
Mycoplasma pneumonia, 69, 71
Myelodysplastic syndrome, 241
Myelofibrosis, 242
Myeloproliferative diseases, 240, 241–242
Myocardial infarction, 17–21, 50Q/58A
  clinical presentation, 17
  complications, 19–20
  ECG, 12
  investigations, 17–18
  management, 18–19
  pathology, 17
  postinfarction prophylaxis, 20–21
Myocarditis, 39–40
Myopathies, 213
Myositis, 189, 213, 302
Myotomes, 210
Myotonia, 212
Myxoedema coma, 261–262
Myxoma, cardiac, 40

N

Naproxen, 303
Natriuretic peptides, 151, 167
Nebulisers, 68, 80, 84
Neck, infectious diseases, 355
Necrotising fasciitis, 361
Neglect, definition, 182
Neisseria gornorrhoeae, 304, 368
Neisseria meningitidis (meningococcus),
      189, 190, 332, 358
Nelson's syndrome, 270
Neostigmine, 213

Nephritis, acute, 155, 160
Nephroblastoma, 162
Nephron, 150
Nephropathy
  diabetic, 281
  interstitial, 161
Nephrotic syndrome, 155, 159–160,
      174Q/177A
Nerve conduction tests, 188–189
Neuralgia, post-herpetic, 363–364
Neurological disease
  AIDS, 340, 341
  cerebrovascular disease, 195–200
  clinical aspects, 182–189
  degenerative, 200–205
  infections, 189–194
  inflammatory, 207–208
  investigations, 187–189, 216Q/222A
  muscle, 212–213
  peripheral nervous system, 210–212
  spinal cord, 208–210
  symptoms, 182–187,
      215Q/220A:221–222A,
      218Q/224A
  terminology, 182
  tumours, 194–195
  see also specific diseases
Neuroma, acoustic, 186, 194, 214Q/219A
Neuropathy
  peripheral, 211–212
    AIDS, 341
  rheumatoid disease, 308
Neutropenia, 239–240, 249Q/252A, 333,
      334–335
  signs, 229
Neutrophils, 230, 238–239, 249Q/252A
  normal values, 4
Nicorandil, 16
Nicotinic acid, 273
Nifedipine, 44
Nimodipine, 200
Nitrates, cardiovascular disease, 16, 17,
      25
Non-Hodgkin's lymphoma, 242–243,
      250Q/253A
Non-steroidal anti-inflammatory drugs
      (NSAIDs), 68, 159, 303,
      322Q/326A
Norfloxacin, 376
Nose, infectious diseases, 355
Notifiable diseases, 138Q/144A, 375,
      379Q/384A

O

Obesity, 274, 291Q/296A
  hypertension and, 42
Occupational disease, respiratory, 82, 85, 89
Octreotide, 264, 268
Oculomotor nerves, 184–185
Oedema, 166, 167, 168
Oesophageal candidiasis, 339
Oesophageal varices, 132
Oesophagitis, reflux, 102, 106
Oesophagus
  Barrett's, 106
  diseases, 105–107
  motility, 105
Ofloxacin, 376
Oligaemia, 64
Oliguria, 156, 167
Olsalazine, 120
Omeprazole, 108
Opthalmopathy, thyroid-asscociated, 259
Optic nerve damage, 184
Osmolality, 151, 166
  disorders, 170–171
Osteitis fibrosa et cystica, 318
Osteoarthritis, 303, 313–315, 322Q/326A,
      325Q/329A